# SALEM HEALTH

# INFECTIOUS DISEASES & CONDITIONS

# SALEM HEALTH

## INFECTIOUS DISEASES & CONDITIONS

Volume 3

Editor
H. Bradford Hawley
Wright State University

SALEM PRESS, INC.
Ipswich, Massachusetts          Hackensack, New Jersey

**Note to Readers**

The material presented in *Salem Health: Infectious Diseases and Conditions* is intended for broad informational and educational purposes. Readers who suspect that they or someone they know has any disorder, disease, or condition described in this set should contact a physician without delay. This set should not be used as a substitute for professional medical diagnosis. Readers who are undergoing or about to undergo any treatment or procedure described in this set should refer to their physicians and other health care providers for guidance concerning preparation and possible effects. This set is not to be considered definitive on the covered topics, and readers should remember that the field of health care is characterized by a diversity of medical opinions and constant expansion in knowledge and understanding.

**Library of Congress Cataloging-in-Publication Data**

Infectious diseases and conditions / editor, H. Bradford Hawley.
    p. ; cm. – (Salem health)
    Includes bibliographical references and indexes.
    ISBN 978-1-58765-776-4 (set : alk. paper) — ISBN 978-1-58765-777-1 (v. 1 : alk. paper) —
ISBN 978-1-58765-778-8 (v. 2 : alk. paper) — ISBN 978-1-58765-779-5 (v. 3 : alk. paper)
    1. Communicable diseases–Encyclopedias.  I. Hawley, H. Bradford.  II. Series: Salem health (Ipswich, Mass.)
    [DNLM: 1. Communicable Diseases–Encyclopedias–English.  WC 13]
    RC112.I4577 2012
    616.003–dc23

                                                                                            2011020526

PRINTED IN THE UNITED STATES OF AMERICA

# Contents

# Complete List of Contents

## Volume 1

# Volume 2

Complete List of Contents

xi

# Volume 3

# Complete List of Contents

# SALEM HEALTH

## INFECTIOUS DISEASES
## & CONDITIONS

# Q

## Q fever

CATEGORY: Diseases and conditions
ANATOMY OR SYSTEM AFFECTED: All
ALSO KNOWN AS: *Coxiella burnetii* fever, Q fever pneumonia, query fever

### DEFINITION

Q fever is an uncommon febrile, pneumonia-like illness that is most often contracted by people whose occupations bring them in contact with infected farm animals. First described as a disease among workers in a meat packing plant, the letter *Q* in the name of the disease derives from the word "query," meaning "unknown origin," although the *Q* probably also refers to Queensland, the Australian province in which the packing plant was located.

### CAUSES

The tiny gram-negative bacterium *Coxiella burnetii* is the causative agent of Q fever. Usually classified with other obligate intracellular parasites known as *Rickettsia*, *Coxiella* is the only member of this group that does not need an arthropod vector for transmission. Ticks transmit the bacteria between animals, but most human transmission results from inhalation of dust containing bacteria from dried animal feces or urine or from the consumption of unpasteurized milk.

### RISK FACTORS

Workers in slaughterhouses and meat processing facilities have the highest risk, although veterinarians, textile workers handling raw wool, and others whose occupations put them in direct contact with cattle, sheep, and goats are also at risk. Transplant recipients, persons with cancer, and persons with chronic kidney disease have an increased risk of developing the more serious chronic form of the disease.

### SYMPTOMS

The acute form of the illness is most often characterized by the sudden onset of severe headache, high

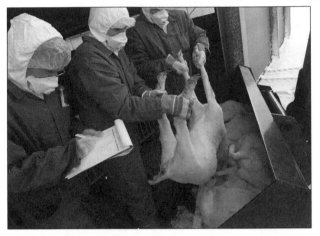

*As a preventive measure, pregnant goats and sheep were killed in the Netherlands in 2009 after an outbreak of Q fever, which the animals transmitted to more than two thousand persons in that country.* (AP/Wide World Photos)

fever, chills, sweats, confusion, nausea, muscle pain, or general malaise. Pneumonia or hepatitis may develop in serious cases, and in a small percentage of infected persons, the infection will persist for many months as chronic Q fever. The majority of persons with the chronic form of the disease will develop endocarditis, a serious complication in which the bacteria establish additional sites of infection in the aortic heart valves.

### SCREENING AND DIAGNOSIS

Diagnosis of infection with *C. burnetii* requires an immunological or serological laboratory test designed to measure host antibodies to the pathogen. The indirect immunofluorescence assay (IFA) is widely used and considered the most dependable, but immunohistochemical staining of infected tissue and deoxyribonucleic acid (DNA) isolation and identification by the polymerase chain reaction (PCR) are also utilized.

### TREATMENT AND THERAPY

Starting the patient on an immediate antibiotic regimen of doxycycline is the preferred treatment. It is typically prescribed as a dosage of 100 milligrams, twice per day, for two to three weeks. Tetracycline and hydroxychloroquine have also proven useful. Treatment of chronic Q fever with endocarditis requires a combination of doxycycline and quinolone antibiotics, and the course of therapy may take three to four years.

## PREVENTION AND OUTCOMES

An effective vaccine against Q fever has been developed, and it is recommended for use by those with occupational risks for infection. The vaccine is not commercially available in the United States, but it can be obtained through government agencies such as the U.S. Army Medical Research Institute of Infectious Diseases. Pasteurization of milk usually kills the bacteria, but *Coxiella* can survive at 60° Fahrenheit (pasteurization temperature normally is set at 62.9° Fahrenheit, leaving a relatively small margin of error).

*Jeffrey A. Knight, Ph.D.*

## FURTHER READING

Lacasse, Alexandre, et al. "Q Fever." eMedicine. Available at http://emedicine.medscape.com/article/227156-overview.

Madigan, Michael T., and John M. Martinko. *Brock Biology of Microorganisms.* 12th ed. Upper Saddle River, N.J.: Pearson/Prentice Hall, 2010.

Marrie, T. J., and D. Raoult. "*Coxiella burnetii* (Q Fever)." In *Mandell, Douglas, and Bennett's Principles and Practice of Infectious Diseases*, edited by Gerald L. Mandell, John F. Bennett, and Raphael Dolin. 7th ed. New York: Churchill Livingstone/Elsevier, 2010.

Parker, N. R., J. H. Barralet, and A. M. Bell. "Q Fever." *The Lancet* 367 (February 25, 2006): 679-688.

Shakespeare, Martin. *Zoonoses.* 2d ed. London: Pharmaceutical Press, 2009.

Willey, Joanne M., Linda M. Sherwood, and Christopher J. Woolverton. *Prescott, Harley, and Klein's Microbiology.* 7th ed. New York: McGraw-Hill, 2008.

## WEB SITES OF INTEREST

*Genetic and Rare Diseases Information Center*
http://rarediseases.info.nih.gov/gard

*National Organization for Rare Disorders*
http://www.rarediseases.org

**See also:** Atypical pneumonia; Brucellosis; Food-borne illness and disease; Leptospirosis; Respiratory route of transmission; *Rickettsia*; Soilborne illness and disease; Zoonotic diseases.

# Quarantine

CATEGORY: Prevention

## DEFINITION

Quarantine is a state of compulsory or enforced isolation, confinement, or segregation to contain the spread of disease or other form of contamination. Quarantine can be applied to people, animals, and imported goods. The word "quarantine" comes from the Latin term *quaranta* ("forty"), which referred in this case to the numbers of days of confinement for ships coming into European ports in the fourteenth century.

Human quarantine periods vary according to the time necessary to prove that a person is no longer able to transmit a given disease. The quarantine may range from five days, in the case of measles, to forty days in cases of poliomyelitis and whooping cough.

## QUARANTINE CONDITIONS

Persons with leprosy were once exiled to leper colonies to isolate them from general populations. Persons with tuberculosis were once confined in sanatoriums and, later, in locked wards of hospitals for six months. Today, persons under quarantine must remain in their homes, hospitals, or other designated health care facilities until cleared by a public health official or by a health care provider.

## PRESENT QUARANTINE USE

Quarantine is still used in cases of emerging and infectious diseases that are difficult to treat. Diseases for which people may be quarantined include cholera, diphtheria, tuberculosis, smallpox, yellow fever, and Ebola and Marburg viruses. In 2003, a ten-day period was used in Canada and China to limit the spread of severe acute respiratory syndrome (SARS). Quarantine plans were prepared but not implemented for the swine influenza A (H1N1) outbreak in the United States in 2008.

Quarantine is ineffective, however, for diseases in

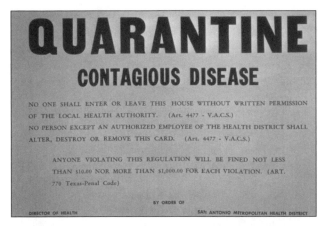

*An undated sign announces a disease-related quarantine in San Antonio, Texas.* (CDC)

which the carrier is contagious before showing symptoms. In addition, lengthy quarantine periods raise human rights concerns, and the confinement of infected persons who refuse medical treatment remains controversial.

## IMPACT

In November, 2005, after debating the ethical and practical considerations of quarantine, the American Medical Association adopted guidelines, which are specified in "The Use of Quarantine and Isolation as Public Health Interventions." These guidelines include the promotion of least-restrictive measures, timely detection and treatment, and education of the population. In October, 2006, the World Health Organization developed similar guidelines for addressing ethical issues in the planning of responses to pandemic influenza.

*Bethany Thivierge, M.P.H.*

## FURTHER READING

American Medical Association. "The Use of Quarantine and Isolation as Public Health Interventions." Available at http://www.cdc.gov/ncidod/sars/isolationquarantine.htm.

Bauerle, Bass S., et al. "If You Ask Them, Will They Come? Predictors of Quarantine Compliance During a Hypothetical Avian Influenza Pandemic: Results from a Statewide Survey." *Disaster Medicine and Public Health Preparedness* 4 (2010): 135-144.

Hodge, James G., Jr. "Protecting the Public's Health in an Era of Bioterrorism: The Model State Emergency Health Powers Act." *Accountability in Research* 10 (2003): 91-107.

Hunter, Nan D. *The Law of Emergencies: Public Health and Disaster Management.* Burlington, Mass.: Butterworth-Heinemann, 2009.

## WEB SITES OF INTEREST

*Centers for Disease Control and Prevention*
http://www.cdc.gov/quarantine

*Emerging and Reemerging Infectious Diseases Resource Center*
http://www.medscape.com/resource/infections

*World Health Organization: Global Alert and Response*
http://www.who.int/csr/don

**See also:** Bioterrorism; Centers for Disease Control and Prevention (CDC); Epidemiology; Outbreaks; Psychological effects of infectious disease; Public health; Social effects of infectious disease; World Health Organization (WHO).

# Quinolone antibiotics

CATEGORY: Treatment

## DEFINITION

Quinolone is a synthetic antibacterial (antibiotic) drug that is not of microbial origin. Its synthetic origin stems from nalidixic acid, a by-product of the antimalaria compound quinine. The original quinolones consisted of nalidixic acid, cinoxacin, and oxolinic acid but were of limited use. Chemical modifications of these antibiotics produced an improved class of potent antibiotics known as fluoroquinolones. Fluoroquinolones are divided into several groups based on their broad spectrum of activity and their pharmacological properties. The best-known fluoroquinolones include ciprofloxacin (Cipro), moxifloxacin (Avelox), and levofloxacin (Levaquin).

## MODE OF ACTION

Quinolones generally exhibit concentration-dependent bactericidal tendencies. These agents interfere with bacterial deoxyribonucleic acid (DNA) replica-

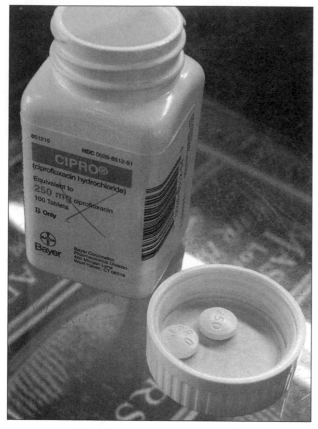

*Ciprofloxacin is a quinolone antibiotic that was used during the anthrax bioterrorism scare in October, 2001.* (AP/Wide World Photos)

tion and cause cell death. During this process, the antibiotic binds to and induces a conformational change in complexes created by bacterial DNA and the enzymes essential for their DNA replication, gyrase and topoisomerase. The bactericidal mechanism occurs at high antibiotic concentrations with the release of free DNA ends from the antibiotic-gyrase-DNA complexes.

### PHARMACOLOGY

The ability of an antibiotic to successfully inhibit infectious bacteria depends on its pharmacological profile. The most important attribute of the quinolones is their high bioavailability. These antibiotics are rapidly distributed into bodily fluids, show increased tissue absorption, have shorter dosing regimens, and are equally effective as either oral or intravenous therapy.

### INDICATIONS

The quinolone antibiotics are active against a broad range of pathogens, including gram-positive and gram-negative bacteria, mycobacteria, atypical pathogens, and some anaerobes. Clinical applications of these antibiotics include the treatment of urinary tract infections, including bacterial prostatitis; gynecological infections; sexually transmitted diseases; gastrointestinal infections, such as bacterial diarrhea; and respiratory tract infections. Several fluoroquinolones are established as ophthalmic agents used to treat bacterial eye infections such as conjunctivitis. One of the best-known fluoroquinolones, ciprofloxacin, is known for its use against anthrax infections.

### SIDE EFFECTS

Quinolones are relatively safe with mild side effects that include nausea, headache, dizziness, and confusion. Serious side effects are uncommon but can occur and include seizures, convulsions, hallucinations, phototoxicity, heart arrhythmias, and hepatotoxicity (liver damage). Quinolones are not recommended for persons with central nervous system disorders or epilepsy. Quinolones have also been linked to tendinitis and tendon rupture and their use is limited among children because of a risk of joint abnormalities. These agents also have an increased association with a severe secondary infection of the colon caused by the bacterium *Clostridium difficile* following antibiotic use.

### IMPACT

The emergence of quinolone-resistant strains of bacteria continues to be a worldwide concern. Although quinolones have evolved into a highly effective and valuable class of antibacterial agents, their continued overuse in clinical and veterinary medicine has limited their future effectiveness. Because of this likelihood of resistance, newer quinolones have been developed and are usually reserved for serious infections.

*Rose Ciulla-Bohling, Ph.D.*

### FURTHER READING

Ball, Peter. "Adverse Drug Reactions: Implications for the Development of Fluoroquinolones." *Journal of Antimicrobial Chemotherapy* 51 (2003): 21-27.

Emmerson, A. M., and A. M. Jones. "The Quinolones: Decades of Development and Use." *Journal of Antimicrobial Chemotherapy* 51 (2003): 13-20.

King, Dana E., Robb Malone, and Sandra H. Lilley.

"New Classification and Update on the Quinolone Antibiotics." *American Family Physician* 61 (2000): 2741-2748.

Oliphant, Catherine M., and Gary M. Green. "Quinolones: A Comprehensive Review." *American Family Physician* 65 (2002): 455-465.

**WEB SITES OF INTEREST**

*Alliance for the Prudent Use of Antibiotics*
http://www.tufts.edu/med/apua

*Centers for Disease Control and Prevention*
http://www.cdc.gov

*U.S. Food and Drug Administration*
http://www.fda.gov

**See also:** Alliance for the Prudent Use of Antibiotics; Aminoglycoside antibiotics; Antibiotics: Types; Bacteria: Classification and types; Cephalosporin antibiotics; Glycopeptide antibiotics; Ketolide antibiotics; Lipopeptide antibiotics; Macrolide antibiotics; Oxazolidinone antibiotics; Penicillin antibiotics; Prevention of bacterial infections; Reinfection; Secondary infection; Superbacteria; Tetracycline antibiotics; Treatment of bacterial infections.

# R

## Rabies

CATEGORY: Diseases and conditions
ANATOMY OR SYSTEM AFFECTED: Brain, central nervous system, spinal cord

### DEFINITION

Rabies is a viral infection that infects the brain and spine. Rabies is almost always fatal unless treated before symptoms appear.

### CAUSES

Rabies is caused by a virus that is found in infected warm-blooded animals. Animals that commonly carry the virus include bats, raccoons, skunks, foxes, and coyotes. The virus that causes rabies is in the saliva, brain, or nerve tissue of infected animals. Humans most often contract rabies through a bite or scratch from an infected animal. The virus may also be passed if infected tissue comes into contact with human mucous membranes. This tissue is found in the eyes, nose, or mouth.

### RISK FACTORS

The only risk factor for rabies is contact with an infected animal. In most parts of the United States, any contact with a bat may be considered a rabies risk factor. One should seek medical advice if a bat is found anywhere inside the home.

### SYMPTOMS

Symptoms often start within three to seven weeks. In some cases, the virus can incubate up to one or more years. Death usually occurs within a week after symptoms appear. The symptoms in humans include pain, tingling, or itching at the site of the bite wound or other site of viral entry; stiff muscles; increased production of thick saliva; flulike symptoms, such as headache, fever, fatigue, and nausea; painful spasms and contractions of the throat when exposed to water (called hydrophobia); erratic, excited, or bizarre behavior; and paralysis. Symptoms in animals include erratic behavior that is often overly aggressive or vicious,

---

### Facts: Rabies

- Rabies occurs in more than 150 countries and territories.

- Worldwide, more than 55,000 people die of rabies infection each year.

- Forty percent of persons who are bitten by suspect rabid animals are children younger than age fifteen years.

- Dogs are the source of 99 percent of human rabies deaths.

- Wound cleansing and immunization within a few hours after contact with a suspect rabid animal can prevent the onset of rabies, and possible death.

- Every year, more than 15 million people worldwide receive a postexposure treatment regimen to avert the disease; this is estimated to prevent 327,000 rabies deaths annually.

*Source:* World Health Organization.

---

and disorientation (for example, nocturnal animals such as bats or foxes appearing during daylight hours).

### SCREENING AND DIAGNOSIS

Any person who has possibly been exposed to rabies should contact a doctor or public health official immediately. To diagnose rabies, the suspect animal, if available and if it appears well, is kept under observation for ten days. If no symptoms develop in the animal, then the reporting person is not at risk for rabies. If the animal is first found sick or dead, its head will be shipped to a special facility, where its brain will be examined for the presence of the virus. In the meantime, the patient may be advised to begin treatment.

If the animal cannot be found, the person bitten may begin treatment as a preventive measure. This decision to treat depends on the animal's species, where the encounter took place, and other factors.

cine will be injected into the patient's upper arm muscles. Certain medicine may interfere with the response to the rabies vaccine.

## PREVENTION AND OUTCOMES

To help prevent rabies, one should vaccinate house pets, avoid contact with wild animals, and avoid touching wild animals, even if they appear dead. Also, one should seal basement, porch, and attic openings to prevent animals from entering the home, and should report animals to local animal control if they are acting strange or appear sick. If a person must contact potentially rabid animals, such as in a work environment, he or she should get a rabies vaccine before exposure. Booster doses are often needed too.

*Michelle Badash, M.S.; reviewed by David L. Horn, M.D., FACP*

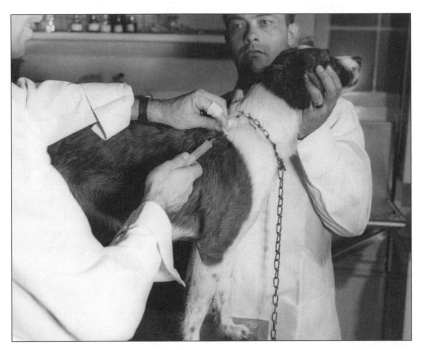

*A veterinarian and colleague with the Centers for Disease Control and Prevention administer a rabies vaccine.* (CDC)

## TREATMENT AND THERAPY

If bitten by an animal, one should wash the wound with soap and water. Doing so will remove saliva, the most critical first step in preventing rabies. One should then consult a doctor or seek care in an emergency room.

If rabies exposure is likely, a doctor will recommend postexposure prophylaxis, treatment to prevent illness. This treatment involves two injections. The first is the human rabies immunoglobulin (HRIg), which ideally should be given within twenty-four hours after exposure. HRIg contains large amounts of antibodies to the rabies virus. In most cases, one-half of the dose should be injected into the wound and surrounding tissue. The rest is injected into a muscle. If the patient has previously received a rabies vaccine, he or she may not need the HRIg shot.

Another type of injection makes the immune system create antibodies against the virus. These antibodies will live in the body for many years. There are three types of rabies vaccines available, including the human diploid cell vaccine (HDCV), rabies vaccine adsorbed (RVA), and purified chick embryo cell culture (PCEC). The doctor will administer five shots of one of these vaccines, which will be given over four weeks. The vac-

## FURTHER READING

Baer, George M., ed. *The Natural History of Rabies.* 2d ed. Boca Raton, Fla.: CRC Press, 1991.

Blanton, Jesse D., et al. "Rabies Surveillance in the United States During 2007." *Journal of the American Veterinary Medical Association* 233 (2008): 884-897.

Centers for Disease Control and Prevention. "Rabies." Available at http://www.cdc.gov/rabies.

Dietzschold, Bernhard, et al. "Concepts in the Pathogenesis of Rabies." *Future Virology* 3, no. 5 (2008): 481-490.

EBSCO Publishing. *DynaMed: Rabies.* Available through http://www.ebscohost.com/dynamed.

Hankins, D. G., and J. A. Rosekrans. "Overview, Prevention, and Treatment of Rabies." *Mayo Clinic Proceedings* 79, no. 5 (May, 2004): 671-676.

Jackson, Alan C., and William H. Wunner, eds. *Rabies.* 2d ed. San Diego, Calif.: Academic Press, 2007.

Krauss, Hartmut, et al. *Zoonoses: Infectious Diseases Transmissible from Animals to Humans.* 3d ed. Washington, D.C.: ASM Press, 2003.

Manning, S. E., et al. "Human Rabies Prevention: United States, 2008." *Morbidity and Mortality Weekly Report* 57 (2008): 1.

Morgan, Marina, and John Palmer. "Dog Bites." *British Medical Journal* 334 (2007): 413-417.

Parker, James N., and Philip M. Parker, eds. *The Official Patient's Sourcebook on Rabies.* San Diego, Calif.: Icon Health, 2002.

### WEB SITES OF INTEREST

*Alliance for Rabies Control*
http://www.rabiescontrol.net

*Centers for Disease Control and Prevention*
http://www.cdc.gov/rabies

*Companion Animal Parasite Council*
http://www.capcvet.org

*Public Health Agency of Canada*
http://www.phac-aspc.gc.ca

**See also:** Antibodies; Cat scratch fever; Dogs and infectious disease; Encephalitis; Rabies vaccine; Rhabdoviridae; Saliva and infectious disease; Transmission routes; Vaccines: Types; Viral infections; Zoonotic diseases.

# Rabies vaccine

CATEGORY: Prevention

### DEFINITION

Rabies vaccines are made from the killed rabies virus and are administered as a series of shots as soon as possible after a potential exposure. Rabies is a serious viral infection of the central nervous system. The virus is transmitted through the saliva of an infected animal through a bite or scratch. Licking alone rarely transmits the disease unless the infected saliva enters an open sore or a mucous membrane. All mammals, such as raccoons, skunks, ferrets, dogs, and cats, are susceptible to infection, but bats are the most commonly infected animals in the United States.

Although earlier administration of the rabies vaccine is preferred, it may be given at any time during the incubation phase. Once symptoms begin, however, it is too late for vaccination.

### DISEASE COURSE

Rabies infection begins slowly with an incubation period of one to three months. The virus travels from the site of the bite through the nerves to the brain, where it replicates. The first symptoms are mild and vague, consisting of headaches, fatigue, and fever. The disease then progresses rapidly. Symptoms of advanced rabies infection include the characteristic hydrophobia, or fear of water, where the presence or even the thought of water causes muscle spasms in the throat. The infected person may become hyperactive and aggressive. As the disease progresses, the person becomes completely paralyzed and dies, often from respiratory failure.

### TYPES

After exposure to rabies, the infected person will receive two types of vaccine. First, rabies immunoglobulin (RIg) is given at a dose based on the weight of the infected person. Part of the RIg is delivered at the site of the bite, if possible, and the remainder is injected into a muscle. The amount of RIg delivered to the wound depends on the size of the wound. Next, a series of five shots of either human-diploid-cell rabies vaccine (HDCV) or purified chick-embryo cell vaccine (PCEC) is administered intramuscularly immediately and then again at three, seven, fourteen, and twenty-eight days. All doses must be administered without interruption.

Pre-exposure vaccines are given to those at high risk for rabies exposure, such as veterinarians or anyone who frequently comes in contact with wild animals. These consist of either HDCV or PCEC, delivered intramuscularly for the initial dose then again at seven, fourteen, twenty-one, and twenty-eight days. After a rabies exposure, two doses of HDCV or PCEC are still required, but RIg is unnecessary.

The vaccines are recommended also for pregnant women who may have been exposed to the rabies virus. Infants and children receive the vaccines on the same schedule as adults, although the dose of RIg is proportionately smaller.

### SIDE EFFECTS

The most common vaccine side effects are swelling, redness, and itching at the vaccine site and headaches, nausea, abdominal pain, dizziness, or muscle aches in general. In rare cases, the person may develop hives or malaise.

### IMPACT

Rabies cannot be treated, but it can be prevented with vaccination. The rabies vaccine is highly effective

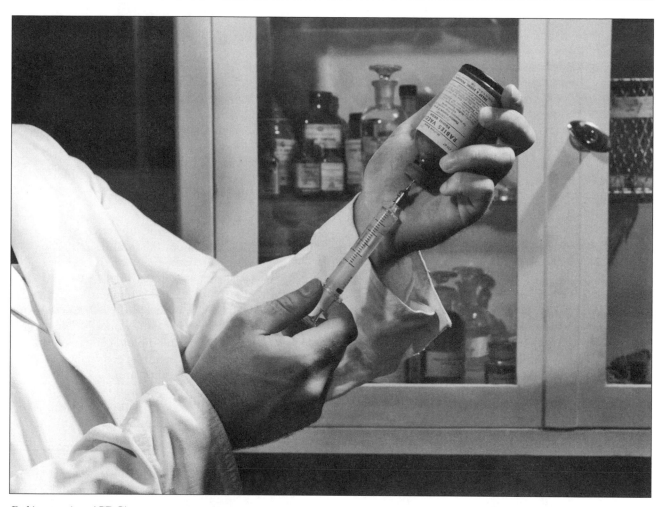

*Rabies vaccine.* (CDC)

when administered as soon as possible after a possible exposure to the rabies virus. The disease is always fatal in unvaccinated people. No case of rabies has occurred in any person who has received the vaccine after exposure to animals proven to be rabid.

*Cheryl Pokalo Jones*

**FURTHER READING**

Atkinson, W., et al., eds. *Epidemiology and Prevention of Vaccine-Preventable Diseases.* 11th ed. Washington, D.C.: Public Health Foundation, 2009.

Hankins, D. G., and J. A. Rosekrans. "Overview, Prevention, and Treatment of Rabies." *Mayo Clinic Proceedings* 79, no. 5 (May, 2004): 671-676.

Jackson, Alan C., and William H. Wunner, eds. *Rabies.* 2d ed. San Diego, Calif.: Academic Press, 2007.

Kienzle, Thomas E. *Rabies.* Philadelphia: Chelsea House, 2006.

Klosterman, Lorrie. *Rabies.* Tarrytown, N.Y.: Marshall Cavendish Benchmark, 2008.

Krauss, Hartmut, et al. *Zoonoses: Infectious Diseases Transmissible from Animals to Humans.* 3d ed. Washington, D.C.: ASM Press, 2003.

Pace, Brian, and Richard M. Glass. "Rabies." *Journal of the American Medical Association* 284, no. 8 (August 30, 2000): 1052.

Parker, James N., and Philip M. Parker, eds. *The Official Patient's Sourcebook on Rabies.* San Diego, Calif.: Icon Health, 2002.

Playfair, J. H. L., and B. M. Chain. *Immunology at a Glance.* 9th ed. Hoboken, N.J.: Wiley-Blackwell, 2009.

**See also:** Antibodies; Bats and infectious disease; Cat scratch fever; Cats and infectious disease; Dogs and infectious disease; Encephalitis; Immunity; Plague; Rabies; Rat-bite fever; Rhabdoviridae; Rodents and infectious disease; Saliva and infectious disease; Vaccines: Types; Viral infections; Zoonotic diseases.

---

# Rat-bite fever

CATEGORY: Diseases and conditions
ANATOMY OR SYSTEM AFFECTED: All
ALSO KNOWN AS: Epidemic arthritic erythema, Haverhill fever, Sodoku, spirillary fever, streptobacillary fever, streptobacillosis

## DEFINITION

Rat-bite fever (RBF) is an infectious disease caused by two strains of bacteria, *Streptobacillus moniliformis* and *Spirillum minus*. The bacteria are spread through the bite of rodents or through the secretion of rodent fluids.

## CAUSES

RBF primarily develops when rats bite or scratch humans, but infection can also occur simply by touching live or dead rats and by being exposed to secretions

---

### Mouse and Rat Facts

TAXONOMIC CLASSIFICATION
**Kingdom:** Animalia
**Subkingdom:** Bilateria
**Phylum:** Chordata
**Subphylum:** Vertebrata
**Class:** Mammalia
**Subclass:** Theria
**Order:** Rodentia
**Suborder:** Myomorpha
**Family:** Muridae (15 subfamilies, 241 genera, and
   1,082 species)

**Geographical location:** Worldwide, through
   introduction by humans
**Habitat:** Occurs in highly varied habitats, usually in
   association with humans
**Gestational period:** Nineteen to twenty-two days,
   although this may be lengthened in nursing
   females because of delayed implantation
**Life span:** Around one year in the wild; laboratory
   rats and mice may live three to four years or
   longer
**Special anatomy:** The scantily haired tail helps to
   distinguish house mice and Norway rats from
   most other types of mice and rats

---

from their eyes, nose, or mouth. Additionally, cleaning rat cages and coming in contact with rat urine or feces can cause RBF. Living in rat-infested environments, such as impoverished areas, often leads to RBF, inadvertently ingesting food or water contaminated with rat feces or urine. Breathing in desiccated particles of rat feces may also result in RBF. Gerbils, squirrels, and weasels also carry RBF; furthermore, animals that hunt and ingest rodents, such as cats and dogs, may also infect humans with RBF through a bite, scratch, or secretions.

## RISK FACTORS

Those who live in rat-infested environments are at greatest risk for RBF. Persons living in Asian countries, such as Japan, where the farming of rice attracts large numbers of rats, are more likely to be infected. However, RBF is also present in impoverished North American cities, which often provide a haven for rodent populations. Sanitation and sewage workers are also at high risk of RBF because of daily rodent contact. Laboratory staff are equally vulnerable to RBF because they regularly handle rats and clean their cages; pet store staff are also susceptible to RBF because of increased exposure to pet rats.

## SYMPTOMS

Symptoms of RBF include a rash, headache, chills, fever, vomiting, swelling of the lymph nodes, skin irritation, wounds that do not heal, and muscle, joint, and back pain. In particular, the area around the rat bite sometimes becomes reddish purple and swollen and ulcerated.

## SCREENING AND DIAGNOSIS

After a physical examination, blood and culture tests are performed to confirm a diagnosis of RBF. The tests determine if *S. moniliformis* or *S. minus* bacteria are in the person's blood, skin, joint fluid, or lymph nodes. Polymerase chain reaction tests and blood antibody tests aid in the diagnosis of RBF.

## TREATMENT AND THERAPY

RBF can be treated successfully in early stages of the disease with seven to fourteen days of antibiotics, primarily penicillin, doxycycline, and erythromycin. If left untreated, RBF is extremely dangerous and can damage the heart, brain, and other vital organs; it can sometimes lead to death.

## PREVENTION AND OUTCOMES

Avoiding rat-populated environments is the best way to prevent RBF; however, if contact with rats cannot be avoided, one should always wear gloves when handling them or their droppings; one should also wash his or her hands often. Persons who have been bitten by a rat should treat the wound with antiseptic immediately to help prevent infection and should contact a physician for further care.

*Mary E. Markland, M.A.*

## FURTHER READING

Dvorak, Glenda, Anna Spickler, and James Roth. *Handbook for Zoonotic Diseases of Companion Animals.* Ames: College of Veterinary Medicine, Iowa State University, 2008.

Gratz, Norman. *The Vector- and Rodent-Borne Diseases of Europe and North America: Their Distribution, Public Health Burden, and Control.* New York: Cambridge University Press, 2006.

Hayashimoto, N., et al. "Isolation of *Streptobacillus moniliformis* from a Pet Rat." *Journal of Veterinary Medical Science* 70 (2008): 493-495.

Peters, C. J. "Infections Caused by Arthropod- and Rodent-Borne Viruses." In *Harrison's Principles of Internal Medicine*, edited by Joan Butterton. 17th ed. New York: McGraw-Hill, 2008.

Suckow, Mark, Steven Weisbroth, and Craig Franklin. *The Laboratory Rat.* 2d ed. Burlington, Mass.: Academic Press/Elsevier, 2006.

## WEB SITES OF INTEREST

*Centers of Disease Control and Prevention*
http://www.cdc.gov/rodents

*Rat Behavior and Biology*
http://www.ratbehavior.org

*University of California, San Francisco*
http://www.iacuc.ucsf.edu/safe/awohsmrhr.asp

**See also:** Bacterial infections; Rodents and infectious disease; Vectors and vector control; Zoonotic diseases.

---

Reemerging infectious diseases. *See* Emerging and reemerging infectious diseases.

---

# Reinfection

CATEGORY: Epidemiology

## DEFINITION

A reinfection occurs when a bacterium, virus, or fungus reemerges to infect a person after he or she has recovered from an initial infection. Some persons are more prone to reinfections than others, such as those with impaired immune systems or those who must take immunosuppressant medications. In addition, some types of infections are more likely to occur as reinfections. For example, simple urinary tract infection (UTI) in women will reoccur in up to 50 percent of cases within a few months; the rate can be higher in more complex cases. In another example, research indicates that those persons who are cured of an infection with *Helicobacter pylori*, bacteria that infect the stomach, are reinfected with *H. pylori* at a rate of about 9 percent per year.

## IMMUNOSUPPRESSANT MEDICATIONS

People who must take immunosuppressive drugs, or immunosuppressants, for autoimmune diseases that attack the body are at risk for reinfection. For example, persons with rheumatoid arthritis are at increased risk for reinfection because they take immunosuppressive medications, such as methotrexate, to decrease pain and other symptoms. These drugs may need to be discontinued if the sick person is hospitalized for a serious infection, such as pneumonia. Others who must take immunosuppressants to treat disease symptoms include persons with inflammatory bowel disease or psoriasis and persons who have received a transplanted organ. Transplant recipients take immunosuppressant drugs so that their bodies will not reject the transplanted organ; these drugs must be taken for life.

## CANCER

Cancer can cause an immune deficiency, particularly among those persons who must have chemotherapy treatment. This treatment can significantly reduce the number of white blood cells produced and can thus leave the person more prone to both infections and reinfections. Persons with cancer who are receiving chemotherapy should be sure to contact their physician or nurse if they have a fever of 100.5° Fahrenheit or greater. An infection may be causing the fever, and it is necessary to determine if immediate treatment is needed.

## ACQUIRED IMMUNE DISORDERS AND INHERITED IMMUNE DEFICIENCIES

People with the acquired immunodeficiency syndrome (AIDS) have an elevated risk for reinfection because their immune systems work poorly. AIDS is caused by infection with the human immunodeficiency virus, which is primarily contracted during unprotected sex with an infected person or when sharing needles in intravenous drug use.

Some people are born with an impaired immune system called common variable immune deficiency (CVID); others are born with related immune deficiency disorders. These disorders are genetic, thus they cannot be transmitted to others. Most people with CVID have pneumonia a minimum of one time in their lives, and many have repeated bouts. These disorders are generally more likely to be linked to males rather than females because many genetic disorders that impair the immune system are X-linked; that is, they are linked to the X chromosome. In many cases, the disorder is not diagnosed until adulthood. About 1 in 50,000 people in the United States has CVID.

## IMPACT

Reinfection, which can cause serious pain and discomfort, can also lead to further complications. For example, reinfection of the urinary tract may lead to kidney infection if it is not treated, and reinfection with *H. pylori* bacteria can lead to the development of peptic ulcers and stomach cancer.

The use of antibiotics for infections can lead to antibiotic resistance if the person taking the medication does not follow through with the treatment plan. Also, reinfection exacerbates the problem of antibiotic resistance if that person has developed resistance to that particular antibiotic.

*Christine Adamec, M.B.A.*

## FURTHER READING

National Institutes of Health, Genetics Home Reference. "Common Variable Immune Deficiency." Available at http://ghr.nlm.nih.gov/condition/common-variable-immune-deficiency. This article provides general information on the genetic causes and on the impact of common variable immune deficiency in the United States.

Parker, James N., and Philip M. Parker, eds. *The Official Patient's Sourcebook on Urinary Tract Infection.* San Diego, Calif.: Icon Health, 2002. Draws from public, academic, government, and peer-reviewed research to provide a wide-ranging handbook for persons with recurring urinary tract infections.

Ryu, Kum Hei, et al. "Reinfection Rate and Endoscopic Changes After Successful Eradication of *Helicobacter pylori*." *World Journal of Gastroenterology* 16, no. 2 (2010): 251-255. Discussion of the rates of reinfection in cases involving *H. pylori* infection of the gastrointestinal tract.

Weiner, I. David, and Christine Adamec. *The Encyclopedia of Kidney Diseases and Disorders.* New York: Facts On File, 2011. This book discusses kidney transplants, the drugs that must be taken to prevent rejection of the transplanted kidney, and the accompanying risks that are associated with transplants, such as reinfection.

## WEB SITES OF INTEREST

*Immune Deficiency Foundation*
http://www.primaryimmune.org

*National Institute of Allergy and Infectious Diseases*
http://www.niaid.nih.gov/topics/antimicrobialresistance

*Todar's Online Textbook of Bacteriology*
http://www.textbookofbacteriology.net

**See also:** AIDS; Alliance for the Prudent Use of Antibiotics; Antibiotics: Types; Drug resistance; HIV; Hospitals and infectious disease; Iatrogenic infections; Immunity; Immunodeficiency; Infection; Microbiology; Primary infection; Public health; Secondary infection; Superbacteria; Wound infections.

---

# Reiter's syndrome

CATEGORY: Diseases and conditions
ANATOMY OR SYSTEM AFFECTED: Bones, eyes, joints, musculoskeletal system, urinary system
ALSO KNOWN AS: Reactive arthritis

## DEFINITION

Reiter's syndrome is an inflammatory reaction to an infection in the body. The syndrome usually follows a urogenital or intestinal infection. Symptoms of the disorder primarily involve three body systems: the joints, eyes, and urinary tract or genitals.

## CAUSES

Reiter's syndrome is triggered by certain infections in genetically susceptible persons. The infection often starts in the urinary tract or genitals and is usually caused by the bacterium *Chlamydia trachomatis. Chlamydia* is passed from person to person through sexual activity.

The infection can also begin in the digestive system. In these cases, the infection occurs after eating food tainted with bacteria, usually *Shigella, Salmonella, Yersinia,* or *Campylobacter.*

About one to four weeks after the infection, a susceptible person may develop Reiter's syndrome. Doctors do not know why some people develop the disease and others do not, but most persons with the condition carry a specific genetic factor called HLA-B27 (or the B27 gene).

## RISK FACTORS

Risk factors for Reiter's syndrome include having family members who have had the syndrome; having inherited the genetic trait associated with Reiter's syndrome; having a sexually transmitted disease (STD); having a recent, new sexual partner; and eating improperly handled food. Also at higher risk are males in general, persons age twenty to forty years, and gay and bisexual males.

## SYMPTOMS

Symptoms occur in three main areas of the body: the joints, the eyes, and the urinary tract and genitals. Men and women may experience different symptoms, and symptoms may come and go. The disease may be milder in women. In rare cases, heart problems may develop later in the disease.

In the joints, specific symptoms include swelling, pain, and redness, especially in the knees, ankles, and feet; heel pain; shortening and thickening of fingers and toes; and back pain and stiffness. In the eyes, the symptoms are redness, pain, irritation, blurred vision, tearing, discharge, and, sometimes, sun sensitivity or swollen eyelids.

Symptoms in the urinary tract and reproductive system includes (in men) frequent urination, a burning sensation when passing urine, penal discharge, sores at the end of the penis, fever, and chills. In women, the symptoms include a burning sensation when passing urine, and an inflamed vagina and cervix. Other symptoms for both men and women include a rash, especially on the palms or soles; ulcers in the mouth or on the tongue; weight loss; poor appetite; fatigue; and fever.

Rare complications may include heart conduction defects (for example, arrhythmias), a heart murmur (aortic insufficiency), and pericarditis (inflammation of outer lining of heart); pneumonia, pulmonary fibrosis, and fluid on the lung (pleural effusion); nervous system problems such as neuropathy, including tingling or loss of sensation; and behavior changes.

## SCREENING AND DIAGNOSIS

A doctor will ask about symptoms and medical history and will perform a physical exam. The doctor's findings will be used to help make a diagnosis. There is no specific test to check for Reiter's syndrome, but other tests may check for a variety of conditions. Blood tests will check for signs of inflammation (the blood's sedimentation rate), signs of infection (with a complete blood count), and the genetic factor associated with Reiter's syndrome (HLA-B27).

Other tests include a culture and a Gram's stain to look for bacteria that commonly cause infections associated with Reiter's syndrome; the removal of synovial fluid from around the joints to check for infection; X rays of the joints; an ultrasound; a magnetic resonance imaging (MRI) scan (a scan that uses radio waves and a powerful magnet to produce detailed computer images); and a computed tomography (CT) scan (a detailed X-ray picture that identifies abnormalities of fine tissue structure).

## TREATMENT AND THERAPY

There is no cure for Reiter's syndrome. However, early treatment of the infection may slow or stop the course of the disease. Most people recover from the initial episode within six months, but some develop a mild, chronic arthritis and others suffer from additional bouts of the disorder.

Treatment aims to relieve symptoms and may include bed rest (short-term bed rest to take strain off the joints), exercise such as gentle range-of-motion to improve flexibility, strengthening to build muscles that can better support the joints, and physical therapy, with specific exercises to keep muscles strong and joints moving. Other treatment options are to protect the joints with assistive devices as recommended by a doctor and occupational therapy to learn how to gently use the joints during daily activities.

The doctor may prescribe medications, including nonsteroidal anti-inflammatory drugs (NSAIDs) such as aspirin, ibuprofen (such as Motrin and Advil), sulfasalazine (Azulfidine); steroids that are injected into the inflamed joint; topical steroid creams that are applied to skin lesions; antibiotics to treat the triggering infection; immunosuppressive drugs (drugs that decrease the immune system's ability to function) such as azathioprine (Azasan, Imuran) and methotrexate; and eye drops.

## PREVENTION AND OUTCOMES

The key to preventing Reiter's syndrome is to avoid the triggering infection. To do so, one should avoid infection with an STD, either by abstaining from sex or by practicing safer sex. Safer sex includes always using a latex condom during sexual intercourse, asking sex partners about their history of sexual disease, having monogamous sex, and getting regular checkups for STDs. One should also take steps to prevent chlamydia urogenital infections, especially if one is age twenty-five years or younger, and should be tested for chlamydia annually. Females who are pregnant also should be tested for chlamydia.

Another preventive measure against developing a triggering infection is to avoid intestinal infections. One can do this by washing one's hands before eating or handling food and by eating only those foods that have been stored and prepared properly.

*Debra Wood, R.N.; reviewed by Jill D. Landis, M.D.*

## FURTHER READING

Bellenir, Karen, ed. *Genetic Disorders Sourcebook*. 3d ed. Detroit: Omnigraphics, 2004.

Harris, Edward D., Jr., et al., eds. *Kelley's Textbook of Rheumatology*. 7th ed. Philadelphia: Saunders/Elsevier, 2005.

Icon Health. *Reiter's Syndrome: A Medical Dictionary, Bibliography, and Annotated Research Guide to Internet References*. San Diego, Calif.: Author, 2004.

Isenberg, David A., et al., eds. *Oxford Textbook of Rheumatology*. 3d ed. New York: Oxford University Press, 2004.

McCance, Kathryn L., and Sue M. Huether. *Pathophysiology: The Biologic Basis for Disease in Adults and Children*. 6th ed. St. Louis, Mo.: Mosby/Elsevier, 2010.

Schrier, Robert W., ed. *Diseases of the Kidney and Urinary Tract*. 8th ed. Philadelphia: Wolters Kluwer Health/Lippincott Williams & Wilkins, 2007.

Toivanen, Auli. "Reactive Arthritis: Clinical Features and Treatment." In *Practical Rheumatology*, edited by Marc C. Hochberg. 3d ed. Philadelphia: Mosby, 2006.

## WEB SITES OF INTEREST

*American Congress of Obstetricians and Gynecologists*
http://www.acog.org

*Arthritis Foundation*
http://www.arthritis.org

*Arthritis Society*
http://www.arthritis.ca

*Genetic Alliance*
http://www.geneticalliance.org

*National Institute of Arthritis and Musculoskeletal and
    Skin Diseases*
http://www.niams.nih.gov

*Spondylitis Association of America*
http://www.spondylitis.org

**See also:** Autoimmune disorders; Bacterial infections; *Campylobacter*; Chlamydia; *Chlamydia*; Food-borne illness and disease; Inflammation; Intestinal and stomach infections; Pelvic inflammatory disease; Prostatitis; *Salmonella*; Sexually transmitted diseases (STDs); *Shigella*; Urethritis; Urinary tract infections; *Yersinia*.

---

> ### Taxonomic Classification
> ### for Reoviridae
>
> **Order:** Unassigned
> **Family:** Reoviridae
> **Subfamily:** Sedoreovirinae
> **Genus:** *Orbivirus*
> **Species:**
> Lipovnik virus
> Tribec virus
> Changuinola virus
> **Genus:** *Rotavirus*
> **Species:** Rotaviruses A, B, and C
> **Genus:** *Seadornavirus*
> **Species:** Banna virus
> **Subfamily:** *Spinareovirinae*
> **Genus:** *Coltivirus*
> **Species:** Colorado tick fever virus

# Reoviridae

CATEGORY: Pathogen
TRANSMISSION ROUTE: Direct contact, ingestion, inhalation

## DEFINITION

The Reoviridae is a ubiquitous and diverse family of viruses. Family members infect plants, insects, humans, and other animals. The Reoviridae family comprises the only viruses known to have double-stranded RNA (ribonucleic acid) genomes. Reovirus infections in humans affect the gastrointestinal and respiratory tracts. Illnesses caused by reoviruses are common but generally mild.

## NATURAL HABITAT AND FEATURES

The reovirus family is represented worldwide, with many species isolated to particular geographic areas. Five genera of reoviruses cause disease in humans. Three of these five genera, *Coltivirus*, *Seadornavirus*, and *Orbivirus*, are composed entirely of arboviruses. Arboviruses infect insects, which then transmit the virus to humans as vectors.

All reovirus family members have a symmetrical structure composed of two concentric icosahedral capsids. Virions measure 60 to 80 nanometers (nm) in diameter and have no outer envelope. The double-stranded RNA genome, located in the viral core, is segmented into ten to twelve separate molecules. The total genome is 16 to 27 kilobase pairs in size, and individual RNA molecules range in size from 680 to 3900 base pairs. Viral replication takes place only in the host cell cytoplasm; the virion core thus carries all the enzymes required for RNA transcription.

## PATHOGENICITY AND CLINICAL SIGNIFICANCE

Rotavirus is the most significant reovirus because of the number of people it infects and because of the severity of the resulting illness. Rotavirus is the leading cause of acute vomiting and severe diarrhea among infants and young children worldwide. Rotavirus accounts for 50 to 80 percent of all cases of viral gastroenteritis. It is more frequent in winter, during cold and dry conditions. Most cases resolve on their own within three to eight days of the start of symptoms.

Rotavirus infections are most severe in infants eleven months of age and younger. Dehydration is a serious complication of rotavirus, leading to high mortality rates in developing countries. Worldwide, one-half million children age five years and younger die each year from rotavirus infection. Before the introduction of a rotavirus vaccine in 2006, nearly all children in the United States, for example, had been infected with rotavirus by their fifth birthday.

Orthoreovirus infection is generally benign in humans, causing no disease symptoms. In rare cases, respiratory or gastrointestinal symptoms may be present.

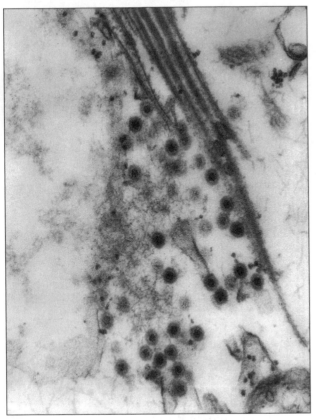

*The Colorado tick fever virus, a member of the Reoviridae family of viruses.* (CDC)

Coltiviruses, orbiviruses, and seadornaviruses are all spread by insects and cause infections only rarely in humans. Symptoms of infection are similar for all viruses in these genera and include fever, muscle aches, and headache. Neurological complications, such as meningitis or encephalitis, may occur but are very rare.

Colorado tick fever (CTF) is caused by a coltivirus found only in the western United States and Canada. Transmitted by the *Dermacentor andersoni* wood tick, CTF is the most serious of the insect-borne reoviruses. Several hundred cases are reported each year in the United States. CTF can be serious in children, with hospitalization required in 20 percent of cases. The illness lasts five to ten days, and fatalities are very rare. A similar human coltivirus is Eyach virus, found in central Europe. As with CTF, Eyach virus is spread by ticks.

Human diseases caused by orbiviruses are extremely rare, with about fifty cases reported worldwide. Orungo virus and Lebombo virus are both transmitted by mosquitoes in Africa, and they have been isolated from humans. Kemovoro, Lipovnik, and Tribec viruses are tickborne and are associated with encephalitis in central Europe and Russia. Meningitis and possibly the autoimmune disorder Guillain-Barré syndrome have been attributed to Lipovnik virus in the area of the Czech Republic.

In South America, serum antibodies against Changuinola virus are common, indicating frequent infection. This virus is transmitted by *Phlebotomous* flies. However, only one case of human disease due to this virus, in Panama, has been reported.

Seadornaviruses are spread by mosquitoes and are endemic to China and Indonesia. The only seadornavirus known to infect humans is Banna virus. The prevalence of Banna virus is unknown because it may be confused with Japanese encephalitis, which is common in Banna virus-endemic areas. Symptoms of Banna virus infection are similar to other arboviruses in the reovirus family and include muscle aches, headache, and, in some cases, encephalitis.

### DRUG SUSCEPTIBILITY

No drugs exist for the treatment of reovirus infection. One possible exception is the drug ribavirin, which has shown promising results against CTF in studies. A vaccine against rotavirus is available.

*Kathryn Pierno, M.S.*

### FURTHER READING

Attoui, Houssam, et al. "Coltiviruses and Seadornaviruses in North America, Europe, and Asia." *Emerging Infectious Diseases* 11, no. 11 (2005): 1673-1679. Also available at http://www.cdc.gov/ncidod/eid/vol11no11/pdfs/05-0868.pdf. Detailed summary of the history, epidemiology, transmission, and molecular biology of these viruses.

Crum-Cianflone, Nancy F. "Orbivirus." Available at http://emedicine.medscape.com/article/224420-overview. Overview, diagnosis, and treatment of orbivirus infections.

Madigan, Michael T., and John M. Martinko. *Brock Biology of Microorganisms.* 12th ed. Upper Saddle River, N.J.: Pearson/Prentice Hall, 2010. An introductory microbiology textbook for students of medicine and microbiology, with simplified descriptions of pathogenic organisms.

Rasouli, Gholamreza, and John W. King. "Reoviruses." Available at http://emedicine.medscape.com/article/227348-overview. Overview of *Rotavirus*, *Coltivirus*, and *Orbivirus*. Covers epidemiology, molecular biology, clinical aspects of disease, and treatment.

**WEB SITES OF INTEREST**

*American Society for Microbiology*
http://www.microbeworld.org

*Big Picture Book of Viruses*
http://www.virology.net/big_virology

*Centers for Disease Control and Prevention*
http://www.cdc.gov/vaccines/vpd-vac/rotavirus/default.htm

**See also:** Children and infectious disease; Colorado tick fever; Encephalitis; Fecal-oral route of transmission; Intestinal and stomach infections; Rotavirus infection; Travelers' diarrhea; Viral infections; Virology; Viruses: Structure and life cycle; Viruses: Types.

---

Repellants. *See* Insecticides and topical repellants.

---

# Reptiles and infectious disease

CATEGORY: Transmission
ALSO KNOWN AS: Reptilian zoonoses

**DEFINITION**

Reptiles, including snakes, lizards, crocodilians, turtles, and tortoises, can act as hosts and reservoirs for many infectious disease agents. Some of these agents, particularly bacteria, can be transmitted to humans through direct contact with reptiles or their environments.

**BACTERIAL INFECTIONS**

Many common bacterial species normally occur in reptiles and generally cause few problems for their hosts. When these bacteria are transmitted to humans, however, through contact with reptiles and their environments, serious illness can result.

*Campylobacter jejuni* and *C. coli* are gram-negative, spiral, microaerophilic bacteria that may be present in the feces and contaminated water of pet reptiles. A *Campylobacter* infection in humans causes vomiting, diarrhea, and other gastroenteritis symptoms. Most cases involving *Campylobacter* resolve within a week with either no treatment or with a course of antibiotics. A rare but serious complication of this type of bacterial infection is Guillain-Barré syndrome, a neurological disorder in which the body's immune system attacks the peripheral nervous system.

*Edwardsiella tarda*, a gram-negative enterobacteria residing in some reptilian species, has occasionally caused gastroenteritis and wound infections in humans who either handled infected reptiles or received bites from pets such as iguanas. *Enterobacter* spp., frequently part of the normal bacterial flora of reptiles, can cause human genitourinary infections and primary bloodstream infections.

*Proteus* spp., *Staphylococcus* spp., *Acinetobacter* spp., and *Shigella* spp. are all common bacteria of the oropharyngeal cavities of snakes and can cause multiple health problems for owners of pet snakes or for those working with snakes in laboratory settings.

A number of species of the bacterial genus *Pseudomonas* are fairly common in the oral cavities of reptiles. These bacteria, perhaps best known for causing what is commonly called hot tub rash and swimmer's ear, grow well in poorly disinfected water and can also be transmitted to humans through wound contamination from bites and scratches.

Species of the genus *Mycobacterium* cause a number of diseases in humans, most notably tuberculosis and leprosy. *M. marinum* is found in salt water and fresh water throughout the world. Although generally found in aquarium fish and their tanks, *M. marinum* has also been isolated from captive lizards, turtles, snakes, and caimans and thus may be a hazard to reptile hobbyists and zoological facility workers.

The rickettsial bacterium *Coxiella burnetii*, which causes Q fever, is usually carried by cattle, sheep, goats, and other domesticated livestock and pets. Reptiles, however, can occasionally carry ticks infected by *Coxiella*; this is a possible source of transmission to humans. Reptiles also serve as a reservoir for another rickettsial bacterium, *Rickettsia marmionii*, which causes Australian spotted fever.

By far the most common bacterial disease transmitted by reptiles is salmonellosis. *Salmonella* spp.

infections afflict approximately 70,000 people in the United States each year. According to the Centers for Disease Control and Prevention (CDC), the number of cases may actually be thirty times that number because many are unreported. The symptoms of a *Salmonella* infection include the onset of fever, one to three days after initial infection, and vomiting, diarrhea, stomach pain, and abdominal cramps. Most persons with salmonellosis recover completely, but some develop complications, including sepsis and meningitis. At greatest risk are infants and children younger than five years of age, organ transplant recipients, immunocompromised persons (such as those with human immunodeficiency virus infection), and the elderly.

Among the various reptiles kept as pets, the primary *Salmonella* hosts are turtles, snakes, and lizards. For many years, most reptile-transmitted salmonellosis cases were contracted from newborn and young turtles. Since 1975, it has been illegal in the United States to sell turtles that have shells less than four inches in length, but enforcement of this law is poor and inadequate. Since 2006, there have been three large multistate outbreaks of *Salmonella* infections because of the selling of young turtles, primarily at flea markets and tourist shops and by street vendors. In 1996, an outbreak of *S. enterica* at a Komodo dragon exhibit at a zoo in Colorado led to sixty-five confirmed cases of salmonellosis.

### FUNGI AND PENTASTOMIDS

Although rarely documented, fungal zoonotic transmission from reptiles can occur through the inhalation of spores, ingestion of fungal material, or contamination of wounds. The fungi genera most likely to be transferred from reptiles to humans include *Mucor, Rhizopus, Candida, Trichosporon, Trichophyton, Aspergillus, Basidobolus,* and *Geotrichum.*

The pentastomids, or tongue-worms, are parasites of reptilian respiratory systems. As adults, most pentastomids, of which there are approximately sixty species, live in the lungs of snakes, lizards, and crocodilians. Visceral pentastomiasis occurs in humans when pentastomid eggs are consumed with the meat of reptiles or by accidental ingestion of feces or body secretions. Nymphs develop in various internal organs, causing damage to the spleen, liver, lungs, eyes, and mesentery. Pentastomiasis cases have been reported in many parts of the world, including Africa, Malaysia, the Philippines, Java, and China.

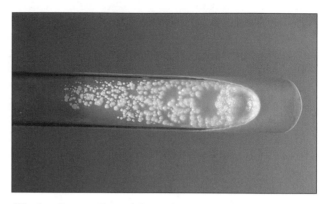

*The fungi genus* Geotrichum *is commonly transferred from reptiles to humans.* (CDC)

### PREVENTION AND OUTCOMES

The most straightforward way to avoid bacterial and fungal infections from reptiles is good hand-washing technique. Children and adults should wash hands and any other body parts exposed to reptiles immediately after any contact. Sensible precautions for those who keep reptiles include not allowing the animals to have free range of living quarters, keeping water dishes and aquariums clean and disinfected, and not washing animals and their artificial habitats in the kitchen sink, bathtubs, or showers, unless these areas are completely disinfected after use.

In countries where pentastomids are a problem, good hygiene is again the primary preventive measure, although this may be difficult in areas in which people do not have access to soap, disinfectants, and clean water. In those cultures in which the eating of reptiles is common, one should thoroughly cook the meat at a temperature high enough to kill parasitic organisms.

*Lenela Glass-Godwin, M.S.*

### FURTHER READING

Austin, C. C., and M. J. Wilkins. "Reptile-Associated Salmonellosis." *Journal of the American Veterinary Medical Association* 212, no. 6 (1998): 866-867. Discusses the transmission of *Salmonella* by various reptile species.

Centers for Disease Control and Prevention. "Turtle-Associated Salmonellosis in Humans: United States, 2006-2007." *Morbidity and Mortality Weekly Report* 56, no. 26 (July 6, 2007): 649-652. Provides a summary of *Salmonella* cases transmitted by turtles in several state outbreaks.

Jacobson, Eliot R. *Infectious Diseases and Pathology of Reptiles: Color Atlas and Text.* Boca Raton, Fla.: CRC Press, 2009. A complete treatise on infectious diseases that affect reptiles. Includes more than one thousand color photographs of reptile species with an emphasis on anatomy and histology.

Roberts, Larry S., and John Janovy, Jr. *Gerald D. Schmidt and Larry S. Roberts' Foundations of Parasitology.* 8th ed. Boston: McGraw-Hill, 2009. A classic work focusing on the parasites of humans and domestic animals.

Romich, Janet A. *Understanding Zoonotic Diseases.* Clifton Park, N.Y.: Thomson Delmar, 2008. A good introduction to zoonotic diseases, including those caused by reptiles, in humans.

## WEB SITES OF INTEREST

*Centers for Disease Control and Prevention*
http://www.cdc.gov

*Clean Hands Coalition*
http://www.cleanhandscoalition.org

*National Center for Emerging and Zoonotic Infectious Diseases*
http://www.cdc.gov/ncezid

**See also:** Bats and infectious disease; Birds and infectious disease; Cats and infectious disease; Dogs and infectious disease; Fleas and infectious disease; Flies and infectious disease; Insect-borne illness and disease; Mites and chiggers and infectious disease; Mosquitoes and infectious disease; Parasitic diseases; Parasitology; Pigs and infectious disease; Protozoan diseases; Rodents and infectious disease; Ticks and infectious disease; Transmission routes; Vectors and vector control; Zoonotic diseases.

# Respiratory route of transmission

CATEGORY: Transmission
ALSO KNOWN AS: Aerosol transmission, droplet contact, droplet transmission

## DEFINITION

In the respiratory route of transmission, a sick person who coughs or sneezes emits airborne droplets of respiratory secretions that contain pathogens (bacteria or viruses). These droplets may be breathed in by another person, who can then become infected. In addition, droplets that land on another person's face may be absorbed through the mucous membranes of the eyes, nose, and mouth, thus infecting that person. Droplets may also be expelled when a person talks, sings, laughs, or vomits. Droplets containing pathogens and respiratory mucus are too large to remain in the air for long and quickly settle on nearby surfaces, where the pathogens can survive up to three hours.

Bacterial diseases commonly transmitted by droplet transmission are bacterial meningitis, strep throat, tuberculosis, and whooping cough (pertussis). Viral diseases transmitted by droplet transmission include the common cold, influenza, mumps, measles, rubella (German measles), and chickenpox. These pathogens thrive in the warm, moist environment of the upper respiratory tract. Some viruses can replicate only in respiratory epithelial cells.

An upper respiratory infection is highly contagious. As many as three thousand droplets can be expelled in a single cough. This could result in the release of as many as twenty thousand viruses. A sneeze releases droplets at a speed of 373 miles (600 kilometers) per second. In cases of influenza, a person can infect others beginning one full day before the onset of symptoms and up to one week after symptoms appear. In cases of measles, 90 percent of unvaccinated or immunocompromised persons living with an infected person will become infected. Human rhinovirus, which causes the common cold, is the most common infective virus, perhaps because of its minimal size; less common infective viruses are ten times larger.

## RESPIRATORY HYGIENE

"Respiratory hygiene" is a term coined by the Centers for Disease Control and Prevention to describe measures that can be taken to decrease the risk of spreading respiratory pathogens. A minimum of three feet of space should be maintained between an infected person and others. When it is necessary to work within three feet of another person, the infected person should wear a disposable medical-procedure mask.

Persons not wearing a mask should cough or sneeze into tissues, dispose of the tissues promptly, and wash their hands with antiseptic soap or an alcohol-based hand sanitizer. Hands should be washed with soap for a minimum of fifteen seconds in warm water and then dried with a disposable towel or a heated blower. Hand sanitizer should not be used on hands that are visibly soiled because it may not reach all pathogens effectively. Tissues and paper towels should be discarded in a no-touch receptacle.

If tissues are not available, one should cough or sneeze into his or her sleeve or elbow. An August, 2009, observational study by medical students at Otago University in Wellington, New Zealand, found that 1 in 77 people covered sneezes and coughs with the arm, while 1 in 30 people used a tissue or handkerchief. Most of the people observed sneezing and coughing in public still covered their mouth with their hands. However, 1 in 4 people failed to cover their cough or sneeze with anything.

## IMPACT

The respiratory route of transmission was brought to increased public attention in 2003 with the outbreak of severe acute respiratory syndrome (SARS), which is caused by a previously unknown coronavirus, and again in 2009 with the pandemic caused by the influenza A (H1N1) virus. News reports showed people wearing disposable medical masks in schools and businesses and when using public transportation. The mortality rate of nearly 10 percent and the more than twelve thousand flu-related deaths in the United States alone prompted funding for research into the respiratory transmission of diseases, particularly the transmission of viruses.

The use of alcohol-based hand sanitizers has become more common, and people are learning to cover their coughs and sneezes with something other than their hands. Annual flu vaccines are becoming more popular. Nasal sprays of live attenuated virus are alternatives to vaccines of killed virus. Treatment with the antiviral drugs Tamiflu (oseltamivir) or Relenza (zanamivir) is recommended for people with influenza who require hospitalization.

*Bethany Thivierge, M.P.H.*

## FURTHER READING

Abraham, Thomas. *Twenty-first Century Plague: The Story of SARS*. Baltimore: Johns Hopkins University Press, 2007. Discusses how the emergence of SARS had effects on global politics, economics, public health practices, and the leadership role of the World Health Organization.

Albert, Ross H. "Diagnosis and Treatment of Acute Bronchitis." *American Family Physician* 82 (2010): 1345-1350. A discussion of viral and bacterial triggers of coughing and the appropriate treatments to reduce pathogenic spread.

Cao, Bin, et al. "Clinical Features of the Initial Cases of 2009 Pandemic Influenza A (H1N1) Virus Infection in China." *New England Journal of Medicine* 361 (2009): 2507-2517. Discusses how the observation of hospitalized patients led to the determination of the incubation period of this then-new strain of flu.

Gralton, Jan, et al. "The Role of Particle Size in Aerosolised Pathogen Transmission: A Review." *Journal of Infection* 62 (2011): 1-13. Discusses research into the mechanisms of respiratory transmission, including particle size, mucous properties, and relative air humidity.

Wald, Priscilla. *Contagious: Cultures, Carriers, and the Outbreak Narrative*. Durham, N.C.: Duke University Press, 2007. Examines how the practice of epidemiology using the Internet and Web is shaping how people view emerging infections and global health.

## WEB SITES OF INTEREST

*Centers for Disease Control and Prevention*
http://www.cdc.gov

*National Institute of Allergy and Infectious Diseases*
http://www.niaid.nih.gov

**See also:** Airborne illness and disease; Anthrax; Bacterial infections; Bacterial meningitis; Biological weapons; Botulism; Chickenpox; Common cold; Contagious diseases; Fungal infections; Immunization; Influenza; Measles; Mumps; Outbreaks; Pneumonia; Public health; Rubella; SARS; Strep throat; Transmission routes; Tuberculosis (TB); Viral infections; Whooping cough.

---

# Respiratory syncytial virus infections

CATEGORY: Diseases and conditions
ANATOMY OR SYSTEM AFFECTED: Lungs, respiratory system

## DEFINITION

Respiratory syncytial virus (RSV) is a common cause of many types of infections of the respiratory system (lungs and breathing passages), including the common cold, bronchitis, bronchiolitis, pneumonia, and croup. Although these infections can happen at any age, they occur most commonly and are usually most severe in infants, young children, and the elderly. In severe cases, RSV infections can cause death.

## CAUSES

RSV is spread through infected fluids of the mouth and nose. The contagious virus most often enters the body from touching the mouth, nose, or eyes. It can also be spread by inhaling droplets from a sneeze or cough.

RSV can survive on surfaces and objects for hours and is easily passed from person to person. Virus shedding (contagiousness) usually lasts for three to eight days, but may last up to four weeks.

## RISK FACTORS

Infants and young children, especially those under two years of age, and the elderly are at higher risk for RSV. Risk factors include exposure to a person infected with the virus or an object contaminated with the virus; premature birth; problems with the heart, lungs, or immune system; present or recent treatment with chemotherapy; having had an organ or bone marrow transplant; and having problems associated with muscle weakness.

## SYMPTOMS

The symptoms of RSV infection vary and usually differ with age and previous exposure to RSV. Young children, the elderly, and people with chronic diseases are more likely to have severe symptoms. In children younger than age three years, RSV can cause illnesses such as bronchiolitis and pneumonia. Symptoms may include stuffy or runny nose, high fever, severe cough, wheezing, shortness of breath, very fast rate of breathing, bluish color of the lips or fingernails, lethargy or irritability, lack of appetite, and discharge from the eyes.

In children older than age three years and in healthy adults, RSV typically causes an upper respiratory infection or cold. Symptoms commonly include a runny or stuffy nose, sore throat, mild cough, headache, low-grade fever, and discharge from the eyes.

## SCREENING AND DIAGNOSIS

A doctor will ask about symptoms and medical history and will perform a physical exam. A variety of tests are available to diagnose RSV. Lab tests called antigen detection assays are commonly done using secretions from the nose.

## TREATMENT AND THERAPY

Mild infections, such as colds, do not need special treatment. The goal is to ease symptoms so that the patient feels more comfortable while the body fights the virus. For symptom relief, one should drink increased amounts of liquids, especially water and fruit juice, to help keep nasal fluid thin and easy to clear; use a cool-mist vaporizer to humidify the air, which may help reduce coughing and soothe irritated breathing passages; use saline (salt water) nose drops to loosen mucus in the nose; and use nonaspirin fever medicine, such as acetaminophen, as needed to reduce fever.

People of all ages can develop severe infections from RSV, but it is most common in the young. Such infections include pneumonia and bronchiolitis and may require treatment in a hospital. This treatment is aimed at opening up breathing passages and may include humidified air, supplemental oxygen, treatments to improve breathing, and, in certain cases, mechanical ventilation (a breathing machine).

## PREVENTION AND OUTCOMES

Basic healthful practices are the best form of protection from RSV for most people. These include washing one's hands often, especially after touching someone who may have a cold or other RSV infection; avoiding touching one's face or rubbing one's eyes; avoiding sharing items such as cups, glasses, silverware, or towels with people who may have a cold or other RSV infection; and avoiding smoke exposure. A monoclonal antibody drug (palivizumab) directed against RSV that is injected monthly can significantly decrease the risk of severe infection in high-risk infants, such as those born prematurely or those who have chronic lung disease.

*Laurie Rosenblum, M.P.H.;*
*reviewed by Christine Colpitts, M.A., CRT*

## FURTHER READING

Busselen, S. "Respiratory Syncytial Virus (RSV)." In *Ferri's Clinical Advisor 2011: Instant Diagnosis and*

*Treatment*, edited by Fred F. Ferri. Philadelphia: Mosby/Elsevier, 2011.

Chernick, Victor, et al., eds. *Kendig's Disorders of the Respiratory Tract in Children*. 7th ed. Philadelphia: Saunders/Elsevier, 2006.

Ham, Richard, et al., eds. *Primary Care Geriatrics: A Case-Based Approach*. 5th ed. St. Louis, Mo.: Mosby/Elsevier, 2007.

Mason, Robert J., et al., eds. *Murray and Nadel's Textbook of Respiratory Medicine*. 5th ed. Philadelphia: Saunders/Elsevier, 2010.

Peters, T. T., et al. "Respiratory Syncytial Virus." In *Principles and Practice of Pediatric Infectious Diseases*, edited by Sarah S. Long, Larry K. Pickering, and Charles G. Prober. 3d ed. Philadelphia: Churchill Livingstone/Elsevier, 2008.

"Respiratory Syncytial Virus." In *Red Book: 2009 Report of the Committee on Infectious Diseases*, edited by L. K. Pickering et al. 28th ed. Elk Grove Village, Ill.: American Academy of Pediatrics, 2009.

## WEB SITES OF INTEREST

*American Lung Association*
http://www.lungusa.org

*KidsHealth*
http://www.kidshealth.org

**See also:** Adenovirus infections; Airborne illness and disease; Atypical pneumonia; Bronchiolitis; Bronchitis; Children and infectious disease; Common cold; Contagious diseases; Croup; Influenza; Laryngitis; Nocardiosis; Paramyxoviridae; Pharyngitis and tonsillopharyngitis; Pneumonia; Respiratory route of transmission; Rhinovirus infections; Saliva and infectious disease; Sinusitis; Strep throat; Viral infections; Viral upper respiratory infections; Whooping cough.

# Retroviral infections

CATEGORY: Diseases and conditions
ANATOMY OR SYSTEM AFFECTED: All

## DEFINITION

A retroviral infection is a disease state caused by a retrovirus that incorporates into a host cell. A retrovirus is composed of ribonucleic acid (RNA) that has the ability to replicate itself in a host cell. Retroviruses are associated with a variety of diseases, including malignancies, immunodeficiencies, and neurologic disorders.

There are seven genera of retroviruses divided into two categories, simple and complex. Perhaps the best known retrovirus is human immunodeficiency virus (HIV), which is the virus that causes acquired immunodeficiency syndrome (AIDS). Other examples of common retroviruses include human T-cell leukemia virus, Raus sarcoma virus in chickens, and murine and feline leukemia viruses in mice and cats. Retroviruses also exist among other host species, ranging from plants to invertebrates, fish, birds, and many mammalian species.

## CAUSES

The cause of an infection in general is the detrimental colonization of a host organism by a foreign pathogenic species. These foreign organisms can interfere with the normal functioning of the host cell, which can lead to chronic wounds, illness, and death.

More specifically, viral infections, for example, are caused by viral particles, which are not considered organisms because they lack metabolism and reproduction (when no host cell is present). In the case of a retroviral infection, the genome carried by a virus is RNA, which can be used directly as messenger RNA to convert the coded message into viral proteins that have specific functions.

One specific protein produced by the retrovirus is the enzyme known as reverse transcriptase, which can then be used to convert RNA into a deoxyribonucleic acid (DNA) molecule. This new DNA molecule is then used to produce more genetic material for new viral particles; it can also incorporate its genetic material in the host cell's genome. These new viruses can remain in the host cell's genome for long periods, without causing disease. However, the viruses are continuously copying the viral genome in the host. At some point, the viral particles leave this quiescent stage and become pathogenic, causing a disease state.

## RISK FACTORS

Because retroviral infection in humans is caused by the incorporation of viral particles into a human host cell, the risk factor for this type of infection is exhibited by the secretion of fluids containing the virus from one person to another. The primary factors con-

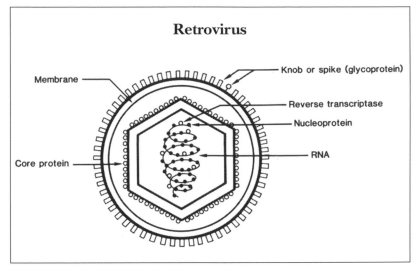

## Retrovirus

Membrane

Knob or spike (glycoprotein)

Reverse transcriptase

Nucleoprotein

Core protein

RNA

*An illustration of the structure of a retrovirus.*

tributing to this spread of viral particles include transmission through sexual intercourse, blood transfusion, or contaminated needles, and transmission by a woman to her fetus or newborn.

Sexual activity is the most widely known transmission factor for HIV infection. Chronic retroviral infection, also common, involves a primary infection that can lead to recurring infections. Once retroviruses are incorporated into host cells, the host immune system is compromised, which further exasperates the risk of future infections. Thus, low immune response has been a major factor in developing a high risk for chronic retroviral disease.

### SYMPTOMS

Because of the severe weakening of the normal functioning host cell after retroviral infection, most symptoms reflect the loss of function of these cells. These symptoms include chronic fatigue, continuous weight loss, low-grade or spiking fever, night sweats and chills, and chronic body aches and pain. These are somewhat vague symptoms, but they reflect the reach of how a host's normal functioning cells become impaired (compromised); these wide-ranging symptoms also reflect the lack of a proper immune response to eradicate the retrovirus from the body. Typically, retroviral infections are systemic, involving many different parts of the body; therefore, symptoms tend to include many organ systems. As the body weakens, symptoms become more severe.

### SCREENING AND DIAGNOSIS

Infection by a retrovirus is generally detected by the presence of specific antibodies to the virus, because antibodies to viruses persist for life. Screening from blood or blood products using the enzyme-linked immunosorbent assays (ELISA) are generally used for diagnosis. A positive serum level that is found repeatedly by ELISA screening is then further tested to confirm the presence of specific antibodies.

Screening for HIV infection, in particular, is most commonly done by collecting secretions from between the cheek and gum and then evaluating them for HIV antibodies. This test is nearly as accurate as a blood test, and because it does not involve a needle stick, it is favored by many persons. Finally, a newer urine test is available for screening. However, if the test is positive, blood tests need to be performed to confirm the presence of HIV.

### TREATMENT AND THERAPY

Antiviral therapy (ART) is the use of drugs to control the retrovirus by interfering with the virus's invasion of cells and multiplication in the host. Although ART can successfully control a retroviral infection, it is not a cure for the disease; also, ART drugs need to be taken for life to maintain their effect.

The most common ART is that used for AIDS, mainly because the disease is so widespread (global) and because of its fatality rate. The most common form of ART for HIV and AIDS is highly active antiretroviral therapy (HAART), a group of three to four drugs taken in combination.

Different classes of drugs effect different stages of the retroviral life cycle. Nucleoside and nucleotide reverse transcriptase inhibitors block (inhibit) reverse transcription of RNA to DNA in a host cell by preventing the elongation of the DNA molecule. Nonnucleoside reverse transcriptase inhibitors inhibit the virility of retroviruses and cause cell death.

### PREVENTION AND OUTCOMES

The best way to prevent infection by a retrovirus is to avoid contact with that virus. Because one of the most common retroviruses is HIV, mainly transmitted either sexually, through a contaminated needle, or through blood transfusions, the only way to protect against HIV infection is to abstain from sex outside a mutually faithful relationship with a partner whom the person knows is not infected with HIV, to abstain from sharing drug needles, and to be aware of blood transfusion origins. No antiretroviral vaccine exists.

*Susan M. Zneimer, Ph.D., FACMG*

## FURTHER READING

Coffin, J. M., S. H. Hughes, and H. E. Varmus, eds. *Retroviruses*. Cold Spring Harbor, N.Y.: Cold Spring Harbor Laboratory Press, 2002. A good discussion of retroviruses.

Kurth, R., and N. Bannert, eds. *Retroviruses: Molecular Biology, Genomics, and Pathogenesis*. Norwich, England: Caister Academic Press, 2010. A comprehensive discussion of retroviruses and related infections.

Levy, Jay A. *HIV and the Pathogenesis of AIDS*. 3d ed. Washington, D.C.: ASM Press, 2007. Provides a review of the research, explains the history of the disease, and examines how scientists, clinicians, and public health workers have responded to HIV and AIDS.

Norkin, Leonard. *Virology: Molecular Biology and Pathogenesis*. Washington, D.C.: ASM Press, 2010. The author provides a detailed account of virus structure and replication and of the basis for disease pathology.

## WEB SITES OF INTEREST

*AIDSinfo*
http://aidsinfo.nih.gov

*Universal Virus Database*
http://www.ictvdb.org

*Viral Zone*
http://www.expasy.org/viralzone

**See also:** AIDS; Antibodies; Antiviral drugs: Mechanisms of action; Autoimmune disorders; HIV; Immunity; Integrase inhibitors; Opportunistic infections; Protease inhibitors; Retroviridae; Reverse transcriptase inhibitors; T lymphocytes; Viral infections; Viruses: Structure and life cycle; Viruses: Types.

# Retroviridae

CATEGORY: Pathogen
TRANSMISSION ROUTE: Direct contact

## DEFINITION

The Retroviridae is a family of latent and pathogenic viruses with a positive-sense, single-stranded RNA (ribonucleic acid) genome for replication. Virions contain reverse transcriptase (RT) enzymes within a spherical capsid. The viruses infect vertebrate host cells by incorporating themselves into the host DNA (deoxyribonucleic acid).

---

**Taxonomic Classification for Retroviridae**

**Order:** Unassigned
**Family:** Retroviridae
**Subfamily:** Orthoretrovirinae
**Genera:** *Deltaretrovirus, Lentivirus*
**Species:**
Human T-lymphotropic virus
Human immunodeficiency virus

---

## NATURAL HABITAT AND FEATURES

Retroviruses, like traditional viruses, require a host to reproduce; retroviruses only infect vertebrate hosts and use the host DNA instead of messenger RNA to replicate. A particular feature of the retrovirus is that its viral RNA genome is integrated as proviral DNA into the host DNA and is passed to progeny of the host, endogenously. A minimum of nine endogenous retroviruses are present in vertebrate genomes, accounting for approximately 1 percent of the human genome, and they appear latent, with no effect on the hosts. Exogenous retroviruses, which are passed among vertebrates through blood and bodily secretions, can be more pathogenic.

All seven genera of the two subfamilies of retroviruses share the same mode of replication and basic virion structure, and they spread through host cells rapidly. Retroviruses consist of a lipid envelope that surrounds a spherical and electron-dense protein core, or capsid. Within the 100-nanometer-diameter capsid are two copies of a 10,000-base pair, single-stranded RNA genome that contains repeats of essential *gag-pol-env* genes in the long terminal ends. Enzymes for host DNA incorporation and genome replication (integrase and RT) are found in the core as well. Pathogenic retroviruses also contain more complex genes (such as *tat* and *rev*).

Retrovirus particles infect host cells rapidly and efficiently by attaching to and entering the host cell and converting single-stranded RNA into double-stranded DNA (proviral DNA) to build a double-stranded DNA provirus that inserts itself into the host DNA. Immature viral particles are then released from the infected host cell to spread throughout the body. This viral framework persists for the entire lifetime of the host. Retroviruses can evolve rapidly and repeatedly on the basis of selective needs, resulting from immune attacks or administered drugs. The individual adaptive mutations complicate treatment greatly, because each infected host's virus can vary according to differing antiviral attacks.

Although retroviruses were first discovered in 1908 by Vilhem Ellermann and Oluf Bang, the RT enzyme used for the replication process was not discovered until 1970. Human T-lymphocyte virus (HTLV) was the first pathogenic retrovirus isolated, in 1980, closely followed in 1984 by human immunodeficiency virus (HIV).

## Pathogenicity and Clinical Significance

Outcomes of pathogenic retroviral infections are host specific and may be neurologic, immunodeficient, or wasting. Namely, HIV leads to acquired immunodeficiency syndrome (AIDS) and HTLV causes adult T-cell leukemia.

HIV is transmitted through sexual secretions, shared needles from injection-drug use, blood, placental fluids, mucosal fluids, and breast milk. Symptoms are initially similar to those of influenza, with body aches and fever. Gradually, symptoms disappear as the immune system attacks the virus, despite viral integration into the host; as the virus begins to overwhelm the host's cells, immune deterioration begins. HIV is monitored by measuring the levels of host cells in the plasma (the viral load) infected by the virus and by measuring the immune system cell count (CD4 count).

Because retroviruses can change the host genome, they also can develop oncogenes in the body. Infection with HTLV-1 leads to the formation of tumors that can lead to adult T-cell leukemia. HTLV is spread through perinatal and sexual transmission or through contact with infected blood products. HTLV leukemia is an aggressive disease that has a mortality of approximately one year. In equatorial areas of the world, infection with HTLV-1 may cause tropical spastic paraparesis, with symptoms of neurologic deficiency.

## Drug Susceptibility

HIV is the primary pathogenic retrovirus against which drug treatments have been developed. Since the development of the first antiretroviral (ARV) agent, the nucleoside reverse transcriptase inhibitor zidovudine, in 1987, five classes of ARV drugs have been developed against HIV. All ARV classes attack HIV at different stages of replication, cell entry, or DNA integration to slow the viral assault.

Nucleoside reverse transcriptase inhibitors replace normal genome building blocks to stop virus reproduction, and non-nucleoside reverse transcriptase inhibitors disable the RT enzyme for the same effect. Protease inhibitors prevent action of a replicating enzyme, fusion and entry inhibitors prevent steps needed for entry into host cells, and integrase inhibitors disable the enzyme used for DNA incorporation.

ARV drug treatments are introduced as highly active ARV therapy (HAART) regimens for maximum antiviral attack. The particular drugs used vary around a standard, recommended regimen; medications are added, removed, or replaced as necessary when resistance builds to a certain drug or entire mechanistic class. Atripla, a combination pill that contains efavirenz (an NNRTI), emtricitabine (an NRTI), and tenofovir (another NRTI), is an example of an initial HAART regimen for a person newly diagnosed with HIV.

Because retroviral genomes have the ability to change and adapt to outside pressures rapidly and efficiently, drug susceptibility varies by viral strain and by particular infected host, and it depends on immune system attacks and on treatments administered to the host. Extensive genotypic and phenotypic susceptibility testing may be performed in persons with HIV, and can be analyzed by infectious disease experts to identify specific drug agents or classes that retain effectiveness and suppress HIV replication.

More often, the infected person's viral load is measured every six to eight weeks and compared with earlier measurements to manage a treatment regimen. If HAART is effective, viral load will be reduced, reflecting lower levels of virus in the blood. If, after twenty days on a regimen, viral load is not lowered to undetectable levels, the regimen is considered ineffective and can lead to virologic failure without a change of therapy.

In addition to researching expanded drug options within each ARV class, HiV researchers are studying methods to prevent initial retrovirus infection. These experimental methods include using microbicidal agents as mucosal barriers in sexual contact and using a vaccine against HIV.

*Nicole M. Van Hoey, Pharm.D.*

### FURTHER READING

Boucher, Charles A. B. "Retroviruses and Retroviral Infections." In *Cohen and Powderly Infectious Diseases*, edited by Jonathan Cohen, Steven M. Opal, and William G. Powderly. 3d ed. Philadelphia: Mosby/Elsevier, 2010. A thorough discussion of retroviral families and pathogenicity, with descriptions of the resultant diseases.

"A Brief Chronicle of Retrovirology." In *Retroviruses*, edited by J. M. Coffin, S. H. Hughes, and H. E. Varmus. Cold Spring Harbor, N.Y.: Cold Spring Harbor Laboratory Press, 2002 Also available at http://www.ncbi.nlm.nih.gov/books/nbk19403. A historical description of retroviridae identification and differentiation.

Kurth, R., and N. Bannert, eds. *Retroviruses: Molecular Biology, Genomics, and Pathogenesis*. Norwich, England: Caister Academic Press, 2010. A comprehensive discussion of retroviruses and related infections.

Luzuriaga, Katherine, and John L. Sullivan. "Introduction to Retroviridae." In *Principles and Practice of Pediatric Infectious Diseases*, edited by Sarah S. Long, Larry K. Pickering, and Charles G. Prober. 3d ed. Philadelphia: Churchill Livingstone/Elsevier, 2008. A textbook discussion on retrovirus transmission that is particularly focused on transmission among children.

### WEB SITES OF INTEREST

*AIDSinfo*
http://aidsinfo.nih.gov

*Big Picture Book of Viruses*
http://www.virology.net/big_virology

**See also:** AIDS; Antiviral drugs: Mechanisms of action; Antiviral drugs: Types; Autoimmune disorders; HIV; HIV vaccine; Immunity; Immunodeficiency; T lymphocytes; Viral infections; Viruses: Structure and life cycle; Viruses: Types.

# Reverse transcriptase inhibitors

CATEGORY: Treatment
ALSO KNOWN AS: Non-nucleoside reverse transcriptase inhibitors (non-nukes), nucleoside analogues, nucleoside and nucleotide reverse transcriptase inhibitors (nukes)

### DEFINITION

Reverse transcriptase inhibitors (RTIs) are antiviral drugs that treat human immunodeficiency virus (HIV) infection. Two types of RTIs are discussed here.

### MECHANISM OF ACTION

RTIs incorporate into the deoxyribonucleic acid (DNA) of HIV and stop it from reproducing. More specifically, HIV contains genetic information in the form of ribonucleic acid (RNA); when HIV infects a human T cell (or lymphocyte), it assembles a new HIV DNA chain by combining its own RNA with some of the DNA of the infected human cell. To do this, it uses an enzyme called reverse transcriptase. RTIs prevent the reverse transcriptase enzyme from working. Therefore, incomplete DNA is synthesized and, thus, cannot be used to create a new copy of the virus.

### NRTIS AND NNRTIS

Nucleoside and nucleotide reverse transcriptase inhibitors (NRTIs) and non-nucleoside reverse transcriptase inhibitors (NNRTIs) are two classes of drugs that thwart the function of the reverse transcriptase enzyme in two different ways. NRTIs (or nukes) compete with deoxynucleotides from the human T cell for incorporation into the DNA that the HIV is assembling. NRTIs are analogues of these naturally occurring deoxynucleotides and are classified as competitive substrate inhibitors. In contrast, NNRTIs (or non-nukes) are not incorporated into the new viral DNA chain but physically block the protein domains of reverse transcriptase that are needed for DNA synthesis. NNRTIs are classified as noncompetitive inhibitors of reverse transcriptase.

The following drugs are RTIs: Combivir (lamivudine and zidovudine), Emtriva (emtricitabine), Epivir (lamivudine), Epzicom (abacavir and lamivudine), Hivid (zalcitabine), Rescriptor (delaviridine), Retrovir (AZT, zidovudine), Trizivir (abacavir-lamivudine-zidovudine), Truvada (emtricitabine-tenofovir), Videx (didanosine), Viramune (nevirapine), Viread (tenofovir), Zerit (stavudine), and Ziagen (abacavir).

## IMPACT

In 1981, the Centers for Disease Control and Prevention (CDC) reported five cases of pneumonia of unknown cause in Los Angeles County, sparking widespread medical and media attention and marking awareness of a new disease that would become known as AIDS (acquired immunodeficiency syndrome). By the beginning of 1987, the World Health Organization had been notified of 43,880 cases of AIDS worldwide. AIDS, and the fear and prejudice against people with HIV infection, had spread widely and rapidly. The same year, the U.S. Food and Drug Administration (FDA) approved the first drug indicated for the treatment of HIV infection: the NRTI known as zidovudine, or azidothymidine (AZT). Zidovudine had an enormous effect on the disease; it also had an effect on the way AIDS as a disease was perceived. People began to think of AIDS as a chronic, but manageable disease, and not as a death sentence.

Soon came the need for drugs with better resistance; zidovudine slows HIV significantly, but it does not stop it entirely. NNRTIs became the third class of HIV drugs indicated for the treatment of HIV infection (after protease inhibitors). The first NNRTI, nevirapine, was approved by the FDA in 1996. There are now six different classes of HIV drugs that act on different targets. The most popular target remains the reverse transcriptase enzyme, and both nukes and non-nukes remain central to HIV drug therapy.

Drug resistance develops quickly with monotherapy, and NRTIs and NNRTIs are always used in conjunction with other drugs, either as an ingredient (as in Combivir and Trizivir) or as part of combination therapy. This combination therapy is called highly active antiretroviral therapy (HAART), for which a minimum of three drugs from different classes are combined.

*Stephanie Eckenrode, B.A.*

## FURTHER READING

De Béthune, Marie-Pierre. "Non-Nucleoside Reverse Transcriptase Inhibitors (NNRTIs), Their Discovery, Development, and Use in the Treatment of HIV-1 Infection." *Antiviral Research* 85, no. 1 (2010): 75-90.

De Clercq, Erik. "Antiviral Drug Discovery and Development: Where Chemistry Meets with Biomedicine." *Antiviral Research* 67, no. 2 (2005): 56-75.

Skowron, Gail, and Richard Ogden, eds. *Reverse Transcriptase Inhibitors in HIV/AIDS Therapy.* New York: Humana Press, 2006.

## WEB SITES OF INTEREST

*AIDSinfo*
http://aidsinfo.nih.gov

*Avert.org*
http://www.avert.org

**See also:** AIDS; Antibodies; Antiviral drugs: Mechanisms of action; Antiviral drugs: Types; Autoimmune disorders; Blood-borne illness and disease; HIV; Immunity; Integrase inhibitors; Maturation inhibitors; Protease inhibitors; Quinolone antibiotics; Retroviral infections; T lymphocytes; Treatment of viral infections; Viral infections.

# Rheumatic fever

CATEGORY: Diseases and conditions
ANATOMY OR SYSTEM AFFECTED: All

## DEFINITION

Rheumatic fever is an inflammatory condition. It involves the connective tissue in the body. The most severe complication is rheumatic heart disease, which may permanently damage the heart valves, which affect the flow of blood to and from the heart. Often, the symptoms of valve damage appear ten to thirty years after the initial event.

## CAUSES

Rheumatic fever is caused by the immune system responding to group A *Streptococcus* pharyngitis (strep throat). In this case, the immune system not only fights the bacteria but also attacks its own tissue, often heart tissue.

## RISK FACTORS

Factors that may increase the risk of rheumatic fever include previously having rheumatic fever, being malnourished, and living in overcrowded conditions. At higher risk are children ages five to fifteen years.

## SYMPTOMS

Symptoms usually appear two to four weeks after a strep infection and include pain and swelling in large joints; fever; weakness; muscle aches; shortness of breath; chest pain; nausea and vomiting; hacking cough; circular rash; lumps under the skin; and abnormal, sudden movements of arms and legs.

## SCREENING AND DIAGNOSIS

A doctor will ask about symptoms and medical history and will perform a physical exam that includes a careful examination of the heart. The doctor may take a throat culture and order a blood test to check for streptococcal antibodies.

Further examination includes testing the blood's erythrocyte sedimentation rate to measure inflammation in the body; blood cultures for bacteria in the blood; an electrocardiogram (a test that records the heart's activity by measuring electrical currents through the heart muscle); an echocardiogram (a sonogram that visualizes the heart valves and measures the contractile function of the heart muscle); and chest X rays (a test that uses radiation to take a picture of structures inside the body, in this case the heart).

## TREATMENT AND THERAPY

The goals of treatment are to kill the strep bacteria, treat the inflammation caused by the rheumatic fever, and prevent future cases of rheumatic fever. Treatment includes medication to treat the strep infection (such as penicillin or other antibiotics, including erythromycin and azithromycin). Antibiotics may need to be taken for several years to prevent recurrence. These medications may be given by mouth or by injection.

Medications to help with joint pain and swelling include aspirin or other nonsteroidal anti-inflammatory drugs (NSAIDs), and corticosteroids may be used if NSAIDs are not effective.

In some cases the inflammation can be severe. The patient may have to be on bed rest or restricted activity for a period of time.

## PREVENTION AND OUTCOMES

One should treat strep throat with antibiotics promptly to help prevent the onset of rheumatic fever. Persons with a sore throat and fever that last more than twenty-four hours should consult a doctor.

*Reviewed by Jill D. Landis, M.D.*

## FURTHER READING

Bonow, R. O., et al. "ACC/AHA 2006 Guidelines for the Management of Patients with Valvular Heart Disease." *Journal of the American College of Cardiology* 48 (2006).

Carapetis, J. R., et al. "Acute Rheumatic Fever." *The Lancet* 366 (2005): 155-168.

Durack, David T., and Michael H. Crawford, eds. *Infective Endocarditis*. Philadelphia: W. B. Saunders, 2003.

English, Peter C. *Rheumatic Fever in America and Britain: A Biological, Epidemiological, and Medical History*. New Brunswick, N.J.: Rutgers University Press, 1999.

Gerber, M. "*Streptococcus pyogenes* (Group A *Streptococcus*)." In *Principles and Practice of Pediatric Infectious Diseases*, edited by Sarah S. Long, Larry K. Pickering, and Charles G. Prober. 3d ed. Philadelphia: Churchill Livingstone/Elsevier, 2008.

Hahn, R. G., et al. "Evaluation of Poststreptococcal Illness." *American Family Physician* 71 (2005): 1949-1954.

Robertson, K. A., J. A. Volmink, and B. M. Mayosi. "Antibiotics for the Primary Prevention of Acute Rheumatic Fever." *BMC Cardiovascular Disorders* 5 (2005): 11.

Spagnuolo, M., B. Pasternack, and A. Taranta. "Risk of Rheumatic Fever Recurrences After Streptococcal Infections: Prospective Study of Clinical and Social Factors." *New England Journal of Medicine* 285 (1971): 641-647.

Steeg, Carl N., Christine A. Walsh, and Julie S. Glickstein. "Rheumatic Fever: No Cause for Complacence." *Patient Care* 34, no. 14 (July 30, 2000): 40-61.

## WEB SITES OF INTEREST

*American Heart Association*
http://www.heart.org

*Heart and Stroke Foundation of Canada*
http://www.heartandstroke.com

*National Library of Medicine*
http://www.nlm.nih.gov

*Public Health Agency of Canada*
http://www.phac-aspc.gc.ca

**See also:** Bacterial endocarditis; Bacterial infections; Behçet's syndrome; Bloodstream infections; Endocarditis; Epiglottitis; Group A streptococcal infection; Inflammation; Mononucleosis; Myocarditis; Myositis; Pericarditis; Pharyngitis and tonsillopharyngitis; Septic arthritis; Strep throat; Streptococcal infections; *Streptococcus*.

# Rhinosporidiosis

CATEGORY: Diseases and conditions
ANATOMY OR SYSTEM AFFECTED: Eyes, nose, skin

## DEFINITION

Rhinosporidiosis is a fungal infection that causes reddish-purple, tumorlike masses on the nasal mucous membrane, the conjunctiva of the eye, or the urethra. Such masses can extend to the lips, palate, uvula, epiglottis, larynx (voice box), trachea (windpipe), bronchi, ears, scalp, genitals, rectum, and the skin.

## CAUSES

Rhinosporidiosis is caused by the organism *Rhinosporidium seeberi*, which has features of both fungi and protozoa. Genetic analysis has determined that *R. seeberi* is a member of a group of aquatic parasites of the class Mesomycetozoea. It is theorized that *R. seeberi* is a parasite of fish.

## RISK FACTORS

The greatest number of rhinosporidiosis cases has been reported in India and Sri Lanka, but the infection has been diagnosed in persons from the Americas, Europe, Africa, and Asia. It is most common in tropical areas. The reservoir of this microorganism and the mode of transmission are unknown, although *R. seeberi* appears to be associated with drinking contaminated water or with bathing or swimming in contaminated water. Rhinosporidiosis is more common in children and in boys and men.

## SYMPTOMS

The tumors of rhinosporidiosis grow from a stem and bleed easily. The tumors have whitish spots, which are its spores. These tumors can obstruct the nose and cause increased nasal drainage, cough, sneezing, and postnasal discharge. The tumors in the eye can cause excessive tearing, redness, photophobia, and infection. The tumors are not painful, but their presence is felt as pressure. The condition can be chronic, but it is rarely fatal.

## SCREENING AND DIAGNOSIS

There is no routine screening for rhinosporidiosis, but because of the external location of the growths, they are easy to see. Diagnosis is based on viewing tissue smears of the growths under a microscope. *R. seeberi* resembles *Coccidioides immitis*, so infection with *C. immitis* must be ruled out. *C. immitis* has smaller endospores and cannot be stained with the same fungal stains as *R. seeberi*.

## TREATMENT AND THERAPY

The treatments for infection with *R. seeberi* are intravenous antifungal medications such as amphotericin B and dapsone and surgical removal of the growth using cauterization. Antifungal drugs have not been particularly effective, and they must be administered for a minimum of one year. Surgery is the treatment of choice. The growth must be removed at its base with a wide excision to prevent a recurrence of the tumor.

## PREVENTION AND OUTCOMES

Because there appears to be a correlation with swimming and bathing in contaminated fresh water, one should avoid swimming or bathing in waters in tropical countries where *R. seeberi* is endemic. Also, one should avoid drinking from contaminated water sources in these countries. Any fresh-water body that is associated with rhinosporidiosis should be avoided.

*Christine M. Carroll, R.N.*

## FURTHER READING

Fredricks, David N., et al. "*Rhinosporidium seeberi*: A Human Pathogen from a Novel Group of Aquatic Protistan Parasites." *Emerging Infectious Disease* 6 (March/April, 2000): 3. Also available at http://www.cdc.gov/ncidod/eid/vol6no3/fredricks.htm.
Kumari, Rashmi, Chandrashekar Laxmisha, and Devinder M. Thappa. "Disseminated Cutaneous Rhinosporidiosis." *Dermatology Online Journal* 11 (2005): 19. Available at http://dermatology.cdlib.org/111.
Richardson, Malcolm D., and Elizabeth M. Johnson.

*The Pocket Guide to Fungal Infection.* 2d ed. Malden, Mass.: Blackwell, 2006.

Weedon, David. *Skin Pathology.* 3d ed. New York: Churchill Livingstone/Elsevier, 2010.

## WEB SITES OF INTEREST

*Centers for Disease Control and Prevention*
http://www.cdc.gov

*Global Network for Neglected Tropical Diseases*
http://globalnetwork.org

**See also:** *Coccidioides*; Coccidiosis; Developing countries and infectious disease; Emerging and reemerging infectious diseases; Fungal infections; Fungi: Classification and types; Parasites: Classification and types; Parasitic diseases; Tropical medicine; Waterborne illness and disease.

# Rhinovirus infections

CATEGORY: Diseases and conditions
ANATOMY OR SYSTEM AFFECTED: Lungs, nose, throat, upper respiratory tract
ALSO KNOWN AS: Common cold

## DEFINITION

A rhinovirus infection is a viral infection that usually affects the nose and throat. In rare cases, a rhinovirus infection is seen in croup and pneumonia, and it may contribute to asthma conditions. Rhinovirus infection is commonly referred to as a common cold.

## CAUSES

Rhinovirus infections are caused by small viruses belonging to the Picornaviridae family. Approximately one hundred types of rhinoviruses have been identified. Exposure to the virus by direct contact with an infected person or with an infected shared object (fomite), or exposure through contact with droplets from the sneeze or cough of an infected person, can cause rhinovirus infection. The rhinovirus is highly contagious.

## RISK FACTORS

Exposure to a person infected with the rhinovirus causes the infection, but several risk factors may in-crease a person's chance of becoming ill. Children and infants are more at risk because their immune systems have not yet developed resistance to most viruses. Hygiene plays a role in disease transmission, and children are less likely to wash their hands carefully. Although children are taught to cough into their arms, forgetting to do so, and sharing toys or other items, may lead to infection. Any time the immune system is weakened, infection with the rhinovirus is more likely to occur. Rhinovirus infections are more common when people spend time indoors, such as in the fall and winter, because of close contact with others.

## SYMPTOMS

Signs and symptoms of infection with the rhinovirus usually occur two to three days after exposure to the virus. Runny nose, sore throat, difficulty swallowing, mild fever, cough, and a general feeling of uncomfortableness are the most common symptoms of a cold. Severe symptoms include swollen glands, sinus pain, vomiting, pain in the abdomen, difficulty breathing, excessive fatigue or sleepiness, ear pain, and severe headache. Persistent crying may occur in children. When symptoms are severe or last more than one week, or if one has difficulty breathing or is unable to drink adequate fluids, a physician should be consulted.

## SCREENING AND DIAGNOSIS

There are no screening tests for rhinovirus infection. Diagnosis is based on reported contact with an infected person and signs and symptoms. Rhinovirus infection may not require a visit to a doctor unless symptoms increase in severity.

## TREATMENT AND THERAPY

The most common treatment for rhinovirus infection includes rest, drinking plenty of fluids, and the careful use of over-the-counter (OTC) pain relievers or cold medicines. All OTCs have side effect risks that should be considered. Children should not be given cough and cold medicines unless directed by a physician. Decongestant nasal sprays should be used on a limited basis in adults and should not be used in children. Saline drops and a suction bulb may be used in infants and children to clear a stuffy nose. Chicken soup has been shown in scientific studies to help relieve cold (and flu) symptoms. There is no cure for

## Rhinovirus Gene Studies May Help Find a Treatment for the Common Cold

Genomic mapping has been completed for the human rhinovirus (HRV). In a collaborative effort among four research institutions, all ninety-nine strains of the common cold virus, HRV, have been genetically sequenced. This data set provides an important baseline framework for future analysis of new HRVs that may be identified, according to the study authors Ann C. Palmenberg from the University of Wisconsin and her colleagues at the University of Maryland School of Medicine and the J. Craig Venter Institute in Rockville, Maryland. The database will help inform future research of the development of antiviral agents and vaccines.

Rhinovirus can alter human genes. A University of Calgary study published in the *American Journal of Respiratory and Critical Care* in 2008 found that the rhinovirus causes cold symptoms not by triggering an immune response in the host, but by altering the host cellular genes that control inflammation and antiviral responses. The randomized study involved nasal scrapings from thirty-five healthy volunteers, half of whom were inoculated with rhinovirus. Changes in gene expression were analyzed for nasal scrapings taken at eight and forty-eight hours after inoculation. While eight-hour samples found no differences in cellular genes between groups, the forty-eight-hour sample found more than 6,500 genes altered in the inoculation group compared with control group. Two groups of genes were of special interest: affected genes involved in the inflammatory process and antiviral genes, according to study authors David Proud and colleagues. A faulty visperin gene, known to play a role in other viral infections, such as influenza, hepatitis, and cytomegalovirus, was identified. The identification of altered human genes associated with rhinovirus infection provides potential new direction for therapeutic research.

*Sandra Ripley Distelhorst*

and should practice good hygiene by washing hands carefully and frequently, especially when in public places. One should not share personal items with persons who have a cold and should keep shared areas clean. Finally, one should sneeze and cough into tissues to avoid spreading the virus to others.

*Patricia Stanfill Edens, R.N., Ph.D., FACHE*

### FURTHER READING

Eccles, Ronald, and Olaf Weber, eds. *Common Cold.* Boston: Birkhäuser, 2009.

Pappas, D. E., et al. "Symptom Profile of Common Colds in School-Aged Children." *Pediatric Infectious Disease Journal* 27 (2008): 8-11.

Schaffer, Kirsten, Alberto M. LaRosa, and Estella Whimbey. "Respiratory Viruses." In *Cohen and Powderly Infectious Diseases,* edited by Jonathan Cohen, Steven M. Opal, and William G. Powderly. 3d ed. Philadelphia: Mosby/Elsevier, 2010.

Shors, Teri. *Understanding Viruses.* Sudbury, Mass.: Jones and Bartlett, 2008.

### WEB SITES OF INTEREST

*Centers for Disease Control and Prevention*
http://www.cdc.gov

*Clean Hands Coalition*
http://www.cleanhandscoalition.org

**See also:** Adenovirus infections; Airborne illness and disease; Bronchiolitis; Bronchitis; Children and infectious disease; Common cold; Contagious diseases; Coronavirus infections; Coxsackie virus infections; Hygiene; Influenza; Pharyngitis and tonsillopharyngitis; Picornaviridae; Pneumonia; Respiratory route of transmission; Sinusitis; Strep throat; Viral infections; Viral pharyngitis; Viral upper respiratory infections.

---

the common cold, and antibiotics are not used unless a bacterial infection develops during the course of the disease.

### PREVENTION AND OUTCOMES

To help prevent infection with the rhinovirus, one should avoid contact with persons who have a cold

## *Rhizopus*

CATEGORY: Pathogen
TRANSMISSION ROUTE: Direct contact, ingestion, inhalation

### DEFINITION

*Rhizopus* is a genus of saphrocytic filamentous fungi (molds) with species that may cause zygomycosis.

---

**Taxonomic Classification for *Rhizopus***

**Kingdom:** Fungi
**Phylum:** Zygomycota
**Order:** Mucorales
**Family:** Mucoraceae
**Genus:** *Rhizopus*
**Species:**
*R. arrhizus*
*R. microsporus*
*R. rhizopodiform*

## NATURAL HABITAT AND FEATURES

*Rhizopus* is a filamentous fungus found worldwide that lives on dead organic material (as a saphrocyte) in soil, decaying fruit and vegetables, old bread, and animal feces. *Rhizopus* species are common contaminants that can cause serious, even fatal, infections in humans.

Colonies of *Rhizopus* mature in four days at 98.6° to 113° Fahrenheit (37-45° Celsius) on a standard agar medium. The texture is typically dense and cottony. From the front, the colony is initially white, turning to grey or yellowish brown with the release of spores. The reverse is white to pale.

On microscopic observation of the colony, broad, thin-walled hyphae (filaments) are observed. They are either not septate (segmented) or sparsely septate. Sporangiospores, specialized structures on the hyphae, carry sporangia (the spores or sporangiospores). The sporangiospores are mostly brown and unbranched. The sporangia are located at the tip of the sporangiospores and are round with flattened bases. They can be solitary or can form clusters. Swelling or projection (apophysis) of sporangia is absent or rarely seen. The sporangiospores are one-celled, round to ovoid, hyaline (transparent) to brown, and smooth or striated.

Other structures observed are rhizoids, which are rootlike hyphae located at the point where the stolons (stems of hyphae) and sporangiospores meet, and columella, which are small, column-like spherical or elongated structures. After the release of spores, apophyses and columella often collapse to form an umbrella-like structure. Features such as the length of sporangiospores; presence, length, and pigmentation of rhi-zoids; diameter of sporangia; presence and shape of columella, presence of stolons; and the size, shape, and surface texture of sporangiospores help differentiate among the different species of *Rhizopus* and between *Rhizopus* and other fungi of the phylum Zygomycota.

## PATHOGENICITY AND CLINICAL SIGNIFICANCE

*Rhizopus* species are among the fungi that cause zygomycosis, a syndrome of invasive, opportunistic infections. This syndrome was formerly called mucormycosis. Other fungi with species that cause zygomycosis include the genera *Absidia* and *Mucor*. Among all cases of zygomycoses in humans, *R. arrhizus* is the most common cause.

Zygomycosis rarely occurs in healthy persons. It does, however, appear to be on the rise in the United States among persons with predisposing factors. These factors include diabetic acidosis; immunosuppression, such as that caused by bone marrow transplantation or corticosteroid therapy; and immunodeficiency. Other factors that may predispose a person to develop zygomycosis include treatment with desferoxamine (to remove excess iron), renal failure, extensive burns, trauma, prematurity, and intravenous drug abuse. In persons with these conditions or in persons receiving these therapies, the body's natural defense mechanisms against fungal infections have been compromised.

The primary route of infection begins with inhalation of spores that have been released into the air. Initial infection usually occurs in the nasal sinuses or the lungs. Once the infection penetrates the mucosal layer, it invades underlying tissue, nerves, and blood vessels and can disseminate through the circulatory system. Zygomycosis includes mucocutaneous, rhinocerebral, pulmonary, gastrointestinal, and disseminated infections. In rhinocerebral disease, the most common form of zygomycosis, the infection rapidly disseminates from the paranasal sinuses. If untreated, it can reach the brainstem, leading to coma and even death within a few days.

*Microsporus* and *rhizopodiformis* are associated with cutaneous infections traced to contaminated surgical dressings and splints in hospital settings. Burn patients are especially vulnerable to these infections, which can lead to gangrene. Gastrointestinal infection can develop after ingestion of spores on spoiled food.

## DRUG SUSCEPTIBILITY

Little data are available on the susceptibility profile of *Rhizopus* species, even in the laboratory (in vitro) setting. In one study, the minimum inhibitory concentration for amphotericin B was lower than that of the azoles itraconazole, ketoconazole, and voriconazole against strains of *arrhizus*. Amphotericin B remains the drug of choice when treating zygomycosis caused by *Rhizopus* species.

Early detection and aggressive treatment are critical if there is to be success in treating zygomycosis. The first step is to reverse or control the underlying disease, immunosuppression, or other factors facilitating the infection. Amphotericin B at high intravenous doses must be administered. No other antifungal agents are effective against invasive infections caused by *Rhizopus*. Surgery is usually required to remove infected dead tissue.

*Ernest Kohlmetz, M.A.*

## FURTHER READING

Brown, J. "Zygomycosis: An Emerging Fungal Infection." *American Journal of Health-System Pharmacy* 62 (2005): 2593-2596. Discusses the growing frequency of zygomycosis cases in the United States

Richardson, Malcolm D., and David W. Warnock. *Fungal Infection: Diagnosis and Management.* New ed. Malden, Mass.: Wiley-Blackwell, 2010. Chapter 13 contains valuable information related to *Rhizopus* and other fungi that cause zygomycosis.

Ryan, Kenneth J., and George Ray. *Sherris Medical Microbiology: An Introduction to Infectious Diseases.* 5th ed. New York: McGraw-Hill Medical, 2010. A first text in microbiology for students in medicine and medical science, with a focus on infectious diseases. Margin notes and a glossary help make the information more accessible. Chapter 45, on opportunistic infections, discusses zygomycosis.

St. Georgiev, Vassil. *Opportunistic Infections: Treatment and Prophylaxis.* Totowa, N.J.: Humana Press, 2003. Examines zygomycosis as an opportunistic infection. Covers prevention and treatment.

## WEB SITES OF INTEREST

*Centers for Disease Control and Prevention, Division of Foodborne, Bacterial, and Mycotic Diseases*
http://www.cdc.gov/nczved/divisions/dfbmd

*Doctor Fungus*
http://www.doctorfungus.org

*Mycology Online*
http://www.mycology.adelaide.edu.au

**See also:** *Aspergillus*; Coccidiosis; Cryptococcosis; Diagnosis of fungal infections; Fungal infections; Fungi: Classification and types; *Histoplasma*; Microbiology; Mold infections; Mucormycosis; Mycoses; Opportunistic infections; Paracoccidioidomycosis; Prevention of fungal infections; Treatment of fungal infections; Zygomycosis.

---

# *Rickettsia*

CATEGORY: Pathogen
TRANSMISSION ROUTE: Blood

## DEFINITION

*Rickettsia* are obligate, intracellular, parasitic, gram-negative coccobacilli. Their ATP transport system allows them to be energy parasites. Humans are usually accidental hosts, while other mammals and arthropods serve as reservoirs. Rickettsial-type organisms also have been linked to plant diseases.

---

**Taxonomic Classification for *Rickettsia***

**Kingdom:** Bacteria
**Phylum:** Proteobacteria
**Class:** Alphaproteobacteria
**Order:** Rickettsiales
**Family:** Rickettsiaceae
**Genus:** *Rickettsia*
**Species:**
*R. africae*
*R. akari*
*R. australis*
*R. connorii*
*R. japonica*
*R. prowazekii*
*R. rickettsi*
*R. sibirica*
*R. typhi*

---

## NATURAL HABITAT AND FEATURES

Because they are small, obligate, intracellular, parasites, *Rickettsia* spp. were originally thought to be viruses. Further studies showed them to be true bacteria. All have a gram-negative-type cell wall, and all are normally visualized by Giemsa staining. Their genomes are made of deoxyribonucleic acid (DNA) and are incomplete, lacking genes for enzymes of anaerobic metabolism and for production of most amino acids and nucleotides. They do possess the enzymes for aerobic metabolism, but normally use a unique ATP transport system to absorb ATP from their hosts instead of making it themselves. This allows them to be energy parasites.

The genome of one of these bacteria, *prowazekii*, is the most closely related bacterial genome to the genome of mitochondria. No *Rickettsia* spp. can be grown on artificial media; instead, they must be cultured in living tissue, usually a chick embryo. In infected humans, *Rickettsia* spp. usually induce their own phagocytosis by the endothelial cells lining blood vessels. Inside the cells, they escape from the phagosome into the cytoplasm, where they replicate. Many species escape the cell by causing lysis, which destroys the host cell. Other species exit by extrusion through filipodia, finger-like projections on the cell surface.

Serology and DNA studies have separated these bacteria into two main groups: the typhus group (*prowazekii* and *typhus*) and the spotted fever group (all others). Another group, formerly called the *Rickettsia* scrub typhus group, has been separated into the related genus *Orientia*. The genera *Ehrlichia*, *Anaplasma*, and *Coxiella* are similar but only distantly related small intracellular parasites.

The most common reservoirs for *Rickettsia* are ticks, fleas, and mites. Rodents and other mammals also serve as reservoirs. *Prowazekii*, the causative agent of epidemic typhus, has a human reservoir and is transmitted from human to human through body lice.

## PATHOGENICITY AND CLINICAL SIGNIFICANCE

Transmission and the course of the disease are slightly different between the typhus and spotted fever groups. In the typhus group, *prowazekii*, the causative agent of epidemic typhus, are deposited on the host's skin in the feces of human body lice. Irritation caused by the louse's saliva causes humans to scratch; the louse feces, with the bacteria, can then enter through the scratch-abraded skin.

Symptoms appear suddenly after about eight days of incubation and include fever, chills, headache, and muscle and joint pain. One week later, a rash appears in some infected persons. This rash starts on the trunk and spreads toward the extremities. Stupor and delirium may follow. Mortality can be up to 70 percent of those infected, and full recovery can take several months.

Humans are the main reservoir of the disease; however, other mammals can serve as reservoirs. In the Eastern United States, flying squirrels are important reservoirs. The lice themselves are not reservoirs because they die soon after becoming infected; thus, crowded conditions are needed for epidemic spread.

*Typhi*, the causative agent of endemic typhus, is deposited on humans in the feces of rat or cat fleas. The course of the disease is much like epidemic typhus, but the disease is much milder, and humans recover in less than three weeks, even when not treated.

In the spotted fever group, the bacteria are released into the arthropod's saliva and then enter the mammalian host. The arthropods may emerge from the egg already infected because there is transovarian transfer of bacteria from the female to her eggs. Uninfected arthropods also may become infected when they take a blood meal from an infected mammal. *R. rickettsia* causes Rocky Mountain spotted fever, the most common rickettsial disease in the United States. Several species of tick, including the dog tick, are able to transmit this disease. Ticks must remain attached for some time for disease transmission because the bacteria are in a dormant state and must become active before they can enter the saliva and then the mammal, a process that may take up to forty-eight hours. The ticks themselves are the main reservoirs, while wild rodents serve as secondary reservoirs.

The onset of symptoms is sudden, two to twelve days after the tick bite, and includes fever, chills, headache, and muscle pain. A rash appears in almost all infected persons two or three days later. This rash begins on the hands and feet, often includes the palms and soles, and spreads toward the trunk. Complications include respiratory and renal failure, seizures, and coma. Mortality is about 20 percent in untreated persons. Other spotted fevers are transmitted by ticks or mites and show similar infection patterns and symptoms, although the symptoms may be milder.

## DRUG SUSCEPTIBILITY

Doxycycline, a tetracycline-type antibiotic, is the drug of choice for treating rickettsial diseases. Tetracycline and chloramphinicol also are used. They are taken orally for one week or more, although fever usually disappears in two to three days. The antibiotics can be administered intravenously in severe cases.

*Richard W. Cheney, Jr., Ph.D.*

## FURTHER READING

Didier, Raoult, and Phillipe Parola, eds. *Rickettsial Diseases.* New York: Informa Health Care, 2007. After a brief introduction to the organisms, this book explains many rickettsial diseases in detail.

Hechemy, Karim E., et al., eds. *Rickettsiology and Rickettsial Diseases.* Boston: Wiley-Blackwell, 2009. This brings together current research on all phases of *Rickettsia* and rickettsial diseases.

Madigan, Michael T., and John M. Martinko. *Brock Biology of Microorganisms.* 12th ed. Upper Saddle River, N.J.: Pearson/Prentice Hall, 2010. A comprehensive college textbook that provides broad coverage of microbiology and bacterial diseases.

## WEB SITES OF INTEREST

*Centers for Disease Control and Prevention, Division of Vector Borne Infectious Diseases*
http://www.cdc.gov//ncidod/dvbid

*National Center for Emerging and Zoonotic Infectious Diseases*
http://www.cdc.gov/ncezid

**See also:** Arthropod-borne illness and disease; Blood-borne illness and disease; Fleas and infectious disease; Lyme disease; Mediterranean spotted fever; Mites and chiggers and infectious disease; Rickettsial diseases; Rocky Mountain spotted fever; Ticks and infectious disease; Tularemia; Typhus; Typhus vaccine; Vectors and vector control; Zoonotic diseases.

# Rickettsial diseases

CATEGORY: Diseases and conditions

## DEFINITION

Rickettsial diseases include infections caused by bacteria of the genera *Rickettsia* (which causes spotted fevers and epidemic and endemic typhus), *Orientia* (which causes scrub typhus), and *Coxiella* (which causes Q fever). Some authorities also include as rickettsial diseases members of the more distantly related genera *Ehrlichia* and *Anaplasma*.

## CAUSES

When an arthopod vector (such as a tick, louse, flea, or mite) obtains a blood meal from an infected animal, bacteria in the blood are inoculated directly into the arthropod, where they subsequently multiply within its gastrointestinal tract and appear later in its feces. When the arthropod next feeds on an uninfected individual (animal or human), the *Rickettsia* are transmitted to the new host either directly or by contamination of the bite with fecal material from the arthropod.

## RISK FACTORS

With the exception of Q fever (which can be transmitted as an aerosol), all rickettsial diseases are spread through the bite of an arthropod vector. Wild animal populations serve as the natural reservoir for most species of *Rickettsia*, and humans are often incidental hosts. Epidemic typhus is unique in that it is the only rickettsial disease for which there is no wild animal reservoir. The disease is spread only by the human body or by head lice. Epidemic typhus has played perhaps a more important role than any other disease in shaping world history. It has been said, for example, that French emperor Napoleon I's retreat from Russia in the early nineteenth century was started by a louse, and that lice have defeated the most powerful armies of Europe and Asia. The typhus epidemic during World War I spread throughout Eastern Europe and led to almost three million deaths. Because of the crowded and often unsanitary conditions that characterize land-based military operations during wartime, the spread of lice between soldiers has always been a problem. In all wars involving the United States before World War II, more soldiers died from typhus than from combat-related injuries.

## SYMPTOMS

After an incubation period of one to three weeks, symptoms of epidemic typhus include an abrupt onset of high fever, chills, headache, and myalgia. Several days later, a characteristic rash will appear, beginning on the trunk and spreading to the extremities, except

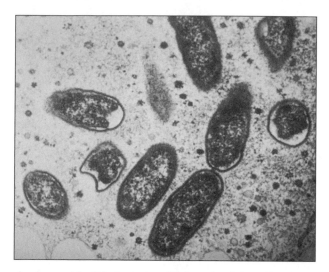

*A micrograph of the bacterium* Rickettsia rickettsii.

for the face, palms, and soles of the feet. Mortality rates in untreated cases are 10 to 30 percent.

Endemic typhus, which is maintained in the wild rat population and transmitted by the bite of the rat flea, is like epidemic typhus, although its onset is less abrupt and the symptoms are generally less severe. The disease can be mild in children, and the illness rarely lasts more than two weeks.

Rocky Mountain spotted fever (RMSF) was first reported in the Western United States but is now most prevalent in the southeastern United States. The rickettsial pathogens are maintained in populations of many dogs and small wild animals, and the disease is transmitted by the bite of wood or dog ticks.

RMSF is a systemic infection triggered by rickettsial growth in cells lining small blood vessels throughout the body. Symptoms include high fever, severe headache, myalgia, nausea, and vomiting. The rash will develop within three to five days, appearing first on the wrists and ankles and then spreading within hours to the trunk, covering the entire body. The illness can last up to three weeks, and in severe cases significant complications are not uncommon (hearing loss, neuropathy, incontinence, motor dysfunction, and occasionally shock and death).

The bacteria responsible for Q fever is widespread in domestic animal populations (such as cattle, sheep, and goats), and the disease can be spread either from the bite of an infected tick or, more commonly, from inhalation of dust containing bacteria from dried animal feces or urine; Q fever also can be spread through the consumption of unpasteurized milk. The symptoms and course of infection are similar to RMSF, although a rash usually fails to develop.

## SCREENING AND DIAGNOSIS

Diagnosis of the various rickettsial diseases may be difficult because their early signs and symptoms are often nonspecific or may resemble benign viral infections.

## TREATMENT AND THERAPY

The drug of choice for treating all rickettsial diseases is doxycycline, administered as early in the infection cycle as possible. In persons who are intolerant of tetracycline antibiotics, intravenous chloramphenicol or fluoroquinolones have been effective.

## PREVENTION AND OUTCOMES

For disease prevention, vector control is of utmost importance. The use of insect repellants containing NN-diethyl metatoluamide (DEET) generally prevents tick attachment.

*Jeffrey A. Knight, Ph.D.*

## FURTHER READING

Brachman, Philip S., and Elias Abrutyn, eds. *Bacterial Infections of Humans: Epidemiology and Control.* 4th ed. New York: Springer, 2009. A college-level introduction to principles of epidemiology and public health, with a useful chapter on RMSF.

Didier, Raoult, and Phillipe Parola, eds. *Rickettsial Diseases.* New York: Informa Health Care, 2007. After a brief introduction to the organisms, this book explains many rickettsial diseases in detail.

Hechemy, Karim E., et al., eds. *Rickettsiology and Rickettsial Diseases: Fifth International Conference.* Boston: Wiley-Blackwell, 2009. Written for advanced readers, this symposium volume is devoted exclusively to rickettsial diseases.

Madigan, Michael T., and John M. Martinko. *Brock Biology of Microorganisms.* 12th ed. Upper Saddle River, N.J.: Pearson/Prentice Hall, 2010. A comprehensive college textbook that provides broad coverage of microbiology and bacterial diseases.

Shakespeare, Martin. *Zoonoses.* 2d ed. London: Pharmaceutical Press, 2009. Designed primarily for health care professionals, this is an accessible introduction to diseases transmitted between animals and humans.

## WEB SITES OF INTEREST

*Centers for Disease Control and Prevention, Division of Vector Borne Infectious Diseases*
http://www.cdc.gov//ncidod/dvbid

*National Center for Emerging and Zoonotic Infectious Diseases*
http://www.cdc.gov/ncezid

**See also:** Arthropod-borne illness and disease; Fleas and infectious disease; Lyme disease; Mediterranean spotted fever; Mites and chiggers and infectious disease; *Rickettsia*; Rocky Mountain spotted fever; Ticks and infectious disease; Tularemia; Typhus; Typhus vaccine; Vectors and vector control; Zoonotic diseases.

# Rift Valley fever

CATEGORY: Diseases and conditions
ANATOMY OR SYSTEM AFFECTED: All

## DEFINITION

Rift Valley fever (RVF) is an infectious disease with flulike symptoms that affects livestock (mostly) and humans in the Rift Valley region of eastern Africa. RVF comes from the RVF virus. Humans and animals get RVF either from a bite by RVF-infected mosquitoes or by close contact with livestock infected with the RVF virus. While RVF is deadly in animals, the virus in humans is usually treated by helping to alleviate symptoms.

## CAUSES

Both people and animals, such as goats, sheep, cattle, and other livestock, get RVF through the bite of a mosquito infected with the RVF virus. The threat of the virus is especially high during the rainy season or in rainier years, when more mosquitoes hatch eggs. The mosquito eggs contain RVF, and then the mosquitoes born from them are infected. Persons, such as farmers, herders, veterinarians, and slaughterers, who work closely with livestock can also contract the disease through contact with blood or other bodily fluids and tissues or organs of infected animals.

## RISK FACTORS

The people at greatest risk of getting RVF are those who work directly or indirectly with livestock, especially persons who handle animal tissues or fluids. Heavy rains also increase the chance of humans and livestock being bitten by mosquitoes infected with the RVF virus. In regions in which there might already be a current outbreak of RVF, persons who sleep outdoors or travelers to the area are also at risk.

## SYMPTOMS

RVF symptoms are flulike and can be marked by a fever, weakness, aches, back pain, nausea, and dizziness. Most people with RVF usually recover on their own within two weeks. In more serious cases, those infected can experience severe bleeding, brain inflammation, and eye complications, such as inflammation of the retina. A small percentage of people who get eye complications may experience some permanent loss of vision. Less than 1 percent of people actually die from RVF. Often, the death rate can be attributed to other factors, such as other illnesses or infections. Infected livestock have higher death rates.

## SCREENING AND DIAGNOSIS

RVF's initial symptoms can be flulike, but a blood test can determine if a person has RVF.

## TREATMENT AND THERAPY

There is no specific treatment for RVF, other than treatment to alleviate any of the flulike symptoms. There are plans to develop an RVF vaccine for humans.

## PREVENTION AND OUTCOMES

The most effective prevention against getting RVF is avoiding mosquito bites by using insect repellent, wearing long pants and long sleeves, and using a bed net while sleeping. Persons working with livestock that may be infected with the RVF virus need to take special precautions when coming into direct or indirect contact with animals and animal parts.

*Micki Pflug Mounce, B.A.*

## FURTHER READING

Davies, F. Glyn, and Vincent Martin. *Recognizing Rift Valley Fever*. 17th ed. Rome: Food and Agriculture Organization of the United Nations, 2003.

Kapoor, Shailendra. "Resurgence of Rift Valley Fever." *Infectious Diseases in Clinical Practice* 16, no. 1 (2008): 9-12.

Marquardt, William C., ed. *Biology of Disease Vectors*. 2d ed. New York: Elsevier Academic Press, 2005.

## WEB SITES OF INTEREST

*American Society of Tropical Medicine and Hygiene*
http://www.astmh.org

*Centers for Disease Control and Prevention, Division of Vector Borne Infectious Diseases*
http://www.cdc.gov/ncidod/dvbid

*Neglected Tropical Diseases Coalition*
http://www.neglectedtropicaldiseases.org

**See also:** Arthropod-borne illness and disease; Developing countries and infectious disease; Malaria; Mosquitoes and infectious disease; Sleeping nets; Vectors and vector control; Viral infections.

# Ringworm

CATEGORY: Diseases and conditions
ANATOMY OR SYSTEM AFFECTED: Nails, scalp, skin
ALSO KNOWN AS: Dermatomycosis, dermatophytosis, tinea infection

## DEFINITION

Ringworm is a fungal infection of the skin, including the nails, hands, feet, and scalp. Despite its name, ringworm has nothing to do with worms. Both adults and children can be affected, but ringworm occurs most commonly in children. A fungal infection of the feet is sometimes called athlete's foot.

## CAUSES

Ringworm is caused by microscopic skin fungi that live on the outer layer of the skin. A person can get ringworm from direct skin-to-skin contact with infected people or pets. Ringworm is also transmitted by sharing hats and personal hair-grooming items (such as brushes and combs), and through contact with locker room floors, shower stalls, seats, or clothing used by an infected person.

## RISK FACTORS

Risk factors for developing ringworm include contact with surfaces (such as seat backs and shower stalls), clothing, or personal grooming items used by an infected person; skin-to-skin contact with an infected person or pet; and spending time in nurseries, schools, day-care centers, or locker rooms. At higher risk are children age twelve years or younger. Ringworm of the scalp rarely occurs in children after puberty or in adults.

## SYMPTOMS

When ringworm appears on the skin, it makes circular, reddish patches with raised borders. Eventually, the patches grow larger, and the centers of the patches turn clear, giving a ringlike appearance. Symptoms of ringworm vary, depending on the part of the body affected. On the scalp (tinea capitis), the infection begins with small bumps on the head that grow larger and form a circular pattern. Hair may become brittle and break, forming scaly, hairless patches. On the hands (tinea manus), the infection affects the palms and spaces between the fingers. On the feet (tinea pedis, or athlete's foot), the infection may cause scaling between the toes or thickening and scaling on the heels or soles. Infection of the nails (tinea unguium) causes fingernails and toenails to become yellow, thick, and crumbly. Infection of the groin area (tinea cruris, or jock itch) causes a chafed, reddish, itchy, sometimes painful rash. Infection of the skin around the entire body (tinea corporis) produces flat, scaly, round spots. Infection on the face (tinea faciei) produces red, scaly patches.

Ringworm symptoms on the body usually appear four to ten days after exposure. Scalp symptoms will appear in ten to fourteen days.

## SCREENING AND DIAGNOSIS

A doctor will ask about symptoms and medical history and will examine the patient's skin. Ringworm is often easily diagnosed by appearance. However, symptoms may be like other conditions. A sample of the affected area may be taken for testing.

## TREATMENT AND THERAPY

Treatment for ringworm may include a topical treatment. This type of treatment is used for ringworm of the skin or body and includes antifungal creams and powders. It usually takes at least two weeks for the ringworm to clear. After ringworm clears, treatment is usually continued for at least two more weeks.

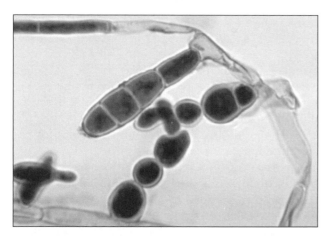

Epidermophyton floccosum, *a fungus that causes ringworm and other fungal infections.* (CDC)

For ringworm involving the body, hands, or feet, nonprescription treatment is highly effective. The following are some of the available treatments that can cure ringworm: tolnaftate, undecylenic acid, miconazole, and terbinafine. Terbinafine is more effective than the other medications. It usually needs to be used for only one week instead of four weeks. Terbinafine, however, is more expensive than the alternatives.

Oral treatment is used for ringworm of the nails and scalp. Early treatment for scalp ringworm is critical in preventing permanent hair loss. Prescription pills are given for scalp ringworm (four to eight weeks, and occasionally longer) and nail ringworm (four to nine months, and occasionally longer). If the patient developed ringworm from a pet, the pet should be treated too.

## PREVENTION AND OUTCOMES

To help prevent ringworm, one should avoid contact with any infected person, animal, surface, or object; avoid sharing personal hair-grooming items or clothing or shoes; wear sandals in locker room areas; avoid scratching during infection, to prevent ringworm from spreading to other areas; wear clothing that minimizes sweating and moisture buildup; wear breathable shoes or sandals; and keep moisture-prone areas of the body clean and dry.

*Michelle Badash, M.S.;*
*reviewed by David L. Horn, M.D., FACP*

## FURTHER READING

American Academy of Family Physicians. "Tinea Infections: Athlete's Foot, Jock Itch, and Ringworm." Available at http://www.aafp.org/afp/980700ap/980700b.html.

Berger, T. G. "Dermatologic Disorders." In *Current Medical Diagnosis and Treatment 2011*, edited by Stephen J. McPhee and Maxine A. Papadakis. 50th ed. New York: McGraw-Hill Medical, 2011.

Burns, Tony, et al., eds. *Rook's Textbook of Dermatology.* 8th ed. 4 vols. Hoboken, N.J.: Wiley-Blackwell, 2010.

EBSCO Publishing. *DynaMed: Tinea Capitis.* Available through http://www.ebscohost.com/dynamed.

Higgens, E. M., L. C. Fuller, and C. H. Smith. "Guidelines for the Management of Tinea Capitis." *British Journal of Dermatology* 143 (2000): 53-58.

Richardson, Malcolm D., and Elizabeth M. Johnson. *The Pocket Guide to Fungal Infection.* 2d ed. Malden, Mass.: Blackwell, 2006.

## WEB SITES OF INTEREST

*American Academy of Dermatology*
http://www.aad.org

*American Academy of Family Physicians*
http://familydoctor.org

*College of Family Physicians of Canada*
http://www.cfpc.ca

*DoctorFungus.org*
http://doctorfungus.org

**See also:** Antifungal drugs: Types; Athlete's foot; Chromoblastomycosis; Dermatomycosis; Dermatophytosis; Diagnosis of fungal infections; *Epidermophyton*; Fungal infections; Fungi: Classification and types; Jock itch; Onychomycosis; Prevention of fungal infections; Skin infections; Tinea capitis; Tinea corporis; Tinea versicolor.

# Rocky Mountain spotted fever

CATEGORY: Diseases and conditions
ANATOMY OR SYSTEM AFFECTED: Blood, cardiovascular system

## DEFINITION

Rocky Mountain spotted fever (RMSF) is a severe disease that is potentially fatal. The disease, which is spread by ticks, was first recognized in the Rocky Mountains area of the United States. RMSF is now found in most U.S. states.

## CAUSES

RMSF is caused by the bacterium *Rickettsia rickettsii*, which is carried by the American dog tick and the Rocky Mountain wood tick. When an infected tick bites a human, the disease is passed through the person's skin into the bloodstream. The bacteria multiply inside cells of the inner lining of small arteries, causing inflammation. The inflammation is known as vasculitis.

## RISK FACTORS

Factors that increase the chance of getting RMSF include exposure to tick-infested areas, contact with pets that roam in tick-infested areas, being outdoors often during the months of April to September, and residing in or visiting states where RMSF occurs most commonly. These states include, but are not limited to, Arkansas, Georgia, Kentucky, North Carolina, South Carolina, Oklahoma, Tennessee, and Virginia. At higher risk are men, children, and young adults.

## SYMPTOMS

The first symptom of RMSF is a sudden high fever that often occurs within one to fourteen days of a tick bite. Other symptoms may include nausea, vomiting, muscle pain, a lack of appetite, and a severe headache. Later signs may include a rash, abdominal pain, joint pain, diarrhea, a cough, irritability, insomnia, lethargy, confusion, delirium (or, in severe cases, coma), and an enlarged liver, spleen, and lymph nodes. In severe cases, symptoms include low blood pressure and shock.

## SCREENING AND DIAGNOSIS

A doctor will ask about symptoms and medical history and will perform a physical exam. RMSF can be difficult to diagnose because it resembles other diseases. Three indicators that the doctor will look for are a fever, a rash (which may not be present early), and a history of a tick bite (which is not always known by the patient). Blood tests may be done to confirm the diagnosis. Treatment is often started based on a best guess. Doctors sometimes fail to consider RMSF as a diagnosis when adults or children present with only a high fever. One should be sure the doctor knows if the patient has been outdoors.

## TREATMENT AND THERAPY

RMSF is treated with antibiotics, and it is important to start this treatment early. The most commonly used antibiotics in treating RMSF are doxycycline and tetracycline.

## PREVENTION AND OUTCOMES

The best way to prevent RMSF is to limit one's exposure to ticks. Persons who live in areas that are prone to ticks should take the following precautions: wear light-colored clothing; tuck pants into socks; apply insect repellents containing NN-diethyl meta-

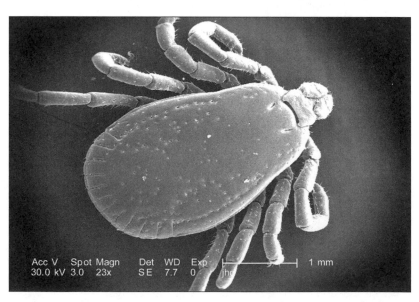

*A male* Dermacentor *tick, a vector for Rocky Mountain spotted fever.* (CDC)

toluamide, or DEET, to exposed skin; and apply permethrin to clothing. For young children, DEET should be avoided or used sparingly. After returning from outdoor areas, one should carefully check for ticks and should also check pets for ticks.

*Michelle Badash, M.S.;*
*reviewed by David L. Horn, M.D., FACP*

**FURTHER READING**

Bratton, R. L., and G. R. Corey. "Tick-Borne Disease." *American Family Physician* 71 (2005): 2323.

Chen, Luke F., and Daniel J. Sexton. "What's New in Rocky Mountain Spotted Fever?" *Infectious Disease Clinics of North America* 22 (2008): 415-432.

EBSCO Publishing. *DynaMed: Rocky Mountain Spotted Fever.* Available through http://www.ebscohost.com/dynamed.

Goddard, Jerome. *Physician's Guide to Arthropods of Medical Importance.* 4th ed. Boca Raton, Fla.: CRC Press, 2003.

Schlossberg, David, ed. *Infections of Leisure.* 4th ed. Washington, D.C.: ASM Press, 2009.

Vanderhoof-Forschner, Karen. *Everything You Need to Know About Lyme Disease and Other Tick-Borne Disorders.* 2d ed. Hoboken, N.J.: John Wiley & Sons, 2003.

Walker, David H. "*Rickettsia rickettsii* and Other Spotted Fever Groups." In *Principles and Practice of Infectious Diseases,* edited by Gerald L. Mandell, John F. Bennett, and Raphael Dolin. 7th ed. Philadelphia: Churchill Livingstone/Elsevier, 2009.

**WEB SITES OF INTEREST**

*Centers for Disease Control and Prevention*
http://www.cdc.gov/ticks

*Public Health Agency of Canada*
http://www.phac-aspc.gc.ca

**See also:** Anaplasmosis; Arthropod-borne illness and disease; Behçet's syndrome; Bubonic plague; Cat scratch fever; Colorado tick fever; Ehrlichiosis; Encephalitis; Fever; Giardiasis; Hemorrhagic fever viral infections; Inflammation; Lyme disease; Mediterranean spotted fever; Plague; *Rickettsia*; Ticks and infectious disease; Tularemia; Vectors and vector control; Zoonotic diseases.

# Rodents and infectious disease

**CATEGORY:** Transmission

## DEFINITION

Rodent-transmitted diseases are responsible for severe and deadly illnesses in human populations. These diseases include hantavirus pulmonary syndrome, murine typhus, rat-bite fever, leptospirosis, and eosinophilic meningitis.

## HANTAVIRUS PULMONARY SYNDROME (HPS)

Humans contract HPS by inhaling dried rat or mouse secretions. Though rare, HPS is a public concern because its affect on the human body is severe and can lead to death. HPS manifests in two stages of symptoms, which first appear about one to five weeks following exposure to the hantavirus.

With the first stage, an infected person experiences fever, fatigue, body ache, headache, lung congestion, nausea, diarrhea, and abdominal pain. With the second stage, known as the cardiopulmonary stage, the congestion in the lungs progresses to a cough, shortness of breath, a worsening buildup of fluid in the lungs, low blood pressure, rapid heartbeat, multiple organ failure, and respiratory distress.

HPS can be diagnosed with a blood test. Persons with HPS are treated with assisted respiration, often in a hospital's intensive care unit.

## MURINE TYPHUS

Humans contract murine typhus, a rickettsial infection caused by *Rickettsia typhi*, by being bitten by infected rat fleas. Domestic cats may also carry these infected fleas. Active in warm climates, murine typhus infection may last as long as two weeks. However, if left untreated, the disease can be fatal in severe cases. Following an incubation period of six to fourteen days, symptoms include headache, myalgia, and rash. A bacterial disease, murine typhus is treated with antibiotics.

*Rat-bite fever.* Rat-bite fever is transmitted to humans through a bite, scratch, or ingestion of food or water contaminated with infected rat feces or other secretions. It is a bacterial illness caused by *Streptobacillus moniliformis* and *Spirillum minus.* Symptoms include fever, body ache, nausea, and rash, and they may progress to arthralgia, pneumonia, or meningitis.

## Rodent Facts

### TAXONOMIC CLASSIFICATION

**Kingdom:** Animalia
**Subkingdom:** Bilateria
**Phylum:** Chordata
**Subphylum:** Vertebrata
**Class:** Mammalia
**Order:** Rodentia
**Suborders:** Sciurognathi (squirrel-like rodents), Myomorpha (mouselike rodents)
**Families:** Sciuridae (squirrels), Anomaluridae (scaly-tailed squirrels), Heteromyidae (pocket mice), Muridae (rats and mice), Gliridae and Selevinidae (dormice), Zapodidae (jumping mice and birchmice), Abrocomidae (chinchilla rats), Echimyidae (spiny rats), Thryonomyidae (cane rats), Petromyidae (African rock rats), Bathyergidae (African mole rats)

**Geographical location:** Every continent except Antarctica
**Habitat:** Mostly on land or underground, in forests, plains, and deserts
**Gestational period:** Varies greatly, though generally two weeks in a mouse and about one month in a rat
**Life span:** Most smaller species live for one to three years, while large rodents survive for more than ten years
**Special anatomy:** All rodents possess incisor teeth designed for gnawing; these teeth grow continuously from the roots and wear away at their tips, giving them chisel-like edges that can gnaw through very hard materials; however, they lack cuspids (tearing teeth) that are seen in carnivores

Rat-bite fever is diagnosed by testing for the presence of the infectious bacteria on the skin or in the blood or the lymph nodes. It is treated with antibiotics.

*Leptospirosis.* The bacterium *Leptospira* is found in the urine of infected wild and domestic rodents. Humans can contract leptospirosis by handling infected rodents or by ingesting water that is contaminated with infected rodent urine. An infected person will show signs of illness two to four days after exposure. Symptoms include headache, fever, abdominal pain, diarrhea, and rash. In severe cases, infected persons may have kidney or liver damage, meningitis, or breathing difficulty. Leptospirosis is diagnosed by testing a person's blood or urine, and the infection is treated with antibiotics.

*Eosinophilic meningitis.* Humans can get eosinophilic meningitis, an invasion of the central nervous system by parasites, from ingesting the larvae of the rat lungworm (*Angiostrongylus cantonensis*), which can be hosted by snails and slugs. Eating infected snails or vegetables will make a person vulnerable to contracting eosinophilic meningitis. Symptoms, including headache, fever, and nausea, may last several weeks or months. Treatment includes headache-control measures and antifungal therapy.

### PREVENTION

The best prevention of rodent-transmitted infectious diseases is indoor and outdoor rodent control. Indoor rodent-control measures include maintaining a clean kitchen, storing food and garbage in rodent-proof containers, throwing away uneaten pet food daily, setting rodent traps, and sealing entry holes larger than one-quarter-inch in diameter. Outdoor rodent-control measures include clearing brush and stored items from a building's foundation and removing woodpiles and other potential nesting sites.

Flea control is another preventive measure against rodent-transmitted infectious disease. Flea-control medicine should be administered to pets. To avoid contact with feral, and potentially infective, animals, one should not provide food for birds or wild animals. Fallen fruit from trees should be picked up and discarded. One should use a flea-killer spray around sites that are vulnerable to rodent nesting.

Other measures include not swimming in water that may be contaminated with rodent urine. Also, for walking through shallow water or on ground inhabited by rodents, one should wear protective footwear and clothing.

### RESPONSE

Rodent infestation in the home, marked by droppings (feces), nests, or gnawed food packaging, requires disinfection of the suspected areas of infestation. Because dried rodent urine and feces will aerosolize during removal, a mask or respirator should be worn while cleaning an area known or suspected to have rodent infestation. One should wear rubber gloves when cleaning, and instead of sweeping or vac-

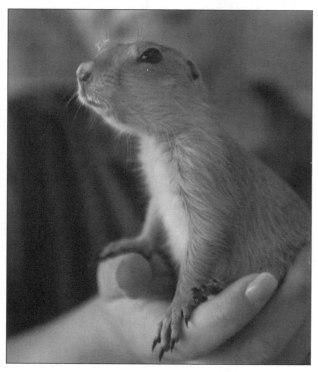

*The prairie dog is a type of rodent.* (AP/Wide World Photos)

uuming droppings and nests, one should wipe the contaminated areas with detergent or a hypochlorite solution. After wiping up the droppings or nesting materials, the area should be disinfected. Dead rodents should be sprayed with disinfectant, bagged with cleaning materials, and discarded in a waste disposal system recommended by a local or state health department.

## IMPACT

Rodents are the cause of many bacterial, rickettsial, and viral infections impacting humans. The control of rodent populations is critical to public health and health management.

*Melissa Walsh*

## FURTHER READING

Committee on Infectious Diseases of Mice and Rats. *Companion Guide to Infectious Diseases of Mice and Rats.* Washington, D.C.: National Academies Press, 1991.

Gratz, Norman. *Vector- and Rodent-Borne Diseases in Europe and North America: Distribution, Public Health Burden, and Control.* New York: Cambridge University Press, 2006.

Padovan, Dennis. *Infectious Diseases of Wild Rodents.* Anacortes, Wash.: Corvus, 2006.

## WEB SITES OF INTEREST

*Centers of Disease Control and Prevention*
http://www.cdc.gov/rodents

*National Center for Emerging and Zoonotic Infectious Diseases*
http://www.cdc.gov/ncezid

**See also:** Airborne illness and disease; Bacterial meningitis; Fleas and infectious disease; Hantavirus infection; Insect-borne illness and disease; Leptospirosis; Parasitic diseases; Plague; Rat-bite fever; Respiratory route of transmission; *Rickettsia*; Transmission routes; Typhus; Zoonotic diseases.

---

Rosea. *See* Pityriasis rosea.

---

# Roseola

CATEGORY: Diseases and conditions
ANATOMY OR SYSTEM AFFECTED: Skin
ALSO KNOWN AS: Exanthem subitum, roseola infantum

## DEFINITION

Roseola is an infection caused by a virus. It is characterized by a sudden onset of high fever followed by a rash. This disorder usually resolves on its own with no complications. Roseola can occur year-round, but it is most common in the spring and fall months.

## CAUSES

Roseola is usually caused by a virus called human herpesvirus-6 (HHV-6). It can also be caused by human herpesvirus-7 (HHV-7). These viruses are not the same as the herpesviruses that cause cold sores or genital herpes.

## RISK FACTORS

Persons who are at high risk for roseola are children six months to three years of age. The infection is most common in infants between six and fifteen months of age.

## SYMPTOMS

Symptoms of roseola include a fever (103° to 105° Fahrenheit) that begins suddenly, is not associated with other symptoms, and lasts three days (and occasionally a day or two longer); convulsions, which may occur in association with high fever in up to 5 to 10 percent of children; and a rash that develops typically twelve to twenty-four hours after the fever, appears first on the chest and the abdomen, is rose-colored, which may spread to arms, legs, neck, and face and lasts for a few hours to a few days, and does not itch. The characteristic sign of roseola is the appearance of a rash after the fever disappears.

Other symptoms or signs may include swelling of lymph nodes in the neck and behind the ears, irritability, and a poor appetite. Symptoms of an upper respiratory tract infection may be present before the onset of a fever.

## SCREENING AND DIAGNOSIS

A doctor will ask about symptoms and medical history and will perform a physical exam. The symptoms and physical findings of roseola are so distinctive that, most often, no other tests are needed. In most cases, however, there is a history of other children with roseola in the patient's community.

## TREATMENT AND THERAPY

No treatment is needed for roseola unless the child is immunocompromised. One should, however, keep the child's fever down and should maintain good hydration with fluids. Medications to reduce the fever include acetaminophen (such as Tylenol) or ibuprofen (such as Advil and Motrin). The fever also can be reduced with lukewarm sponge baths.

Aspirin is not recommended for children or teens with a current or recent viral infection because of the risk of Reye's syndrome. One should consult a doctor about medicines that are safe for children. Consult a doctor too if the child has a seizure or if the fever persists, or both.

## PREVENTION AND OUTCOMES

To help prevent the spread of roseola, one should avoid contact with an infected child. The incubation period for roseola is five to fifteen days. The virus is thought to be spread by contact with infected saliva, with adults forming the main reservoir for the virus.

One should carefully and frequently wash hands to help prevent the spread of roseola.

*Reviewed by Kari Kassir, M.D.*

## FURTHER READING

Behrman, Richard E., Robert M. Kliegman, and Hal B. Jenson, eds. *Nelson Textbook of Pediatrics.* 18th ed. Philadelphia: Saunders/Elsevier, 2007.

Beers, Mark H., et al. *The Merck Manual of Diagnosis and Therapy.* 18th ed. Whitehouse Station, N.J.: Merck Research Laboratories, 2006.

## WEB SITES OF INTEREST

*About Kids Health*
http://www.aboutkidshealth.ca

*American Academy of Dermatology*
http://www.aad.org

*American Academy of Family Physicians*
http://familydoctor.org

*Centers for Disease Control and Prevention*
http://www.cdc.gov

*KidsHealth*
http://www.kidshealth.org

**See also:** Chickenpox; Children and infectious disease; Contagious diseases; Erythema infectiosum; Erythema nodosum; Fever; Herpesviridae; Herpesvirus infections; Hygiene; Impetigo; Measles; Molluscum contagiosum; Pityriasis rosea; Rubella; Saliva and infectious disease; Scarlet fever; Skin infections; Viral infections.

# Rotavirus infection

CATEGORY: Diseases and conditions
ANATOMY OR SYSTEM AFFECTED: Abdomen, gastrointestinal system, intestines, stomach
ALSO KNOWN AS: Stomach flu, stomach virus

## DEFINITION

Rotavirus infection is an intestinal inflammation transmitted by a ribonucleic acid (RNA) virus that results in extreme diarrhea, especially in young children.

## Causes

Rotavirus infection is primarily caused when fecal germs on a person's hands are transmitted to the mouth and ingested. However, because rotavirus infection is extremely contagious, it also can be contracted by inhaling infected sputum in a sneeze or cough. Rotavirus germs also can be ingested in food or water contaminated with fecal particles.

## Risk Factors

Young children are at greatest risk of contracting rotavirus infection, and almost all children have suffered a rotavirus infection by their fifth birthday. Child-care staff and children who attend day-care centers are even more prone to rotavirus infection because they are regularly exposed to children in close proximity. The elderly, especially those in nursing homes, also are susceptible to rotavirus infection, as are those with weakened immune systems. Frequent travelers to developing countries also risk greater exposure because of contaminated food and water sources.

## Symptoms

The symptoms of rotavirus infection include diarrhea, nausea, abdominal pain, vomiting, dehydration, fever, chills, and loss of appetite.

## Screening and Diagnosis

After conducting a physical exam, a physician will question the affected person about his or her symptoms. Confirmation of a rotavirus infection may be obtained through a rapid antigen test applied to the person's stool sample in the laboratory and examined through electron microscopy.

## Treatment and Therapy

No cure exists for rotavirus infection, but the most serious symptom, dehydration, is treatable by drinking large amounts of liquids, especially liquids that contain electrolytes (such as Gatorade). Severely dehydrated persons will require the intravenous administration of liquids in a hospital setting. Stomach cramps and diarrhea may be slightly mitigated by eating bland food, such as soda crackers, and a fever can be reduced by using a damp cloth on the forehead.

## Prevention and Outcomes

Complete prevention of rotavirus infection is impossible, but one can take steps to greatly reduce the likelihood of infection. First and foremost is vaccination. In 2006, two vaccines, RotaTeq and Rotarix, became available for infants, and they are extremely effective in preventing rotavirus infection or in lessening the severity of infection if it occurs. Additionally, because tests have shown that the rotavirus survives for several hours on hands, vigilant handwashing is highly effective in reducing transmission. Children should consistently wash their hands, especially after using the toilet and before eating. Child-care workers and all persons associated with children also should practice rigorous handwashing. Dirty diapers should be disposed of immediately after changing, and diaper changing areas should be regularly disinfected. Because rotavirus survives for days on hard surfaces, all toilets, counters, and children's toys should also be cleaned regularly with disinfectant. Persons traveling in developing countries should boil all drinking water before ingesting.

*Mary E. Markland, M.A.*

## Further Reading

Chadwick, Derek, and Jamie A. Goode, eds. *Gastroenteritis Viruses.* New York: John Wiley & Sons, 2001.

Gray, James, and Ulrich Desselberger, eds. *Rotaviruses: Methods and Protocols.* Totowa, N.J.: Humana Press, 2000.

Kirschner, Barbara S., and Dennis D. Black. "The Gastrointestinal Tract." In *Nelson Essentials of Pediatrics*, edited by Karen J. Marcdante et al. 6th ed. Philadelphia: Saunders/Elsevier, 2011.

Matson, David O. "Rotaviruses." In *Principles and Practice of Pediatric Infectious Diseases*, edited by Sarah S. Long, Larry K. Pickering, and Charles G. Prober. 3d ed. New York: Churchill Livingstone/Elsevier, 2008.

## Web Sites of Interest

*American Society of Tropical Medicine and Hygiene*
http://www.astmh.org

*Rotavirus Vaccine Program*
htto://www.rotavirus.org

**See also:** Children and infectious disease; Developing countries and infectious disease; Fecal-oral route of transmission; Inflammation; Intestinal and stomach infections; Reoviridae; Rotavirus vaccine; Travelers' diarrhea; Tropical medicine; Viral infections; Waterborne illness and disease.

# Rotavirus vaccine

CATEGORY: Prevention

## DEFINITION

The rotavirus vaccine prevents infection with rotavirus, a pathogen that invades the gastrointestinal system and can cause severe disease accompanied by vomiting, diarrhea, and fever. Many children acquire rotavirus and manifest only mild vomiting and diarrhea, but often, affected children require hospitalization to manage the resultant dehydration.

## MECHANISM OF ACTION

The mechanism of action of the rotavirus vaccine depends upon the brand administered. The RotaTeq vaccine is a combination of a bovine strain of the virus that does not cause disease in humans and a component of the human rotavirus that cannot cause active infection. These components are then administered together in an oral dose and elicit an immune response without actually causing the disease, therefore providing protection from future illness.

The Rotarix brand of the vaccine is derived from a strain of human rotavirus that has been weakened enough to not cause active disease, while still eliciting an immune response from the patient.

## HISTORY

The vaccine against rotavirus was first licensed in 1998. In 1999, the recommendation that the rotavirus vaccine be administered to all children was withdrawn because of reports of an association with intussusception, an illness that causes one segment of the bowel to telescope into another, sometimes requiring surgical repair. In 2006 and 2008, new, safer forms of the vaccine were licensed under the names RotaTeq and Rotarix, respectively.

## ADMINISTRATION

It is recommended that the rotavirus vaccine be administered to all children in two or three doses depending on which brand of vaccine is to be given. RotaTeq is the three-dose form of the vaccine and is given at two, four, and six months of age. Rotarix is the two-dose form and is given at two and four months of age. Both forms of the vaccine are oral and, therefore, do not require an injection for administration.

## IMPACT

Rotavirus is the most common cause of acute gastrointestinal disease worldwide, with increased mortality in developing countries. Since the rotavirus vaccine was developed, concentrated efforts have been made by public health organizations to immunize the children of developing countries. In the United States, uniform administration of the vaccine has led to greatly decreased incidence of rotavirus disease.

*Jennifer Birkhauser, M.D.*

## FURTHER READING

Behrman, Richard E., Robert M. Kliegman, and Hal B. Jenson, eds. *Nelson Textbook of Pediatrics.* 18th ed. Philadelphia: Saunders/Elsevier, 2007.

Loehr, Jamie. *The Vaccine Answer Book: Two Hundred Essential Answers to Help You Make the Right Decisions for Your Child.* Naperville, Ill.: Sourcebooks, 2010.

Matson, David O. "Rotaviruses." In *Principles and Practice of Pediatric Infectious Diseases*, edited by Sarah S. Long, Larry K. Pickering, and Charles G. Prober. 3d ed. New York: Churchill Livingstone/Elsevier, 2008.

Sears, Robert. *The Vaccine Book: Making the Right Decision for Your Child.* New York: Little, Brown, 2007.

## WEB SITES OF INTEREST

*Centers for Disease Control and Prevention*
http://www.cdc.gov/vaccines

*Children's Hospital of Philadelphia, Vaccine Education Center*
http://www.chop.edu/service/vaccine-education-center

*Rotavirus Vaccine Program*
http://www.rotavirusvaccine.org

**See also:** Children and infectious disease; Developing countries and infectious disease; Fecal-oral route of transmission; Reoviridae; Rotavirus infection; Travelers' diarrhea; Waterborne illness and disease.

# Roundworms

CATEGORY: Pathogen
TRANSMISSION ROUTE: Blood, ingestion

## DEFINITION

Roundworm infestations of the intestines or other body tissues are among the most common of human parasitic infections worldwide. Humans are the definitive hosts of several species of roundworms and accidental hosts of roundworm larvae that normally infect other animal species.

## NATURAL HABITAT AND FEATURES

Roundworms have a complex life cycle, involving eggs, immature larvae, and mature worms. The life stages of roundworms typically involve different host species and environments. For example, the egg and larval stages of various human intestinal roundworms mature in soil. These intestinal roundworms include common roundworms (*Ascaris lumbricoides*), hookworms (*Ancylostoma duodenale* and *Necator americanus*), pinworms (*Enterobius vermicularis*), *Strongyloides stercoralis*, and *Trichuris trichiura*. Infections with intestinal roundworms are most common in tropical and subtropical regions. Notably, pinworm eggs can mature without a soil phase, which explains the high incidence of this roundworm infection in cold climates throughout the world, including the United States.

Roundworms that live their larval stage in biting insects spread disease to humans through injection of larvae during a bite. Because the species of insects that carry roundworm larvae typically live in warm climates, the associated parasitic diseases are also seen in these locales. The diseases include filariasis (*Wuchereria bancrofti*, *Brugia malayi*, and *B. timori*), loiasis (*Loa loa*), onchocerciasis or river blindness (*Onchocerca volvulus*), and infections with *Mansonella*.

Guinea worm disease, caused by ingesting water contaminated with *Dracunculus medinensis*-infected copepods, is a tropical disease commonly found in the Middle East, India, and Africa. Trichinellosis occurs throughout the world, caused by ingestion of raw or undercooked meat contaminated with larvae from various *Trichinella* species. *T. spiralis* and *T. pseudospiralis* have worldwide distribution, infecting pigs, birds, and rats.

Parasitic roundworms vary in size, life cycle, site of human infestation, and physical characteristics. Most species include male and female worms, which have cylindrical, nonsegmented bodies. Intestinal roundworms are typically diagnosed by microscopic examination of the stool. A microscopist trained in parasitology can visually distinguish various roundworms and their eggs based on size and characteristic features. Tissue roundworm infections are diagnosed based on clinical signs and symptoms and on recovery and identification of worms or larvae from tissue or blood.

## PATHOGENICITY AND CLINICAL SIGNIFICANCE

The pathogenicity and clinical significance of human roundworms vary according to the species, intensity of infestation (worm burden), and health status of the host. For example, hosts with a low to moderate worm burden with *A. lumbricoides* are commonly asymptomatic. Persons with a heavy infestation may develop impaired digestion or malabsorption, leading to malnutrition. This clinical scenario is most likely in persons with preexisting marginal nutrition. Heavy *A. lumbricoides* infestation may lead to small bowel or common-bile-duct obstruction, which is caused by the mass effect of the worms.

Hookworm larvae burrow into the skin, travel through the circulatory system to the lungs, migrate to the trachea, and are swallowed. Larvae attach to the wall of the small intestine and mature into adult worms. Dermatologic symptoms are common during the migratory phase of the illness, which may be followed by respiratory symptoms. Abdominal pain, diarrhea, protein malnutrition, and iron-deficiency anemia may develop in persons with a well-established hookworm infection.

Symptoms of pinworm infestation are typically limited to nocturnal, perianal pruritus and related sleep disruption. Rarely, pinworms migrate to other body sites, potentially causing bowel ulceration, appendicitis, or salpingitis.

Humans are accidental hosts of *Trichinella* worms. Larvae mature in the intestine and migrate to muscle tissue, where they encyst. Trichinellosis is usually subclinical. Rarely, complications such as myocarditis, pneumonia, or encephalitis may become life-threatening.

With filariasis, roundworm larvae injected during an insect bite migrate to the lymphatic system, mature, and then produce microfilariae, which are released into the bloodstream. The presence of adult

## Taxonomic Classification for Roundworms

**Kingdom:** Animalia
**Phylum:** Nemata
**Class:** Chromadorea
**Order:** Ascaridida
**Superfamily:** Ascaridoidea
**Family:** Anisakidae
**Genera:** *Anisakis, Pseudoterranova*
**Species:**
*A. simplex*
*P. decipiens*
**Family:** Ascarididae
**Genus:** *Ascaris*
**Species:** *A. lumbricoides*
**Order:** Oxyurida
**Superfamily:** Oxyuroidea
**Family:** Oxyuridae
**Genus:** *Enterobius*
**Species:** *E. vermicularis*
**Order:** Rhabditida
**Suborder:** Strongylida
**Superfamily:** Ancylostomatoidea
**Family:** Ancylostomatidae

**Subfamily:** Ancylostomatinae
**Genus:** *Ancylostoma*
**Species:**
*A. duodenale*
*A. caninum*
*A. braziliense*
**Subfamily:** Bunostominae
**Genus:** *Necator*
**Species:** *N. americanus*
**Superfamily:** Panagrolaimoidea
**Family:** Strongyloididae
**Genus:** *Strongyloides*
**Species:** *S. stercoralis*
**Order:** Spirurida
**Superfamily:** Filarioidea
**Family:** Onchocercidae
**Genera:** *Brugia, Loa, Mansonella,*
*Onchocerca, Wuchereria*
**Species:**
*B. malayi*
*B. timori*
*L. loa*

*M. ozzardi*
*M. perstans*
*O. volvulus*
*W. bancrofti*
**Superfamily:** *Dracunculoidea*
**Family:** Dracunculidae
**Genus:** *Dracunculus*
**Species:** *D. medinensis*
**Class:** Enoplea
**Subclass:** Enoplia
**Order:** Trichocephalida
**Family:** Trichinellidae
**Genus:** *Trichinella*
**Species:**
*T. spiralis*
*T. pseudospiralis*
*T. nelson*
*T. britovi*
*T. nativa*
**Family:** Trichuridae
**Genus:** *Trichuris*
**Species:** *T. trichiura*

worms in the lymphatic system may cause acute and chronic inflammation, potentially leading to lymphadenitis, lymphangitis, chronic lymphadenopathy, lymphedema, hydrocele, and elephantiasis.

Onchocerciasis, another filarial roundworm disease, remains a major cause of blindness in parts of Central Africa and West Africa. The microfilariae have an affinity for the eyes, in addition to other body sites. Secondary choroiditis, glaucoma, iridocyclitis, and optic atrophy can lead to significant visual impairment or blindness.

### DRUG SUSCEPTIBILITY

Anthelmintic drugs, including mebendazole, albendazole, ivermectin, and pyrantel pamoate, are generally effective for intestinal roundworm infections, including trichuriasis, enterobiasis, ascariasis, strongyloidiasis, hookworm infestation, and the intestinal phase of trichinellosis. Diethylcarbamazine and ivermectin are used to treat dracunculiasis, loiasis, and lymphatic filariasis. These drugs clear microfilariae from the peripheral blood but generally do not

eradicate adult worms. Ivermectin is the treatment of choice for onchocerciasis.

*Tina M. St. John, M.D.*

### FURTHER READING

Kazura, James W. "Tissue Nematodes, Including Trichinellosis, Dracunculiasis, and the Filariases." In *Mandell, Douglas, and Bennett's Principles and Practice of Infectious Diseases*, edited by Gerald L. Mandell, John F. Bennett, and Raphael Dolin. 7th ed. New York: Churchill Livingstone/Elsevier, 2010. Infectious disease textbook with referenced discussion of tissue roundworms, including epidemiology, life cycle, clinical manifestations, diagnosis, and treatment.

Maguire, James H. "Intestinal Nematodes (Roundworms)." In *Mandell, Douglas, and Bennett's Principles and Practice of Infectious Diseases*, edited by Gerald L. Mandell, John F. Bennett, and Raphael Dolin. 7th ed. New York: Churchill Livingstone/Elsevier, 2010. Infectious disease textbook with referenced discussion of intestinal roundworms, including epidemiology, life cycle, clinical manifestations, diagnosis, and treatment.

Saviolia, Lorenzo, and Albis F. Gabrielli. "Helminthic Diseases: Intestinal Nematode Infection." In *International Encyclopedia of Public Health*, edited by Kristian Heggenhougen and Stella Quah. Burlington, Mass.: Academic Press/Elsevier, 2008. Public health reference including a review of the epidemiology, biology, disease burden, diagnosis, treatment, and public health management of intestinal roundworm infections.

### WEB SITES OF INTEREST

*Centers for Disease Control and Prevention*
http://www.cdc.gov/parasites

*Microbiology and Immunology On-line: Parasitology*
http://pathmicro.med.sc.edu/book/parasit-sta.htm

*Partners for Parasite Control*
http://www.who.int/wormcontrol

**See also:** Ascariasis; Capillariasis; Cholera; Developing countries and infectious disease; Dracunculiasis; Elephantiasis; Enterobiasis; Filariasis; Flukes; Giardiasis; Hookworms; Lymphadenitis; Parasitic diseases; Pinworms; Soilborne illness and disease; Strongyloidiasis; Taeniasis; Tapeworms; Travelers' diarrhea; Trichinosis; Tropical medicine; Waterborne illness and disease; Whipworm infection; Worm infections.

# Rubella

CATEGORY: Diseases and conditions
ANATOMY OR SYSTEM AFFECTED: All
ALSO KNOWN AS: German measles, three-day measles

### DEFINITION

Rubella is a contagious but usually mild childhood disease caused by the rubella virus. The virus can lead to congenital disease of newborns if a pregnant woman is exposed to the virus during her first trimester.

### CAUSES

The rubella virus is a member of the *Rubivirus* genus of the Togaviridae family. The transmission route is through the respiratory system by direct contact with discharge from the nose or mouth of an infected person, as might occur during a cough or sneeze. The average incubation period for rubella is sixteen days. The infected person is contagious from about one week before the rash appears to two to three weeks after the onset of the rash. Humans are the only hosts for this virus.

### RISK FACTORS

With early immunizations, 99 percent of children never contract rubella. Exposure of nonimmunized children in close spaces such as schools could pose a risk, but this is unlikely. The main risk is to pregnant women or to women of childbearing age who have low rubella titers. The success of the immunization program in the United States has significantly decreased the risk of rubella for pregnant women.

### SYMPTOMS

Rubella is usually a mild illness. The affected person may feel fatigued for a few days. Typical symptoms include malaise with painful enlargement of the lymph nodes behind the ear (postauricle) and neck (suboccipital and cervical lymph nodes). Usually, red macular spots appear on the face; the rash spreads to the trunk and then to the arms and legs. Some people with rubella do not have a rash; even in those who develop a rash, the pattern may vary.

Other symptoms of rubella include a low-grade fever of 101° Fahrenheit or lower. About 10 to 15 percent of older youth and young adults experience joint pain or arthralgia. Coldlike symptoms with congestion and cough may be present. Complications are rare, but extreme cases may result in rubella encephalopathy with headache and seizures; neuritis, or irritated nerves; and orchitis, or inflamed testes.

### SCREENING AND DIAGNOSIS

The health care provider will take a medical history and perform a physical examination. Diagnosis will be made by assessment of physical symptoms such as enlarged and painful cervical and postauricle lymph nodes, coupled with a low-grade temperature and a macular rash on the face, trunk, and limbs. Most cases are mild and may go undiagnosed. Confirmation of the rubella diagnosis is obtained by measuring the presence or increased antibody titer of IgM (rubella-specific immunoglobulin M) through blood or culture testing. In the United States, rubella immunizations are mandated for all children before they start attending school, so the occurrence of this disease is rare.

Rubella is dangerous to pregnant women in the first trimester and up to twenty weeks of pregnancy; about 80 percent of babies born to infected mothers will experience the adverse effects of congenital rubella syndrome. Severe abnormalities include cataracts, blindness, mental retardation, microcephaly, deafness, heart defects and disorders, hepatomegaly, pneumonitis, and bone disorders. The later a pregnant woman is exposed, the less chance her illness will affect her unborn fetus. Young women of childbearing age with low rubella titers may choose to receive vaccinations before their first pregnancy. The rubella vaccine should not be given to pregnant women.

### TREATMENT AND THERAPY

Symptoms are usually mild and need minimal supportive treatment. Acetaminophen or ibuprofen can be taken for relief of pain, fever, and joint aches. Maintaining adequate fluid intake is recommended but no isolation of the infected person is necessary.

### PREVENTION AND OUTCOMES

After a rubella outbreak in the mid-1960's, vaccines for immunization against rubella were developed. Getting vaccinated is the best way to prevent rubella. Rubella immunizations are required by most states in the United States. A live virus is usually given in a combination vaccine for measles, mumps, and rubella (MMR) to infants at twelve to fifteen months of age and through a booster shot at age four to six years (or at age eleven to twelve years). These two immunizations usually provide lifetime immunity to rubella. The vaccine can be given to women of childbearing age.

In general, one should avoid the vaccine if he or she has had severe allergic reactions to vaccines or vaccine components, is pregnant (a woman should avoid pregnancy for one to three months after receiving the vaccine), has a weakened immune system, or has a high fever or severe upper respiratory tract infection.

Women who are not sure if they have been vaccinated should be tested. This is especially important if they are in occupations, such as health care, teaching,

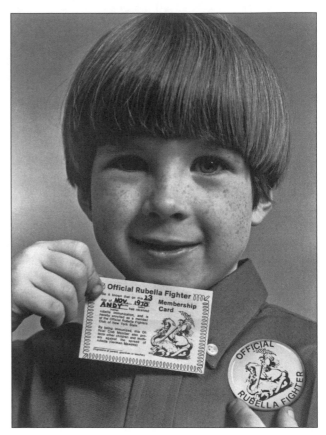

*Rubella immunization programs in the United States in the 1960's and 1970's encouraged children's participation in the campaign with membership cards and buttons.* (CDC)

and child care, with a high risk of exposure to rubella. The vaccine offers most people a lifelong protection against rubella infection.

Immunizations remain the primary method of prevention of rubella. Risks related to taking the vaccine are minor for most people but can be severe for those who have an allergic reaction. Some parents are concerned that immunization with rubella vaccine may be related to autism, but epidemiological studies do not confirm this belief.

*Marylane Wade Koch, M.S.N., R.N.*

### FURTHER READING

Behrman, Richard E., Robert M. Kliegman, and Hal B. Jenson, eds. *Nelson Textbook of Pediatrics.* 18th ed. Philadelphia: Saunders/Elsevier, 2007.

Centers for Disease Control and Prevention. "MMR

Vaccines: What You Need to Know." Available at http://www.cdc.gov/vaccines/pubs/vis/downloads/vis-mmr.pdf.

"Congenital Rubella." *The New York Times* Health Guide. Available at http://health.nytimes.com/health/guides/disease/congenital-rubella/overview.html.

DeStafano, Frank. "Vaccines and Autism: Evidence Does Not Support a Causal Association." *Clinical Pharmacology and Therapeutics* 82, no. 6 (December, 2007): 756-759.

Hawkins, Trisha. *The Need to Know Library: Everything You Need to Know About Measles and Rubella.* New York: Rosen, 2001.

Peter, G., and P. Gardner. "Standards for Immunization Practice for Vaccines in Children and Adults." *Infectious Disease Clinics of North America* 15 (2001): 9-19.

## WEB SITES OF INTEREST

*About Kids Health*
http://www.aboutkidshealth.ca

*American Academy of Pediatrics*
http://www.healthychildren.org

*Centers for Disease Control and Prevention*
http://www.cdc.gov/rubella

*National Foundation for Infectious Diseases*
http://www.nfid.org

*Viral Zone: Rubivirus*
http://www.expasy.org/viralzone/all_by_species/626.html

**See also:** Acne; Airborne illness and disease; Chickenpox; Children and infectious disease; Contagious diseases; Immunity; Immunization; Impetigo; Measles; MMR vaccine; Mononucleosis; Mumps; Pityriasis rosea; Pregnancy and infectious disease; Respiratory route of transmission; Roseola; Scarlet fever; Skin infections; Vaccines: Types; Viral infections.

# S

## Saliva and infectious disease

CATEGORY: Transmission

### DEFINITION

Saliva, a derivative of blood plasma that is necessary for optimal chewing, swallowing, and speaking, can carry microbes such as streptococci, cytomegalovirus, and hepatitis types A, B, and C. Thus, infectious diseases can be transferred from one person to another in saliva.

Saliva normally keeps the tissues of the oral cavity moistened and cleared of food particles. Although saliva is 98 percent water, it also contains mucus, enzymes, electrolytes, and antibacterial agents that keep natural oral flora in check.

### CAUSES

Saliva can spread an infectious disease by many means, including through spit, bites, kisses, sneezes and coughs, and sharing food, beverages, and personal items.

*Spit.* The forcible ejection of saliva is called spitting. A person may spit to remove phlegm, or he or she may spit to show contempt. Depending on weather conditions, spit that lands on a sidewalk, paved street, or other outdoor surface may sustain live pathogens for six to eight hours, creating a public health hazard. Countries such as Australia, Brazil, China, and India have addressed this health issue.

When saliva containing bacteria or viruses makes contact with another person, the microorganisms can enter the recipient's body through wounds in the skin or through the mucous membranes of the mouth, nose, and eyes. Diseases such as tuberculosis, influenza, and hepatitis may be passed this way. To deter spitting and biting and, thus, to reduce the risk of getting infected, police and other law enforcement officers are now placing mesh hoods over the heads of combative detainees, arrestees, and prisoners as protection. Also, contemptuous spitters, in some locales, may face a criminal charge of felonious assault.

*Bites.* When a person's teeth create a wound in another person's skin, the biter's saliva also enters that wound. There are two forms of contact: striking a person with a clenched fist that hits that person's mouth and catches on that person's teeth and biting another person hard enough to break his or her skin and draw blood. Of these wounds, 10 to 15 percent become infected; the pathogens may be aerobic or anaerobic. Diseases that may result from this transference of saliva include tetanus, tuberculosis, syphilis, and hepatitis types B and C.

*Kisses.* Saliva is exchanged during kissing, which can lead to diseases such as infectious mononucleosis and meningococcal disease, both of which are transmitted through the oral mucous membranes.

*Sneezes and coughs.* Droplets of saliva containing influenza virus or other microbes are ejected from a person's mouth during sneezing and coughing. Another person standing within three feet of the sick person is at risk of inhaling these droplets or receiving the spray on the skin. Even if the sick person covers his or her sneeze or cough with his or her hands, the microbe-containing saliva will be transferred to whatever surface is subsequently touched, including door knobs, writing implements, and money. Some kinds of microbes live longer than others on these surfaces and may be picked up by the next person to come in contact. Public health officials urge persons to cover their sneezes and coughs with tissue or with their own elbow.

*Sharing beverages.* Saliva and infectious diseases can be passed by sharing beverages. Bacteria, viruses, and fungi that live in the mucous lining of the mouth, tongue, and throat may be shed in saliva that is washed back into a beverage after drinking, thus contaminating it for the next drinker. For this reason, beverages that come in containers should be poured into individual cups or glasses when serving more than one person.

*Sharing food.* The microorganisms in saliva may contaminate food if a utensil or piece of food (such as a carrot stick or potato chip) that has had contact with saliva or has been in the mouth is returned to a shared food supply, such as a container of dip. For this reason, one should use a spoon to place dip or sauce onto a plate for personal consumption and should not eat from a shared serving utensil.

Alaskan Natives have a cultural practice of chewing solid foods before feeding them to infants, incidentally transmitting cavity-causing bacteria and other oral pathogens to infants. To prevent the transmission of disease-causing bacteria and other pathogens, one should use a chlorhexidine mouthwash before each feeding.

*Sharing personal items.* Saliva is left behind on items such as eating utensils, toothbrushes, drinking glasses, and oral thermometers. When these items are put into another person's mouth without cleaning, the pathogens in the saliva may be transferred. Dental caries, or cavities, and other microbes may be transmitted from an adult to a child when the adult puts a pacifier in his or her mouth to clean or moisten it before giving it to the child.

## IMPACT

Saliva has important physiological functions, including the cleansing, moisturizing, and buffering of mucous membranes in the mouth, pharynx, and esophagus. The measurement of enzyme levels in saliva is the basis of new diagnostic tools for many diseases, including type 2 diabetes and hormone deficiencies. However, one milliliter of saliva may contain 100 billion microorganisms of 190 different types. Researchers are studying the addition of antimicrobial agents to toothpastes, mouthwashes, and artificial saliva solutions to determine their protective effects in the mouth and rest of the body. They are also studying the preventive effects of these agents in the propagation of microbes and infectious diseases.

*Bethany Thivierge, M.P.H.*

## FURTHER READING

Gorbach, Sherwood L., John G. Bartlett, and Neil R. Blacklow, eds. *Infectious Diseases.* 3d ed. Philadelphia: W. B. Saunders, 2004. A thorough discussion of infectious diseases. Includes a brief history, an account of the mechanisms of disease, and a concise discussion of a broad range of infectious agents.

Mandell, Gerald L., John E. Bennett, and Raphael Dolin, eds. *Mandell, Douglas, and Bennett's Principles and Practice of Infectious Diseases.* 7th ed. New York: Churchill Livingstone/Elsevier, 2010. A complete and practical reference book with a worldwide per-

spective and information about new and emerging infectious diseases.

Pretty, Iain, et al. "Human Bites and the Risk of Human Immunodeficiency Virus Transmission." *American Journal of Forensic and Medical Pathology* 20, no. 3 (1999): 232-239. A literature review of articles examining HIV in saliva and its transmission via human bites. Includes an evaluation of the risk of infection and seroconversion for those who have been bitten.

Tenovuo, Jorma. "Antimicrobial Agents in Saliva: Protection for the Whole Body." *Journal of Dental Research* 81, no. 12 (2002): 807-809. An extensive literature review that identifies the antimicrobial agents in saliva and discusses their clinical implications.

## WEB SITES OF INTEREST

*American Dental Association*
http://www.ada.org

*American Medical Association*
http://www.ama.org

*Centers for Disease Control and Prevention*
http://www.cdc.gov

*National Institute of Dental and Craniofacial Research*
http://www.nidcr.nih.gov

**See also:** Arthropod-borne illness and disease; Cat scratch fever; Cytomegalovirus infection; *Eikenella* infections; Epstein-Barr virus infection; Food-borne illness and disease; Hepatitis A; Hepatitis B; Hepatitis C; Herpesviridae; Horizontal disease transmission; Mononucleosis; Mouth infections; Oral transmission; Rat-bite fever; Respiratory route of transmission; Sexually transmitted diseases (STDs); *Streptococcus*; Transmission routes.

---

# *Salmonella*

CATEGORY: Pathogen
TRANSMISSION ROUTE: Direct contact, ingestion

## DEFINITION

*Salmonella* are gram-negative, motile, non-spore-forming, nonencapsulated, facultative-anaerobic rods that cause several diseases, primarily enteric (intestinal), in humans and other animals.

## Tips for Consumers of Eggs and Egg Products

- Avoid eating recalled eggs or products containing recalled eggs. Recalled eggs might still be in grocery stores, restaurants, and homes. Consumers who have recalled eggs should discard them or return them to their retailer for a refund. Persons who think they might have become ill from eating recalled eggs should consult their health care providers.

- Keep shell eggs refrigerated at or below 45° Fahrenheit (at or below 7° Celsius) at all times.

- Discard cracked or dirty eggs.

- Wash hands, cooking utensils, and food preparation surfaces with soap and water after contact with raw eggs.

- Eggs should be cooked until both the white and the yolk are firm and should be eaten promptly after cooking.

- Avoid keeping eggs warm or at room temperature for more than two hours.

- Refrigerate unused or leftover egg-containing foods promptly.

- Avoid eating raw eggs.

- Avoid restaurant dishes made with raw or undercooked, unpasteurized eggs. Restaurants should use pasteurized eggs in any recipe (such as hollandaise sauce or caesar salad dressing) that calls for raw eggs.

- Consumption of raw or undercooked eggs should be avoided, especially by young children, elderly persons, and persons with weakened immune systems or with debilitating illness.

*Source:* U.S. Food and Drug Administration

## NATURAL HABITAT AND FEATURES

The genus *Salmonella* was named for Daniel E. Salmon, an American veterinary pathologist and bacteriologist. The type strain, originally named *S. choleraesuis*, was discovered by Salmon's research associate, Theobald Smith. The genus is closely related to *Escherichia coli* (*E. coli*) and was initially subdivided into hundreds of species named for the diseases it caused and for the host organism: for example, *S. typhi* (typhoid fever), *S. enteritidis* (gastroenteritis), *S. typhimurium* (mouse typhoid), and *S. choleraesuis* (hog cholera).

After further genetic testing and after scientists determined that most *Salmonella* spp. are not very host specific, most of the original species were combined into a single species, *S. enterica*. This species was then divided into five subspecies and more than two thousand strains or serovars; for example, *S. enterica* subsp. *enterica serovar Typhi* has replaced *S. typhi*, *S. enterica* subsp. *enterica serovar Enteritidis* has replaced *S. enteritidis*, and *S. enterica* subsp. *arizonae* has replaced *S. arizonae*. Only *S. bongori* was deemed distinct enough to stand alone as a different species. The older designations are still frequently used in both professional journals and the popular press.

## PATHOGENICITY AND CLINICAL SIGNIFICANCE

Of the hundreds of *Salmonella* strains, fewer than twenty cause human disease. *S. enterica* subsp. *enterica* contains the majority of disease-causing strains. Salmonellosis is the second most common cause of gastroenteritis, surpassed only by *Campylobacter* spp. infections. Infections caused by *Salmonella* spp. are considered zoonotic because many strains of this bacterium can be transferred from humans to animals and from animals to humans.

Most cases of salmonellosis are the result of fecal to oral contamination caused by ingestion of fecal-contaminated food. Because *Salmonella* spp. are so widespread and can survive several weeks in water or on vegetation and more than two years in soil, transmission is relatively easy. For example, during butchering and processing, raw meats can become contaminated with the intestinal contents of the butchered animals. Shellfish are easily contaminated when raw sewage makes its way into aquatic habitats. An infected chicken can deposit *Salmonella* into her eggs before shell deposition or on the shell as the egg is laid. Irrigating or washing crop plants in water contaminated by *Salmonella* can contaminate the crops. Food preparers with poor hygiene can also contaminate food.

In addition to food contamination, pets, especially birds, reptiles, and amphibians, can harbor *Salmonella*, which can easily be transferred from their cloacae to their feathers or skin.

The best way to prevent salmonellosis is to always wash one's hands after using the toilet, handling raw meat, cleaning up feces, and handling a bird, reptile,

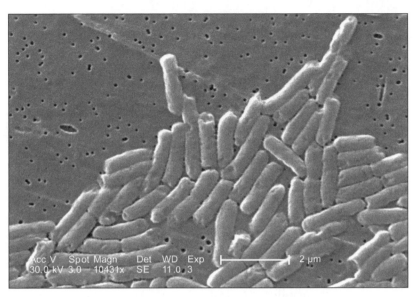

*A micrograph of a colony of* Salmonella *bacteria.* (CDC)

fever, headache, rose-colored spots on the upper chest, and organ inflammation. Humans heterozygous for cystic fibrosis may have lowered susceptibility to typhoid fever because the changes in the cell membrane of heterozygotes decrease the likelihood of bacterial invasion.

Fewer than four hundred cases of typhoid fever occur in the United States each year, and most of these cases are contracted outside the country. In the developing world, nearly 22 million cases of typhoid are seen each year and lead to more than 6 million deaths. Most of these deaths are caused by dehydration, so rehydration therapy is critical in treating this or any other salmonellosis.

or amphibian. In addition, cooking all food to an internal temperature of 167° Fahrenheit (75° Celsius) and boiling water for a minimum of one minute kills *Salmonella*. Freezing, however, will usually not kill all *Salmonella* in contaminated food or water. Cutting boards used for raw meat should also be cleaned thoroughly, preferably with bleach.

In humans, the most serious salmonellosis is typhoid fever caused by *S. enterica* sub. *enterica serovar Typhi*, also called *S. typhi*. This bacterium is highly adaptable and can produce stress-related proteins that allow the bacterium to survive better under environmental stresses (such as increased temperatures, acidic conditions, and the presence of antibiotics). Unlike many *Salmonella* strains, this bacterium has only one animal reservoir: humans. It is usually transmitted through contaminated water and undercooked, contaminated food. Because of this, it causes most problems in developing countries with poor sanitation.

*S. typhi* can also be transmitted by food-service workers who were previously infected. About 5 percent of all persons who had typhoid fever retain infective bacteria and can pass these along. In the United States, food service workers who have had typhoid fever are required to be free of the typhoid bacterium (as measured by fecal swabs) before they can return to work.

Diarrhea is the most common symptom of salmonellosis, but bacteria can enter the intestinal epithelium and migrate to other areas of the body, causing

## DRUG SUSCEPTIBILITY

Bacterial strains resistant to ampicillin, chloramphenicol, trimethoprim/sulfamethoxazole, and streptomycin are so common that these antibiotics are no longer used. Ciprofloxacin is the drug of choice, but strains resistant to it are on the rise. Cephtriaxone and cephotaxime are being used more often, especially in areas with multiple resistance. Both oral and injectable vaccines are available, but these are only 50 to 70 percent effective. A very similar, but less common disease is paratyphoid fever, which is caused by the Paratyphoid serovar.

*S. enterica serovar Enteritidis* is the most frequent cause of *Salmonella* gastroenteritis in humans. Many other serovars can also cause gastroenteritis. The most common symptoms are diarrhea, abdominal cramps, and nausea. Unlike typhoid fever, gastroenteritis in healthy persons rarely lasts more than one week, although in rare cases it can become systemic. It is usually treated with rehydration therapy and is not always treated with antibiotics unless it is severe.

*Richard W. Cheney, Jr., Ph.D.*

## FURTHER READING

Braden, Christopher R. "*Salmonella enterica* Serotype *Enteritidis* and Eggs: A National Epidemic in the United States." *Clinical Infectious Diseases* 43 (2006): 512-517. Discusses the increase in *Enteritidis* outbreaks in the United States since the 1970's and the deposition of *Salmonella* in the eggs while still in the ovary.

Garrity, George M., ed. *The Proteobacteria*. Vol. 2 in *Bergey's Manual of Systematic Bacteriology*. 2d ed. New York: Springer, 2005. This volume describes the proteobacteria in detail.

Madigan, Michael T., and John M. Martinko. *Brock Biology of Microorganisms*. 12th ed. Upper Saddle River, N.J.: Pearson/Prentice Hall, 2010. This text outlines many common bacteria and describes their natural history, pathogenicity, and other characteristics.

Romich, Janet A. *Understanding Zoonotic Diseases*. Clifton Park, N.Y.: Thomson Delmar Learning, 2008. This book has a good section on salmonellosis and its causes and treatments.

## WEB SITES OF INTEREST

*Canadian Partnership for Consumer Food Safety Education*
http://www.canfightbac.org

*Centers for Disease Control and Prevention, Division of Foodborne, Bacterial, and Mycotic Diseases*
http://www.cdc.gov/nczved/divisions/dfbmd

*U.S. Department of Agriculture, Food Safety Information Center*
http://foodsafety.nal.usda.gov

**See also:** Amebic dysentery; Bacteria: Classification and types; *Enterobacter*; *Escherichia*; Fecal-oral route of transmission; Food-borne illness and disease; Intestinal and stomach infections; Microbiology; Pathogens; Salmonellosis; *Shigella*; Travelers' diarrhea; Waterborne illness and disease.

---

# Salmonellosis

CATEGORY: Diseases and conditions
ANATOMY OR SYSTEM AFFECTED: All
ALSO KNOWN AS: Enteric fever, paratyphoid fever, salmonella enterocolitis, salmonella food poisoning, salmonella gastroenteritis, typhoid fever

## DEFINITION

Salmonellosis is an infection caused by the *Salmonella* genus of the bacterial family Enterobacteriaceae. Acute gastroenteritis is the most common form of sal-

---

**Taxonomic Classification
for *Salmonella***

**Kingdom:** Bacteria
**Phylum:** Proteobacteria
**Class:** Gammaproteobacteria
**Order:** Enterobacteriales
**Family:** Enterobacteriaceae
**Genus:** *Salmonella*
**Species:**
*S. bongori*
*S. enterica*

---

monellosis. Other clinical manifestations of salmonellosis include enteric fever and bacteremia. Hematogenous seeding of other organs may lead to secondary manifestations of salmonellosis, including endocarditis, pneumonia, pyelonephritis, septic arthritis, and osteomyelitis.

## CAUSES

*Salmonella* bacteria live in the intestinal tracts of humans and of a variety of wild and domestic animals throughout the world. Poultry, cattle, dairy cows, pigs, sheep, goats, and other agricultural livestock commonly carry *Salmonella*. Pet birds, lizards, turtles, iguanas, dogs, and cats may also carry disease-causing *Salmonella* species. Bacteria pass in the feces of infected animals. Fecal contamination of food or water, unsanitary food-handling practices, and infection of egg-laying hens can lead to salmonellosis.

In the developing world, lack of sewage systems, inadequate water treatment, and inconsistent or inadequate sanitation practices may lead to *Salmonella* contamination of drinking water or agricultural fields. Most salmonellosis outbreaks involve acute gastroenteritis, although typhoid fever remains a significant health threat in impoverished parts of the world, including areas of Asia, Africa, Central America, and South America. *S. enterica* sub. *enterica serovar* Typhi (or *S. typhi*) and *S. enterica* sub. *enterica serovar* Paratyphi (or *S. paratyphi*), the causative agents of typhoid and paratyphoid fever, respectively, live exclusively in the human intestine. These illnesses pass from one person to another through human fecal contamination of foodstuffs. *S. typhi* carriers can cause community outbreaks, as in the infamous case of Typhoid Mary in New York City in the early twentieth century.

Infection of egg-laying hens is a common cause of

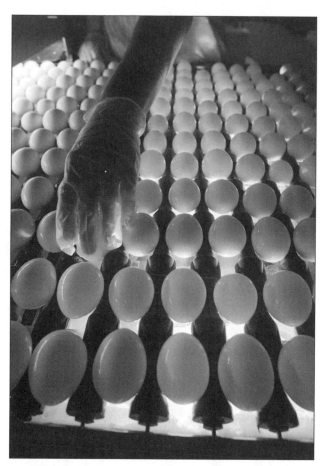

*A U.S. Department of Agriculture inspector checks eggs at an egg farm in Maine, following allegations the eggs may have been contaminated with* Salmonella. *(AP/Wide World Photos)*

salmonellosis outbreaks. The bacteria infect the ovaries of hens, contaminating the eggs before shell formation. Infected hens commonly appear healthy, complicating detection of *Salmonella*-contaminated eggs. Breaks in sanitation or hygiene protocols during food cultivation, processing, and packaging can also lead to salmonellosis outbreaks.

### RISK FACTORS

Ingestion of raw or undercooked eggs is a significant risk factor for eggborne salmonellosis. Unpasteurized milk can also transmit *Salmonella*. Inadequate handwashing and cross-contamination between meats and uncooked produce during food preparation can potentially lead to salmonellosis.

Because livestock and pets may carry *Salmonella* bacteria, the failure to wear gloves or thoroughly wash the hands after handling animals or their feces is a risk factor for salmonellosis. Cattle, dairy cows, poultry, turtles, lizards, and snakes are common sources of infection.

Young children, persons with human immunodeficiency virus infection or acquired immunodeficiency syndrome, organ transplant recipients, and those undergoing cancer treatments have an increased risk for salmonellosis because of their immature or weakened immune systems.

### SYMPTOMS

*Salmonella* gastroenteritis symptoms begin twelve to seventy-two hours after ingestion of water or food and include nausea, vomiting, diarrhea, and abdominal cramps, which may be accompanied by a fever of 100° to 102° Fahrenheit (38° to 39° Celsius), chills, and headache. Fever typically resolves within two to three days; gastrointestinal symptoms usually abate within seven days. Immunocompromised persons may develop severe symptoms, bacteremia, and dehydration.

Symptoms of typhoid and paratyphoid fever develop more gradually than those associated with salmonella gastroenteritis. Approximately six to thirty days after infection, a low-grade fever, headache, anorexia, fatigue, and abdominal pain develop, typically accompanied by constipation or diarrhea. Symptoms intensify over three to four days, with fevers typically reaching 101° to 104° F (38.5° to 40° C). Some persons will develop a maculopapular, rose-colored rash on the trunk. Although uncommon, persons with enteric fever may develop neuropsychiatric symptoms, including lethargy, confusion, frank delirium, seizures, and coma.

### SCREENING AND DIAGNOSIS

Routine screening is not conducted for salmonellosis, except in outbreak situations wherein carrier identification becomes critical. Isolation of *Salmonella* from body tissues, fluids, or excretions remains the cornerstone of diagnosis. For acute gastroenteritis, diagnosis is confirmed by isolation of *Salmonella* from the stool. In persons with bacteremia, isolation of *Salmonella* from the blood confirms the diagnosis.

Definitive diagnosis of enteric fever is often challenging because of the limited sensitivity of blood and stool cultures with this form of salmonellosis. Isolation of *S. typhi* or *S. paratyphi* from the blood, stool, bone marrow, intestinal secretions, urine, or secondary infection sites confirms the diagnosis; bone marrow cultures are the most sensitive. Serologic tests for antibodies to *S. typhi* antigens may also aid in the diagnosis of typhoid fever. Polymerase chain reaction testing for *Salmonella* is used in some locales.

## TREATMENT AND THERAPY

In an otherwise healthy person, nontyphoidal, gastrointestinal salmonellosis is typically a self-limited illness, resolving spontaneously without antibiotic therapy. Oral or intravenous fluid replacement may be necessary for persons with severe symptoms. Antibiotic therapy is commonly prescribed for immunocompromised persons with gastrointestinal salmonellosis and for those who are otherwise at high risk for complications. Salmonella bacteremia and enteric fever are treated with antibiotic therapy, commonly a fluoroquinolone or a third-generation cephalosporin.

## PREVENTION AND OUTCOMES

Proper food handling and handwashing are key to preventing gastrointestinal salmonellosis. One should wash hands with soap and running water before and after handling food, especially raw meats. Thoroughly cooking meat and eggs kills *Salmonella* contaminants that may be present. Handwashing after using the toilet, changing diapers, and handling animals also helps prevent salmonellosis.

The Centers for Disease Control and Prevention recommends typhoid immunization for travelers visiting areas with a high incidence of *S. typhi*. Oral and intramuscular vaccines effectively protect approximately 50 to 80 percent of persons immunized against typhoid fever.

*Tina M. St. John, M.D.*

## FURTHER READING

Fischer Walker, Christa L., David Sack, and Robert E. Black. "Etiology of Diarrhea in Older Children, Adolescents, and Adults." *PLoS Neglected Tropical Diseases* 4 (2010): e768. Systematic review of twenty-two studies from around the world, examining the causative agents of infectious diarrhea and demonstrating the ongoing, high incidence of salmonellosis in community settings.

Pegues, David A., and Samuel I. Miller. "*Salmonella* Species, Including *Salmonella typhi*." In *Mandell, Douglas,*

*and Bennett's Principles and Practice of Infectious Diseases*, edited by Gerald L. Mandell, John F. Bennett, and Raphael Dolin. 7th ed. New York: Churchill Livingstone/Elsevier, 2010. Infectious disease text with referenced discussion of salmonellosis epidemiology, microbiology, pathogenesis, treatment, and prevention.

Thaver, Durrane, et al. "A Comparison of Fluoroquinolones Versus Other Antibiotics for Treating Enteric Fever." *British Medical Journal* 338 (2009): b1865. Meta-analysis of twenty randomized, controlled trials examining clinical and microbiological failures and relapse rates associated with antibiotics for the treatment of enteric fever.

## WEB SITES OF INTEREST

*Centers for Disease Control and Prevention*
http://www.cdc.gov/salmonella

*PathoSystems Resource Integration Center*
http://www.patricbrc.org

*U.S. Department of Agriculture, Food Safety Information Center*
http://foodsafety.nal.usda.gov

**See also:** Birds and infectious disease; Cats and infectious disease; Dogs and infectious disease; *Escherichia*; Fecal-oral route of transmission; Food-borne illness and disease; Intestinal and stomach infections; *Salmonella*; Typhoid fever; Waterborne illness and disease; *Yersinia*; Yersiniosis; Zoonotic diseases.

---

Sanitizers. *See* Disinfectants and sanitizers.

---

# Sarcoidosis

CATEGORY: Diseases and conditions
ANATOMY OR SYSTEM AFFECTED: Immune system, lungs, lymph nodes, respiratory system, skin

## DEFINITION

Sarcoidosis is a rare inflammatory disease characterized by the formation of granulomas (small, abnormal clumps of immune cells) in different parts of the body, most commonly the lungs, skin, eyes, liver, and lymph nodes.

Sarcoidosis is classified into five stages, generally based on the level of disease in the lungs. Stages progress from stage 0, in which the person has a normal chest X ray, to stage 4, which features the scarring of lung tissue, or pulmonary fibrosis.

### CAUSES

The cause of sarcoidosis is not known. It is thought to result from an abnormal immune response to bacteria or viruses or to be genetic. An environmental factor, such as a drug or an airborne pathogen, may trigger the disease.

### RISK FACTORS

Sarcoidosis occurs most often at age twenty-five to forty, but can occur at any age. Men and blacks are at higher risk than are women and Caucasians. Sarcoidosis is most commonly reported in people of Asian, German, Irish, Puerto Rican, and Scandinavian origin, indicating an ethnic or geographic component.

### SYMPTOMS

The severity of the disease varies and ranges from mild with no symptoms to severe with lasting organ damage. Symptoms can develop gradually and last many years, or they can appear suddenly and disappear just as quickly. Typical symptoms include a persistent cough; shortness of breath; a vague feeling of fatigue and general unwellness; a fever; weight loss; small red bumps on the face, arms, or buttocks; red watery eyes; and arthritis in the ankles, elbows, wrists, and hands.

If left untreated, sarcoidosis can lead to pulmonary fibrosis, eye disease, skin disease, and problems of the nervous system, heart (arrhythmia or cardiomyopathy), and liver.

### SCREENING AND DIAGNOSIS

The symptoms of sarcoidosis often mimic other diseases. Thus, diagnosis is often made by ruling out diseases with similar features, diseases such as lymphoma, tuberculosis, rheumatoid arthritis, rheumatic fever, and fungal infections.

To diagnose and determine the severity of the disease, the following tests may be performed: physical exam, chest X ray, lung function tests, blood tests (to look for abnormal liver function, elevated calcium in the blood, and elevated levels of angiotensin-converting enzyme), bronchoscopy, biopsy, mediastinoscopy (a biopsy of mediastinum lymph nodes), slit-lamp examination (to look for eye damage using a high-intensity lamp), and an electrocardiogram.

### TREATMENT AND THERAPY

Mild sarcoidosis may not require treatment. For more severe cases, therapy is aimed at reducing inflammation, preventing fibrosis, and decreasing symptoms. Corticosteroids (an anti-inflammatory drug) are generally preferred for treatment. Alternate treatments that also suppress the immune system include methotrexate and azathioprine (Imuran). Hydroxychloroquine (Plaquenil) may be beneficial for skin diseases, nervous system involvement, and elevated blood-calcium levels. For the majority of cases, sarcoidosis goes into remission within three years of diagnosis and in less than five years in most other cases.

### PREVENTION AND OUTCOMES

Because the cause of sarcoidosis is not known, there are no recommendations for prevention. However, to reduce the risk of symptoms, one should protect his or her lungs (by, for example, not smoking).

*Anita P. Kuan, Ph.D.*

### FURTHER READING

Barr, Gilbert. *Living with Sarcoidosis and Other Chronic Health Conditions.* Bloomington, Ind.: iUniverse, 2004.

Bowers, B., S. Hasni, and B. L. Gruber. "Sarcoidosis in World Trade Center Rescue Workers Presenting with Rheumatologic Manifestations." *Journal of Clinical Rheumatology* 16, no. 1 (January, 2010): 26-27.

Boyer, Thomas D., Teresa L. Wright, and Michael P. Manns, eds. *Zakim and Boyer's Hepatology: A Textbook of Liver Disease.* 5th ed. Philadelphia: Saunders/Elsevier, 2006.

National Library of Medicine. "Sarcoidosis." Available at http://www.nlm.nih.gov/medlineplus/sarcoidosis.html.

Nunes, H. "Sarcoidosis." *Orphanet Journal of Rare Diseases* 2 (November 19, 2007): 46.

Parker, James N., and Philip M. Parker. *The Official Patient's Sourcebook on Sarcoidosis.* San Diego, Calif.: ICON Health, 2002.

**See also:** Allergic bronchopulmonary aspergillosis; Erythema nodosum; Herpesvirus infections; Mold infections; Mycetoma; Mycoses; Skin infections.

# Sarcosporidiosis

CATEGORY: Diseases and conditions
ANATOMY OR SYSTEM AFFECTED: Gastrointestinal system, intestines, muscles, musculoskeletal system
ALSO KNOWN AS: Sarcocystosis

## DEFINITION

Sarcosporidiosis is a rare intestinal or muscular infection caused by various species of the genus *Sarcocystis*, an intracellular protozoan parasite that infects humans and, mostly, nonhuman animals. Humans may (rarely) serve as intermediate hosts or (accidentally) as definitive hosts for various *Sarcocystis* species that have an obligatory two-host life cycle.

## CAUSES

There are more than one hundred species of *Sarcocystis*, and they have worldwide distribution. The most common species that cause sarcosporidiosis in humans include *S. bovihominis* and *S. suihominis*. Humans acquire intestinal sarcosporidiosis after eating raw or undercooked beef and pork that contain mature sarcocysts. The ingested infective sporozoites replicate and discharge in the stool as sporocysts. Once shed, sporocysts are typically ingested by an intermediate host (usually a cow or pig). Muscular sarcocystosis is probably caused by ingestion of sporocysts excreted by various definitive hosts.

## RISK FACTORS

At increased risk of infection are persons who ingest undercooked beef or pork and persons who practice poor hand-hygiene (and, thus, increase their risk of exposure to the bacteria). Human sarcosporidiosis is distributed worldwide, but most cases have been documented in Southeast Asia. Fewer than one hundred cases have been reported.

## SYMPTOMS

Infection with *Sarcocystis* in healthy persons causes intestinal or muscular sarcosporidiosis (based on whether the person is serving as a definitive or intermediate host). Intestinal sarcosporidiosis most commonly manifests with nausea, abdominal pain, diarrhea, and generalized myalgia. Serious complications are rare and may include dehydration, eosinophilic enteritis, and ulcerative obstructive entercolitis. Intestinal sarcosporidiosis is transient and usually self-limited. Muscular sarcosporidiosis is mostly asymptomatic and found incidentally, though painful muscle swellings, generalized muscle weakness, fever, myositis (that may persist for many years), vasculitis, or periarteritis are possible.

## SCREENING AND DIAGNOSIS

Intestinal sarcosporidiosis can be diagnosed in the lamina propria of the small bowel and by fecal examination. Oocysts with two sporocysts or individual sporocysts in human feces are diagnostic for intestinal infection. Muscular sarcosporidiosis is diagnosed by microscopic examination of muscle biopsies.

## TREATMENT AND THERAPY

Specific antiparasitic therapy for intestinal sarcosporidiosis is not indicated, as the infection in humans represents the fully formed terminal stage of the parasite. In muscular sarcosporidiosis, metronidazole and cotrimoxazole (antibacterial and antiprotozoal drugs) can be used. Corticosteroids can be used to reduce inflammation associated with muscular involvement. Persons with intestinal sarcosporidiosis will need a six-month follow-up after infection that includes testing to document the clearance of the sarcocyst from the stool.

## PREVENTION AND OUTCOMES

Prevention of the disease in humans consists of avoiding the consumption of raw or undercooked beef and pork. Because sarcocysts can be found in a large percentage of the world's beef cows, and to a lesser extent in pigs, camels, sheep, horses, and other domesticated animals, all associated meat products should be properly cooked or frozen before consumption. Also, one can prevent infestation in domesticated animals by feeding them deep-frozen or processed meat products only. A person can destroy sarcocysts by cooking meat at 158° Fahrenheit (70° Celsius) for fifteen minutes, by freezing meat at 25° F (–4° C) for two days, or by freezing meat at –4° F (–20° C) for one day.

*Katia Marazova, M.D., Ph.D.*

## FURTHER READING

Fayer, Ronald. "*Sarcocystis* spp. in Human Infections." *Clinical Microbiology Reviews* 17 (October 2004): 894-902.

Ondrasik, Nicholas R., Gunther Hsue, and Raphael J Kiel. "Sarcosporidiosis." Available at http://emedicine.medscape.com/article/228279-overview.

Velásquez, J.N., et al. "Systemic Sarcocystosis in a Patient with Acquired Immune Deficiency Syndrome." *Human Pathology* 39 (2008): 1263-1267.

## WEB SITES OF INTEREST

*Center for Food Security and Public Health*
http://www.cfsph.iastate.edu/factsheets/pdfs/sarcocystosis.pdf

*Microbiology and Immunology On-line: Parasitology*
http://pathmicro.med.sc.edu/book/parasit-sta.htm

**See also:** Diagnosis of protozoan diseases; Food-borne illness and disease; Immune response to protozoan diseases; Intestinal and stomach infections; Myositis; Parasites: Classification and types; Parasitic diseases; Pathogens; Prevention of protozoan diseases; Protozoa: Structure and growth; Protozoan diseases.

---

# SARS

CATEGORY: Diseases and conditions
ANATOMY OR SYSTEM AFFECTED: Lungs, respiratory system
ALSO KNOWN AS: Severe acute respiratory syndrome

## DEFINITION

SARS, or severe acute respiratory syndrome, is a highly contagious, life-threatening respiratory disease caused by a coronavirus (known as SARS-CoV). Coronavirus is in the same family that contains the influenza virus. SARS is associated with flulike symptoms that progress to pneumonia and can lead to respiratory failure and death. SARS is believed to have originated in Guangdong Province in southern China. It is spread by close person-to-person contact.

## CAUSES

SARS is caused by a strain of the same virus that causes the common cold. Previous to the outbreak of the SARS pandemic in early 2003, influenza virus was not serious or fatal in humans. It is believed that the specific strain of virus responsible for the SARS outbreak originated from one or more animal viruses and evolved into a completely new strain. SARS is mainly spread through direct contact with infected persons and is transmitted by airborne droplets produced when an infected person sneezes or coughs. Contaminated droplets can also land on various surfaces and objects. Therefore, SARS can also be spread by contact with contaminated objects.

## RISK FACTORS

The greatest risk for infection with SARS-CoV is direct, close contact with another infected person, especially in close quarters such as airplanes or trains. People of Southeast Asian descent who possess a particular genetic variation in an immune system gene have a greater risk of developing SARS. This gene variation is rare in other populations. Unprotected health care workers are at significant risk of infection.

## SYMPTOMS

Symptoms of SARS are like those of the common cold or flu. They include fever, muscle aches, headache, fatigue, decreased appetite, diarrhea, a dry cough, shortness of breath, runny nose, and sore throat. Pneumonia, which can develop within a few days, can lead to respiratory failure and death.

## SCREENING AND DIAGNOSIS

SARS is difficult to diagnose, especially in its early stages because the symptoms are like those of colds, the flu, and pneumonia. Suspicion of SARS can be confirmed with specific laboratory tests to detect SARS antibodies or with deoxyribonucleic acid (DNA) tests to isolate the presence of viral DNA in secretions. These tests, however, are not standardized,

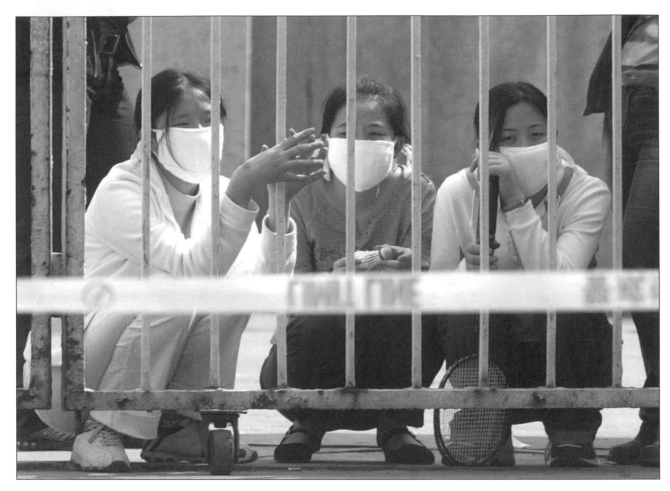

*Three women are quarantined at a hospital in Beijing, China, during the SARS outbreak of 2003.* (AP/Wide World Photos)

nor are they rapid enough to be used for diagnosis. Without laboratory confirmation, the diagnosis of SARS is based on clinical evaluation of atypical pneumonia and a history of exposure to the SARS virus. Detection of other agents that cause atypical pneumonia or influenza can be useful in ruling out SARS, but the possibility of dual infection still exists. X ray of the lungs and a pulse oximetry, to test oxygen levels in the blood, are useful to monitor lung involvement.

### TREATMENT AND THERAPY

If SARS is suspected, the infected person should be isolated and put on mechanical ventilation. There is no effective treatment for SARS. In some clinical studies, serious complications and death from SARS have been prevented by a combination of antiviral drugs normally used to treat acquired immunodefi-

ciency syndrome (AIDS). Antibiotics have no effect on coronavirus. A protein isolated from red algae was shown to have antiviral activity against the SARS-CoV in mice.

### PREVENTION AND OUTCOMES

The World Health Organization and the Centers for Disease Control and Prevention offer prevention guidelines for stopping the spread of SARS. These guidelines include the following: staying home and avoiding public places for a minimum of ten days after the associated fever has ended and the respiratory symptoms have begun to improve; general hygiene including washing hands frequently with soap and water and using hand sanitizers; using disposable gloves and face masks when coming in contact with an infected person or contaminated fluids; covering one's nose and mouth when sneezing or coughing; not sharing bedding, towels, and eating utensils and washing those items thoroughly; and using household disinfectant on any surface (such as doorknobs, counter tops, and light switches) thought to be contaminated.

*Joan Letizia, Ph.D.*

### FURTHER READING

Fowler, R. A., et al. "Critically Ill Patients with Severe Acute Respiratory Syndrome." *Journal of the American Medical Association* 290 (2003): 367-373.

Johnston, Robert. "A Candidate Vaccine for Severe Acute Respiratory Syndrome." *New England Journal of Medicine* 351 (2004): 827-828.

Joseph, S. M., et al. "The Severe Acute Respiratory Syndrome." *New England Journal of Medicine* 349 (2003): 2431-2441.

Kamps, Bernd Sebastian, and Christian Hoffmann, eds. *SARS Reference*. Available at http://sarsreference.com/sarsref/treat.htm.

Kleinman, Arthur, and James L. Watson, eds. *SARS in China: Prelude to Pandemic?* Stanford, Calif.: Stanford University Press, 2006.

Peiris, M., et al., eds. *Severe Acute Respiratory Syndrome.* Malden, Mass.: Blackwell, 2005.

Yang, Z. Y., et al. "A DNA Vaccine Induces SARS Coronavirus Neutralization and Protective Immunity in Mice." *Nature* 428 (2004): 561-564.

### WEB SITES OF INTEREST

*American Lung Association*
http://www.lungusa.org

*American Public Health Association*
http://www.apha.org

*Centers for Disease Control and Prevention*
http://www.cdc.gov/ncidod/sars

*World Health Organization*
http://www.who.int/csr/resources/publications/sarsnewguidance

**See also:** Airborne illness and disease; Anthrax; Atypical pneumonia; Contagious diseases; Coronaviridae; Coronavirus infections; Epidemics and pandemics: History; Outbreaks; Pneumonia; Public health; Respiratory route of transmission; Respiratory syncytial virus infections; Viral infections.

# Scabies

CATEGORY: Diseases and conditions
ANATOMY OR SYSTEM AFFECTED: Skin
ALSO KNOWN AS: The itch

### DEFINITION

Scabies is an infestation of the skin. It is most commonly caused by a tiny mite.

### CAUSES

An infestation results when a female mite burrows into a person's skin and lays its eggs. The scabies mite does not suck blood, and it does not transmit any disease between people other than scabies.

Scabies is highly contagious. Most often, it is passed from person to person through close and generally prolonged physical contact, including sexual contact. Scabies can also spread by persons who share clothing, towels, and bedding. Scabies can occasionally also be acquired from certain mammals. It is most common in dogs with sarcoptic mange. Scabies from dogs differs somewhat from human scabies and rarely passes from person to person.

### RISK FACTORS

Factors that increase the chance of getting scabies include sexual contact with new or multiple partners; close, physical contact with a person who has scabies; living in close quarters with others (such as in a nursing home or in military barracks); a weakened immune system; and close contact with animal scabies. At higher risk are children younger than age fifteen years and adults older than age sixty-five years.

### SYMPTOMS

Symptoms of scabies include intense itching, usually worse at night, and small red bumps, pimples, or lines on the skin. In more severe cases, the infested area may appear crusty and may become infected and discharge pus.

Scabies rarely affects the face or head. Any body area, or even the whole body, may be involved, but areas most often affected include the hands, especially between the fingers; wrists and elbows; feet; genitals and pubic area (especially in men); buttocks; around the nipples (especially in women); waistline; belly-button and lower abdomen; areas where clothing is tight; and under rings, watches, or jewelry.

### SCREENING AND DIAGNOSIS

A doctor will ask about symptoms and medical history and will perform a physical exam. Scabies can often be diagnosed based on these steps, but the doctor might scrape off some skin to be examined under a microscope to confirm the diagnosis.

### TREATMENT AND THERAPY

One should first remove scabies from the living environment to avoid reinfestation after treatment. It is recommended that all bedding and clothing be thoroughly laundered. Also, other members of one's household or institution should be treated for scabies.

Scabies is usually treated by applying permethrin cream 5 percent. It is applied to the skin from the neck down. The cream is left on the skin for eight to twelve hours. Excessive use of this medication can be harmful. One should carefully read and follow the directions and should not repeat treatments unless instructed to do so by a doctor. If new, itchy bumps continue to appear in the days following treatment, one should alert the doctor.

It may take several weeks for itching to disappear following successful treatment. Itching can be temporarily relieved with antihistamine, corticosteroid cream (such as Lotrisone), antihistamines, and corticosteroids. Some severe cases may respond poorly to other treatments. In this case, an oral medication called ivermectin (Stromectol) is sometimes prescribed. It is given as a single dose. Alternative topical creams include crotamiton 10 percent (Eurax) and lindane 1 percent. Lindane is a second-line treatment. It should be given only to those patients who are unable to take other medications or who have not responded to these other medications. Lindane can be toxic and should not be overused.

### PREVENTION AND OUTCOMES

To reduce the risk of getting scabies, one should avoid close physical contact with anyone who has scabies or an undiagnosed itchy rash, and should avoid sharing that person's clothing, towels, or bedding. To prevent the spread of scabies from one person to an-other, those who share living quarters with an infected person should be considered for treatment. Also, one should wash or dry clean all clothing, bedding, and towels that may have become infested. Mites, which cause scabies infestation, can live for two to five days after they leave a human body and are likely to remain infectious during this time.

*Rick Alan; reviewed by David L. Horn, M.D., FACP*

### FURTHER READING

Andrews, R. M., et al. "Skin Disorders, Including Pyoderma, Scabies, and Tinea Infections." *Pediatric Clinics of North America* 56 (2009): 1421.

Hu, S., and M. Bigby. "Treating Scabies: Results from an Updated Cochrane Review." *Archives of Dermatology* 144 (2008): 1638-1640.

Levy, Sandra. "The Scourge of Scabies: Some Ways to Treat It." *Drug Topics* 144, no. 22 (November 20, 2000): 56.

McPhee, Stephen J., and Maxine A. Papadakis, eds. *Current Medical Diagnosis and Treatment 2011.* 50th ed. New York: McGraw-Hill, 2011.

"Scabies." In *Clinical Dermatology: A Color Guide to Diagnosis and Therapy*, edited by T. P. Habib. 4th ed. Philadelphia: Mosby 2004.

Sheorey, Harsha, John Walker, and Beverly Ann Biggs. *Clinical Parasitology.* Carlton South, Vic.: Melbourne University Press, 2000.

Stewart, Kay B. "Combating Infection: Stopping the Itch of Scabies and Lice." *Nursing* 30, no. 7 (July, 2000): 30-31.

Turkington, Carol, and Jeffrey S. Dover. *The Encyclopedia of Skin and Skin Disorders.* 3d ed. New York: Facts On File, 2007.

Weedon, David. *Skin Pathology.* 3d ed. New York: Churchill Livingstone/Elsevier, 2010.

### WEB SITES OF INTEREST

*American Academy of Dermatology*
http://www.aad.org

*American Academy of Family Physicians*
http://familydoctor.org

*Centers for Disease Control and Prevention*
http://www.cdc.gov/parasites

*National Institute of Allergy and Infectious Diseases*
http://www.niaid.nih.gov

**See also:** Acariasis; Arthropod-borne illness and disease; Body lice; Chickenpox; Contagious diseases; Crab lice; Dogs and infectious disease; Head lice; Impetigo; Mites and chiggers and infectious disease; Parasitic diseases; Pityriasis rosea; Sexually transmitted diseases (STDs); Skin infections.

# Scarlet fever

CATEGORY: Diseases and conditions
ANATOMY OR SYSTEM AFFECTED: Skin, throat, upper respiratory tract
ALSO KNOWN AS: Scarlatina

## DEFINITION

Scarlet fever is a bacterial infection that produces a sore throat, upper respiratory symptoms, and a characteristic rash. It was once a serious childhood ailment, but it is quite treatable now with antibiotics.

## CAUSES

Scarlet fever is caused by group A beta-hemolytic *Streptococcus pyogenes*. This type of bacteria produces a toxin that causes a rash. Scarlet fever usually develops in conjunction with strep throat.

## RISK FACTORS

Risk factors for scarlet fever include untreated strep infection; close contact with someone who has an untreated strep infection; and overcrowded environments, or being especially close to others, such as at a day-care facility, school, or nursing home. At higher risk are children ages three to fifteen years.

## SYMPTOMS

The first signs of strep throat are a red, swollen throat and a fever higher than 101° Fahrenheit. If strep is diagnosed and treated with antibiotics, the infection may progress to scarlet fever. Additional symptoms include vomiting, a headache, swollen glands in the neck, a white or yellow coating on the tongue, a bright red tongue (known as strawberry tongue), a loss of appetite, abdominal pain, body aches, and chills.

Scarlet fever has a characteristic rash. Small red spots usually appear on the neck and chest within twenty-four to forty-eight hours after onset of the illness. This rash will spread quickly over the body to the

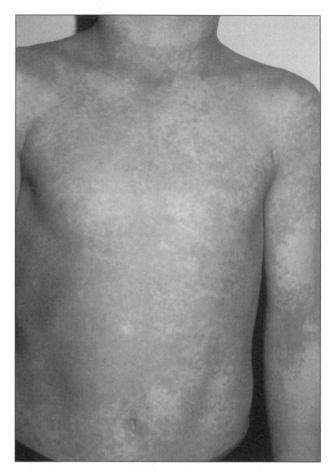

*A boy with a scarlet fever rash.*

abdomen, arms, and legs. The rash feels rough, like sand paper, and the redness blanches with pressure. There may also be flushing in the face with paleness around the mouth. Elbows, underarms, and other body-crease areas may show red streaks called Pastia's lines. In seven to ten days the rash will peel off.

## SCREENING AND DIAGNOSIS

A doctor will ask about symptoms and medical history and will perform a physical exam. The doctor also will swab the back of the throat for testing. The sample may be sent to a lab for a throat culture or a rapid strep-antigen test (also called a rapid strep test) may be done in the office.

## TREATMENT AND THERAPY

Scarlet fever can be treated with antibiotics, such as penicillin or amoxicillin. It is usually taken for about ten days. Erythromycin or azithromycin can be used for those with penicillin allergy. One should take all the prescribed medication to prevent recurrence or complications. A person with an active strep infection is usually contagious until the antibiotic has been taken for a minimum of twenty-four hours.

In rare cases, untreated strep throat infection may cause permanent damage to the heart and joints (rheumatic fever), permanent damage to the kidneys (glomerulonephritis), streptococcal toxic shock syndrome, and a local abscess.

## PREVENTION AND OUTCOMES

There is no vaccine against scarlet fever, but many have been under development. However, there are steps one can take to help prevent scarlet fever. These include getting early treatment for strep infections; avoiding school or work until the prescribed antibiotics have been taken for a minimum of twenty-four hours or until the doctor has given the approval to return to work or school; avoiding contact with people who have untreated strep infections; avoiding sharing cups, utensils, towels, bed linen, or personal items with infected people; and washing one's hands often, especially after touching someone who may have an infection.

*Michelle Badash, M.S.; reviewed by Kari Kassir, M.D.*

## FURTHER READING

Behrman, Richard E., Robert M. Kliegman, and Hal B. Jenson, eds. *Nelson Textbook of Pediatrics.* 18th ed. Philadelphia: Saunders/Elsevier, 2007.

EBSCO Publishing. *DynaMed: Scarlet Fever.* Available through http://www.ebscohost.com/dynamed.

Icon Health. *Scarlet Fever: A Medical Dictionary, Bibliography, and Annotated Research Guide to Internet References.* San Diego, Calif.: Author, 2004.

Jaggi, P., and S. T. Shulman. "Group A Streptococcal Infections." *Pediatrics in Review* 27 (2006): 99-104.

McKinnon, H. D., Jr., and T. Howard. "Evaluating the Febrile Patient with a Rash." *American Family Physician* 62 (2000): 804.

Weedon, David. *Skin Pathology.* 3d ed. New York: Churchill Livingstone/Elsevier, 2010.

## WEB SITES OF INTEREST

*About Kids Health*
http://www.aboutkidshealth.ca

*American Academy of Family Physicians*
http://familydoctor.org

*College of Family Physicians of Canada*
http://www.cfpc.ca

*KidsHealth*
http://www.kidshealth.org

**See also:** Bacterial infections; Contagious diseases; Erythema infectiosum; Erythema nodosum; Group A streptococcal infection; Hygiene; Pharyngitis and tonsillopharyngitis; Pityriasis rosea; Roseola; Rubella; Skin infections; Staphylococcal infections; *Staphylococcus*; Strep throat; Streptococcal infections; *Streptococcus.*

---

# Schistosomiasis

CATEGORY: Diseases and conditions
ANATOMY OR SYSTEM AFFECTED: Digestive system, gastrointestinal system, urinary system
ALSO KNOWN AS: Bilharziasis, Katayama fever

## DEFINITION

Schistosomiasis is a chronic parasitic infection of the digestive or urinary tract caused by digenetic trematode worms (*Platyhelminthes, Trematoda*) of the genus *Schistosoma* (called *Bilharzia* in some earlier literature).

## CAUSES

Most human schistosomiasis is caused by infection by three species: *S. haematobium*, which affects the bladder and is prevalent in Africa and the Middle East; *S. mansonii*, an intestinal parasite found in Africa and tropical areas of the Western Hemisphere, where it was introduced during the slave trade; and *S. japonicum*, an intestinal parasite common in East Asia. Human species also infect other animals. Contact with cercaria of species infecting waterfowl causes the allergic condition known as swimmer's itch. The disease is contracted through immersion in water contaminated by sewage and containing snails capable of acting as alternate hosts in the complex life cycle of *Schistosoma*.

## Risk Factors

The World Health Organization classifies schistosomiasis as a neglected tropical disease, one that has historically attracted little attention because it mainly affects people in poor tropical countries, usually is not dramatic in its manifestations, and does not spread directly from human to human. People who work in irrigated agriculture or bathe and wash clothes in polluted water are most at risk. Areas near the Aswan High Dam in Egypt, for example, where dam building allowed expansion of irrigation and attracted in-migration from endemic regions, have become foci for schistosomiasis.

In common with other helminth (worm) infections, susceptibility to schistosomiasis appears to be related to allergic response, which is triggered by initial infection and prevents reinfection once the parasite has become established. Adults from outside endemic regions who come into contact with high infestations often develop schistosomiasis because of the massive colonization during a single exposure.

## Symptoms

The disease commences when swimming larvae known as cercaria penetrate skin through the pores and migrate through the bloodstream to the portal blood of the liver, where they mature into adults. Except in massive infection, this phase is usually asymptomatic. Adult schistosome pair and migrate to peripheral venules of the bladder or intestine, where they lodge and begin producing eggs. Some eggs are excreted and hatch into larvae that infect snails, but many enter the host's bloodstream and are carried to other parts of the body. Although nonviable, the eggs contribute to pathology. Most of the symptoms of the disease are caused either by granuloma formation around worms or their eggs, or from mechanical blockage of blood vessels by eggs.

Symptoms of schistosomiasis include fever, cough, abdominal pain, diarrhea, enlargement of the liver and spleen, and eosinophilia. Symptoms of chronic schistosomiasis include colonic polyposis with bloody diarrhea, portal hypertension hematemesis and splenomegaly, cystitis and ureteritis with hematuria, pulmonary hypertension, glomerulonephritis, and (rarely) central nervous system lesions. Many infections are asymptomatic or nearly so, and the severity of symptoms declines with time.

## Screening and Diagnosis

Examining stool or urine samples for eggs is the most common diagnostic method. Techniques for concentrating eggs may be employed; even so, low-level infections may be missed because few eggs are being released. Serological tests are useful in determining the level of exposure in a population, but they do not distinguish active cases from those cases in which the person has recovered. Biopsies and imaging can be used to assess damage and detect the parasite in situ, but these tests are unavailable in most areas where the disease is prevalent. The availability of safe and effective chemotherapeutic agents for the condition make extensive testing to obtain a definitive diagnosis unnecessary in the case of persons who are known to have been exposed and who present the usual symptoms.

## Treatment and Therapy

Two or three oral doses of praziquantel are sufficient to kill adult schistosome. The drug is inexpensive, and major side effects are extremely rare. Except in severe long-standing cases, symptoms caused by granulomas can be expected to subside. In endemic areas, schistosomiasis often accompanies and exacerbates the effects of childhood malnutrition; treatment programs that also address this have better outcomes.

The governments of Nigeria and Madagascar, in collaboration with the World Health Organization, have adopted programs to treat all schoolchildren in high-incidence areas with praziquantel. Because a high percentage of these children are infected and are immune to reinfection, praziquantel use is an effective way of reducing both the incidence of the disease and its ill effects, which include poor learning because of chronic ill health.

## Prevention and Outcomes

Vaccines have been developed for schistosomiasis, but they are of limited effectiveness and are not widely used. Where feasible, reduction of water contamination by urine and feces can break the infection cycle. Complete elimination from irrigation water is not possible, however, even in developed countries, especially because domestic animals are possible hosts.

The control of the snail vectors has been explored, with mixed results. Poisoning with molluscicides is

## Cycle of Schistosomiasis Infection

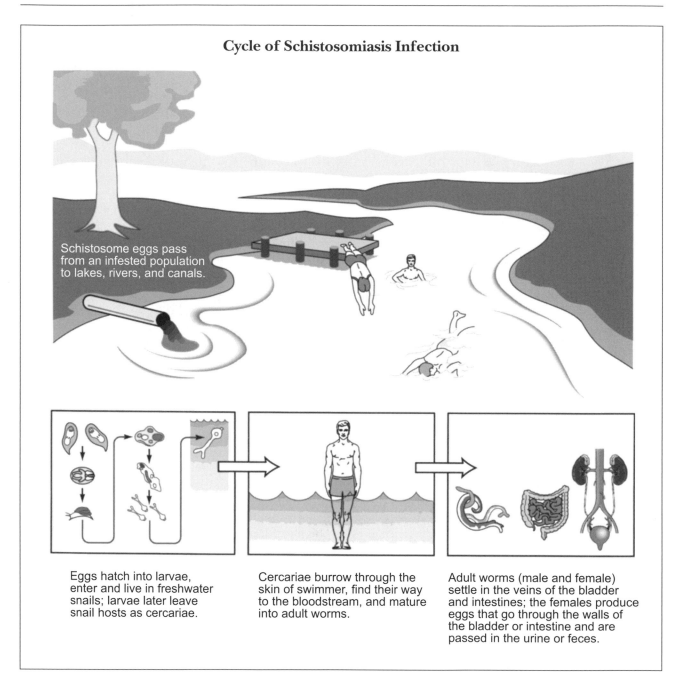

Schistosome eggs pass from an infested population to lakes, rivers, and canals.

Eggs hatch into larvae, enter and live in freshwater snails; larvae later leave snail hosts as cercariae.

Cercariae burrow through the skin of swimmer, find their way to the bloodstream, and mature into adult worms.

Adult worms (male and female) settle in the veins of the bladder and intestines; the females produce eggs that go through the walls of the bladder or intestine and are passed in the urine or feces.

not recommended because nontarget species are affected and an area's overall ecology is disrupted. Some success has been achieved in Puerto Rico through introducing predators and nonhost competing species. One concern of global warming is the possible expansion of tropical snails into warm temperate areas such as the southeastern United States. A combined approach involving education about sewage disposal and water use, managing irrigation systems to reduce snail habitat, and promptly treating infected humans holds the best prospect for reducing schistosomiasis worldwide so that it is no longer a serious threat to human health.

*Martha A. Sherwood, Ph.D.*

## FURTHER READING

Mahmoud, Adel A. F., ed. *Schistosomiasis*. London: Imperial College Press, 2001.

Roberts, Larry S., and John Janovy, Jr. *Gerald D. Schmidt and Larry S. Roberts' Foundations of Parasitology*. 8th ed. Boston: McGraw-Hill, 2009.

Secor, W. Evan, and Daniel G. Colley, eds. *Schistosomiasis*. Vol. 10 in *World Class Parasites*, edited by Samuel J. Black and J. Richard Seed. New York: Springer Science, 2005.

World Health Organization. *Neglected Tropical Diseases: Hidden Successes, Emerging Opportunities*. Geneva: Author, 2009.

_____. *Prevention and Control of Schistosomiasis and Soil-Transmitted Helminthiasis*. Geneva: Author, 2001.

## WEB SITES OF INTEREST

*Centers for Disease Control and Prevention*
http://www.dpd.cdc.gov/dpdx/html/schistosomiasis.htm

*Neglected Tropical Diseases Coalition*
http://www.neglectedtropicaldiseases.org

*World Health Organization*
http://www.who.int/topics/schistosomiasis

**See also:** Developing countries and infectious disease; Flukes; Intestinal and stomach infections; Parasites: Classification and types; Parasitic diseases; Tropical medicine; Waterborne illness and disease; Worm infections.

---

# Schistosomiasis vaccine

CATEGORY: Prevention

## DEFINITION

Several vaccines have been developed for the prevention of schistosomiasis, a snail-transmitted, waterborne, parasitic disease that infects about 200 million people worldwide. No vaccine, however, has been able to produce consistent immunity. Antigens from schistosomules and schistosomes show some promise.

Clinical trials by the Pasteur Institute have resulted in good immune response for volunteers in Niger and Senegal. The late discovery of several *Schistosoma* genomes continues to expand opportunities for schistosomiasis vaccine research. Cocktails (combination therapies) of recombinant antigens also offer hope for a vaccine.

## IMMUNIZATION

The control of schistosomiasis infection depends on drug treatment, which has effectively reduced morbidity. Immunization is still much needed to complement drug therapy because of a high reinfection rate. Hope for successful immunization through vaccination is based on some degree of natural protection seen in endemic human populations and the partial success of prototype vaccines.

## PATHOLOGY

*Schistosoma* is a parasitic helminth (worm) carried by snails and is transmitted to humans through contact with contaminated fresh-water sources. There are three major species. *S. mansoni* is found in North Africa, Arabia, and parts of South America. *S. haematobium* is found in the Middle East and Africa. *S. japonicum*, which causes the most severe infections, is endemic to China and Southeast Asia. Children who play in contaminated water and women who wash in contaminated water are most at risk. Chronic infections may cause anemia, kidney failure, liver damage, growth retardation in children, and bladder cancer.

## PATHOGENICITY

Fresh-water snails infected with schistosomiasis release larvae that enter the body through breaks in human skin. The free-swimming larvae then lose their tails and become schistosomules that migrate through the venous system and lay their eggs. Eggs that remain in the body stimulate the formation of scar tissue in the form of fibrosis or granulomas that may lead to organ failure. Other eggs exit the body through urine or feces to hatch in fresh water and continue the cycle of infection and reinfection.

## IMPACT

There is a definite need to develop a vaccine to complement drug therapy for schistosomiasis. Schistosomiasis continues to be a major health problem in endemic areas around the world and is second only to malaria in disease occurrence. Estimates are that *Schistosoma* infects 280 million people and causes 280,000 deaths each year. The treatment drug of choice, praziquantel, reverses pathology, but it comes with concerns of the emergence of drug-resistant strains of schistosomiasis.

*Christopher Iliades, M.D.*

**FURTHER READING**

Bergquist, Robert. "Prospects for Schistosomiasis Vaccine Development." Special Program for Research and Training in Tropical Diseases, World Health Organization. Available at http://www.who.int/tdrold/publications/tdrnews/news71/schisto.htm.

Driguez, Patrick, et al. "Schistosomiasis Vaccine Discovery Using Immunomics." *Parasites and Vectors* 3, no. 4 (2010). Also available at http://www.parasitesandvectors.com/content/3/1/4.

McManus, D. P., and A. Loukas. "Current Status of Vaccines for Schistosomiasis." *Clinical Microbiology Reviews* 21 (2008): 225-242.

Plotkin, Stanley A., Walter A. Orenstein, and Paul A. Offit. *Vaccines.* 5th ed. Philadelphia: Saunders/Elsevier, 2008.

**WEB SITES OF INTEREST**

*Centers for Disease Control and Prevention, Parasites and Health*
http://www.dpd.cdc.gov/dpdx/html/schistosomiasis.htm

*Emerging and Reemerging Infectious Diseases Resource Center*
http://www.medscape.com/resource/infections

*Vaccine Research Center*
http://www.niaid.nih.gov/about/organization/vrc

*World Health Organization, Parasitic Diseases*
http://www.who.int/vaccine_research/diseases/soa_parasitic/en/index5.html

**See also:** Cholera vaccine; Developing countries and infectious disease; Disease eradication campaigns; Emerging and reemerging infectious diseases; Epidemiology; Globalization and infectious disease; Immunity; Immunization; Malaria vaccine; Microbiology; Parasitic diseases; Polio vaccine; Public health; Schistosomiasis; Vaccines: Experimental; Vaccines: History; Vaccines: Types; Virology; Waterborne illness and disease; Worm infections.

# Schools and infectious disease

CATEGORY: Epidemiology

## DEFINITION

Infectious diseases are rarely the top concern of school and public health officials in the United States. Instead, of central concern are obesity, diabetes, asthma, smoking, substance abuse, eating disorders, and bullying behaviors. Now-routine immunization requirements for school entrance have reduced the occurrence of infectious diseases in schools in industrialized nations. However, these diseases have not been completely eradicated, and seasonal infections such as influenza require ongoing school readiness.

## CONTAGIOUS DISEASES OF THE SKIN, HAIR, AND EYES

Particularly in the preschool and elementary school years, infections that visibly affect the skin, hair, and eyes are fairly common. These diseases may be caused by viruses, bacteria, fungi, or lice; they may be mild and self-limited with no other symptoms outside the skin, or they may cause significant illness.

*Chickenpox.* Although it is seen less commonly since the varicella vaccine was licensed in 1995, chickenpox still occurs in localized outbreaks in children who are not immunized. Chickenpox is caused by the varicella virus, which spreads easily by inhaling infected droplets released when a child sneezes or coughs. The virus can also be spread though direct contact with chickenpox skin blisters. Varicella vaccine is now required for school entrance in nearly every state, and it is about 90 percent effective in preventing the illness. For the small percentage of children who still develop chickenpox, even after being vaccinated, the illness is usually mild and, generally, comes with fewer than fifty skin lesions.

For nonimmunized children, chickenpox is more severe and may result in pneumonia, infection of the brain (encephalitis), and other complications. For this reason, one should never deliberately expose a child to chickenpox to "get the infection over with." An infected child may be contagious for one or two days before any skin blisters appear, and the child will remain contagious (and should be kept home from school) until all of the blisters have dried up and crusted over.

*Impetigo.* Impetigo is an infection of the skin caused

by *Staphylococcus* or *Streptococcus* bacteria. Both types of this disease are highly contagious by direct contact, and both spread easily among young children in preschool settings. Impetigo develops as an area of redness and blistering of the skin that quickly weeps (oozes) yellowish fluid and becomes covered with honey-colored crusts. This often occurs on the face or arms and begins in an area of irritated skin, such as a patch of eczema or a scratch. Treatment is with either oral antibiotics or an antibiotic cream, and the child should be kept from school until twenty-four hours after treatment is begun.

*Erythema infectiosum.* Also called fifth disease, erythema infectiosum is a mild illness often seen in school outbreaks in the late winter and spring months. Generally, the only symptoms are reddened cheeks followed by a fine, lacy, red rash over the trunk that may be slightly itchy. This infection is caused by parvovirus B19; about one-half of adults are immune. However, adults and older children not previously exposed may also have painful and swollen joints, and there can be some risk of miscarriage for nonimmune pregnant women exposed to the virus. Children with fifth disease are contagious only before they break out in the rash, and they are no longer contagious by the time the rash appears. For this reason, most school systems do not advise keeping an otherwise asymptomatic child with fifth disease at home.

*Head lice.* Head lice (pediculosis capitis) has long been associated with school-related infectious diseases, and it is most common in preschool and elementary school children. Infestation of the hair with these 2 millimeter parasitic insects generally causes more anxiety than actual physical discomfort, as the lice do not carry disease and tend to cause only minor itching. In many countries, cases of head lice appear in nearly all children.

Lice treatments involve the application of one of several approved treatments (available over the counter and by prescription), with repeat treatments either on day nine or in a three-dose regimen with repeat treatments on days seven and fourteen. In the past, undergoing treatment meant that children would be refused readmission to school until treatment was completed and there were no remaining visible "nits" (eggs and dead egg-casings) clinging to the hair shaft. However, the difficulty in removing all nits even after successful treatment, and the frequent misidentification of dandruff, skin particles, and scabs as

nits, led to many uninfested children being excluded from school for an average of twenty days.

Many school policies are changing. Head lice are most commonly spread by direct head-to-head contact, which is not commonplace in the classroom beyond the preschool years. Lice are much less likely to be spread by the shared use of brushes, combs, and headgear. In the United States, most head lice are probably transmitted during close sleeping arrangements, such as the sharing of beds at sleepovers and summer camps, rather than at school. The American Academy of Pediatrics (AAP) recommends that school nurses be well trained in proper diagnosis of head lice, particularly in recognizing nits, mainly to avoid diagnostic confusion. At the same time, the AAP recommends that school districts abandon their "nonit" policies for a child's return to school, and that children should return to school the day after their first treatment, even if nits remain visible in the hair.

*Conjunctivitis.* The most common cause of conjunctivitis, or pinkeye, is a viral infection of the clear membrane covering the white of the eye and lining the eyelids. Viral conjunctivitis causes reddened, itchy eyes with a clear watery discharge, and it is spread by contact with secretions (tears and nasal discharge) that often are spread from the fingers. Children may remain contagious for ten to twelve days. Bacterial conjunctivitis also causes reddened eyes, but it is more likely to result in thick, puslike, yellow or green eye secretions, and it responds quickly to antibiotic drops. Students with bacterial conjunctivitis can usually return to school twenty-four hours after beginning treatment, but students with viral conjunctivitis should remain home until they are symptom free or until cleared by a physician.

*Methicillin-resistant* Staphylococcus aureus *(MRSA).* MRSA has become a problem in schools, particularly in physical education classes and high school athletic programs. This type of bacteria mainly causes skin infections, usually of open wounds, and is resistant to many common antibiotics that were previously able to treat *Staphyloccocus* (staph) infections. MRSA causes redness, swelling, pain, and pus, and it must be diagnosed by a bacterial culture. It spreads by direct skin-to-skin contact or by contact with a used bandage, towel, or surface in a locker room or other athletic facility. Athletes who have a break in the skin should clean the area and cover it to prevent infection. Those who already have an MRSA-infected wound

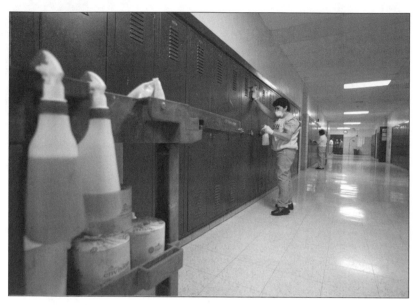

*A worker disinfects lockers at a high school in Fort Worth, Texas, during the H1N1, or swine, influenza outbreak of 2009.* (AP/Wide World Photos)

should always keep the area completely covered to prevent spreading the infection to another person. As long as the infected area is not draining and can be completely covered, infected athletes, according to the CDC, do not need to be excluded from athletic participation. It also is not necessary to close or completely disinfect a school if a student has been diagnosed with MRSA.

## RESPIRATORY INFECTIONS

*Common cold.* The most common respiratory illness in schools is the viral infection known as the common cold. Caused by a variety of viruses and spread by coughs, sneezes, and contaminated surfaces such as doorknobs, colds affect otherwise healthy young children up to six times per year. Chances are that each classroom will have a minimum of one child with a cold. Although some preschools and day-care centers may exclude children from attending if they exhibit cold symptoms, no medical reason exists for doing so, because these illnesses are mild, self-limited, and ubiquitous.

*Influenza.* Another respiratory illness, influenza, is of much greater concern in schools. Influenza, commonly referred to as the flu, is characterized by respiratory symptoms more severe than those of the common cold. Flu symptoms also include high fever,

headache, and muscle aches, and the flu has the potential for complications, including pneumonia and, rarely, death. The illness is contagious and is transmitted through inhaling or contacting the droplets of an infected person's cough or sneeze.

Influenza occurs in predictable seasonal outbreaks during the winter months in both the Northern (peaking in January and February) and Southern (peaking in July and August) hemispheres. Several slightly different influenza viruses circulate each year, and these viruses tend to change year to year. Each year's flu vaccine is tailored to prevent the viruses that are predicted for that year by virologists. These predictions are not always completely correct, meaning that in some years, even those persons who get that season's vaccine will not be well protected.

Schools have three main strategies at their disposal for preventing large outbreaks of influenza among students and staff. The primary tool is immunization. The CDC recommends that all children older than age six months receive an annual seasonal influenza vaccine, and schools often encourage this by means of letters and other reminders to parents. Particularly in years in which a new strain of flu is causing a pandemic, such as the 2009 H1N1 virus pandemic, schools may provide in-school vaccinations with parental approval.

The second strategy available to schools for the prevention of influenza outbreaks is attention to basic hygiene measures. Schools are teaching children to cover their mouths and noses with a tissue when coughing or sneezing and to discard the tissue in the trash immediately afterward. Alternatively, children are being taught to sneeze into their arms near their elbows, instead of into their bare hands, if no tissue is available. Handwashing is emphasized as a means to prevent transmission after coughing, sneezing, blowing one's nose, or touching an object that has been used by a sick person. In preschools and elementary schools, children should be given frequent opportunities for handwashing, and when no water is available, children should have access to a gel-based hand sanitizer. These concepts can be reinforced as part of morning announcements, in handouts, and through frequent review.

The third tool available to schools to manage influenza is attendance policy. Children and staff who display flulike symptoms should not attend school. However, because persons with influenza are contagious for about twenty-four hours before showing any symptoms, and will remain contagious until about the fifth day of illness, this type of attendance policy cannot completely protect students and staff. During the 2009 pandemic flu season, some schools closed when a significant number of students became ill. In general, however, this practice is not recommended for a variety of reasons, including that when schools are closed, parents often bring younger children to a babysitter, a neighbor, or even to the workplace. Older children, especially teenagers, often use this time away from school to congregate with their friends, often in public places. Overall, it appears that a school closure because of a flu scare aids in spreading the virus into the community, rather than keeping it contained. However, if absenteeism among teachers and staff is so high that the school cannot function appropriately, school closures may be inevitable.

*Strep throat.* Streptococcal pharyngitis, or strep throat, is another common respiratory illness in school-age children. The majority of sore throats are caused by some of the many viruses that cause the common cold, but up to 30 percent may be caused by the bacterium *Streptococcus pyogenes.* Children with a sore throat, fever, swollen lymph nodes (glands) in the neck, headache, and, sometimes, abdominal pain and vomiting are most likely to have strep throat, which is spread by infected droplets from coughing and sneezing and from contaminated hands. Strep throat should be diagnosed either by a rapid screening test or a throat culture, so that antibiotics are not used unnecessarily for a viral infection. Antibiotics should be given for a minimum of twenty-four hours before an infected child returns to school, and they are critical for the prevention of later complications from *S. pyogenes.* These complications include scarlet fever, heart valve damage, and kidney damage.

*Bacterial meningitis.* Bacterial meningitis is a serious illness that is life-threatening, may begin during the school day, and may progress in severity in a matter of hours. Any child who develops a headache, along with a stiff neck, fever, confusion, or rash or discoloration of the skin, should be taken to a hospital for emergency treatment. If a certain type of bacterial meningitis (meningococcal meningitis) is diagnosed, health officials will contact the school and identify students and staff who were in direct contact with the infected child so that prophylactic (preventive) antibiotics can be administered to all who had contact.

Bacterial meningitis spreads by infected droplets from a cough or sneeze. A vaccine called meningococcal conjugate vaccine (MCV4) is routinely recommended at ages eleven and twelve years. Meningitis is also caused by a wide variety of viruses and is generally less severe. It is not prevented by or treated with antibiotics.

## GASTROINTESTINAL INFECTIONS

*Gastroenteritis.* Diarrhea and vomiting (gastroenteritis) is usually a more serious problem among preschool and early elementary age students, who are more likely to have poor restroom hygiene and more likely to put their hands, toys, and other items in or near their mouths. Infections causing these symptoms can be classified as being waterborne, food-borne, or acquired from another person or animal through contact with their feces or body secretions.

A sudden, large outbreak of gastroenteritis in a school is often caused by a food-borne illness from cafeteria food. In this case, school officials should alert local or state health officials. Health officials will conduct an investigation of the outbreak to determine the cause. The investigation will include extensive questioning of students and staff, microbiological testing of food remnants and kitchen surfaces, and medical testing of cafeteria staff.

Other sudden, large outbreaks in a school may prove to be caused by noroviruses, which can be food-borne but are more often spread quickly and easily from person to person through either direct contact with contaminated feces or vomit or from touching contaminated surfaces such as restroom doors or another person's towel. A norovirus infection tends to cause a day or two of severe diarrhea in children, and then clears on its own.

## IMPACT

Given that fifty-five million children age eighteen years and younger attend schools each day in the United States, an infectious disease affecting one child could potentially affect (and infect) many more. Many of the worst infectious diseases are rarely, if ever, seen in today's schools because of stringent, compulsory school immunization laws. Today's schools, however, face other potential infectious disease challenges.

Some students remain unimmunized because of their parent's religion, or because of other reasons, providing an opening for disease outbreaks. Antibiotic resistance, such as that seen with MRSA infections, is likely to become a more widespread problem. Immigrant populations in some areas increase a student's potential exposure to tuberculosis. As teens engage in oral and genital sex at earlier ages, herpes infections, gonorrhea, human immunodeficiency virus infection, and other sexually transmitted infections will likely become more prevalent among teen social networks, which tend to revolve around school activities. School nurses and administrators, and public health officials, should continue to devote time and attention to infectious disease in the schools.

*Lindsey Marcellin, M.D., M.P.H.*

### FURTHER READING

Aronson, Susan S., and Timothy R. Shope. *Managing Infectious Diseases in Child Care and Schools: A Quick Reference Guide.* 2d ed. Elk Grove Village, Ill.: American Academy of Pediatrics, 2009. A reference on infectious disease management and prevention in school and child-care settings.

Centers for Disease Control and Prevention. "Questions and Answers About Methicillin-Resistant *Staphylococcus aureus* (MRSA) in Schools." Available at http://www.cdc.gov/features/mrsainschools.

Fisher, Margaret C. *Immunizations and Infectious Diseases: An Informed Parent's Guide.* American Academy of Pediatrics, 2006. A pediatrician explains childhood infection and its prevention.

Frankowski, Barbara L., and Joseph A. Bocchini, Jr. "Clinical Report: Head Lice." *Pediatrics* 126 (August, 2010): 392-403. A report from the American Academy of Pediatrics' Council on School Health and the Committee on Infectious Diseases includes a clinical overview of head lice diagnosis and treatment and expert opinion on school policies related to head lice.

Lee, Marilyn B., and Judy D. Greig. "A Review of Gastrointestinal Outbreaks in Schools: Effective Infection Control Interventions." *Journal of School Health* 80 (2010): 588-598. A review of documented gastrointestinal illness outbreaks in schools since 2000.

### WEB SITES OF INTEREST

*American School Health Association*
http://www.ashaweb.org

*Centers for Disease Control and Prevention*
http://www.cdc.gov/healthyyouth/infectious

*KidsHealth*
http://www.kidshealth.org

*National Association of School Nurses*
http://www.nasn.org

*Pediatric Infectious Diseases Society*
http://www.pids.org

**See also:** Bacterial infections; Bacterial meningitis; Chickenpox; Children and infectious disease; Common cold; Conjunctivitis; Contagious diseases; Epidemics and pandemics: Causes and management; Epidemiology; Erythema infectiosum; Hygiene; Impetigo; Influenza; Measles; Methicillin-resistant staph infection; Mumps; Outbreaks; Parasitic diseases; Public health; Rubella; Strep throat; Vaccines: Types; Viral infections.

---

# Seasonal influenza

CATEGORY: Diseases and conditions
ANATOMY OR SYSTEM AFFECTED: Eyes, gastrointestinal system, lungs, nose, respiratory system, stomach, throat
ALSO KNOWN AS: The flu

### DEFINITION

Seasonal influenza (the flu) is a viral infection that affects the respiratory system. It can cause mild to severe illness and sometimes death. To avoid getting the flu, one should get vaccinated every year.

### CAUSES

The flu is caused by the influenza virus. Each winter, the virus spreads around the world. The strains usually differ from one year to the next. The two main kinds of influenza virus are type A and type B.

A person who is infected with the virus may sneeze or cough, releasing droplets into the air. If another person breathes in infected droplets, he or she can become infected. A person can also become infected by touching a contaminated surface, which risks the transfer of the virus from one's hand to one's mouth or nose.

## RISK FACTORS

Factors that increase the chance of getting the flu include living or working in crowded group conditions, such as in nursing homes, schools, day-care centers, and the military. Factors that increase the risk of developing complications from flu include being pregnant; having recently given birth; having diabetes or chronic lung, heart, kidney, liver, nerve, or blood conditions; and being in a chronic care facility. Other persons at risk are those who have a weakened immune system, such as people infected with the human immunodeficiency virus and people taking immuno-suppressive drugs.

Also at higher risk are children younger than five years of age, adults ages sixty-five years and older, and people younger than the age of nineteen years (and who are on a long-term aspirin regimen).

## SYMPTOMS

A person with the flu is infectious beginning one day before his or her own symptoms start and up to five days (sometimes more) after becoming sick. This means that a person who has the flu could infect others before knowing that he or she is sick.

Symptoms usually start abruptly and include a high fever and chills; severe muscle aches; severe fatigue; a headache; decreased appetite or other gastrointestinal symptoms, such as nausea, vomiting, and diarrhea (more common in children than in adults); a runny nose and nasal congestion; sneezing; watery eyes or conjunctivitis; a sore throat; a cough (that lasts for two or more weeks); and swollen lymph nodes in the neck. The ill person might start to feel better in seven to ten days but may still have a cough and feel tired.

## SCREENING AND DIAGNOSIS

A doctor will ask about symptoms and medical history to determine a person's diagnosis of the flu. In some cases, the doctor may take samples from the person's nose or throat to confirm the diagnosis.

## TREATMENT AND THERAPY

Treatment for the flu includes antiviral prescription medicines. Most people with the flu do not need antiviral medicine, but persons who do are those who are in a high-risk group or who have a severe illness (such as breathing problems). Antiviral medicines, which generally help relieve symptoms and shorten the time a person is sick, should be taken within forty-eight hours of the first symptoms. These medicines include zanamivir (Relenza), which may worsen a patient's asthma or chronic obstructive pulmonary disease (COPD), and oseltamivir (Tamiflu), amantadine (Symmetrel), and rimantadine (Flumadine), all three of which are ineffective against some kinds of seasonal influenza viruses. Furthermore, oseltamivir (and perhaps zanamivir) may increase the risk of self-injury and confusion shortly after being ingested, especially by children. One should monitor children closely for signs of unusual behavior.

Other forms of treatment include rest, which will help the body fight the flu; fluids, including water, juice, and caffeine-free tea; over-the-counter pain relievers, which are used to control fever and to treat aches and pains (adults can use acetaminophen or ibuprofen); and decongestants, which are available as pills or as nasal sprays. One should not use a nasal spray for more than three to five days. When stopping, the patient may experience an increase in congestion called a rebound.

Prescription cough medicines and cough drops also are available, as are over-the-counter cough and cold medicines. These include decongestants, expectorants, antihistamines, and cough suppressants. However, these should not be used to treat infants or children less than two years of age. Rare but serious side effects have been reported, including death, convulsions, rapid heart rates, and decreased levels of consciousness. Serious side effects have also been reported in children between the ages of two and eleven years.

Herbal treatments, such as elderberry extract, may reduce flu symptoms. Researchers have found that products such as Sambucol and ViraBLOC, which contain elderberry, decrease symptoms in some studies. Herbal remedies, however, are not regulated by the government, so care should be taken in using them. The herbal supplements may not have the same ingredients as those studied and may contain impurities.

## PREVENTION AND OUTCOMES

To prevent getting the flu, one should get vaccinated and do so each year because the virus changes every season. The best time to get vaccinated is between the months of September and January (or later, because the flu season can last longer). Two forms of the vaccine are available: a flu shot (injection) and a nasal spray (FluMist). The nasal spray is approved for healthy (and nonpregnant) people between the ages of two and forty-nine years.

People who care for others with severely weakened immune systems should not get the nasal spray; instead they should get the flu shot. The flu shot is not effective against H1N1 flu, however, which has its own vaccine.

Persons who want to reduce their risk of the flu should consider the vaccine. It takes about two weeks for the vaccination to protect against the flu. Those who should get a yearly flu vaccine include children ages six months to eighteen years; parents, babysitters, and caretakers of children less than six months of age (because these children are too young to be vaccinated); adults older than fifty years of age (because vaccination in this age group likely reduces hospitalizations and deaths); those living or working in nursing homes and long-term care facilities; those with chronic medical conditions such as asthma; those with diabetes, kidney problems, hemoglobin abnormalities, or immune system problems; women who are pregnant; health care workers; and those living with someone who is at high risk for complications from the flu.

People who should not be vaccinated are those who are severely allergic to chicken eggs, those who had a severe reaction to vaccination in the past, and children less than six months of age. Persons who are sick and have a fever should discuss vaccination with a medical provider.

There are general measures one can take to reduce the risk of getting the flu. These measures include washing one's hands often, especially after contacting someone who is sick (rubbing alcohol-based cleaners on one's hands is also helpful), and avoiding close contact with people who have respiratory infections. The flu can spread starting one day before and ending seven days after symptoms appear.

Other preventive measures are to cover one's mouth and nose with a tissue when coughing or sneezing, and then throwing away the tissue after use; avoid spitting; avoid sharing drinks or personal items; avoid biting one's nails; and avoid putting one's hands near one's eyes, mouth, or nose. Another measure is to keep surfaces clean by wiping them with a household disinfectant.

One should consult a doctor about lowering the risk of getting the flu (also about lowering the risk for children who are one year of age or older) with antiviral medications (such as zanamivir). Antiviral medications are helpful for persons at high risk for the flu and for those who were only recently vaccinated (within the past two weeks), especially if the flu is spreading in one's community; for persons at high risk for the flu and who cannot have the vaccine; and for persons not vaccinated and who have repeated close contact with persons (such as family members) who are at high risk for the flu. Persons (such as the elderly, infants, and persons with cancer) who are at risk for complications of the flu and who live with someone who has the flu should get antiviral medications.

Persons who have the flu should take the following steps to avoid spreading the virus to others: Before returning to school or work, one's fever should be gone for at least twenty-four hours without the help of fever-reducing medicine. This could take up to seven days after symptoms first appear. A sick person who cannot avoid close contact should cover his or her mouth and nose with a face mask.

*Rosalyn Carson-DeWitt, M.D.;*
*reviewed by David L. Horn, M.D., FACP*

**FURTHER READING**

Belshe, R. B., et al. "Live Attenuated Versus Inactivated Influenza Vaccine in Infants and Young Children." *New England Journal of Medicine* 356 (2007): 685-696. Available through *DynaMed Systematic Literature Surveillance* at http://www.ebscohost.com/dynamed.

Centers for Disease Control and Prevention. "Home Care Guidance: Physician Directions to Patient/Parent." Available at http://www.cdc.gov/h1n1flu/guidance_homecare_directions.htm.

_____. "Key Facts About Seasonal Influenza (Flu) and Flu Vaccine." Available at http://www.cdc.gov/flu/keyfacts.htm.

Cowling, B. J., et al. "Facemasks and Hand Hygiene to Prevent Influenza Transmission in Households: A Cluster Randomized Trial." *Annals of Internal Medicine* 151, no. 7 (2009): 437-446. Available through *DynaMed Systematic Literature Surveillance* at http://www.ebscohost.com/dynamed.

EBSCO Publishing. *DynaMed: Influenza.* Available through http://www.ebscohost.com/dynamed.

_____. *Health Library: Flu.* Available through http://www.ebscohost.com.

Mandell, Gerald L., John E. Bennett, and Raphael Dolin, eds. *Mandell, Douglas, and Bennett's Principles and Practice of Infectious Diseases.* 7th ed. New York: Churchill Livingstone/Elsevier, 2010.

Nichol, K. L., et al. "Effectiveness of Influenza Vaccine in the Community-Dwelling Elderly." *New England Journal of Medicine* 357 (2007): 1373-1381. Available through *DynaMed Systematic Literature Surveillance* at http://www.ebscohost.com/dynamed.

Smith, N. M., et al. "Prevention and Control of Influenza: Recommendations of the Advisory Committee on Immunization Practices." *Morbidity and Mortality Weekly Report* 55 (2006): 1-42.

U.S. Food and Drug Administration. "Public Health Advisory: FDA Recommends that Over-the-Counter (OTC) Cough and Cold Products Not Be Used for Infants and Children Under Two Years of Age." Available at http://www.fda.gov/safety/medwatch.

_____. "2008 Safety Alerts for Drugs, Biologics, Medical Devices, and Dietary Supplements: Tamiflu (Oseltamivir Phosphate)." Available at http://www.fda.gov/safety/medwatch.

World Health Organization. "Influenza Vaccines." *Weekly Epidemiological Record* 28, no. 77 (2002): 229-240.

Zakay-Rones, Z., et al. "Inhibition of Several Strains of Influenza Virus In Vitro and Reduction of Symptoms by an Elderberry Extract (*Sambucus nigra l.*) During an Outbreak of Influenza B Panama." *Journal of Alternative and Complementary Medicine* 1 (1995): 361-369.

_____. "Randomized Study of the Efficacy and Safety of Oral Elderberry Extract in the Treatment of Influenza A and B Virus Infections." *Journal of International Medical Research* 32, no. 2 (2004): 132-140.

**WEB SITES OF INTEREST**

*American Lung Association*
http://www.lungusa.org

*Centers for Disease Control and Prevention*
http://www.cdc.gov/flu

*Flu.gov*
http://www.flu.gov

*National Institute of Allergy and Infectious Diseases*
http://www.niaid.nih.gov/topics/flu

*Public Health Agency of Canada*
http://www.phac-aspc.gc.ca

**See also:** Airborne illness and disease; Common cold; Contagious diseases; Fever; H1N1 influenza; Influenza; Influenza vaccine; Pharyngitis and tonsillopharyngitis; Respiratory route of transmission; Vaccines: History; Vaccines: Types; Viral infections; Viral pharyngitis; Viral upper respiratory infections; Viruses: Types.

---

# Secondary infection

CATEGORY: Transmission
ALSO KNOWN AS: Superinfection

## DEFINITION

A secondary infection is a simultaneous infection or one that follows a treated initial (primary) infection. Also, a secondary infection can occur after reactivation of the initial infection. The secondary infection may be bacterial or viral, and it is often described as a superinfection.

## CAUSES

Antibiotics taken to eliminate harmful bacteria from the body also eliminate necessary healthy (commensal) bacteria. Thus, a secondary infection can be caused by drug treatment of a primary infection that leaves the body immunocompromised and susceptible to more illnesses and infections; immunosuppression leads to secondary infection. A common example of secondary infection is superimposed bacterial pneumonia that is caused by a primary infection with influenza; the influenza damaged the lining of the lungs and nose, making the person more susceptible to bacterial infection of the respiratory tract.

## ROUTES OF TRANSMISSION

In addition to being transmitted by direct contact with a pathogen, secondary infections also can occur by nosocomial routes. A nosocomial infection is one that is acquired in a hospital or other medical setting during the course of a patient's care. Infection can occur through contact with infected medical personnel and visitors or through surgery or other medical procedure. In this case, the specific organ focused on in surgery already may have abnormal tissue, leading to decreased immunity and a greater chance of secondary infection.

Pregnancy is a natural immunosuppressed state, and viral infections acquired by a woman during this time could cause birth defects, birth disorders, and other adverse pregnancy outcomes. Medical staff should distinguish between a secondary infection that occurred by reinfection with a different strain of a virus and reactivation of an initial infection, as the latter poses less risk for fetal transmission than does the former.

## PREVENTION AND TREATMENT

Preventive measures include proper hygiene techniques, such as handwashing, and avoiding contact with sick persons. Vaccinations, such as for influenza, are recommended to decrease the rate of primary infections that begin this pathway.

A secondary infection may present with symptoms more severe than those with a primary infection, mainly because of compromised immunity. The treatment of a secondary infection depends on the type of infection, and the need for antibiotics depends on the severity of symptoms.

## IMPACT

Recognizing the risk factors for acquiring a secondary infection and implementing preventive measures reduce the morbidity and mortality associated with these infections. One study estimated that the secondary bacterial infections acquired after an H1N1 influenza outbreak, for example, were factors in up to 55 percent of all H1N1 influenza deaths. The economic implications of reducing these infections are significant too, especially in hospital settings.

*Janet Ober Berman, M.S., CGC*

## FURTHER READING

Brachman, Philip S., and Elias Abrutyn, eds. *Bacterial Infections of Humans: Epidemiology and Control.* 4th ed. New York: Springer, 2009.
Downie, Fiona, et al. "Barrier Dressings in Surgical Site Infection Prevention Strategies." *British Journal of Nursing* 19 (2010): S42-S46.
Ornoy, Asher, et al. "Effects of Primary and Secondary Cytomegalovirus Infection in Pregnancy." *Reproductive Toxicology* 21 (2006): 399-409.
Stewart, Bruce, et al. "Imaging and Percutaneous Treatment of Secondarily Infected Hepatic Infarctions." *Interventional Radiology* 190 (2008): 601-607.

## WEB SITES OF INTEREST

*Association for Professionals in Infection Control and Epidemiology*
http://www.knowledgeisinfectious.org

*Centers for Disease Control and Prevention*
http://www.cdc.gov

*Community and Hospital Infection Control Association*
http://www.chica.org

**See also:** Antibiotics: Types; Bacterial infections; Bacteriology; Bloodstream infections; Childbirth and infectious disease; Disinfectants and sanitizers; Epidemiology; Fungal infections; Hospitals and infectious disease; Hygiene; Iatrogenic infections; Immunity; Infection; Microbiology; Opportunistic infections; Parasitic diseases; Pathogens; Pregnancy and infectious disease; Primary infection; Public health; Superbacteria; Viral infections; Virology; Wound infections.

# Sepsis

CATEGORY: Diseases and conditions
ANATOMY OR SYSTEM AFFECTED: All

## DEFINITION

Sepsis is a systemic inflammatory response to infection. In the United States, about 750,000 persons develop sepsis each year, and 215,000 die from the infection. In the past, the term "septicemia" (or "blood poisoning") was often used interchangeably with sepsis, but that practice has fallen out of favor because the disease description, "blood poisoning," is considered imprecise.

## CAUSES

Sepsis often begins when there is an infection in the body. In this situation, the body frequently has trouble delivering oxygen to all the organs and cells that need it. The lungs, abdomen, urinary tract, skin, brain, and bone are common starting points for sepsis. Sepsis can also affect the intestine, where bacteria thrive, and already-infected areas after surgery. A foreign object (such as a catheter or drainage tube) inserted into the body also can cause sepsis.

### RISK FACTORS

Sepsis has become more common, especially among hospitalized persons. People at risk include the elderly, neonatal patients, immunocompromised persons, and persons who use injectable drugs. The widespread use of antibiotics encourages the growth of drug-resistant microorganisms. There is a higher incidence of sepsis when a person is already weakened by a condition such as malnutrition, alcoholism, liver disease, diabetes, a malignant neoplasm, organ transplantation, bone marrow transplantation, or human immunodeficiency virus (HIV) infection.

Of persons with end-stage renal disease, 75 percent will die of sepsis. Sepsis also causes high rates of mortality in persons undergoing dialysis and in renal transplant recipients. Systemic inflammatory response syndrome and acute respiratory distress syndrome are closely related to sepsis.

Among persons who already have sepsis, blacks are 80 percent more likely to die than are whites. Preliminary studies have identified socioeconomic status, educational level, genetics, and the number of other chronic diseases a person has as areas for further research into whether race has any effect on the mortality of people with sepsis.

### SYMPTOMS

Symptoms of sepsis include shaking, chills, fever, weakness, rapid heart rate, rapid breathing, low blood pressure, decreased urine output, nausea, vomiting, and diarrhea. Sepsis can cause infections that attack crucial body systems, such as the lining of the brain, the sac around the heart, the bones, or the large joints. Sepsis can also bring about impaired intestinal function.

Sepsis can attack the endothelium, the thin layer of cells within the blood vessels, which affects the circulation, the heart, and, ultimately, the organs of the body. Multiple organ failure is a common effect of sepsis. Apoptosis, also known as suicide of the cells, is closely linked to multiple organ failure and sepsis.

### SCREENING AND DIAGNOSIS

Because sepsis is so lethal, early diagnosis is crucial. Some of the signs are a temperature above 101° or below 96° Fahrenheit, a heart rate above ninety beats per minute, or a breathing rate faster than twenty beats per minute. Additional signs include having a white blood cell count greater than 12,000 cubic millimeters or having pus-forming or other pathogenic organisms. Blood cultures are drawn to determine the source of the infection. Diagnostic tests may also be performed on wound secretions or on cerebrospinal fluid. Imaging scans may be done too.

A number of factors can complicate diagnosis. Doctors often do not see persons with sepsis until those persons are in the later stages of illness and who tend to have several complex diseases. Sepsis may be one component of a larger disease process, such as systemic inflammatory response syndrome or multiple organ dysfunction syndrome.

If there is damage to vital organs, the diagnosis becomes severe sepsis. The most serious form of sepsis is septic shock, with the complication of low blood pressure that does not respond to standard treatment.

### TREATMENT AND THERAPY

Because sepsis spreads so quickly, treatment may start before the results of blood cultures are available. More potent antibiotics are available, covering a broader spectrum. Immunosuppressive agents may also be used. Other treatments include insulin, painkillers, sedatives, and surgery. One strategy is to attempt invasive treatment of inflammatory, infectious, and neoplastic diseases.

Clinical trials have shown some success with steroid treatment or activated protein C. Anti-inflammatory agents have not worked. In some clinical trials, researchers have used agents to counteract cell death.

Respiratory failure is treated with gas exchange and oxygen. To treat liver failure, therapy involves stimulating beta 2 receptors. For cardiac dysfunction, the patient is treated with volume therapy and vasoactive drugs. Ventilator support is used for neurological problems. Most survivors of sepsis regain renal function over time.

### PREVENTION AND OUTCOMES

The best protection against sepsis is frequent handwashing, staying current on immunizations, and seeking prompt care for infections. Skin that has redness, swelling, or pus should be examined by a doctor. In hospitals, the best prevention is identifying sepsis early and treating it with the correct antibiotic, a protocol that will help to reduce organ dysfunction. In many cases, however, sepsis strikes persons who are already vulnerable.

*Merrill Evans, M.A.*

**FURTHER READING**

Baue, Arthur, et al., eds. *Sepsis and Organ Dysfunction: Epidemiology and Scoring Systems: Pathophysiology and Therapy.* New York: Springer, 1998.

Bone, R. C., et al. "Definitions for Sepsis and Organ Failure and Guidelines for the Use of Innovative Therapies in Sepsis." *Chest* 101 (1992): 1644-1655.

Dellinger, R. Phillip, et al. "Surviving Sepsis Campaign: International Guidelines for Management of Severe Sepsis and Septic Shock: 2008." *Critical Care Medicine* 36 (2008): 296-327.

Evans, Timothy, and Mitchell P. Fink, eds. *Mechanisms of Organ Dysfunction in Critical Illness.* New York: Springer, 2002.

Folstad, Steven G. "Soft Tissue Infections." In *Emergency Medicine: A Comprehensive Study Guide*, edited by Judith E. Tintinalli. 6th ed. New York: McGraw-Hill, 2004.

Klein, Deborah G. "Shock and Sepsis." In *Introduction to Critical Care Nursing*, edited by Mary Lou Sole, Deborah G. Klein, and Marthe J. Moseley. 5th ed. St. Louis, Mo.: Saunders/Elsevier, 2009.

Mayr, Florian B., et al. "Infection Rate and Acute Organ Dysfunction Risk as Explanations for Racial Difference in Severe Sepsis." *Journal of the American Medical Association* 24 (2010): 2495-2503.

Sarnak, Mark J., and Bertrand L. Jaber. "Mortality Caused by Sepsis in Patients with End-Stage Renal Disease Compared with the General Population." *Kidney International* 58 (2000): 1758-1764.

Zucker-Franklin, D., et al. *Atlas of Blood Cells: Function and Pathology.* 3d ed. Philadelphia: Lea & Febiger, 2003.

**WEB SITES OF INTEREST**

*National Heart, Lung, and Blood Institute*
http://www.nhlbi.nih.gov

*Sepsis Alliance*
http://www.sepsisalliance.org

*Surviving Sepsis Campaign*
http://www.survivingsepsis.org

**See also:** Bacterial infections; Bloodstream infections; Disseminated intravascular coagulation; Infection; Neonatal sepsis; Osteomyelitis; Prosthetic joint infections; Septic arthritis; Septic shock.

# Septic arthritis

CATEGORY: Diseases and conditions
ANATOMY OR SYSTEM AFFECTED: Bones, joints, musculoskeletal system
ALSO KNOWN AS: Bacterial arthritis, infectious arthritis, prosthetic joint infection, pyogenic arthritis

## DEFINITION

Septic arthritis is a serious infection of the joints caused by bacteria. This infection causes a joint to be filled with pus cells, which in turn release substances directed against the bacteria. However, this action can damage the bone and surrounding cartilage.

Septic arthritis is a medical emergency. If left untreated, it causes loss of function in the affected joint and can lead to septic shock, a potentially fatal condition. With early treatment, however, recovery is usually good.

## CAUSES

Septic arthritis develops when bacteria spreads from the source of infection through the bloodstream to a joint. This condition can result from direct infection through an injection or a penetration wound, during surgical procedures, or from an injury that directly contaminates the joint.

Septic arthritis can strike at any age but occurs most often in children younger than age three years. In infants, the hip is a frequent site of infection; in toddlers, common sites of infection are the shoulders, knees, and hips. In these young persons, the most common bacterial causes are staphylococci (which cause staph infections), streptococci (which triggers strep throat), and *Streptococcus pneumoniae*, the bacterium responsible for most identified cases of pneumonia.

Septic arthritis rarely occurs from early childhood through adolescence. After this time, its incidence increases. In adults, it most commonly affects weight-bearing joints such as the knees. *Mycobacterium*, which causes tuberculosis, and *Borrelia*, the bacterium that causes Lyme disease, can also lead to septic arthritis.

### Risk Factors

The following increase one's chances of developing septic arthritis: diseases that weaken the immune system, such as human immunodeficiency virus infection, or taking drugs that suppress immunity; a history of joint problems or having other types of arthritis, gout, or lupus; a history of intravenous drug use; chronic illnesses such as anemia, diabetes, sickle cell disease, or kidney failure; joint replacement or organ transplant surgery; and skin conditions such as psoriasis or eczema that could allow for infections to penetrate through the skin.

### Symptoms

Symptoms of septic arthritis, in newborns or infants, include crying when the infected joint is moved (such as during a diaper change), immobility of the limb of the infected joint, irritability, fever, and persistent crying for any reason. In children and adults, the symptoms include intense joint pain, joint swelling and redness, fever, chills, and immobility of the infected joint or its limb.

### Screening and Diagnosis

A doctor, who will ask about symptoms and medical history and will perform a physical exam, may refer the patient to a rheumatologist or an orthopedics specialist. Tests may include withdrawing a sample of synovial fluid (fluid that lubricates the joint) from the affected joint to test it for white blood cells and bacteria, performing a culture of blood and urine to rule out other causes (such as gout), X rays to assess joint damage, and draining fluid from the infected joint. Severe cases may require surgery.

### Treatment and Therapy

Antibiotic therapy, which is started as soon as a diagnosis is made, is sometimes initially given intravenously to ensure the infected joint receives medication to kill the bacteria. The specific medications used depend on the type of bacteria determined to cause the infection. The remaining course of antibiotics may be given orally. Rest, immobilizing the joint, and warm compresses may be used to manage pain. Physical therapy or exercises may also speed recovery.

### Prevention and Outcomes

To help reduce the chance of getting septic arthritis, one should get prompt treatment for bacterial infections that could lead to septic arthritis. Persons in a high-risk group may be given antibiotics as a preventive measure.

*Sid Kirchheimer;*
*reviewed by David L. Horn, M.D., FACP*

### Further Reading

Forbes, Betty A., Daniel F. Sahm, and Alice S. Weissfeld. *Bailey and Scott's Diagnostic Microbiology.* 12th ed. St. Louis, Mo.: Mosby/Elsevier, 2007.

Górski, Andrzej, Hubert Krotkiewski, and Michał Zimecki, eds. *Inflammation.* Boston: Kluwer, 2001.

Klein, Deborah G. "Shock and Sepsis." In *Introduction to Critical Care Nursing*, edited by Mary Lou Sole, Deborah G. Klein, and Marthe J. Moseley. 5th ed. St. Louis, Mo.: Saunders/Elsevier, 2009.

Melvin, Jeanne L., and Virginia Wright, eds. *Pediatric Rheumatic Diseases.* Vol. 3. Bethesda, Md.: American Occupational Therapy Association, 2000.

Seibel, M. J., P. Robin Simon, and John P. Bilezikian, eds. *Dynamics of Bone and Cartilage Metabolism.* 2d ed. San Diego, Calif.: Academic Press, 2006.

### Web Sites of Interest

*Arthritis Foundation*
http://www.arthritis.org

*Arthritis Society*
http://www.arthritis.ca

*National Arthritis and Musculoskeletal and Skin Diseases Information Clearinghouse*
http://www.niams.nih.gov

**See also:** Bacterial endocarditis; Bacterial infections; Bloodstream infections; *Borrelia*; Children and infectious disease; Iatrogenic infections; Inflammation; *Mycobacterium*; Osteomyelitis; Prosthetic joint infections; Rheumatic fever; Sepsis; Septic shock; *Staphylococcus*; *Streptococcus*; Wound infections.

# Septic shock

CATEGORY: Diseases and conditions
ANATOMY OR SYSTEM AFFECTED: Blood, cardiovascular system, circulatory system, heart, immune system
ALSO KNOWN AS: Sepsis-associated organ dysfunction

## DEFINITION

Septic shock is acute cardiovascular collapse precipitated by a complex interaction between biochemical agents in the bloodstream and the body's immune system as it attempts to respond to infectious agents. Arterial hypotension persists despite adequate fluid resuscitation. The circulatory system is unable to meet the metabolic demands of cells: delivery of oxygen and nutrients and removal of waste products. Pumping and circulation fail, leading to reduced tissue perfusion and organ dysfunction. Mortality approaches 40 to 70 percent.

## CAUSES

Infectious agents such as gram-positive and gram-negative bacteria, viruses, fungi, and yeast trigger an exaggerated immune inflammatory response. The lipopolysaccharide (LPS) shell on gram-negative bacteria is an extremely strong stimulator of systemic inflammation.

## RISK FACTORS

Substantive risk factors include a compromised immune system, thermal burns, malnutrition, extremes of age, chronic medical conditions, use of invasive medical devices, hospitalization, steroid administration, and urinary tract, respiratory, or abdominal infection. Recent research has demonstrated polymorphisms, mutations, and dysregulation of cellular receptors that negatively affect the body's recognition of and response to pathogens.

## SYMPTOMS

Infection is heralded by fever, tachycardia, tachypnea, and abnormal white blood cell count. Respiratory distress or frank respiratory failure ensues. Myocardial depression, decreased cardiac output, and vasodilation lead to hypotension refractory and fluid resuscitation and may require vasopressor and hydrocortisone support. Peripheral pulses and capillary refill are diminished. A procoagulant state develops in an attempt to prevent the dissemination of pathogens, leading to coagulopathy and dermal petechiae and purpura. Renal and gastrointestinal function diminishes.

## SCREENING AND DIAGNOSIS

Diagnosis is incumbent on history, physical examination, clinical signs and symptoms, hematologic labs (blood culture, complete blood count, differential, immature to total neutrophil ratio, and serum lactate), acute-phase reactants and biomarkers (interleukin-6, adrenomedullin, C-reactive protein, and procalcitonin), and radiological evaluation of suspected source sites.

## TREATMENT AND THERAPY

Elimination of the infection source is vital to survival. Culture and sensitivity testing of infected sites to identify the causative organism allows selection of definitive antimicrobial therapy. Until culture results are known empiric antibiotic therapy is required. Antibiotics should be administered within an hour of a diagnosis of sepsis. Newer microarray testing is allowing earlier identification of pathogens leading to better definitive antibiotic therapy. Cardiovascular support includes adequate ventilation and oxygenation, vasopressor support, corticosteroids, and adequate hematologic parameters (platelets, red blood cells).

## PREVENTION AND OUTCOMES

Adequate nutrition, management of chronic illness, good handwashing technique, aseptic technique for sterile procedures, the avoidance of trauma or exposure to infectious agents, and the removal of unnecessary tubes and catheters in institutionalized and hospitalized persons reduces the incidence of infection and thus lowers the risk of an exaggerated inflammatory response and shock state.

*Wanda Bradshaw, M.S.N., R.N., NNP-BC, PNP, CCRN*

## FURTHER READING

Dellinger, R. Phillip, et al. "Surviving Sepsis Campaign: International Guidelines for Management of Severe Sepsis and Septic Shock: 2008." *Critical Care Medicine* 36 (2008): 296-327.

Evans, Timothy, and Mitchell P. Fink, eds. *Mechanisms of Organ Dysfunction in Critical Illness.* New York: Springer, 2002.

Klein, Deborah G. "Shock and Sepsis." In *Introduction to Critical Care Nursing*, edited by Mary Lou Sole,

Deborah G. Klein, and Marthe J. Moseley. 5th ed. St. Louis, Mo.: Saunders/Elsevier, 2009.

Tissari, Päivi, et al. "Accurate and Rapid Identification of Bacterial Species from Positive Blood Cultures with a DNA-based Microarray Platform." *The Lancet* 375 (January, 2010): 224-230.

## WEB SITES OF INTEREST

*National Heart, Lung, and Blood Institute*
http://www.nhlbi.nih.gov

*Sepsis Alliance*
http://www.sepsisalliance.org

*Surviving Sepsis Campaign*
http://www.survivingsepsis.org

**See also:** Antibodies; Bloodstream infections; Gangrene; Hygiene; Infection; Sepsis; Septic arthritis.

# Seroconversion

CATEGORY: Immune response

## DEFINITION

Seroconversion is the development of specific antibodies in the body in response to an infection or a vaccination. Many people associate seroconversion with human immunodeficiency virus (HIV) infection, in which an HIV-negative person (one who has no antibodies for the virus that causes acquired immunodeficiency syndrome, or AIDS) becomes HIV-positive (has antibodies to HIV, presumably resulting from infection with the virus). Seroconversion, however, is a natural function of the immune system that is not unique to HIV exposure, and it is beneficial in most cases.

## ANTIGENS AND ANTIBODIES

An antigen is a foreign material that enters the body. It can be an infectious organism (a bacterium, for example) or a foreign substance, such as pollen. Antibodies, also known as immunoglobulins (Igs), are molecules that recognize specific parts of an antigen, such as a protein on the surface of the antigen. The part of the antigen that the antibody recognizes is called an epitope. Antibodies bind to antigens because their binding sites fit the epitopes of the antigens. The fit extends beyond shape to other properties. For example, the binding site may have a complementary electrical charge to that of the epitope it recognizes.

Antibodies are produced by specialized white blood cells (lymphocytes) called B cells. Each antibody is specific to antigens that have similar epitopes.

## SEROCONVERSION

B cells produce specific antibodies in response to an entry of a foreign substance (or microorganism) into the body. Seroconversion is the appearance of these specific antibodies. The body's initial immune response, which includes seroconversion, may take time to build, which explains why a person often gets sick when first exposed. The immune system retains a memory of the infection even after it clears from the body, so the production of antibodies and other immune responses happen much quicker for any subsequent infections. If the same infection attacks the body again, the person infected could be asymptomatic or could have only a mild illness.

## IMPACT

Seroconversion is a significant concept in immunity. The production of specific antibodies against an invading microorganism is one in a series of responses that allows humans to overcome many infections that would otherwise overwhelm the body. This system, however, can go awry. In autoimmune diseases, such as AIDS, the body makes antibodies (seroconverts) against its own tissues, producing serious health consequences for the person with the autoimmune disorder.

Seroconversion can be used to test earlier exposure to infections, and it can also assess response to treatments of infectious diseases. In persons with hepatitis B, for example, treatment success can be measured by seroconversion to antibodies against the hepatitis B e antigen, with the corresponding disappearance of the antigen itself from circulation. Studies based on seroconversion and the persistence of antibodies in circulation have also been used to evaluate vaccines such as MMR (measles, mumps, and rubella) to determine how long a person is protected from disease before needing a booster vaccine.

*Adi R. Ferrara, B.S., ELS*

## FURTHER READING

Murphy, Kenneth, Paul Travers, and Mark Walport. *Janeway's Immunobiology*. 7th ed. New York: Garland Science, 2008.

Parham, Peter. *The Immune System*. 3d ed. New York: Garland Science, 2009.

Sompayrac, Lauren M. *How the Immune System Works*. 3d ed. Hoboken, N.J.: Wiley-Blackwell, 2008.

## WEB SITES OF INTEREST

*AIDSinfo*
http://aidsinfo.nih.gov

*Microbiology and Immunology On-line: Immunology*
http://pathmicro.med.sc.edu/book/immunol-sta.htm

**See also:** Agammaglobulinemia; AIDS; Antibiotics: Types; Antibodies; Autoimmune disorders; HIV; Immune response to bacterial infections; Immune response to parasitic diseases; Immune response to viral infections; Immunity; Immunodeficiency; Incubation period; Infection; Neutropenia; Opportunistic infections; Reinfection; T lymphocytes; Virology.

# Serology

CATEGORY: Diagnosis

## DEFINITION

Serology is the scientific study of serum, or body fluids such as blood, semen, and saliva. In serology, serum is tested to identify antibodies that form in response to microorganisms, such as viruses, bacteria, and parasites, that are foreign to the body.

Blood serum, the liquid part of blood that is normally golden yellow, is the substance that remains after blood cells are removed. Serum (naturally) comprises water and a very high number of various proteins. These proteins include albumin, which aids in the proper retention of water in the bloodstream, and globulins, which are proteins produced by antigens that act as antibodies. Serum accumulates on burns, scrapes, or impetigo sores, and as it dries, it produces a characteristic honey-golden crust.

Antibodies usually form from three causes: in response to an infection against a given microorganism; in response to other foreign proteins, such as mismatched blood from a transfusion; and in response to one's own proteins, in cases of autoimmune disease. The search for an explanation for immunity to disease led to the discovery of modified globulins (named antibodies) in blood serum. It was recognized that antibodies protected against disease-causing viruses and bacteria in the same way that they reacted to innocuous substances, and that specific immune antibodies reacted only to specific antigens or closely related ones. This phenomenon of specificity underlies the practical application of serology. Serological reactions were first adapted to laboratory tests used in the diagnosis of disease in the nineteenth century.

## TECHNIQUE

The body site for serological testing is first cleaned with antiseptic. An elastic band is wrapped around, for example, the upper arm to apply pressure to the area and to make the vein swell with blood. Blood is drawn from a vein, usually from the inside of the elbow or the back of the hand. The blood collects into an airtight vial or tube attached to a needle. The elastic band is removed, and once the blood has been collected, the needle is removed and the puncture site is covered to stop any bleeding.

In infants or young children, a lancet may be used to puncture the skin and make it bleed. The blood collects into a small glass tube called a pipette or onto a slide or test strip. A bandage may be placed over the area if there is any bleeding. The blood is then analyzed in a laboratory.

## APPLICATION

A serology test can be used to diagnose a rheumatic or autoimmune disease or an active or previous infection. It is also used to determine if a person is immune to reinfection by an organism and used to determine blood type.

*Blood typing.* Austrian American pathologist Karl Landsteiner recognized several types of antigens when he separated red blood cells from plasma in a centrifuge. When he added red blood cells from other persons, he found two distinct reactions: repelling and clumping. These two reactions were labeled "A" (when antigen A is present, antigen B is absent, and anti-B antibody is present) and "B" (when antigen B is present and antigen A is absent). A third reaction was labeled "O." This labeling system came to be known as the ABO blood-typing system. Modern blood typing includes testing for many types of enzymes and proteins. Scientists have found more than 150 serum proteins and 250 varieties of cellular enzymes.

*Finding an infection.* The use of a particular serological technique is dependent upon the antibodies suspected. A large variety of serological tests are available, including complement-fixation (CFT), hemagglutination-inhibition (HAI), enzyme-linked immunoassay (EIA), radioimmunoassay (RIA), particle agglutination, immunofluorescence, single radial haemolysis, and Western blot. Most techniques will detect all classes of antibody, although some can be made to detect one specific class only. In the case of a current infection, more antibodies will be present as the disease worsens. If a disease is suspected, the test may need to be repeated from ten days to two weeks after the first test.

Some viral infections may be diagnosed by serology but are better diagnosed by an alternative method. These viruses include herpesviruses (that reactivate from time to time) and respiratory and enteroviruses (the illness has passed by the time an antibody is detectable). The following viral infections, however, are likely to remain diagnosable by serology: hepatitis A, B, and C; human immunodeficiency (HIV); rubella; parvovirus; and Epstein-Barr (EBV).

Hepatitis A, B, and C routinely cannot be cultured. However, serological tests, including the test for HBsAg (the surface antigen of the hepatitis B virus), are well established for these viruses. Despite the availability of molecular biological techniques for the detection of viral nucleic acid, serology is unlikely to be challenged as the main means of diagnosis for hepatitis A, B, and C.

HIV can be diagnosed by serology, except in newborns. Rubella and parvovirus can be diagnosed by serology because the onset of clinical symptoms coincides with the appearance of antibodies, and, thus, there is little need for other means of diagnosis. Although EBV serology is reliable, the heterophile antibody test is usually used for diagnosing cases of infectious mononucleosis.

## IMPACT

The impact of serology is wide and deep. Serology is a useful way to monitor the success of treatment of

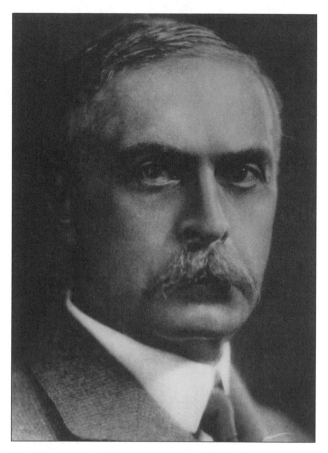

*Karl Landsteiner.* (The Nobel Foundation)

infection without using invasive or more expensive methods. Serology can be used to estimate the proportion of disease caused by a certain pathogen in a specific population. It has been used to describe the movement of populations and has answered other anthropological questions.

Advances in serology have made possible earlier diagnosis and, therefore, earlier initiation of therapy. For example, the diagnosis of tuberculosis in a person with HIV infection had been hampered by the low yield of acid-fast bacilli on smear and culture studies. Serology provides an effective alternative.

The development of the ABO blood-typing system has saved millions of lives by avoiding mismatched blood tranfusions and organ transplantations; likewise, the discovery of the Rh antigen has helped millions of pregnant women avoid miscarriage.

Serology also has been applied to drug testing and has given rise to the industry known as biotech (biotechnology), which is focused on the creation of monoclonal antibodies.

*Stephanie Eckenrode, B.A.*

**FURTHER READING**

James, Stuart H., and Jon J. Nordby. *Forensic Science: An Introduction to Scientific and Investigative Techniques.* Boca Raton, Fla.: CRC Press, 2002. A broad examination of forensic science, which includes serology. Includes illustrations and case studies.

Sachs, Hans. "Some Considerations on the History and Development of Serological Science." *Irish Journal of Medical Science*, no. 185 (May, 1941): 177-185. An early article on the development of serology as a medical science.

Stanley, Jacqueline. *Essentials of Immunology and Serology.* Albany, N.Y.: Delmar, 2002. Comprehensive, yet straightforward; explains how the components of the immune system combine to generate the immune response and how these responses relate to infectious diseases.

Turgeon, Mary Louise. *Immunology and Serology in Laboratory Medicine.* 4th ed. St. Louis, Mo.: Mosby/Elsevier, 2009. A good introductory clinical text that details methodologies, clinical applications, and interpretations of basic serology.

**WEB SITES OF INTEREST**

*Biochemical Society*
http://www.biochemistry.org

*Lab Tests Online*
http://www.labtestsonline.org

*Protocolpedia*
http://www.protocolpedia.com

*Virtual Library of Biochemistry, Molecular Biology, and Cell Biology*
http://www.biochemweb.org

**See also:** Acid-fastness; Antibodies; Bacteriology; Biochemical tests; Gram staining; Immunoassay; Infection; Microbiology; Microscopy; Pathogens; Polymerase chain reaction (PCR) method; Pulsed-field gel electrophoresis; Virology.

---

Severe acute respiratory syndrome. *See* SARS.

# Sexually transmitted diseases (STDs)

CATEGORY: Transmission
ALSO KNOWN AS: Sexually transmitted infections, VD, venereal diseases

**DEFINITION**

Sexually transmitted diseases (STDs) are infections that are primarily contracted through sexual contact. Until the 1980's, STDs were commonly known as venereal diseases, a derivative of the name "Venus," the Roman goddess of love. By the beginning of the twenty-first century, however, another shift in terminology arose. Because a sexually transmitted pathogen may cause an infection that may or may not lead to a disease, some health authorities prefer to distinguish between a sexually transmitted infection (STI) and the potential consequence of that infection, an STD. Nevertheless, "STD" is still preferred by many health agencies, such as the Centers for Disease Control and Prevention, and is typically used synonymously with STI.

**TRANSMISSION AND EPIDEMIOLOGY**

The three most prevalent routes of STD transmission are through mucous membranes, skin breaks or abrasions, and bodily fluids. Mucous membranes, which include the lips, penis head, and vaginal lining, are more easily penetrable by pathogens than is skin. This is one reason sexual activity, more than non-sexual skin-to-skin contact, increases the probability of transmitting an infection. Although the skin is a more effective barrier to pathogens than mucous membranes, sexual activity that tears or abrades the skin will weaken that barrier. Furthermore, some STDs, such as human papillomavirus (HPV) and herpes simplex (HSV), are transmissible by skin-to-skin contact. Most sexual activities involve the exchange of bodily fluids, such as genital fluids or saliva. Bodily fluids may harbor viruses or other potentially harmful microbes, making sexual activity a prime means of disease transmission.

The communicable period for an STD is the time the disease can be transmitted. Many people think that if a person has no symptoms of an STD, then he or she cannot transmit an STD to someone else. This thinking is erroneous, however, because disease carriers may be asymptomatic (without discernable symptoms) yet able to transmit an infection. Additionally, the incubation period, the time between being infected and the appearance of the disease symptoms, varies greatly among STDs. Thus, a person may not appear to be a carrier only because the disease has not progressed to the stage in which symptoms are evident.

STDS have been a scourge on society since ancient times. For example, the Bible describes measures that are used to prevent the spread of what was probably (based on the description of the discharge) gonorrhea. It appears, however, that STDs are more widespread in modern society than they were in ancient times. The extent of STDs in a society is measured in two ways: The incidence of a disease is the number of new cases, whereas the prevalence of an affliction refers to the total number of cases.

Several factors have contributed to the dramatic increase in the prevalence of STDs since the 1970's. These factors include premarital sex, a decrease in the age of sexual activity, the availability of hormonal contraception, and the legalization of abortion.

The actual incidence of STDs can be only roughly estimated because of a lack of comprehensive reporting. Health authorities estimate that between 400 million and 500 million new cases of STDs occur worldwide each year; up to 12 million people in the United States become infected annually. In the United States, the prevalence of STDs has been estimated as follows: 25 percent of the population has a minimum of one STD by age twenty-one years, 33 percent by age twenty-four years, and 50 percent by age thirty-five years.

## RISK FACTORS

Given the prevalence of STDs in the United States, it has been estimated that the probability of being infected with a minimum of one STD during one act of sexual intercourse is approximately 25 percent. This likelihood varies greatly, however, depending on numerous factors, which can be categorized into behavioral and demographic variables.

In general, any interpersonal sexual behavior carries some risk of transmitting an STD. The risk progressively increases, however, as the number of sexual partners increases. Research has also shown that the less familiar one is with a sexual partner and the more promiscuous are those in a person's social network, the greater the risk of STD infection. Additionally,

some types of sexual practices are riskier than others. Overall, anal sex presents the greatest risk for the spread of STDs, followed by vaginal intercourse and oral sex. Using barrier contraceptive methods significantly decreases the risk but does not eliminate it. Latex condoms are more effective than natural membranes in preventing pathogen transmission; however, even latex condoms are not 100 percent effective against viruses, including the human immunodeficiency virus (HIV).

STDs can also be transmitted through nonsexual behaviors. Any skin-to-skin contact can transmit STDs such as syphilis, HPV, and herpes. Intravenous drug use increases the risk for many STDS, such as HIV. STDs can be passed on to offspring through birth and through breast-feeding. For example, a woman who has a genital STD, such as herpes, can pass that on to her fetus if she gives birth vaginally. Also, breast milk may contain HIV or other pathogens. (However, breast milk also contains antibacterial and antiviral substances.)

Infection with one STD increases the risk of infection with another STD. For example, having genital herpes increases the likelihood of getting infected with HIV. Moreover, having an STD may weaken the immune system, making it easier for another STD to establish itself in a person's body.

Several demographic variables are associated with STD risk. A woman's reproductive system provides a better host (because of its greater mucosal surface area) and an easier entry point into the body (such as open ends of the Fallopian tubes) than does a man's reproductive system for diverse pathogens that cause STDs. Consequently, a woman is much more likely to be infected with an STD than is a man. Moreover, women are more likely to be asymptomatic for STDs and more likely to suffer additional adverse effects, such as pelvic inflammatory disease or infertility.

The gender risk factor is often compounded with age. People age fifteen to twenty-five years are the most likely to be infected with an STD, and for females the risk is especially high because the cervical ectropion (which recedes with age) is easily infected by pathogens. Younger people typically engage in riskier sexual practices and are more likely to use drugs (impairing their decision-making abilities). Both practices put younger people at greater risk for STD infection.

Other significant demographic factors for developing

## Trends in Sexually Transmitted Diseases in the United States: Data for Gonorrhea, Chlamydia, and Syphilis (2009)

| | Gonorrhea | Chlamydia | Syphilis |
|---|---|---|---|
| **Disease Burden** | Cases reported: 301,174<br>Rate per 100,000: 99.1 | Cases reported: 1,244,180<br>Rate per 100,000: 409.2 | Cases reported: 13,997<br>Rate per 100,000: 4.6 |
| **Trends over Time** | Reported gonorrhea cases declined steadily (17 percent since 2006) and are now at the lowest level since the CDC began tracking the disease in 1941.<br><br>While gonorrhea is declining for all races and ethnicities, since 2006 the drop has been smaller for blacks (15 percent) than for Hispanics (21 percent) or whites (25 percent). | Chlamydia diagnoses are up 19 percent from 2006. The increase is likely caused by expanded screening and not an increase in disease. From 2000 to 2009, the chlamydia screening rate among young women nearly doubled (from 25 to 47 percent).<br><br>However, data suggest that most young women are still not getting screened. The CDC estimates that there are 2.8 million chlamydia cases annually, more than twice the number actually reported. | Reported syphilis cases overall continue to rise (39 percent since 2006). For the first time in several years, syphilis did not increase among women. There was an 88 percent increase in syphilis among women from 2004 to 2008.<br><br>For the first time in several years, cases of congenital syphilis did not increase in 2009 (427 total cases). Since 1991, which saw 4,424 reported cases, rates have declined. |

Source: Centers for Disease Control and Prevention.

an STD include sexual orientation, race and ethnicity, socioeconomic standing, and geographic location. Gay and bisexual men tend to engage in riskier sexual behaviors and tend to have more sex partners than heterosexuals. African Americans, followed by Hispanic Americans, and persons of lower socioeconomic status tend to engage in sexual activity at younger ages and tend to have more sex partners. Also, the prevalence of STDs is much higher in urban locations than in suburban or rural areas.

## COMMON STDS AND THEIR SYMPTOMS

There are more than thirty different STDs, which are caused by bacteria, viruses, protozoa, fungi, and parasites. Although each STD has a distinctive symptom profile, there are general indicators of STDs. These indicators include genital itching, rashes, sores, and warts; painful sex and urination; genital discharge; and flulike symptoms such as aches, pains, night sweats, and fever.

*Chlamydia.* The most common bacterial STD is chlamydia, which is estimated to affect 50 percent of all sexually active women in the United States by the age of thirty years. Symptoms include genital discharge and burning or painful urination; however, more than 80 percent of women and nearly 50 percent of men are asymptomatic. More than 20 percent of women infected with *Chlamydia* will develop PID, and chlamydia infection is a major cause of miscarriages and tubal pregnancies. Chlamydia also can lead to infertility.

*Gonorrhea.* The second most common bacterial STD is gonorrhea (also known as clap or drip). The symptoms and consequences are like those of chlamydia, and about one-half of all people with gonorrhea have chlamydia. As with chlamydia, approximately 80 percent of women are asymptomatic; however, more than 80 percent of men notice greenish-yellow discharge from the penis.

*Syphilis.* Syphilis is caused by a spirochete bacterium

that invades the bloodstream through the skin and leaves a round, painless chancre sore at the point of entry a few weeks after infection. If untreated by antibiotics, a nonitching skin rash will occur, which will disappear as the disease progresses to an asymptomatic latency stage that often lasts for years. In its final stage, untreated syphilis may lead to blindness, heart failure, or brain damage (or all of these conditions).

Other common bacterial STDs include nongonococcal or nonspecific urethritis, which causes burning urination; chancroid, which results in painful genital sores; and bacterial vaginosis, which is accompanied by vaginal itching and a fishy odor.

*Genital herpes and warts.* The most common viral STDs are genital herpes and warts, caused by herpes simplex and HPV viruses, respectively. Herpes causes painful genital blisters that will recur up to several times a year for the rest of a person's life. HPV causes nonpainful genital warts that may grow to cause painful genital or anal obstructions. HPV is associated with approximately 80 percent of cervical cancer cases and is linked with other cancers.

*HIV infection.* Both herpes and HPV increase the risk of HIV infection, which may lead to acquired immunodeficiency syndrome (AIDS). AIDS weakens the immune system and compromises the body's ability to fight infections and diseases, which may be fatal. HIV infection may lead to flulike symptoms; however, initial infection is typically asymptomatic.

*Hepatitis.* More infectious than HIV are the several viruses that can cause hepatitis, a disease that affects the liver. Symptoms of hepatitis include jaundice, darkened urine, fatigue, diarrhea, and nausea; however, about one-half of all infected people are asymptomatic. Consequences of hepatitis include liver inflammation, which may progress to cirrhosis or cancer.

Several nonbacterial and nonviral STDs have their primary symptom as genital itching. The fungus *Candida albicans* is present in healthy women but can multiply when the chemical balance of the vagina is disturbed, producing a condition known as candidiasis. Candidiasis can be sexually transmitted and result in vaginal irritation and a "cheesy" discharge. Trichomoniasis is a common condition transmitted by a single-celled protozoan that causes a frothy, green-yellow vaginal discharge with a foul odor. Scabies and lice (also known as crabs) are highly contagious parasites that can cause intense itching and rashes. Protozoan and parasitic organisms can live in cloth and can sur-

vive on nonporous surfaces, providing numerous nonsexual means of transmission.

## Prevention and Treatment

There are three main ways to prevent STDs: Limit exposure to carriers of STDs, decrease risky practices, and increase behaviors that may guard against STDs. The best way to prevent STDs is to practice sexual abstinence. The second most effective preventive measure is to practice sexual exclusivity with an uninfected partner. If these two measures fail, then limiting the number of sexual partners and asking potential sexual partners if they have an STD will reduce the risk of infection.

Certain actions increase the likelihood of STD transmission and can be reduced or avoided. Such behaviors include sexual intercourse without a condom; allowing the blood, semen, or vaginal fluid of an infected partner to contact one's genitals, anus, or mouth; and allowing contaminated objects, such as used needles, to penetrate one's skin. Some practices have been demonstrated to decrease the risk of transmitting an STD. Among these are being circumcised, washing with soap before and after sex, urinating before and after sex, and getting vaccinated against viruses that cause warts and hepatitis. There are, however, concerns about the side effects of some of the vaccines. To prevent the maternal transmission of STDs, women can treat an STD before conceiving or early in the course of pregnancy, can give birth by cesarean section instead of vaginally, and can abstain from breast-feeding.

Treatment for a suspected STD begins with proper diagnosis. Diagnostic tests include visual inspection for lesions and parasites, laboratory cultures for discharges, and blood tests. Once the specific infection is identified, a treatment course is determined. Special soaps are first-line treatments for scabies and lice. Antibiotics may also be prescribed for parasitic and protozoan infections. Antibiotics are the main treatment option for bacterial STIs; however, because of acquired resistance by some bacteria, only certain antibiotics may work against the specific bacteria that are causing the particular infection being treated. Antibiotics will exacerbate fungi infections. Other options are vaginal creams, probiotics, and drugs such as nystatin. Viral infections are not curable with antibiotics, but there are numerous antiviral drugs that can decrease the severity and frequency of viral outbreaks.

## IMPACT

The physical consequences of STDs are a double-edged sword. On one hand, the carrier's health is threatened. STDs can cause physical scarring, pain, damaged organs, infertility, cancer, heart disease, and death. On the other hand, a carrier can hurt one's spouse or significant other or can hurt a former romantic partner.

The health consequences exact a staggering financial burden on society too. The American Social Health Association estimated that at the beginning of the twenty-first century, the direct annual medical cost of bacterial and viral STDs in the United States was $8.4 billion. More difficult to estimate is the psychological cost of STDs. A host of negative emotions, such as embarrassment, guilt, shame, regret, depression, and anger, can beset persons with STD infections.

*Paul J. Chara, Jr., Ph.D.*

## FURTHER READING

Aral, Sevgi O., et al., eds. *Behavioral Interventions for Prevention and Control of Sexually Transmitted Diseases.* New York: Springer, 2008. A comprehensive review of diverse social and individual approaches in preventing STDs.

Bolton, M., A. McKay, and M. Schneider. "Relational Influences on Condom Use Discontinuation: A Qualitative Study of Young Adult Women in Dating Relationships." *Canadian Journal of Human Sexuality* 19 (2010): 91-104. Results of a qualitative study that examines "the psycho-social dynamics of condom use discontinuation within dating relationships."

Boston Women's Health Collective. *Our Bodies, Ourselves: A New Edition for a New Era.* 35th anniversary ed. New York: Simon & Schuster, 2005. A popular, classic book dealing with all aspects of women's sexuality, including STDs and safer sex.

Fan, Hung Y., Ross F. Conner, and Luis P. Villarreal. *AIDS: Science and Society.* 5th ed. Sudbury, Mass.: Jones and Bartlett, 2007. A good discussion of the perspectives of science and society regarding HIV infection and AIDS.

Grimes, Jill. *Seductive Delusions: How Everyday People Catch STDs.* Baltimore: Johns Hopkins University Press, 2008. Retelling the stories of persons with STDs, the author provides basic information on the risks of STD infection and on the treatment options available.

Marr, Lisa. *Sexually Transmitted Diseases: A Physician Tells You What You Need to Know.* 2d ed. Baltimore: Johns Hopkins University Press, 2007. A physician who specializes in the treatment of STDs offers a readable introduction to the most common STDs.

Nack, Adina. *Damaged Goods? Women Living with Incurable Sexually Transmitted Diseases.* Philadelphia: Temple University Press, 2008. An informative and insightful examination of women who are living with STDs and how they see themselves as sexual beings facing social stigma.

## WEB SITES OF INTEREST

*American Social Health Association*
http://www.ashastd.org

*Centers for Disease Control and Prevention*
http://www.cdc.gov/std

*National Institute of Allergy and Infectious Diseases*
http://www.niaid.nih.gov

*National Women's Health Information Center*
http://www.womenshealth.gov

*Sex Information and Education Council of Canada*
http://www.sieccan.org

**See also:** AIDS; Bacterial infections; Cervical cancer; Childbirth and infectious disease; Chlamydia; Contagious diseases; Genital herpes; Genital warts; Gonorrhea; Herpesvirus infections; HIV; Human papillomavirus (HPV) infections; Men and infectious disease; Mononucleosis; Oral transmission; Pregnancy and infectious disease; Public health; Saliva and infectious disease; Schools and infectious disease; Social effects of infectious disease; Syphilis; Transmission routes; Viral infections; Women and infectious disease.

---

# *Shigella*

CATEGORY: Pathogen
TRANSMISSION ROUTE: Direct contact, ingestion

## DEFINITION

*Shigella* are gram-negative, nonmotile, non-spore-forming, nonencapsulated, facultative-anaerobic rods

## Taxonomic Classification for *Shigella*

**Kingdom:** Bacteria
**Phylum:** Proteobacteria
**Class:** Gammaproteobacteria
**Order:** Enterobacteriales
**Family:** Enterobacteriaceae
**Genus:** *Shigella*
**Species:**
*S. boydii*
*S. dysenteriae*
*S. flexneri*
*S. sonnei*

that cause bacillary dysentery (shigellosis) in humans and other primates.

### NATURAL HABITAT AND FEATURES

*Shigella* was named for Kiyoshi Shiga, a Japanese physician and bacteriologist, who first isolated *S. dysenteriae* in 1896. There are four recognized species. Other *Shigella* spp. that were named in the first half of the twentieth century have either been moved to other genera (for example, *Shigella galinarum* is now *Salmonella galinarum*) or subsumed into one of the four recognized species (for example, *S. ambigua* is now *S. dysenteriae* type II). These bacteria are closely related to *Escherichia coli* and share most genes with *E. coli* strain K12.

*Shigella* spp. infections occur only naturally in primates. Other animals are not normally infected, but infections have been induced in a few animals used as models for the disease and its treatment. Infection is usually fecal to oral and can occur anytime food or water becomes contaminated with infected feces. Infection also can occur during certain sex practices. Good hygiene, including thorough handwashing with soap and water after fecal elimination, is the best way to prevent shigellosis.

The most common site for bacterial growth is in the large intestine. A dose of as few as ten organisms is enough to cause infection in some persons. Symptoms usually occur twenty-four to forty-eight hours after ingestion of *Shigella*-contaminated food or water. *Shigella* spp. thrive in the large intestine and, because of their virulence plasmid, have the ability to invade intestinal epithelial cells. This invasion leads to the most common symptoms of shigellosis: diarrhea, abdominal cramps, nausea, and vomiting. In addition, blood, pus, and mucus are often present in the stool because invasion often leads to ulceration of the colonic epithelium.

The disease is usually self-limiting and lasts about one week in healthy adults, by which time the immune system disposes of the invading bacteria. In infants, small children, and those debilitated from other illnesses, the disease may last longer; dehydration caused by diarrhea and vomiting can lead to severe problems. Damaging enterotoxins and Shiga toxins are coded by the virulence plasmid and are produced by most strains. Shiga toxins can cause hemolytic uremic syndrome, which leads to anemia and kidney failure. Some non-*Shigella* spp. also contain Shiga toxins because plasmid transfer can occur across species lines. A small percentage of persons with *S. flexneri* may develop Reiter's syndrome, which causes joint pain, eye irritation, and painful urination. Reiter's syndrome can last months or even years and can lead to difficult-to-treat chronic arthritis.

Persons often remain infective for up to two weeks after the dysentery symptoms abate because bacteria remain in the intestine for one to two weeks after recovery. For several years after infection, persons may retain immunity against the particular *Shigella* strain that infected them, but they are susceptible to other strains. Rehydration is the main treatment for shigellosis; however, antibiotic therapy can be used in severe cases. The antibiotics of choice are ampicillin, trimethoprim/sulfamethoxazole, nalidixic acid, ciprofloxacin, and azithromycin. Because resistance plasmids are easily transferred between members of the Enterobacteriaceae, antibiotic resistant *Shigella* strains are becoming more widespread. Various *Shigella* vaccines have been investigated and live attenuated vaccines have been tested; however, no broad-spectrum *Shigella* vaccine is available.

*S. dysenteriae* has twelve serotypes and is the major cause of epidemic dysentery. This disease usually occurs in less developed countries with poor sanitation and is often seen in Africa, Southeast Asia, and the Indian sub-continent. Fecal to oral transmission usually occurs because of sewage-contaminated water. *S. dysenteriae* type I causes the most severe form of shigellosis. It is especially severe in malnourished and otherwise debilitated persons; life-threatening complications often occur. More than 30 percent of dysentery cases worldwide are caused by *S. dysenteriae*.

*S. flexneri*, with six serotypes, is the most common cause of endemic dysentery worldwide and accounts for more than 60 percent of shigellosis in less-developed countries. The main sources are contaminated water and food caused by poor sanitation and the use of human waste to fertilize crop plants. Neither *S. dysenteriae* nor *S. flexneri* are major pathogens in areas where good sanitation leads to the availability of clean water and proper disposal of fecal wastes. In the developed world, less than 15 percent of shigellosis cases can be traced to *S. flexneri* and even less to *S. dysenteriae*. *S. sonnei* has a single serotype and is biochemically different than the other *Shigella* spp. The only known reservoir of *S. sonnei* is the human intestinal tract, and this bacterium does not survive for extended periods in other locations. It is most commonly transmitted by infected food handlers who have poor hygiene and is the most common cause of endemic shigellosis in developed countries. Approximately 77 percent of shigellosis in developed countries and 70 percent in the United States is caused by *S sonnei*, which is less virulent than other *Shigella* spp. and causes a milder form of shigellosis. Occasional outbreaks have occurred in the United States and have been traced to *S. sonnei*-infected food handlers.

*S. boydii*, with twenty-three known serotypes, is the most genetically diverse of the *Shigella* spp. As in other *Shigella* spp., most *S. boydii* serotypes are similar to *E. coli*; however, there are some that seem to share genes with *Vibrio cholerae*. Although *S. boydii* has worldwide distribution, it is most common on the Indian subcontinent. It affects all primates, including humans, and can survive for extended periods in the soil. It is responsible for only a small percentage of human shigellosis in the rest of the world.

*Richard W. Cheney, Jr., Ph.D.*

**FURTHER READING**

Garrity, George M., ed. *The Proteobacteria*. Vol. 2 in *Bergey's Manual of Systematic Bacteriology*. 2d ed. New York: Springer, 2005. This volume describes the Proteobacteria in detail.

Madigan, Michael T., and John M. Martinko. *Brock Biology of Microorganisms*. 12th ed. Upper Saddle River, N.J.: Pearson/Prentice Hall, 2010. This text outlines many common bacteria and describes their natural history, pathogenicity, and other characteristics.

Niyogi, S. K. "Shigellosis." *Journal of Microbiology* 43

(2005): 133-143. This article reviews shigellosis and its effects on human health.

Romich, Janet A. *Understanding Zoonotic Diseases*. Clifton Park, N.Y.: Thomson Delmar Learning, 2008. This book has a good section on shigellosis and its causes and treatments.

**WEB SITES OF INTEREST**

*Canadian Partnership for Consumer Food Safety Education*
http://www.canfightbac.org

*Centers for Disease Control and Prevention, Division of Foodborne, Bacterial, and Mycotic Diseases*
http://www.cdc.gov/nczved/divisions/dfbmd

*U.S. Department of Agriculture, Food Safety Information Center*
http://foodsafety.nal.usda.gov

**See also:** Amebic dysentery; Bacteria: Classification and types; *Enterobacter*; *Escherichia*; Fecal-oral route of transmission; Food-borne illness and disease; Intestinal and stomach infections; Microbiology; Pathogens; Primates and infectious disease; *Salmonella*; Salmonellosis; Shigellosis; Travelers' diarrhea; Waterborne illness and disease.

# Shigellosis

CATEGORY: Diseases and conditions
ANATOMY OR SYSTEM AFFECTED: Gastrointestinal system, intestines, stomach

**DEFINITION**

The microscopic bacterium *Shigella* causes the infectious disease shigellosis. An acute bacterial infection attacks the lining of the intestines, resulting in diarrhea, fever, and stomach cramps.

**CAUSES**

Shigellosis is spread by fecal-oral contact. This can occur when people ingest food or water contaminated with *Shigella*. Shigellosis can spread when food grows in a field that contains contaminated water. Flies can spread shigellosis by breeding in infected feces. Shigellosis can also spread when people drink, swim in, or play in contaminated water. Transmission can be spread through sexual contact, particularly through anal and oral sex.

Shigellosis commonly occurs in developing countries with inadequate sanitation. It thrives in areas with overcrowding, poor handwashing technique, and lack of protocols for safe food and water. The disease also spreads easily in close quarters, such as daycare centers, refugee camps, and jails and prisons.

### RISK FACTORS

About eighteen thousand cases of shigellosis are reported in the United States alone each year. Many milder cases are not diagnosed or reported; public health officials estimate the actual number of cases could be as high as 360,000 annually. The infection is most common in children age two to four years.

Shigellosis is the most common cause of diarrhea among visitors to developing countries. It infects hundreds of millions of people around the world each year, resulting in an estimated one million deaths, mostly among children in countries with inadequate medical resources.

### SYMPTOMS

The symptoms of watery diarrhea, fever, and stomach cramps begin from one to three days after a person comes into contact with the bacterium. In some cases, the incubation period is as short as twelve hours. Often, the diarrhea contains blood and mucus, and the infected person may develop fever. Some experience nausea, vomiting, anorexia, or a cramping rectal pain. The symptoms usually resolve within five to seven days, even without treatment, but the infected person may still be contagious for another week or two.

Some people do not experience symptoms at all, but while infected, they can pass *Shigella* to others. Sometimes, dehydration occurs, which can lead to the death of a person who has severe shigellosis.

In developing countries, infected persons may experience prolonged, acute diarrhea, lasting seven to thirteen days, or persistent diarrhea, lasting fourteen days or more; this leads to malnutrition. These long-term conditions have the potential to be life-threatening.

About 3 percent of persons with shigellosis develop Reiter's syndrome, consisting of pain of the joints, irritation of the eyes, and painful urination. The syndrome can last for months or years, and it can lead to

chronic, treatment-resistant arthritis. Another rare complication is hemolytic-uremic syndrome, a form of kidney failure that includes anemia and clotting problems.

Persons with high fever, confusion, headache with stiff neck, lethargy, or seizures should seek emergency care. These symptoms are most common in children.

### SCREENING AND DIAGNOSIS

A stool culture identifies *Shigella* in the feces of an infected person. Because there are several different strains of *Shigella*, the stool culture will help to determine the correct treatment. A blood test also may be done if symptoms are severe, or to rule out other causes.

### TREATMENT AND THERAPY

Persons with mild cases of shigellosis usually recover quickly, without treatment. However, antibiotics can shorten the course of the illness by a few days. Some *Shigella* bacteria have become resistant to antibiotics.

Infected persons should drink water and electrolyte solutions (such as Gatorade) to replace fluids lost by diarrhea and should follow their normal diet, as much as possible, to ensure nutrition. Doctors recommend that persons with shigellosis avoid foods that are high in fat and sugar, spicy foods, and alcohol and coffee until two days after all symptoms have disappeared.

Because shigellosis is particularly dangerous for children, research is ongoing into *Shigella* vaccines. A person who has recovered from shigellosis is unlikely to be infected with the same strain for several years. Antidiarrheal medicines such as loperamide (Imodium) and atropine (Lomotil) should not be taken by persons with shigellosis, as they can make the illness worse.

### PREVENTION AND OUTCOMES

Handwashing with soap can prevent the spread of shigellosis. Because of contagion, infected persons should be separated from those who are not infected. People with shigellosis should not prepare food or pour water for others. If a child in diapers is infected, all persons who change the diapers should observe strict sanitation and should dispose of the diapers properly. Precautions for food and water safety will prevent shigellosis. Travelers should drink only treated or boiled water and should eat cooked hot foods and self-peeled fruit.

Government agencies in the United States are working to prevent outbreaks of shigellosis. Shigella infections are monitored by the Centers for Disease Control and Prevention and by state and local health departments. These agencies investigate shigellosis, track how it is transmitted, and develop methods of controlling the disease. In addition, these agencies conduct research into ways to identify and treat shigella infection. The U.S. Food and Drug Administration checks imported foods and advocates for improved food-preparation techniques in restaurants and in food-processing plants. The U.S. Environmental Protection Agency checks the safety of drinking water.

*Merrill Evans, M.A.*

## FURTHER READING

Alam, N. H. "Treatment of Infectious Diarrhea in Children." *Pediatric Drugs* 5, no. 3 (2003): 151-165. Discusses three primary diarrheal diseases that impact childhood morbidity and death in developing countries, including shigellosis, and practices for treatment.

Bain, W. B., et al. "Common-Source Outbreak of Waterborne Shigellosis at a Public School." In *An Introduction to Epidemiology*, edited by Thomas C. Timmreck. 3d ed. Sudbury, Mass.: Jones and Bartlett, 2002. Includes a case study of a shigellosis outbreak at a public school in Stockport, Iowa.

Bhattacharya, S. K. "An Evaluation of Current Shigellosis Treatment." *Expert Opinion on Pharmacotherapy* 4, no. 8 (2003): 1315-1320. Surveys the use of antibiotics in the treatment of shigellosis and discusses personal hygiene practices.

Moore, Sean R., Noelia L. Lima, Alberto M. Soares, et al. "Prolonged Episodes of Acute Diarrhea Reduce Growth and Increase Risk of Persistent Diarrhea in Children." *Gastroenterology* 139 (2010): 1156-1164. This article discusses the consequences of prolonged episodes of acute diarrhea in children.

Rebmann, Terri. "Spotlight on Shigellosis." *Nursing* 39 (2009): 59-60. In addition to the standard information about shigellosis, this article includes details about taking a comprehensive patient history and the importance of patient teaching.

Shannon, Joyce Brennfleck, ed. *Contagious Diseases Sourcebook.* Detroit: Omnigraphics, 2010. A chapter

on shigellosis focuses on prevention and on public health considerations.

## WEB SITES OF INTEREST

*Centers for Disease Control and Prevention, Division of Foodborne, Bacterial, and Mycotic Diseases*
http://www.cdc.gov/nczved/divisions/dfbmd

*Neglected Tropical Diseases Coalition*
http://www.neglectedtropicaldiseases.org

*U.S. Department of Agriculture, Food Safety Information Center*
http://foodsafety.nal.usda.gov

**See also:** Amebic dysentery; Bacterial infections; Children and infectious disease; Developing countries and infectious disease; *Escherichia;* Fecal-oral route of transmission; Flies and infectious disease; Food-borne illness and disease; Giardiasis; Intestinal and stomach infections; *Salmonella; Shigella;* Travelers' diarrhea; Tropical medicine; Waterborne illness and disease.

---

# Shingles

CATEGORY: Diseases and conditions
ANATOMY OR SYSTEM AFFECTED: Peripheral nervous system, skin
ALSO KNOWN AS: Herpes zoster infection

## DEFINITION

Shingles is a painful viral infection of the nerves and skin.

## CAUSES

Shingles is caused by the varicella zoster virus, the same virus that leads to chickenpox. Shingles occurs in people who have had chickenpox. After causing the first chickenpox infection, the virus does not leave the body. Instead, it settles in nerve roots near the spinal cord. Once reactivated, the virus travels along nerve paths to the skin, where it causes shingles, manifested as pain and a rash.

## RISK FACTORS

Only 20 percent of people who have had chickenpox eventually develop shingles, so researchers are trying to determine what makes some people more likely than others to develop the condition. Some of the factors that make people more likely to develop shingles include excessive emotional or physical stress and extreme fatigue. People with certain medical conditions, including a weakened immune system, are much more likely to develop shingles. Conditions that increase the risk include a history of childhood cancer; current cancer, especially Hodgkin's disease, lymphoma, and leukemia; and human immunodeficiency virus (HIV) infection or acquired immunodeficiency syndrome (AIDS). People older than sixty years of age are about three times more likely to develop shingles than are younger people, and Caucasians are four times more likely than African Americans to develop shingles.

Certain medications or medical treatments increase the risk for shingles. These include radiation therapy and immunosuppressant drugs (for organ transplants, cancer, and autoimmune diseases), chemotherapy, and steroid medications such as cyclosporine, azathioprine, cyclophosphamide, chlorambucil, and cladribine.

## Symptoms

Shingles usually begins with an unpleasant itching, burning, tingling, or painful sensation in a bandlike area of the skin. The skin rash of shingles begins to appear three to four days after noticing these sensations. The prodromal period is the time (about three to four days) before the rash actually occurs. During this time, one might have the following symptoms: fever, muscle aches, fatigue, anxiety, nervousness, and discomfort in the skin, usually on one side of the face, torso, trunk, back, or buttocks. This discomfort may feel like numbness, itching, burning, stinging, tingling, shooting pain, electric shock, or sharp pain. Another symptom is extreme sensitivity to even light touch.

The period of active shingles begins when the rash is first noticed in the same location where the skin sensations were originally felt. The rash begins as a reddish band or individual bumps running in a line. The bumps develop fluid-filled centers. Within seven to ten days, the bumps begin to dry and crust over. Pain or itching, or both, in the area of the rash may begin, and the pain may be severe. If the rash develops on the side of the nose or elsewhere on the face, which can signal that the eye is affected, one should contact a doctor immediately.

Although the rash of active shingles usually disap-

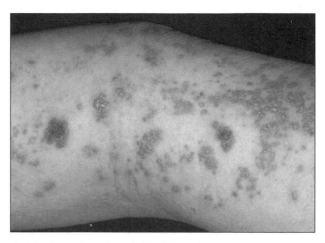

*A shingles rash and associated blistering.*

pears within one week to one month, in about 20 percent of cases, the rash, even if healed, continues to cause pain and discomfort. This syndrome of pain in the area of the previously infected nerve is called postherpetic neuralgia (PHN), and it can be quite severe and debilitating.

## Screening and Diagnosis

Screening tests are usually administered to people without current symptoms, but who may be at high risk for certain diseases or conditions. However, there are no screening tests or screening guidelines for the early detection of shingles.

Generally, shingles is easily diagnosed by its characteristic discomfort and pain and by its distinctive rash. To confirm that one has shingles, a doctor may scrape some skin from a blister or collect some of its fluid. These samples can then be sent to a laboratory for testing. The tests can detect the presence of the varicella zoster virus. These tests include microscopic examination, viral culture, immunofluorescence, and polymerase chain reaction techniques. It may take several weeks to obtain test results.

## Treatment and Therapy

There are no treatments to cure shingles. Rather, treatment involves lifestyle changes, medications, and alternative and complementary therapies to lessen symptoms. Treatment attempts to shorten the length of the illness; prevent shingles by getting the shingles vaccine; prevent complications, such as PHN; relieve and reduce pain and discomfort; and prevent the rash from becoming infected. There are no surgical procedures for the treatment of shingles.

Itching and pain may be relieved with calamine lotion, wet compresses, frequent oatmeal baths, over-the-counter pain relievers (such as acetaminophen, ibuprofen, and naproxen); and capsaicin, a topical substance that comes from hot peppers. The doctor may prescribe drugs to relieve pain that does not respond to over-the-counter remedies.

Certain antiviral medications may control shingles by changing how the virus reproduces in nerve cells. These medications include acyclovir (Zovirax), famciclovir (Famvir), and valacyclovir (Valtrex). Antiviral therapy may shorten a shingles episode, but the therapy must be started within forty-eight to seventy-two hours of the first development of symptoms. These medications can reduce the severity and duration of PHN too and are recommended for patients with the highest risk for this condition (persons who are older than age fifty-five years). Taking antiviral medications before PHN develops is the most effective way to reduce its severity. The doctor may also prescribe a short course of oral steroid medication (such as prednisone) if the patient's immune system is functioning normally.

Other treatments for PHN are available, including capsaicin; tricyclic antidepressants (which may also treat shingles); selective serotonin reuptake inhibitors (SSRIs); Lidoderm patches, a transdermal form of lidocaine, which is a local anesthetic; gabapentin and pregabalin, which are antiseizure medications that also treat PHN; transcutaneous electrical nerve stimulation, a device that generates low-level pulses of electrical current on the skin's surface; and nerve blocks, which are injections near nerves to provide temporary pain relief. Nerve blocks are used as a last resort.

## PREVENTION AND OUTCOMES

There is no proven way to prevent shingles. Stress and fatigue may contribute to an outbreak. Future cases of shingles should decrease as more children are vaccinated against chickenpox.

A vaccine called Zostavax is approved by the U.S. Food and Drug Administration for usage in the prevention of shingles in those persons age sixty years and older. In clinical trials, the vaccine reduced the risk of developing shingles by about 50 percent. The vaccine decreases the likelihood of getting shingles

and the severity of the illness if shingles does occur. Persons with a history of anaphylaxis (a type of allergic reaction) to neomycin should not receive this vaccine.

*Rosalyn Carson-DeWitt, M.D.;*
*reviewed by David L. Horn, M.D., FACP*

## FURTHER READING

Mounsey, Anne L., Leah G. Matthew, and David C. Slawson. "Herpes Zoster and Postherpetic Neuralgia: Prevention and Management." *American Family Physician* 72 (2005): 1075-1080. A clinical guide to preventing and treating shingles and postherpetic neuralgia.

Tyring, S. K. "Management of Herpes Zoster and Postherpetic Neuralgia." *Journal of the American Academy of Dermatology* 57, no. 6, suppl. (2007): S136-S142. Preventing and treating shingles and postherpetic neuralgia from the perspective of dermatology.

Weaver, Bethany A. "Herpes Zoster Overview: Natural History and Incidence." *Journal of the American Osteopathic Association* 109 (2009): S2-S6. An overview of herpes zoster, or shingles.

Whitley, Richard J. "Varicella-Zoster Virus." In *Mandell, Douglas, and Bennett's Principles and Practice of Infectious Diseases*, edited by Gerald L. Mandell, John F. Bennett, and Raphael Dolin. 7th ed. New York: Churchill Livingstone/Elsevier, 2010. This chapter features a discussion of the virus that causes chickenpox and shingles.

## WEB SITES OF INTEREST

*American Academy of Dermatology*
http://www.aad.org

*HealingChronicPain.org*
http://www.healingchronicpain.org/content/neuralgia

*National Institute of Neurological Disorders and Stroke*
http://www.ninds.nih.gov/disorders/shingles

*National Shingles Foundation*
http://www.vzvfoundation.org

**See also:** Aging and infectious disease; Antiviral drugs: Types; Chickenpox; Chickenpox vaccine; Herpes zoster infection; Herpesviridae; Herpesvirus infections; Immunity; Immunization; Postherpetic neuralgia; Reinfection; Scabies; Skin infections; Stress and infectious disease; Vaccines: Types; Viral infections.

# Sinusitis

CATEGORY: Diseases and conditions
ANATOMY OR SYSTEM AFFECTED: Auditory system, ears, nose, throat, upper respiratory tract
ALSO KNOWN AS: Rhinosinusitis, sinus infection

## DEFINITION

Sinusitis is inflammation of the sinus cavities usually associated with infection. The sinus cavities are air-filled spaces in the skull. Acute sinusitis lasts for less than three weeks, and chronic sinusitis is diagnosed when symptoms last a minimum of three months. Persons with repeated bouts of acute sinusitis may have recurrent sinusitis.

## CAUSES

Infectious sinusitis is caused by bacterial or fungal infection of the sinus cavities. The most common bacterial organisms to cause acute sinusitis are *Streptococcus pneumoniae*, *Haemophilus influenzae*, and *Moraxella catarrhalis*.

## RISK FACTORS

It is possible to develop sinusitis with or without the risk factors listed here. However, the more risk factors, the greater the likelihood of developing sinusitis. Risk factors for developing sinusitis include smoking and being exposed to secondhand smoke. In general, elderly people and young people have a higher risk of developing respiratory tract infections, including sinusitis. Women have a greater chance of developing sinusitis than men. Whites and blacks have a higher risk of developing sinusitis than do Hispanics.

Environmental risk factors include traveling to high altitudes, air pollution, and living in the American Midwest or American South. In addition, flying and diving both increase the chance of getting sinusitis.

The following medical conditions increase the chance of getting sinusitis: a recent cold; the prolonged use of decongestant sprays; nasal obstruction caused by polyps, deviated septum, facial bone abnormalities, swollen adenoids, cleft palate, tumor, or allergies; certain chronic illnesses, including cystic fibrosis,

Kartagener's syndrome (a chronic lung disease), Wegener's granulomatosis (a rare disease that causes blood vessel walls to become inflamed), asthma, sarcoidosis, human immunodeficiency virus infection, acquired immunodeficiency syndrome, and diabetes; and head injury or other medical condition that requires insertion of a tube into the nose.

## SYMPTOMS

Symptoms of sinus infection are like those of the common cold. However, when caused by a cold virus, such symptoms typically improve after a few days. Persons who continue to have nasal symptoms ten to fourteen days after having a cold may have developed a sinus infection.

Symptoms of sinus infection include nasal congestion; nasal discharge that may be thick, greenish, or yellowish; headache (in acute sinusitis); ear pain; toothache (dental pain); facial pain and pressure that increases when lying down or bending; facial fullness or congestion; nagging cough that may get worse when lying down; fever; decreased energy or fatigue; bad breath; unpleasant taste in mouth; decreased sense of smell; and fever, especially in children.

Most experts believe that sinus infection does not cause chronic headaches. However, alteration in sinus pressure associated with weather changes might provoke headaches in susceptible people.

## SCREENING AND DIAGNOSIS

The purpose of screening is early diagnosis and treatment. Screening tests are usually administered to people without current symptoms, but who may be at high risk for certain diseases or conditions. However, there are no screening tests or screening guidelines for the early diagnosis of either acute or chronic sinusitis.

Acute sinusitis is a temporary condition that generally is easily treated with medications and often resolves without treatment. Screening for chronic sinusitis might find affected persons who have no symptoms, but there is no evidence that health would be improved by presymptomatic treatment for this condition.

A physical examination may reveal tenderness when a doctor taps or presses over the area of the sinuses or on the teeth in the upper jaw. In many cases of acute sinusitis, a doctor can diagnose sinusitis based on symptoms and the physical examination. However, in recurrent and chronic sinusitis, other tests may be performed. These tests may include the following:

## Balloon Sinuplasty

In late 2005, the Acclarent Company received permission from the U.S. Food and Drug Administration (FDA) to market a device to clear blocked sinuses similar to that used to clear blocked arteries in the heart. A flexible catheter tube inserted into the nostril guides a balloon into the targeted sinus. The balloon is inflated, spreading the bones of the passageway sufficiently to permit accumulated mucus or pus to drain. A minimally invasive outpatient procedure, balloon sinuplasty is performed under local anesthesia and takes one to two hours. Persons report little or no pain and can often return to normal activity within twenty-four hours. The sinuplasty devices are not reusable, and the procedure is covered by some private insurance plans.

The procedure cannot be used if nasal polyps need to be removed. Nevertheless, it provides a possible alternative for persons with sinusitis who do not need, or prefer not to undergo, surgical procedures involving cutting away bone or other tissue to open the blocked sinus.

Surgeons using the devices have praised them. The American Rhinologic Society, however, was more cautious in its October, 2006, position statement, asserting that the technology had limited indication. In November, one health maintenance organization in California labeled the procedure investigational and not medically necessary, noting that because the FDA's clearance was based on the devices' comparability to already approved procedures, it did not require submission of safety or effectiveness data. The American Academy of Otolaryngology–Head and Neck Surgery issued its first position statement on the procedure in March, 2007. The statement said that "the evidence regarding the safety of sinus balloon catheterization has been supportive, and that balloon catheterization is a promising technique for the treatment of selected cases of rhinosinusitis."

*Milton Berman, Ph.D.*

*Transillumination.* This simple procedure involves shining a bright light (as from a flashlight) over the person's cheek in a dark room. If no light illuminates certain areas of the face, then it is likely that the person has a sinus infection. This test, though, is not reliable and is not commonly performed.

*Nasal culture.* The doctor might send a sample of the patient's nasal discharge to a laboratory, where it can be tested for the presence of bacteria. Accurate evaluation of a nasal culture usually requires that the culture be obtained during nasal endoscopy. Some patients with chronic sinusitis may benefit from nasal culture. However, if the patient is otherwise healthy and has acute sinusitis, a nasal culture is usually not done.

*Nasal cytology.* The doctor might send a sample of the patient's nasal discharge to a laboratory to help determine other causes of the sinusitis.

*Sinus X ray.* X rays are of limited use for diagnosing the presence of sinusitis within certain sinuses. Infection in other pairs of sinuses (such as the ethmoid sinuses) may require other types of imaging tests.

*Computed tomography (CT) scan.* A CT scan is a detailed X ray that identifies abnormalities of fine tissue structure. This type of imaging study can be useful for diagnosing sinusitis, including in those areas not well visualized by sinus X rays. CT scans are particularly effective for diagnosing chronic sinusitis.

*Magnetic resonance imaging (MRI) scan.* The doctor may order this test if a tumor or fungal infection is suspected. Overall, MRI is not helpful for diagnosing this condition.

*Sweat chloride test.* This is a test for cystic fibrosis in children who also have polyps or infection, or both, caused by *Pseudomonas* organisms.

*Blood tests for immune function.* These tests may be requested by the doctor if the patient has recurrent or chronic sinusitis.

*Cilary function.* This is a specialized test performed if all other tests fail to identify the cause of recurrent, chronic sinusitis.

*Sinus puncture.* If there is some confusion about the patient's diagnosis, the doctor may choose to send the patient to a specialist to have a sinus puncture performed. This involves using a needle to remove a bit of fluid from within the sinuses. This fluid will then be sent to a lab to identify the infecting bacteria and to determine the most effective type of antibiotic for treatment. In most cases, a nasal endoscopy with culture provides the same amount of information with less discomfort.

*Nasal endoscopy.* This procedure uses a slim, flexible tube with a fiberoptic light at the end (endoscope). It is inserted into the nose. The doctor can inspect the mucosa of the nose and the openings of the sinuses. If indicated, the doctor can also take samples or biopsies through the endoscope for lab examination to look for fungus, tumors, or other uncommon causes of sinusitis.

## TREATMENT AND THERAPY

The goals of treating sinusitis include relieving the discomfort, opening the nasal passages, curing the infection, preventing complications, and preventing recurrence. Treatment includes lifestyle changes, medications, and surgery.

Drinking increased amounts of fluid may help to thin out nasal secretions and to help against plugged nasal passages and sinuses. Salt-water nose sprays or nasal irrigation may also loosen nasal secretions. One could also make a "humidifier" by filling a bowl with steaming water every couple of hours and making a steam tent by placing a towel over the head. The steam tent helps one breathe in the steam.

Another treatment is to use decongestant pills and nasal sprays to shrink nasal passages. One should not use nasal sprays for more than three to four consecutive days. Persons who need longer treatment should consult a doctor, who may prescribe intranasal corticosteroid medications, especially if the patient has had recurrent sinus problems. Allergy medications called antihistamines may help sinusitis symptoms if they are caused by allergies. However, antihistamines also might dry the nasal mucosa.

The doctor may decide to prescribe antibiotics if the infection seems to be caused by bacteria. Medical studies have shown, however, that antibiotics are not effective in treating acute sinusitis. Over-the-counter pain medication, such as acetaminophen, ibuprofen, or aspirin, can be used to treat sinus pain. Aspirin is not recommended for children or teenagers with a current or recent viral infection because of the risk of Reye's syndrome. One should consult the doctor about medicines that are safe for children.

Another treatment is using cough medicines containing guaifenesin. These medicines can help the patient cough up secretions.

Surgery is a last resort for people with troublesome and serious chronic sinusitis. The procedure includes repairing a deviated septum, removing nasal polyps, and functional endoscopic sinus surgery, in which a lighted scope is used to enlarge the sinuses to improve drainage.

## PREVENTION AND OUTCOMES

The following actions may help reduce the risk of developing sinusitis:

*Smoking cessation.* Smoking interferes with the normal defenses in the respiratory tract that protect against infection. Smoking cessation can help the respiratory tract slowly heal itself. Furthermore, exposure to both secondhand smoke and air pollution can make one more prone to sinusitis.

*Avoiding infections.* Although there is no evidence that one can avoid getting sinus infections, there are some basic steps that may help a person avoid infections in general. These basic steps are to wash one's hands frequently and thoroughly and to avoid close contact with people who are ill.

*Filtering and humidifying the air.* Keeping air humidified may help to keep sinuses and the respiratory tract from becoming overly dry. High-efficiency particulate air, or HEPA, filters for home furnaces and vacuum cleaners remove allergens from the air.

*Treating allergies.* Persons who suspect they have an allergy should be tested. Keeping allergy symptoms to a minimum can help decrease susceptibility to respiratory tract infections, including sinusitis.

*Sinus surgery.* Corrective surgery for deviated septum or surgical removal of the blockage in sinuses will prevent future episodes of chronic or recurrent sinusitis.

Finally, persons who have had trouble with sinusitis after flying should consult a doctor about using a nasal decongestant spray fifteen minutes before takeoff and landing. If possible, one should avoid air travel if he or she has a cold or other sinus condition.

*Rosalyn Carson-DeWitt, M.D.;*
*reviewed by Elie Edmond Rebeiz, M.D., FACS*

## FURTHER READING

Bhattacharyya, N. "Clinical and Symptom Criteria for the Accurate Diagnosis of Chronic Rhinosinusitis." *Laryngoscope* 116 (2006): 1-22. A clinical guide for diagnosing chronic sinusitis.

Brook, Itzhak, ed. *Sinusitis: From Microbiology to Management.* New York: Taylor & Francis, 2006. A text that includes a scientific overview of sinusitis and its clinical management.

Ferrari, Mario. *PDxMD Ear, Nose, and Throat Disorders.* Philadelphia: PDxMD, 2003. A clinical yet accessible reference that provides a comprehensive list of disorders, with a summary of the condition, background, diagnosis, treatment, outcomes, prevention, and resources.

Kennedy, David W., and Marilyn Olsen. *Living with Chronic Sinusitis: A Patient's Guide to Sinusitis, Nasal Allergies, Polyps, and Their Treatment Options.* Long Island, N.Y.: Hatherleigh Press, 2004. The author, a top ENT doctor, discusses chronic sinusitis, including causes, newer drug options and surgical procedures, and related respiratory allergies.

Marple, B. F., S. Brunton, and B. J. Ferguson. "Acute Bacterial Rhinosinusitis: A Review of U.S. Treatment Guidelines." *Otolaryngology—Head and Neck Surgery* 135 (2006): 341-348. This review of the treatment guidelines for acute sinusitis comes from a respected journal in the field.

## WEB SITES OF INTEREST

*Allergy/Asthma Information Association*
http://aaia.ca

*American Academy of Otolaryngology—Head and Neck Surgery*
http://www.entnet.org

*Clean Hands Coalition*
http://www.cleanhandscoalition.org

*National Institute of Allergy and Infectious Diseases*
http://www.niaid.nih.gov

**See also:** Airborne illness and disease; Atypical pneumonia; Bacterial infections; Bronchiolitis; Bronchitis; Children and infectious disease; Common cold; Contagious diseases; Epiglottitis; *Haemophilus*; *Haemophilus influenzae* infection; Inflammation; Influenza; Middleear infection; Nasopharyngeal infections; Pharyngitis and tonsillopharyngitis; Pneumococcal infections; Pneumonia; Rhinovirus infections; Seasonal influenza; Strep throat; Streptococcal infections; *Streptococcus*.

# Skin infections

CATEGORY: Diseases and conditions
ANATOMY OR SYSTEM AFFECTED: Skin

## DEFINITION

Infections of the skin can be viral or bacterial in nature or may be caused by a fungus or parasite.

## CAUSES

Skin infections are the result of the body's inability to fight foreign microorganisms that may cause damage or disease if left untreated. Humans are hosts for many bacterial species that colonize the skin as normal flora. *Staphylococcus aureus* and *Streptococcus pyogenes* are infrequent resident flora, but they account for a wide variety of pyodermas (bacterial skin infections). Predisposing factors to infection include minor trauma, preexisting skin disease, poor hygiene, and, rarely, impaired host immunity. Impetigo is one example of a superficial bacterial skin infection. Others are folliculitis and cellulitis.

Dermatophytosis is infection with fungi, organisms with high affinity for keratinized tissue, such as skin, nails, and hair. Three fungal genera (*Trichophyton, Microsporum,* and *Epidermophyton*) account for the vast majority of these infections. Fungal reservoirs for these organisms include soil, animals, and infected humans.

Skin may also be infected with viruses, small pathogens that can replicate only inside the cells of living organisms. A common example of a virus that infects skin is the herpes simplex virus (HSV). This infection causes a painful, self-limited, often recurrent dermatitis characterized by small grouped vesicles on an erythematous base. The disease is often mucocutaneous. HSV type 1 is usually associated with orofacial disease, and HSV type 2 is usually associated with genital infection.

## RISK FACTORS

Poor hygiene habits or injury to the skin provide excellent conditions for bacterial growth. Yeast and other fungal infections are more common in immunocompromised persons, persons with diabetes, the elderly, and persons receiving antibiotics. Fungi grow in moist conditions and in the folds of skin. Studies have shown that tinea pedis, commonly known as athlete's foot, is the most frequent clinical form of dermatophytosis, accounting for 59 percent of fungal skin infections. Viruses can spread easily through contact with contaminated persons or surfaces. About 85 percent of the population has antibody evidence of HSV type 1 infection. HSV type 2 infection is responsible for 20 to 50 percent of genital ulcerations in sexually active persons.

## SYMPTOMS

In general, skin infections usually involve a rash of some type as well as itching, redness, and sometimes blisters (bullae) or other types of lesions. For example, with the bacterial skin infection impetigo, two clinical types exist, nonbullous and bullous. The nonbullous type is more common and typically occurs on the face and extremities, initially with vesicles or pustules on reddened skin. The vesicles or pustules eventually rupture to leave a characteristic honey-colored (yellow-brown) crust. Bullous impetigo, almost exclusively caused by *S. aureus*, exhibits flaccid bullae with clear yellow fluid that rupture and leave a golden yellow crust.

Fungal and yeast infections on the body may give rise to the raised red rings of ringworm or the cracking and redness on the skin of the feet in athlete's foot or in the groin area in jock itch. Involvement of the nails is onychomycosis; the nails may thicken, discolor, and finally crumble and fall off.

Viral infections also tend to cause rashes, itching, and redness. Herpes simplex is characterized by small grouped vesicles on an erythematous base.

### SCREENING AND DIAGNOSIS

The diagnosis of a bacterial infection is by clinical presentation; confirmation of this infection, however, is by laboratory culture. For fungal and yeast infections, a potassium hydroxide preparation or culture helps to establish the diagnosis. A viral culture helps to confirm the diagnosis of viral skin infections, such as those caused by HSV. A direct fluorescent antibody (DFA) is a useful but less-specific test. Serology is helpful only for diagnosing primary viral infection. The Tzanck smear can be helpful in

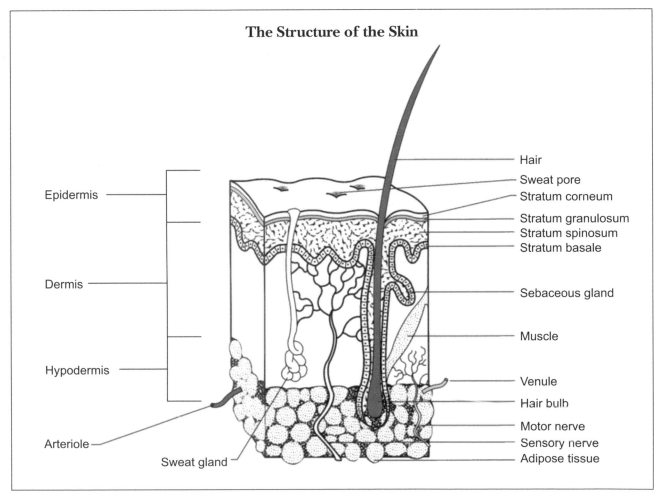

## The Structure of the Skin

- Hair
- Sweat pore
- Stratum corneum
- Stratum granulosum
- Stratum spinosum
- Stratum basale
- Sebaceous gland
- Muscle
- Venule
- Hair bulb
- Motor nerve
- Sensory nerve
- Adipose tissue

- Epidermis
- Dermis
- Hypodermis
- Arteriole
- Sweat gland

*Skin serves as a multilayered protective barrier against invasion by harmful microorganisms. Sometimes, however, infection occurs when that barrier's very complexity fails to prevent disease.*

the rapid diagnosis of herpes viruses infections, but it is less sensitive than culture and DFA.

### TREATMENT AND THERAPY

For bacterial infections such as impetigo, topical treatment is adequate—for example, either with bacitracin (Polysporin) or mupirocin (Bactroban), applied twice daily for seven to ten days. Systemic therapy may be necessary for persons with extensive disease.

For most persons with yeast and other fungal infections, topical treatment with terbinafine (Lamisil), clotrimazole (Lotrimin or Mycelex), or econazole (Spectazole) cream is adequate when applied twice daily for six to eight weeks.

Viral infections may also be difficult to treat. For example, primary HSV treatment may be acyclovir, given as follows: either 200 milligrams (mg) taken orally five times a day or 400 mg taken orally three times a day, both for ten days.

### PREVENTION AND OUTCOMES

Good general health and hygiene help to prevent bacterial skin infection such as impetigo. It is also important to clean minor cuts and scrapes thoroughly with soap and clean water. To prevent yeast and other fungal infections, one should avoid sharing clothing, sports equipment, towels, or sheets; wash clothes in hot water; use fungicidal soap after suspected exposure to ringworm; and avoid walking barefoot, instead wearing appropriate protective shoes in locker rooms and sandals at the beach. For many viral infections, such as HSV, avoidance is the best prevention.

*Margaret Ring Gillock, M.S.*

### FURTHER READING

Swartz, Morton N., and Mark S. Pasternack. "Cellulitis and Subcutaneous Tissue Infection." In *Mandell, Douglas, and Bennett's Principles and Practice of Infectious Diseases*, edited by Gerald L. Mandell, John E. Bennett, and Raphael Dolin. 7th ed. New York: Churchill Livingstone/Elsevier, 2010.

Trent, J. T., D. Federman, and R. S. Kirsner. "Common Bacterial Skin Infections." *Ostomy Wound Management* 47 (2001): 30-34.

Vinh, D. C., and J. M. Embil. "Rapidly Progressive Soft Tissue Infections." *Lancet Infectious Diseases* 5 (2005): 501.

Weedon, David. *Skin Pathology*. 3d ed. New York: Churchill Livingstone/Elsevier, 2010.

### WEB SITES OF INTEREST

*American Academy of Dermatology*
http://www.aad.org

*Centers for Disease Control and Prevention*
http://www.cdc.gov

**See also:** Abscesses; Acne; Athlete's foot; Bacterial infections; Cellulitis; Dermatomycosis; *Epidermophyton*; Fungal infections; Herpes simplex infection; Herpesvirus infections; Impetigo; Jock itch; *Microsporum*; Mouth infections; Onychomycosis; Pityriasis rosea; Ringworm; Roseola; Rubella; Scarlet fever; Staphylococcal infections; Streptococcal infections; Tinea capitis; Tinea corporis; Tinea versicolor; *Trichophyton*; Viral infections.

# Sleeping nets

**CATEGORY:** Prevention
**ALSO KNOWN AS:** Bed nets, insecticide-treated nets

### DEFINITION

Sleeping nets are used to reduce exposure to disease-carrying insects while resting or sleeping.

### GLOBAL DISTRIBUTION

The United Nations Millennium Project is a collaborative worldwide effort to improve the human condition. Reducing the incidence of malaria and other major diseases by 2015 is one of the project's goals. The project distributes heavily subsidized or free, long-lasting, insecticide-treated sleeping nets to children and pregnant females in areas with widespread malaria. Distribution is relatively effective and inexpensive.

### MALARIA

In one area in particular, sub-Saharan Africa, people have received sleeping nets in an effort to fight malaria. A study in Tanzania in 2002 showed a one-third reduction in anemia and parasitemia in pregnant women using insecticide-treated nets (ITNs). The length of time between nets being treated with pesticides was related to their efficacy. The most widely distributed type of net is the long-lasting insecticidal

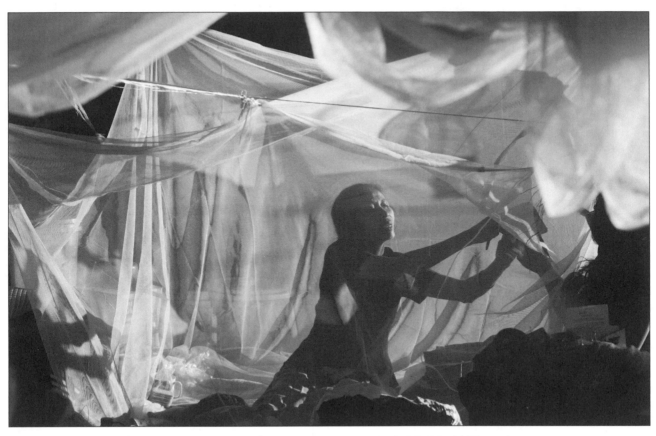

*A woman in East Timor is surrounded by a sleeping, or mosquito, net.* (AP/Wide World Photos)

bed net (LLIN), which is effective for five to seven years. This type of net has pyrethroids (synthetic pesticides), such as permethrin, incorporated into its fibers when manufactured. Pyrethroids are based on derivatives of chrysanthemum flowers.

Untreated nets were traditionally used to reduce exposure to insects, but insects could still get through the nets (either through holes or through an improper seal). The use of pyrethroid kills the insects before entering a net. The mortality rate from malaria in several countries in Africa has been reduced by about 50 percent since these countries started using LLINs instead of untreated sleeping nets.

## DISTRIBUTION ISSUES

A large survey was conducted in Togo, Niger, Kenya, Madagascar, and Sierra Leone to attempt to determine why ITNs were being underused or not used at all by young children (younger than age five years). The study found that many families did not use a net because they still did not have one, even though millions of nets had been distributed earlier. In other cases, a net was used in a household, but that net was used by someone other than young children.

## IMPACT

Sleeping nets can mean the difference between life and death, especially for pregnant women and young children areas such as sub-Saharan Africa. A worldwide effort is ongoing to support the purchase and distribution of insecticide-treated nets in Africa.

*Dawn M. Bielawski, Ph.D.*

## FURTHER READING

Beer, N., et al. "System Effectiveness of a Targeted Free Mass Distribution of Long Lasting Insecticidal Nets in Zanzibar, Tanzania." *Malaria Journal* 9 (2010): 173-181.

Eng, J. L., et al. "Assessing Bed Net Use and Non-use after Long-Lasting Insecticidal Net Distribution: A

Simple Framework to Guide Programmatic Strategies." *Malaria Journal* 9 (2010): 133-141.

Marchant, T., et al. "Socially Marketed Insecticide-Treated Nets Improve Malaria and Anaemia in Pregnancy in Southern Tanzania." *Tropical Medicine and International Health* 7 (2002): 149-158.

Teklehaimanot, Awash, Gordon C. McCord, and Jeffrey D. Sachs. "Scaling Up Malaria Control in Africa: An Economic and Epidemiological Assessment." *American Journal of Tropical Medicine and Hygiene* 77 (2007): 138-144.

## WEB SITES OF INTEREST

*Eradicate Malaria Project*
http://www.gmin.org

*Malaria Foundation International*
http://www.malaria.org

*United Nations Millennium Project*
http://www.unmillenniumproject.org

*World Health Organization*
http://www.who.int/malaria

**See also:** Arthropod-borne illness and disease; Chikungunya; Children and infectious disease; DDT; Dengue fever; Developing countries and infectious disease; Insect-borne illness and disease; Insecticides and topical repellants; Malaria; Mosquito-borne viral encephalitis; Mosquitoes and infectious disease; Rift Valley fever; Tropical medicine; Yellow fever.

# Sleeping sickness

CATEGORY: Diseases and conditions
ANATOMY OR SYSTEM AFFECTED: Brain, central nervous system
ALSO KNOWN AS: Encephalitis lethargica, von Economo's disease

## DEFINITION

Sleeping sickness (encephalitis lethargica, or EL) is a mysterious, atypical form of brain inflammation that occurred as a worldwide epidemic from 1916 to 1928. A true modern plague, it killed or left motionless, in a sleeplike state, millions of people. The epidemic has not recurred, but isolated cases are occasionally reported.

## CAUSES

The cause of EL remains enigmatic. Because of its near concurrence with the Spanish influenza pandemic, an association between the two diseases has been suggested. Many thought influenza did not, in fact, cause encephalitis, and recent reports failed to find the virus in archival EL brains. Even so, because studies on preserved brain tissue have technical limitations, a contribution of influenza virus to disease pathogenesis cannot be excluded. Sleeping sickness may resurface in a future influenza pandemic.

After analyzing sporadic cases, some researchers believe the syndrome is still prevalent and consider it to be secondary to autoimmunity against deep gray-matter neurons, following a streptococcal infection.

## RISK FACTORS

The influenza virus and certain streptococcal infections could constitute risk factors. Young people seemed more susceptible to developing EL. Mortality rates peaked in infants and the elderly.

## SYMPTOMS

Constantin von Economo described the disorder in 1917 and coined the term "encephalitis lethargica." The onset was acute or subacute, with fever, lethargy, headache, and malaise, followed by a state of somnolence. Some patients slipped into a coma that lasted months or years. Additional manifestations included double vision, abnormal eye movements (known as oculogyric crisis), weakness, tremor, muscle twitching, catatonia (unresponsiveness with stereotypy, rigidity, or extreme flexibility), inability to speak (mutism), sleep rhythm reversal, and psychosis. Mortality rates reached 20 to 40 percent.

Sequelae occurred in most survivors, often after an apparent disease-free interval of months or years. An unusual Parkinson's disease-like syndrome, a consequence of dopaminergic system degeneration, emerged as the outstanding motor sequel of EL. Cases of severely impaired, catatonic persons with EL were evoked by Oliver Sacks in his 1973 memoir *Awakenings*. He succeeded in temporarily "awakening" these patients using the anti-Parkinsonian drug L-dopa, after they had spent more than forty years in an immobile state.

## SCREENING AND DIAGNOSIS

The diagnosis relies on clinical symptoms and signs of encephalitis, coupled with visual abnormalities, sleep disturbances, and signs of basal ganglia injury (such as early parkinsonism). Magnetic resonance imaging can reveal basal ganglia lesions.

Pathological studies show inflammation in the gray and white matter of the brain and spinal cord, around blood vessels, and in the meninges. Midbrain and basal ganglia are particularly affected. Neurons undergo degenerative changes.

## TREATMENT AND THERAPY

Treatment is based on symptoms. L-dopa and other anti-Parkinsonian agents can produce dramatic responses in persons treated with these medications.

## PREVENTION AND OUTCOMES

There exists no known preventive measures.

*Mihaela Avramut, M.D., Ph.D.*

## FURTHER READING

Dale, Russel C., et al. "Encephalitis Lethargic Syndrome: Twenty New Cases and Evidence of Basal Ganglia Autoimmunity." *Brain* 127, part 1 (2004): 21-33.

Jubelt, Burk. "Encephalitis Lethargica." In *Merritt's Neurology*, edited by Lewis P. Rowland. 11th ed. Philadelphia: Lippincott Williams & Wilkins, 2005.

McCall, Sherman, et al. "The Relationship Between Encephalitis Lethargica and Influenza: A Critical Analysis." *Journal of Neurovirology* 14 (2008): 177-185.

Von Economo, C. "Die Encephalitis lethargica." *Wiener Klinische Wochenschrift* 30 (1917): 581-585. For a translated version of the full text, see R. H. Wilkins and I. A. Brody, "Neurological Classics IV: Encephalitis Lethargica." *Archives of Neurology* 18 (1968): 324-328.

Woolsey, Thomas A., Joseph Hanaway, and Mokhtar Gado. *Brain Atlas: A Visual Guide to the Human Central Nervous System.* 3d ed. Hoboken, N.J.: John Wiley & Sons, 2008.

## WEB SITES OF INTEREST

*National Institute of Neurological Disorders and Stroke*
http://www.ninds.nih.gov/disorders/encephalitis_lethargica

*National Organization for Rare Disorders*
http://www.rarediseases.org

**See also:** African sleeping sickness; Encephalitis; Inflammation; Influenza; Parasitic diseases; Protozoan diseases; Trypanosomiasis.

# Smallpox

CATEGORY: Diseases and conditions
ANATOMY OR SYSTEM AFFECTED: All

## DEFINITION

Smallpox is a contagious and sometimes deadly viral infection. The disease was eliminated worldwide through global immunization programs. The last known natural-occurring human case was in 1977. However, governments have studied its use as a biological weapon. As a bioweapon, it would be released into the air. Those exposed could develop the disease and then transmit it to other people.

## CAUSES

*Variola major* is the virus that causes smallpox. The virus is spread through the airborne droplets of infected saliva, between people who have direct contact, and through the handling of contaminated bed linens or clothing. Two rare and more serious types of the disease are hemorrhagic and malignant smallpox. They are similarly transmitted.

## RISK FACTORS

The main risk factor for contracting smallpox is exposure to the virus after its release during a biological terrorism attack.

## SYMPTOMS

Symptoms of smallpox usually occur about twelve days after exposure. Hemorrhagic or malignant symptoms, however, usually do not appear until death is near.

Early symptoms of smallpox include high fever, fatigue, severe headache, backache, possible stomach pain or delirium, fatigue, sore throat, and nausea and vomiting. Two to three days later, a rash will appear on the mouth, throat, face, and arms; the rash then spreads to the legs and trunk. Red, flat lesions will appear at the same time, then the lesions will fill with fluid and then pus. Crusts form during the second week, and scabs form and fall off after three to four weeks.

Hemorrhagic symptoms include high fever, fatigue, headache, backache, possible stomach pain, dark red coloration, and bleeding into the skin and mucous membranes. Malignant symptoms include high fever, fatigue, headache, backache, slowly developing lesions that remain soft and flat, skin that looks like reddish-colored crepe rubber, and, if the patient survives, peeling of large amounts of skin.

## SCREENING AND DIAGNOSIS

A doctor will ask the patient about symptoms and medical history and will perform a physical exam. Also, the doctor will consider all possible sources of exposure. Tests may include an examination of saliva and fluid from skin lesions under a microscope, a sampling (a culture) of saliva and fluid from skin lesions, and a blood test to detect antibodies to smallpox.

## TREATMENT AND THERAPY

No effective treatment for smallpox exists, so doctors offer supportive care and take measures to prevent the spread of the infection to other people. Supportive care includes administering fluids and keeping the skin clean. Medications can help control fever and pain. Antibiotics, however, do not work against viruses, so they may be given only if other infections develop.

Smallpox cases are reported to public health officials. A person infected with smallpox should be kept isolated to help prevent the spread of infection. Hospitalized persons will be placed in a special room, and, in some cases, may be quarantined. In most cases, family members can provide care at home. Caregivers should be vaccinated; should wear a mask, gloves, goggles, and a gown; and should disinfect clothing, bed linens, and surfaces.

## PREVENTION AND OUTCOMES

Many people were immunized against smallpox before 1972. This protection has likely worn off or decreased. Routine vaccination is not recommended by health officials in the United States, however, but an emergency supply of the vaccine is kept by the federal government in case of a biological attack.

A vaccination within four days of exposure may prevent the disease and can also make symptoms less severe. Anyone in close contact with a patient after the fever has started should receive the vaccine. Medical and emergency personnel also should be given the vaccine.

If the virus is released in a biological attack, persons infected could see initial symptoms within two weeks or more of the attack. The success of an attack would depend on the dose that was inhaled. Experts predict most of the released viruses could live in dry, cool air, and without sunlight, for one day. Each person infected would likely pass the disease to ten to twenty other people; those people, in turn, could spread it to others. The fatality rate in naturally occurring smallpox is 30 percent or higher.

*Reviewed by David L. Horn, M.D., FACP*

## FURTHER READING

Baciu, Alina, et al., eds. *The Smallpox Vaccination Program: Public Health in an Age of Terrorism.* Washington, D.C.: National Academies Press, 2005.

Breman, J. G., and D. A. Henderson. "Diagnosis and Management of Smallpox." *New England Journal of Medicine* 25 (2002): 1300-1308.

Glynn, Ian, and Jenifer Glynn. *The Life and Death of Smallpox.* New York: Cambridge University Press, 2004.

Hildreth, C. "Smallpox." *Journal of the American Medical Association* 301 (2009): 1086.

Mandell, Gerald L., John E. Bennett, and Raphael Dolin, eds. *Mandell, Douglas, and Bennett's Principles and Practice of Infectious Diseases.* 7th ed. New York: Churchill Livingstone/Elsevier, 2010.

Tucker, Jonathan B. *Scourge: The Once and Future Threat of Smallpox.* New York: Atlantic Monthly Press, 2001.

Working Group on Civilian Biodefense. "Smallpox as a Biological Weapon: Medical and Public Health Management." *Journal of the American Medical Association* 281 (1999): 2127-2137.

World Health Organization. "Smallpox." Available at http://www.who.int/mediacentre/factsheets/smallpox.

## WEB SITES OF INTEREST

*Center for Biosecurity*
http://www.upmc-biosecurity.org

*Centers for Disease Control and Prevention*
http://www.cdc.gov/smallpox

*Emerging and Reemerging Infectious Diseases Resource Center*
http://www.medscape.com/resource/infections

*Public Health Agency of Canada*
http://www.phac-aspc.gc.ca

**See also:** Airborne illness and disease; Anthrax; Biological weapons; Bioterrorism; Botulinum toxin infection; Botulism; Contagious diseases; Disease eradication campaigns; Emerging and reemerging infectious diseases; Monkeypox; Respiratory route of transmission; Saliva and infectious disease; SARS; Smallpox vaccine; Tularemia; Viral infections.

# Smallpox vaccine

CATEGORY: Prevention

## DEFINITION

The development of a smallpox vaccine began with variolation, which was the practice of removing material from the scabbing pustules of infected people and administering that material to healthy people to induce a milder form of smallpox and subsequent immunity. Smallpox, caused by the *Variola major* virus, is thought to have arisen as many as ten thousand years ago in northern Africa and spread to the rest of the world by the seventeenth century, leaving millions dead in its wake.

Although used in Asia and the Middle East as early as the eleventh century, variolation was not in widespread use in Europe until the late eighteenth century. Although variolation was often fatal, the total number of smallpox cases was significantly reduced because of the technique.

## VACCINE DEVELOPMENT

In 1774, an English farmer made the observation that milkmaids who became infected with cowpox, a mild disease caused by the vaccinia virus, seldom became infected with smallpox. The farmer immunized his family against smallpox by infecting them with cowpox taken from a cow's udder.

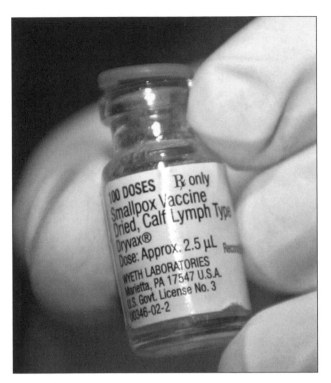

*A vial containing smallpox vaccine.* (AP/Wide World Photos)

Edward Jenner, an English physician, is credited with developing the smallpox vaccine. In 1796, Jenner removed fluid from a cowpox pustule of a milkmaid and inoculated an eight-year-old boy. The boy was exposed to material taken from a fresh smallpox lesion six weeks later but did not develop smallpox. By the early to mid-nineteenth century, inoculation with cowpox replaced variolation. Jenner referred to his preparation as a vaccine because the material came from a cow (*vacca*, in Latin).

The modern vaccine uses an attenuated vaccinia strain. After administration, a pustule develops, eventually scabs over, and falls off. For a few days after vaccination, the patient may have mild symptoms. Rarely do serious side effects develop. Vaccination within three to seven days of exposure to the smallpox virus can result in a significant reduction in the severity of the symptoms.

In 1982, after smallpox had been eradicated and the United States terminated its mandatory vaccination program, production of the smallpox vaccine ceased. In 2007, the U.S. Food and Drug Administration authorized the production of a newer and safer vaccine to be placed in the Strategic National Stockpile to be used in the event of national emergency by the Centers for Disease Control and Prevention.

## IMPACT

The development of the smallpox vaccine led to the eventual eradication of the disease. Although smallpox had been virtually eradicated from developed countries by the 1950's, epidemics continued in developing countries. In 1967, the World Health Organization (WHO) began a worldwide eradication campaign that led to the last endemic case of smallpox, which was reported in 1977. In 1980, WHO announced that the world was free of smallpox.

*Charles L. Vigue, Ph.D.*

## FURTHER READING

Baciu, Alina, et al., eds. *The Smallpox Vaccination Program: Public Health in an Age of Terrorism.* Washington, D.C.: National Academies Press, 2005.

Henderson, D. A., and Richard Preston. *Smallpox: The Death of a Disease—The Inside Story of Eradicating a Worldwide Killer.* Amherst, N.Y.: Prometheus Books, 2009.

Hildreth, C. "Smallpox." *Journal of the American Medical Association* 301 (2009): 1086.

Hopkins, Donald R. *The Greatest Killer: Smallpox in History.* Chicago: University of Chicago Press, 2002.

Koplow, David A. *Smallpox: The Fight to Eradicate a Global Scourge.* Berkeley: University of California Press, 2003.

Plotkin, Stanley A., Walter A. Orenstein, and Paul A. Offit. *Vaccines.* 5th ed. Philadelphia: Saunders/Elsevier, 2008.

Tucker, Jonathan B. *Scourge: The Once and Future Threat of Smallpox.* New York: Atlantic Monthly Press, 2001.

Williams, Gareth. *Angel of Death: The Story of Smallpox.* New York: Palgrave Macmillan, 2010.

## WEB SITES OF INTEREST

*Centers for Disease Control and Prevention*
http://www.cdc.gov/smallpox

*Global Health Council*
http://www.globalhealth.org

*Microbiology and Immunology On-line: Immunology*
http://pathmicro.med.sc.edu/book/immunol-sta.htm

**See also:** Airborne illness and disease; Anthrax; Biological weapons; Bioterrorism; Botulinum toxin infection; Botulism; Contagious diseases; Cowpox; Disease eradication campaigns; Emerging and reemerging infectious diseases; Monkeypox; Respiratory route of transmission; Saliva and infectious disease; SARS; Smallpox; Tularemia; Vaccines: Types; Viral infections.

# Social effects of infectious disease

CATEGORY: Epidemiology

## DEFINITION

The social effects of infectious disease can range from stigmatization to civil unrest and political upheaval. Identifying the source and mode of transmission often involves focusing on people in lower socioeconomic groups, who typically live in overcrowded conditions. Infectious disease control can lead to isolation, discrimination, and violence against those groups and persons who are believed responsible for an outbreak.

Poor regions of the world often have inadequate health care, nutrition, and sanitation, which makes these areas ideal reservoirs for infectious disease. Furthermore, local hygienic practices, cultural traditions, and social behaviors can help perpetuate the transmission of disease.

## QUARANTINE

In the fourteenth century, quarantine was developed to contain the Black Death (bubonic plague) caused by the bacterium *Yersinia pestis.* Although germ theory and modes of disease transmission were unknown, it was commonly accepted that the disease was somehow transported by travelers and goods arriving from plague-infected areas. This understanding led to the establishment of a forty-day isolation period (a quarantine) to identify infected persons, but this did little to stop the spread of plague throughout Europe.

Quarantine was again used around the beginning of the twentieth century in San Francisco to isolate Chinese immigrants believed to be spreading *Y. pestis.* San Francisco was the primary port for incoming Asian immigrants and for exotic goods from the Far

East. Fleas harboring the bacteria were carried by rats aboard the arriving ships. Based on an unconfirmed diagnosis of bubonic plague in a Chinese immigrant, the San Francisco health department quarantined the entire Chinese quarter of the city to satisfy an increasingly fearful and demanding public. Residents of Chinatown were forbidden to leave the area, and the health department began an invasive house-to-house inspection to find any others infected with plague. Chinese community leaders objected to this drastic treatment, but many citizens of San Francisco were calling for more stringent measures. The quarantine was soon lifted because of continuing protests by the Chinese community.

Sporadic deaths from plague continued in Chinatown for the next three months, and the health department began a massive disinfectant campaign. The disease control effort was assumed by the surgeon general of the United States, who reinstated the quarantine and disinfectant programs, prevented Asians from leaving San Francisco, and instituted an inoculation program with an unproven vaccine. The program also led to the burning of personal possessions.

A proposition was then made to move Asian immigrants to a detention camp outside the city. Isolated incidents of violence then erupted in Chinatown, not only against the health department but also against those Chinese people who were cooperating with the health authorities. Chinatown was then enclosed with wooden fences and barbed wire. The quarantine was eventually lifted by a court order. This extreme quarantine response caused more social damage than disease control: In the years 1900 to 1904, there were only 121 reported cases of plague.

Quarantine was used, to a much more productive end, to contain severe acute respiratory syndrome (SARS) during the outbreak of early 2003. Quarantine has also been considered as an option to contain multi-drug-resistant (MDR) and extremely drug-resistant (XDR) tuberculosis. Under this option, passengers on an airliner carrying a person identified as having one of these strains of tuberculosis would be quarantined. Persons who came into contact with the infected passenger would be tested. In the United States, a person who refuses treatment for tuberculosis can be detained until he or she agrees to treatment.

### STIGMA

In the event of an outbreak, identifying the disease source and the success of disease control can depend on how the affected populations are perceived by society at large. The stigma associated with infectious diseases, principally sexually transmitted diseases (STDs), makes it difficult to identify infected persons and their contacts to ensure they receive proper treatment. In some societies, STDs are synonymous with deviant sexual behaviors and a lack of morals. Other diseases, such as typhus and tuberculosis, have historically been associated with certain ethnic groups, thus exacerbating prejudice against these groups. Diseases caused by inadequate and improper sanitation are common in poor neighborhoods, leading to further prejudice against the poor.

Human immunodeficiency virus (HIV) infection is a highly stigmatized infectious disease because it is transmitted primarily through intravenous drug use and sexual activity; HIV, and the disease it causes, acquired immunodeficiency syndrome (AIDS), also is stigmatized because of its early (and still prominent) association with homosexuality. Many people refuse to be tested because of the ramifications of testing positive for HIV infection. In some developing countries, being HIV-positive leads to social isolation and even physical violence for infected persons and their families. As a result, HIV/AIDS prevention programs often remain underfunded or are nonexistent, and people continue to be at risk for HIV infection because of the stigma attached to the disease.

Social stigma has also led to compliance with public health campaigns to control communicable diseases. In the twentieth century, programs to stop the spread of STDs and programs encouraging vaccinations argued that failure to take measures to stop the transmission of infectious diseases was essentially a display of ignorance. The disgrace of having an STD or the stigma of having an unvaccinated child were used to pressure people into compliance with health programs.

### DISENFRANCHISEMENT

Misconceptions surrounding the source of disease can lead to the disenfranchisement of entire ethnic communities. In the 1980's and 1990's, during the early years of the HIV/AIDS epidemic, Haitians around the world were commonly blamed for this disease. Epidemiologists searching for the origin of the virus focused on Haiti because of its reputation as a popular vacation spot for gay men and because of

Haitian voodoo rituals involving blood. Health officials considered intravenous drug users, gay men, and Haitians to be "high-risk" persons. Haitian immigrants in the United States were treated with prejudice and fear and, ultimately, became almost synonymous with HIV/AIDS. Even after being "declassified" as high risk in 1983, they were prohibited by the U.S. Food and Drug Administration (FDA) from donating blood.

The consequences of this distinction were predictable. Reports surfaced of Haitian children being ostracized and even beaten by their classmates. Businesses in Florida were urged not to employ Haitians because their presence would discourage tourists. Pro-Haitian immigrant groups organized protests in Miami and New York City. A small protest outside the FDA office in Miami, a much larger protest in New York City, and several other marches led to the FDA reconsidering and then rescinding its ban on blood donations by Haitian immigrants. However, the association between Haitians and HIV/AIDS was already established, and it persisted for many years.

During the SARS outbreak in early 2003, people in New York's Chinatown were stigmatized. Tourists were encouraged to avoid the area even though not one case of SARS had been reported in that part of the city. There was an influx of Chinese immigrants to New York's Chinatown in the 1990's, leading to the perception that people living in Chinatown had close relationships with mainland China. In addition, the media had so absolutely linked the SARS outbreak with Asians, and Chinese people in particular, that e-mail began to circulate almost immediately, warning people to stay out of Chinatown to avoid being infected. Community groups in Chinatown issued press releases to try to counter these rumors and fears, but businesses still reported losses of 30 to 70 percent. The stigmatization was based on perceptions of the origins of SARS and on fear because the seriousness of the epidemic and the means of transmission were unclear.

## SOCIAL UNREST

The identification of infectious diseases with certain ethnic groups or regions has led to social unrest and violent responses. In 1917, a violent two-day riot erupted in El Paso, Texas, in response to a quarantine imposed to contain typhus. The disease was believed to be spread by Mexican day laborers, who crossed the

border into Texas each day to work. The quarantine applied to Mexicans crossing the border; each day they had to undergo physical examinations, disinfection of their belongings, and disinfecting baths in a mixture of kerosene, vinegar, and gasoline.

The protest, which began when a group of Mexican women attempted to cross the border to work, escalated into a riot. Hundreds of U.S. soldiers were mobilized to the border. Persons who wanted to cross into Texas to work submitted to the examinations. After several months, the disinfection procedures were required weekly only. U.S. health authorities performed nearly 900,000 examinations of Mexicans entering the United States in a five-month period in 1917. Only three cases of typhus were reported in El Paso during that period.

In Africa, the HIV/AIDS epidemic and the smaller hemorrhagic fever outbreaks provide examples of how diseases can cause social and political instability. When the first outbreaks of Ebola hemorrhagic fever occurred in Gabon, Africa, in 1995, international health care workers sent to address the outbreak did so in a culturally insensitive manner, disregarding the local customs and traditions. Sick and deceased persons were kept in tents or body bags. Although this was done for protection against further infection, local residents feared that something appalling was being done to their sick relatives and to their relatives' bodies after death. The autocratic manner in which the disease was managed created hostility and suspicion toward the health care workers. When another outbreak occurred in 2001, health care workers encountered armed villagers opposed to their presence. In contrast, President Robert Mugabe of Zimbabwe attempted to buttress support for his government and preserve social stability in 2008 by proclaiming that he had stopped a cholera epidemic.

## HUMAN RIGHTS

Methods employed to control or eradicate infectious diseases often conflict with basic human rights. During an outbreak, a point is reached where it must be considered whether the rights of a minority of diseased persons outweigh the need to protect the public. Quarantine, mandatory vaccination, and the treatment and reporting of infected persons, while somewhat effective in controlling disease, also are restrictive and invasive.

Quarantine has been used throughout history to

contain communicable diseases, especially those diseases for which the mode of transmission has not been clearly defined. Quarantine is a reasonable measure when substantial proof exists that isolation will be effective in controlling the disease and maintaining public health. Without these assurances, quarantine can have dire social consequences; it also can lead to the exposure of uninfected quarantined persons to the disease. Any quarantine order must be enforced fairly and without singling out any ethnic, racial, or socioeconomic group.

Mandatory vaccinations, like those promoted by the World Health Organization's (WHO) smallpox and polio eradication campaigns, are considered by some to be violations of the rights of persons to determine their own medical care. Again, the issue here is the right of an individual to refuse a possibly harmful vaccination versus the potential to rid the world of a deadly disease. In the 1950's and 1960's, the WHO smallpox eradication campaign in India occasionally involved the military vaccinating people by force.

Similar mandatory vaccination campaigns in Africa led to suspicion among vaccine recipients and community leaders. Cultural and political issues were raised in 2003 regarding the oral polio vaccine. The Nigerian state of Kano suspended oral polio vaccinations for eight months in 2003 and 2004 because of rumors that the vaccines contained traces of HIV and female hormones. The rumors were allegedly started by local Islamic clerics who claimed the vaccines were designed to infect Muslim children with HIV and to sterilize them. Because of this suspension of the vaccination program, Nigeria accounted for 145 of the 201 reported polio cases in Africa in 2004 before resuming the program.

Other types of mandatory actions must also balance a person's right to refuse treatment with the potential to spread the disease to others. Tuberculosis is highly contagious and is quickly reemerging in areas where it has previously been controlled. Tuberculosis is easily cured by an inexpensive course of therapy, but in many cases infected persons do not complete the entire treatment. This has led to the development of MDR and XDR tuberculosis. To help prevent the spread of tuberculosis and the development of these drug-resistant strains, it is now standard procedure worldwide to treat persons under the DOTS (directly observed treatment, short-course) program. The DOTS approach to stopping the spread of tuber-

culosis, while not coercive, is a highly monitored program sponsored by WHO to provide standardized treatment, to provide supervision to ensure persons are taking their medications, and to provide patient support. Since its inception in 1995, approximately thirty-six million persons have been treated under this supervised program and, in 2007, the treatment success rate was 86 percent. While not compulsory, the support and supervision by health care professionals to complete treatment may result in more treatment compliance than would an actual mandate.

A person's right to privacy may also be compromised in the event of an infectious disease outbreak. In some cases, health care workers are required to report infectious diseases to the health authorities to control a potential outbreak and to protect the public. In other cases, third-party notification of anyone the infected person may have come in contact with might be required. This could violate the right to privacy of the infected person; however, it also is necessary to protect those who may have been exposed and to prevent further spread of the disease.

## Impact

In addition to the medical and economic impact of infectious diseases, the social impact can be devastating. It has been repeatedly demonstrated how association of a disease with a particular ethnic, racial, or other minority group can stigmatize an entire community. People can be ostracized and treated with disgust, misjudgment, and even violence based on perceptions regarding how they acquired the disease. An infected person's fear of self-identifying can disrupt disease eradication programs and endanger others who are not infected. In extreme circumstances, epidemics can disrupt disease control programs, cultivate distrust in the health authorities, and result in civil unrest and social instability.

The difficulty of managing infectious disease comes down to this: how to balance programs and medications that will benefit the health of millions with the rights and choices of individual persons. Mandating treatments or vaccinations is a definite infringement on individual human rights. However, doing so protects the rights of others to retain their freedom of movement without being unknowingly exposed to communicable diseases.

*Deborah A. Appello, M.S.*

## FURTHER READING

Bayer, Ronald. "Stigma and the Ethics of Public Health: Not Can We but Should We." *Social Science and Medicine* 67 (2008): 463-472. An examination of the stigmatization of persons in the United States who are identified as having, or being at high risk of acquiring, particular infectious diseases.

Eichelberger, Laura. "SARS and New York's Chinatown: The Politics of Risk and Blame During an Epidemic of Fear." *Social Science and Medicine* 53 (2007): 1284-1295. A sociopolitical study of the stigmatization of residents of New York City's Chinatown during the 2003 SARS epidemic.

Kapp, C. "Nigerian State Promises to End Polio Vaccine Boycott." *The Lancet* 363 (2004): 1876. A report on the northern Nigerian state of Kano's eight-month boycott of the polio vaccine because of suspicion that the vaccine was contaminated.

Leach, Melissa, Ian Scoones, and Andrew Stirling. "Governing Epidemics in an Age of Complexity: Narratives, Politics, and Pathways to Sustainability." *Global Environmental Change* 20 (2010): 369-377. Addresses difficulties encountered by governments when dealing with epidemics while also trying to maintain equality of access to health care.

Markel, Howard. *When Germs Travel: Six Major Epidemics That Have Invaded America Since 1900 and the Fears They Have Unleashed.* New York: Pantheon Books, 2004. Historical examination of tuberculosis, bubonic plague, trachoma, typhus, AIDS, and cholera epidemics introduced into the United States by international travelers. Also looks at the effects these epidemics had on the handling of infectious diseases.

Riley, G. A., and D. Baah-Odoom. "Do Stigma, Blame, and Stereotyping Contribute to Unsafe Sexual Behaviour? A Test of Claims About the Spread of HIV/AIDS Arising from Social Representation Theory and the AIDS Risk Reduction Model." *Social Science and Medicine* 71 (2010): 600-607. A study of youth in Ghana that found that contrary to common expectation, "specific blaming and stereotyping attitudes that constructed HIV/AIDS as a sexual disease were associated with safer intended sexual behaviour."

Selgelid, Michael J. "Pandethics." *Public Health* 123 (2009): 255-259. A review of four ethical issues associated with pandemic influenza: the responsibility to avoid infecting others, the obligation of health care professionals to treat the infected, the allocation of resources, and quarantine measures.

## WEB SITES OF INTEREST

*Centers for Disease Control and Prevention*
http://www.cdc.gov

*Global Health Council*
http://www.globalhealth.org/infectious_diseases

*World Health Organization*
http://www.who.int

**See also:** Aging and infectious disease; Contagious diseases; Developing countries and infectious disease; Disease eradication campaigns; Emerging and re-emerging infectious diseases; Endemic infections; Epidemics and pandemics: History; Epidemiology; Globalization and infectious disease; Men and infectious disease; Outbreaks; Psychological effects of infectious disease; Public health; Quarantine; Schools and infectious disease; Women and infectious disease.

# Soilborne illness and disease

CATEGORY: Diseases and conditions
ANATOMY OR SYSTEM AFFECTED: All
ALSO KNOWN AS: Soil-transmitted diseases

## DEFINITION

Soilborne illnesses and diseases are caused by numerous microorganisms and parasites that live in soils. Soil serves as an ecosystem for diverse microbes that perform various roles and that range from useful organisms in biological and geological processes to dangerous transmitters of diseases. In May, 2001, a resolution of the World Health Assembly of the United Nations emphasized the need for increased medical intervention to minimize the occurrence of soil-transmitted diseases. The next year, the United Nations reiterated the goal of preventing soilborne worm infestations.

## CAUSES

Soilborne, or soil-transmitted, diseases are common, especially in tropical regions, and affect more than two billion people globally in the early twenty-first century, according to the World Health Organization (WHO). In 2010, more than one-half million children internationally suffered sicknesses, particularly helminthiasis infections, contracted from soil. Although most people survive these illnesses, sources indicate approximately 12,000 to 135,000 people die yearly from soilborne helminth infections. Scientists estimate that the life spans of people infected with the most prevalent soilborne diseases and parasites are reduced by 43.5 million life years, more than the lifespan reductions of measles and malaria and exceeded only by tuberculosis.

Most soilborne illnesses are transmitted from soil to humans through the pathogens (such as bacteria, fungi, protozoa, and worms) that are shed in fecal material, which contaminate soil. These pathogens infect people who eat the plants grown in the contaminated soil or who drink water polluted by that soil. Human and nonhuman animals infected with soil-transmitted illnesses perpetuate the cycle when their feces contact soil. Bacteria and viruses associated with enteric diseases, specifically infections in the gastrointestinal tract, often are transmitted to humans in soils that have been used to bury sewage. Landfills that do not have procedures to control leaching enable bacteria and viruses to contaminate soil.

Helminthiasis is a frequently diagnosed disease reported worldwide that is transmitted by contact with soil. Eggs from worms, or helminths, are dormant in soil until they enter human or animal bodies, move through those bodies as larvae, and mature within three months into worms that infest the intestines. Worm infestation is often chronic, as parasites can live several years in their hosts. Soils host numerous types of worms (also referred to as nematodes), including roundworms, hookworms, and whipworms, which transmit diseases to humans.

The roundworm *Ascaris lumbricoides* infects humans with ascariasis. According to WHO, more than one billion humans are infected with this worm. Soils host these parasites' eggs. Roundworms are prolific, producing approximately 200,000 eggs daily. Humans are exposed to these immature worms by touching contaminated soil or by swallowing dirt or food that has not been adequately cleaned. Inside human bodies, roundworm eggs hatch into larvae that then invade essential body parts, including nerves and organs.

Other worms transmitted through soil include the hookworms *Necator americanus* and *Ancylostoma duodenale*. Those larvae enter skin from soil, infecting people with ancylostomiasis. WHO states approximately 740 million people have hookworms. The disease trichuriasis results from eggs from the whipworm, *Trichuris trichiura*, contaminating soil. About 795 million people have this infection, according to WHO.

Humans also are infested with the threadworm *Strongyloides stercorali*, which causes the disease strongyloidiasis as it moves from soil into the feet. Through worm eggs shed in fecal material, infested domestic pets expose humans to parasites and diseases associated with them, including visceral larva migrans and toxoplasmosis infections caused by *Toxoplasma gondii*.

As a cause of anthrax infections, dormant *Bacillus anthracis* bacteria spores often exist in soil for long durations, ranging from several years to decades. Growing grass blades transport anthrax spores from soil when grass-grazing animals ingest them. Associated with listeriosis, the bacterium *Listeria monocytogenes* is frequently found in soils and manure, contaminating livestock and plants used as food sources. The *Brucellosis* bacterium, often associated with livestock, can enter bodies through exposure to touching or breathing dust. The *Leptospira interrogans* bacterium, which causes leptospirosis, is present in soil and muddy areas where rodent urine containing that pathogen soaks into the ground. The *Acinetobacter baumannii* bacterium, which lives in soil, causes acinetobacter.

Most soil-transmitted disease deaths involve the pathogen *Clostridium tetani*, responsible for the deaths of approximately 450,000 infants and 50,000 adults each year. Scientists state that this bacterium's spores can be dormant in soil for almost one-half century and can still infect humans. *C. botulinum* bacteria spores also remain dormant in soils for extended times, causing botulism infections that are spread through foods. Soils in tropical areas often host the bacteria *Burkholderia pseudomallei* and *B. mallei*, which infect people with melioidosis and glanders when they touch or inhale soil or eat foods cultivated in contaminated fields. Nocardiosis infections occur when people breathe *Nocardia* bacteria found in dust or when contaminated soil contacts a person's skin injury.

Rarer, and often more deadly, soil-transmitted diseases occur when *Chromobacterium violaceum* bacteria infect humans by spreading from skin openings through the circulatory system and attacking organs simultaneously, preventing their function. Although Legionnaires' disease is usually transmitted through air or water, the Centers for Disease Control and Prevention (CDC) in 2000 reported cases in which the bacterium *Legionella longbeachae* infected people who had touched potting soil. Scientists have linked poliovirus 1 to soil, noting that the virus can survive more than three months underground and contaminate crops.

Fungi in soils, including the fungi *Mucorales, Aspergillus, Fusarium,* and *Blastomyces dermatitidis,* also transmit diseases. *Cryptococcus neoformans* can infect people who inhale dust containing it, leading to cryptococcal meningitis. Histoplasmosis is another soilborne illness, this time caused by *Histoplasma* fungus, which exists in soils as mold and affects the lung. Fungal *Coccidioides immitis* spores in soil cause coccidioidomycosis infections.

## RISK FACTORS

Socioeconomic factors increase the risk of a person being infected with soilborne diseases. Poor sanitation exposes humans to soils contaminated with microorganisms and parasites. Areas without hygienic toilets or other devices to contain human wastes contribute to soil-transmitted infestations. Inadequate sewage systems result in fecal material being present near houses, schools, and other buildings. Rain washes these soils into water supplies, often rivers and ponds, which people use as a source for drinking water and use for bathing, swimming, fishing, and cleaning of cooking and eating implements.

Impoverished populations often lack access to sufficient preventive medical care. Illiteracy and restricted educational opportunities result in people not having information on preventing soilborne diseases or on treating those conditions if infected. Many people who suffer soil-transmitted diseases do not consume diets with nutritional foods that provide vitamins and minerals. They often eat foods that have not been thoroughly cooked or cleaned, and they do not have access to pasteurized products and boiled water. Pregnant women and people with weak immune systems or other health problems are extra-susceptible to soilborne illnesses and suffer miscarriages and mortality caused by infections.

Populations living in areas where crops are fertilized with feces or irrigated with polluted water risk being infected by diseases transmitted by soil, either by consuming foods, especially vegetables and fruits, grown in those soils or by working in contaminated fields. Runoff from pastures can contaminate communities with pathogens associated with livestock manure. Risks associated with contacting contaminated soils increase with people's proximity to landfills or other sites where sewage is stored in soil and where pathogens seep into the ground.

Dangers associated with exposure to soil depend on how accessible a person's skin is to contacting soils directly. People who work outdoors, performing landscaping, agricultural, forestry, sewage, or other jobs that involve contact with soil are at high risk of acquiring soil-transmitted illnesses. Hikers and others participating in outdoor recreation come into contact with soils and the pathogens they host. Children's risk is increased because they often play in dirt that can be contaminated. People with the disorder called pica (in which they consume, among other non-nutritive substances, soil) are especially vulnerable to soilborne illnesses.

Weather can intensify the occurrence of soilborne diseases. Floods, for example, can force to the surface underground soil layers and the pathogens they host. Violent storms such as hurricanes and typhoons can move soil and pathogens great distances. Soilborne diseases identified as potential biological weapons also present public safety concerns. Terrorists have threatened to use anthrax spores secured from soil sources. The CDC designated *B. pseudomallei* and *B. mallei* to be bioterrorism agents because of their universal availability in soils.

## SYMPTOMS

Various symptoms are exhibited by people infected with soil-transmitted diseases. Probably the most obvious symptom associated with soilborne illness is the shedding of parasites while vomiting or during a bowel movement. People infected with soil-transmitted helminths often suffer gastrointestinal pain and swollen stomachs. Other organs occasionally swell. Infected people frequently experience diarrhea, nausea, bloody bowels, and vomiting, and they can become anemic.

Soil-transmitted infections usually cause people to become weak and listless. Fevers, rashes, headaches, and stiffness are common symptoms too. Infected persons often are not strong enough to attend school or perform labor. Some people with soilborne illnesses exhibit impaired cognition, experiencing problems with memory and language functions. Long-term symptoms include decreased mental and physical development in children. Lung damage from soilborne illness is often exhibited through pneumonia, coughing, or asthma. Although most adults do not exhibit the symptoms of toxoplasmosis infection, children who were infected in utero develop symptoms as they mature. Health problems associated with toxoplasmosis include blindness, deafness, and retardation.

Illnesses associated with soil often weaken immune systems, causing people to develop infections and conditions unrelated to soil. Soil-transmitted diseases are sometimes described as food-borne illnesses, even though pathogens such as *Escherichia coli* O157:H7 and *Salmonella*, which are associated with food poisoning, are present in soil that contaminates foods. Poor agricultural yields, damaged plants, and ill livestock may indicate the presence of pathogens and parasites in soil.

## SCREENING AND DIAGNOSIS

Medical professionals evaluate those with soil-transmitted illnesses according to conditions and physical ailments unique to each person. Examinations usually begin with recording an infected person's medical history and asking where the person lives and if they have traveled to other areas. This geographical information helps clinicians determine the most likely soil-transmitted disease infected the patient.

Health care workers assess various tissue samples to diagnose soilborne diseases associated with microorganisms. Specimens acquired for analysis frequently include blood, sputum, urine, feces, skin, bone marrow, and cerebrospinal fluids. Blood tests reveal the presence of antibodies to bacteria. X rays and biopsies are often used to detect fungal soil-transmitted diseases such as cryptococcosis. Some physicians utilize magnetic resonance imaging or computed tomography scans to assess damage by mucormycosis and other microbe infections.

For diagnosis of helminth infections, patients provide fecal samples for laboratory analysis to detect evidence of parasites and to examine worms. Technicians utilize several methods to evaluate specimens, including formalinethyl acetate sedimentation and Kato-Katz fecal-thick smear to count worm eggs. Medical personnel use imaging procedures and tools, such as endoscopy and ultrasonography, to determine any internal damage to organs and intestines.

## TREATMENT AND THERAPY

Persons diagnosed with soil-transmitted diseases undergo various methods to treat their infection. Many treatments focus on removing worms and include tablets composed of benzimidazole anthelmintics. The drugs most frequently dispensed include albendazole and mebendazole in doses of 400 to 500 milligrams (mg) for children two years of age and older and for adults, including women who have reached their second trimester of pregnancy. Toddlers younger than two years of age receive 200 mg. Amounts of the drug praziquantel are determined by measurements of the patients' height with a dose pole. Helminth-infected persons often receive iron and vitamin A supplements. People at risk of being reinfected receive additional drug doses at later times.

Researchers are developing new pharmaceuticals and methods to control soil-transmitted parasites that have become resistant to standard treatments. Other drugs sometimes used include levamisole, pyrantel pamoate, nitazoxanide, and tribendimidine. Many soilborne infections caused by microbes are treated with antibiotics. These drugs, however, often cannot defeat pathogens that become resistant to antibiotics. Medical researchers have tested the use of recombinant larval antigen ASP2 to create a hookworm vaccination. Scientists have investigated incorporating outer membrane proteins in a leptospirosis vaccine, reporting successes in 2010 in strengthening immunities in test animals.

## PREVENTION AND OUTCOMES

Most people contact soil daily. Interaction with soil varies depending on a person's activities, exposure to the outdoors, and dietary habits. People can minimize the possibility of being infected by avoiding areas most likely to host parasites and pathogens. One should wash his or her hands, feet, or any bare skin that has been in contact with soil. Wearing gloves while gardening lessens hazards associated with handling soils. Wounds, cuts, abrasions, cracks, and other skin damage should be covered with bandages. Shoes prevent soilborne illnesses from being transmitted through the soles of the feet. People should avoid inhaling dust. Masks help block spores in areas where fungi thrive in soil.

Soil contaminant hazards can be minimized through purifying water supplies, cleaning unsanitary sites, and providing sanitary toilet facilities. Other preventive measures include washing soil from raw foods harvested from gardens or bought at markets. Cooking meats thoroughly to destroy parasites helps reduce risks associated with consuming livestock products that might have been infected while animals grazed on forage that grew on contaminated soil.

The transmission of diseases associated with soil can be prevented by not eating soil. Crops fertilized with raw waste or irrigated with wastewater should not be consumed. Agricultural laborers should avoid handling those contaminated soils. People should regularly deworm domesticated pets and not touch any fecal material.

Some schools, particularly in tropical regions or developing countries, sponsor programs to deworm students. Health care personnel provide children medical treatments to purge and prevent further helminth infections. Educational presentations teach children and adults hygienic behavior and discourage contact with hazardous soils. Several charities and shoe manufacturers distribute free shoes in impoverished communities where residents are at risk of contracting soilborne diseases.

*Elizabeth D. Schafer, Ph.D.*

## FURTHER READING

Albonico, Marco, Dirk Engels, and Lorenzo Savioli. "Monitoring Drug Efficacy and Early Detection of Drug Resistance in Human Soil-Transmitted Nematodes: A Pressing Public Health Agenda for Helminth Control." *International Journal of Parasitology* 34, no. 11 (2004): 1205-1210. Reviews pharmaceuticals and techniques to assess which helminths resist chemotherapy, emphasizing the necessity for continued research and development.

Albonico, Marco, et al. *Preventative Chemotherapy in Human Helminthiasis.* Geneva: World Health Organization, 2006. Outlines treatment procedures and drug doses for people representing various age and risk factors. Glossary, charts, appendices.

Ambrosioni, Juan, Daniel Lew, and Jorge Garbino. "Nocardiosis: Updated Clinical Review and Experience at a Tertiary Center." *Infection* 38, no. 2 (2010): 89-97. Presents authors' experiences with this soil-borne disease during a twenty-year period, noting how patients were infected and noting their symptoms, diagnoses, and treatments.

Bethony, Jeffrey, et al. "Soil-Transmitted Helminth Infections: Ascariasis, Trichuriasis, and Hookworm." *The Lancet* 367 (May 6, 2006): 1521-1532. Summarizes information regarding the most prevalent soil-transmitted worm infections, including statistics and prevention and treatment methods.

Brooker, Simon, et al. "Global Epidemiology, Ecology, and Control of Soil-Transmitted Helminth Infections." In *Global Mapping of Infectious Diseases,* edited by Simon I. Hay, Alastair Graham, and David J. Rogers. Amsterdam: Elsevier, 2006. Considers environmental factors that affect the geographical distribution of nematodes and the occurrence of soilborne diseases.

De Siqueira, Isadora Cristina, et al. "*Chromobacterium violaceum* in Siblings, Brazil." *Emerging Infectious Diseases* 11, no. 9 (2005): 1443-1445. Case study of an incident in which three brothers were exposed to soil contaminated with bacteria. Images show microscopic view of bacteria and a scan of organ damage.

"Legionnaires' Disease Associated with Potting Soil— California, Oregon, and Washington, May-June, 2000." *Journal of the American Medical Association* 284, no. 12 (September 27, 2000): 1510. Reports rare incidences in which persons acquired this usually waterborne disease by handling gardening materials.

Santamaría, Johanna, and Gary A. Toranzos. "Enteric Pathogens and Soil: A Short Review." *International Microbiology* 6, no. 1 (2003): 5-9. Examines how disposing solid wastes contaminates soil with microorganisms, noting several soilborne disease outbreaks.

World Health Organization. "Soil-Transmitted Helminthiasis: Number of Children Treated 2007-2008: Update on the 2010 Global Target." *Weekly Epidemiological Record* 85 (April 16, 2010): 141-148. Discusses efforts to prevent worm infections, providing statistics and a map showing locations of the most urgent cases.

## WEB SITES OF INTEREST

*Centers for Disease Control and Prevention*
http://www.cdc.gov/parasites

*Leptospirosis Information Center*
http://www.leptospirosis.org

*Neglected Tropical Disease Initiative*
http://www.neglecteddiseases.gov

*Nematode Net*
http://www.nematode.net

*Wellcome Trust Sanger Institute*
http://sanger.ac.uk/resources/downloads/helminths

*World Health Organization*
http://www.who.int/intestinal_worms

**See also:** Airborne illness and disease; Children and infectious disease; Developing countries and infectious disease; Fecal-oral route of transmission; Foodborne illness and disease; Fungal infections; Intestinal and stomach infections; Parasites: Classification and types; Pathogens; Protozoan diseases; Respiratory route of transmission; Tropical medicine; Waterborne illness and disease; Worm infections.

---

Sore throat. *See* Pharyngitis and tonsillopharyngitis; Strep throat; Viral pharyngitis.

---

# Sporotrichosis

CATEGORY: Diseases and conditions
ANATOMY OR SYSTEM AFFECTED: Lymphatic system, skin

## DEFINITION

Sporotrichosis is an infectious disease caused by the soil fungus *Sporothrix schenckii* that usually affects the skin. Sporotrichosis is commonly acquired through cutaneous inoculation. In rare cases, it can be inhaled. It is not spread from person to person, but zoonotic transmission from infected animals (such as cats and horses) is possible.

## CAUSES

*S. schenckii* is widely distributed in the natural environment and can be found on rose thorns and on twigs, and in sphagnum moss, hay, and soil. The fungus enters the skin through small cuts or punctures, and it spreads from the initial lesion along lymphatic channels. Hematogenous dissemination is rare.

## RISK FACTORS

Persons handling thorny plants, sphagnum moss, or baled hay (such as farmers, nursery workers, landscapers, and gardeners) are at higher risk for the disease. Sporotrichosis resulting from inhalation has been documented in persons with severe chronic obstructive pulmonary disease. Immunosuppressive states and alcoholism predispose to disseminated disease. The disease is most common among adults and slightly more prevalent in males. Sporotrichosis in children may be more common in tropical regions.

## SYMPTOMS

The first symptom is a firm, pink to purple, usually painless skin nodule that resembles an insect bite. It may appear from one to twelve weeks after exposure to the fungus. Over time, the nodule may ulcerate and become chronic. The characteristic infection progresses proximally along lymphatic channels. In the vast majority of cases, disease is limited to the skin. Very rarely, the disease can infect the bones, joints, lungs, and brain. Widespread cutaneous lesions and involvement of multiple visceral organs (including eye, prostate, oral mucosa, paranasal sinuses, and larynx) predominantly occur in persons with compromised immune systems, such as those with human immunodeficiency virus infection, diabetes, alcoholism or other disorders of the immune system.

## SCREENING AND DIAGNOSIS

Diagnosis is based on a nodule biopsy and laboratory identification of the mold.

## TREATMENT AND THERAPY

Skin sporotrichosis is traditionally treated with oral, saturated, potassium iodide solution (three times per day for three to six months until the skin lesions are completely healed). Oral itraconazole (200 milligrams once or twice daily) is the drug of choice for cutaneous and lymphocutaneous forms of the disease. It may also be used to treat bone and joint infections. For persons with severe disease or with pulmonary, brain, or disseminated infection, liposomal amphotericin B is generally recommended; once the person has stabilized, itraconazole can be used for step-down therapy. Infected bone or infected lung areas may need to be surgically removed.

Treating sporotrichosis may take several months or years. With treatment, full recovery can be expected. Spontaneous resolution of cutaneous sporotrichosis has been reported. Disseminated sporotrichosis is associated with significant morbidity and can be life-threatening for people with compromised immune systems.

## PREVENTION AND OUTCOMES

Preventive measures include wearing gloves, long sleeves, heavy boots, and other protective clothing when handling wires, rose bushes, hay bales, conifer (pine) seedlings, or other materials that may cause minor skin breaks. It is also advisable to avoid skin contact with sphagnum moss, which has been implicated as a source of the fungus in a number of outbreaks. When handling animals with skin lesions, the use of gloves minimizes the risk of zoonotic transmission.

*Katia Marazova, M.D., Ph.D.*

## FURTHER READING

Greenfield, Ronald A. "Sporotrichosis." Available at http://emedicine.medscape.com/article/228723-overview.

Kauffman, Carol A. "Sporotrichosis." *Clinical Infectious Diseases* 29 (1999): 231-236.

_____, et al. "Clinical Practice Guidelines for the Management of Sporotrichosis: 2007 Update by the Infectious Diseases Society of America." *Clinical Infectious Diseases* 45 (2007): 1255-1265.

## WEB SITES OF INTEREST

*Centers for Disease Control and Prevention*
http://www.cdc.gov/nczved/divisions/dfbmd/diseases/sporotrichosis

*Microbiology and Immunology On-line: Mycology*
http://pathmicro.med.sc.edu/book/mycol-sta.htm

**See also:** Airborne illness and disease; Allergic bronchopulmonary aspergillosis; Antifungal drugs: Types; Aspergillosis; *Aspergillus*; Blastomycosis; Chromoblastomycosis; *Coccidioides*; Coccidiosis; Fungal infections; *Fusarium*; Histoplasmosis; Mold infections; Mycoses; *Paracoccidioides*; Paracoccidioidomycosis; Respiratory route of transmission; *Rhizopus*; Skin infections; Soilborne illness and disease.

---

# *Stachybotrys*

CATEGORY: Pathogen
TRANSMISSION ROUTE: Ingestion, inhalation, skin

## DEFINITION

The pathogen *Stachybotrys* is a mold that grows on wet cellulose-containing materials. *Stachybotrys* produces a number of mycotoxins, including several trichothecenes and a hemorrhagic protein called hemolysin. *Memnoniella* is a related fungus that has similar growth characteristics and produces similar mycotoxins.

---

**Taxonomic Classification
for *Stachybotrys***

**Kingdom:** Fungi
**Phylum:** Ascomycota
**Class:** Sordariomycetes
**Order:** Hypocreales
**Genus:** *Stachybotrys*
**Species:**
*S. alternans*
*S. chlorohalonata*
*S. cylindrospora*
*S. nephrospora*

---

## NATURAL HABITAT AND FEATURES

*Stachybotrys* is a black or grey fungus (mold) with worldwide distribution. *Stachybotrys* grows on wet cellulose-containing material such as hay, leaves, paper, wood, wall board, textiles, rugs, drywall, and insulating materials. *Stachybotrys* is a fairly slow grower and may be overrun by other molds growing on cellulose-containing substrates.

*Stachybotrys* requires wet conditions to grow; however, *Stachybotrys* spores can remain dormant under dry conditions for several years and can resume active growth and mycotoxin production when water becomes available. The *Stachybotrys* mycotoxins can also retain their potency over several years without active *Stachybotrys* growth. *Stachybotrys* frequently grows in buildings that have been flooded by leaking pipes or toilets, rain infiltration, or natural disasters, including hurricanes.

*Stachybotrys* spores are often hard to grow in culture. Some studies have reported that cellulose-based media or cornmeal media is best for cultured *Stachybotrys* growth.

*Stachybotrys* spores are not as readily spread by air as are most mold spores. Several published studies have been unable to collect any airborne *Stachybotrys* spores, even though the buildings in question may be contaminated with many square meters of *Stachybotrys* growth. Relying on airborne samples only has led many indoor air investigators to falsely conclude that *Stachybotrys* was not growing in the structures under investigation. Because *Stachybotrys* spores are not readily dispersed in the air and are hard to grow in culture, all mold sampling studies that suspect *Stachybotrys* growth should take surface, tape, or building material samples from the building.

## PATHOGENICITY AND CLINICAL SIGNIFICANCE

Localized *Stachybotrys* infections have been reported. Viable *Stachybotrys* was isolated from the lungs of a seven-year-old boy living in a water damaged farmhouse with heavy *Stachybotrys* growth. The boy, who experienced severe fatigue, chronic coughing, and lung hemorrhage, completely recovered after cleanup of his mold-infested home. Unpublished observations have reported *Stachybotrys* growth in nasal sinuses; however, the main health concerns are connected to the mycotoxins and allergens produced by *Stachybotrys*.

The *Stachybotrys* mycotoxins were first reported as contaminants of animal feed and human food. In the 1940's, there were reports of domestic animals dying in the Soviet Union after eating *Stachybotrys*-infested hay. In later years, attention has been focused on humans who are exposed to high levels of *Stachybotrys* and its mycotoxins in indoor air and dust.

*Stachybotrys* produces a wide range of mycotoxins, including the trichothecenes satratoxin, roridan, and deoxynivalenol. The amounts and types of triochothecenes produced vary considerably depending on environmental conditions and the *Stachybotrys* strain. The trichothecene mycotoxins damage the immune

and nervous systems, inhibit protein synthesis, and can cause vomiting. Animal studies have reported that exposure to small amounts of trichothecenes can damage brain cells.

*Stachybotrys* also produces a protein called hemolysin, which causes lung hemorrhage in nonhuman animals and may be linked to human lung hemorrhage. In the 1990's, life-threatening lung hemorrhage was reported in ten infants in Cleveland, Ohio, who lived in water-damaged homes. Airborne levels of *Stachybotrys*, *Aspergillus*, and other molds were much higher in the homes of the infants with lung hemorrhage than in the control homes.

The allergens and mycotoxins from *Stachybotrys* can also worsen asthma and nasal problems. Several studies have reported that heavy indoor exposure to *Stachybotrys* and other molds is associated with significantly poorer lung function and significant deficits in many neuropsychiatric parameters, such as reaction times, color vision, memory, concentration, grip strength, and vocabulary.

The ideal way to control *Stachybotrys* and its mycotoxins is to prevent exposure to the mold. The best way to control *Stachybotrys* growth is to prevent indoor water damage. All cases of indoor water damage, standing water, or visible mold growth should be cleaned within twenty-four hours to prevent growth of *Stachybotrys* and other fungi and bacteria. For large cases of water damages, one should contact a flood remediation company. Several guides are available for mold remediation, including the U.S. Environmental Protection Agency's "Guide to Mold Remediation in Schools and Commercial Buildings" (available at http://www.epa.gov/mold/mold_remediation.html).

Several studies have reported that clean up and water remediation of homes with heavy *Stachybotrys* growth are associated with less asthma, fatigue, and concentration and memory problems in the occupants of the contaminated home.

## DRUG SUSCEPTIBILITY

Because *Stachybotrys* does not appear to cause human infection, antifungal drugs are generally not used to treat persons who have been exposed to *Stachybotrys*. However, some studies have reported that the use of the bile-binding drug cholestryamine may be useful in speeding human excretion of trichothecene mycotoxins. Other research has suggested that eating a well-balanced diet that is high in antioxidants (vitamins A, C, and E, and l-carnitine and coenzyme Q10) can reduce the toxic effects of many myco-toxins.

*Luke Curtis, M.D.*

## FURTHER READING

Elidemir, Okam, et al. "Isolation of *Stachybotrys* from the Lung of a Child with Pulmonary Hemosider-osis." *Pediatrics* 104 (1999): 964-966. A case report of viable *Stachybotrys* growing in the lungs of a seven-year-old boy.

Etzel, Ruth, et al. "Acute Pulmonary Hemorrhage in Infants Associated with Exposure to *Stachybotrys atra* and Other Fungi." *Archives of Pediatric and Ado-lescent Medicine* 152 (1998): 757-762. This study re-ports on ten previously healthy infants who experi-enced sudden pulmonary hemorrhage. Airborne levels of *Stachybotrys* and *Aspergillus* were much higher in case homes versus control homes.

Kilburn, Kaye. "Neurobehavioral and Pulmonary Im-pairment in 105 Adults with Indoor Exposure to Molds Compared to 100 Exposed to Chemicals." *Toxicology and Industrial Health* 25 (2009): 681-692. This paper provides thorough documentation that a group of 105 mold-exposed persons experienced significant deficits in lung function, reaction times, color vision, memory, grip strength, and vocabu-lary.

Samson, Robert, Ellen Hoesktra, and Jens Frisvad. *In-troduction to Food and Airborne Fungi*. 7th ed. Utrecht, the Netherlands: Central Bureau for Fungal Cul-tures, 2004. This guide provides much information about *Stachybotrys* and many other indoor fungi. Includes useful identification keys, photographs, and diagrams.

## WEB SITES OF INTEREST

*American Lung Association*
http://www.lungusa.org

*British Mycological Society*
http://fungionline.org.uk

*Canadian Lung Association*
http://www.lung.ca

*Systematic Mycology and Microbiology Laboratory*
http://www.ars.usda.gov

**See also:** *Aspergillus*; *Bordetella*; Fungal infections; Fungi: Classification and types; *Fusarium*; Histoplas-mosis; Mycoses; Respiratory route of transmission; *Rhizopus*; Soilborne illness and disease.

---

# Staphylococcal infections

CATEGORY: Diseases and conditions
ANATOMY OR SYSTEM AFFECTED: All
ALSO KNOWN AS: Staph infections, *Staphylococcus au-reus* infection

## DEFINITION

Staphylococcal infections are caused by the bacte-rium *Staphylococcus*, of which there are more than thirty types. The most common infective form of *Staphyloccocus* is *S. aureus*, a gram-positive coccus bac-teria with a grapelike appearance. The bacterium is found in the nasal passages and on the skin of humans and animals and is considered normal flora. Under certain conditions, however, these opportunist bac-teria can cause minor to life-threatening infections.

## CAUSES

Although much is known about staphylococcal infections, much remains unknown. The bacteria causing these infections are considered part of the normal flora or usual bacteria occurring in the nose or on the skin. When staphylococci invade the human body through a break in the skin or through the bloodstream, lungs, or digestive tract, the bacteria may become purulent and cause disease.

## RISK FACTORS

The virulence (ability to make a person ill) of staphylococci is considered low in most cases. The risk of severe infections by staphylococci occurs when the host has an immune system weakened by hospitaliza-tion, by a chronic disease such as diabetes, and by treatments with drugs such as chemotherapy and ste-roids. In hospitals, staphylococci may be contracted in surgical or burn units and in general medical-surgical units. Breast-feeding women and the elderly may be at risk for this condition.

Another risk factor is having an internal medical device, such as a urinary tube, inside one's body, pro-viding bacterial access to tissues. Other entry points

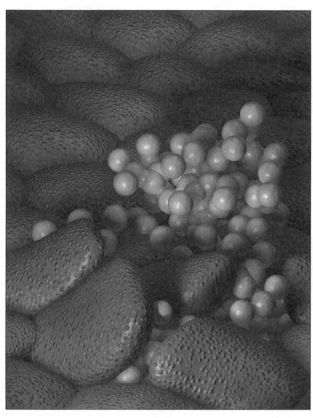

*Staphylococcal bacteria infect the cells lining the nose and mouth.*

for bacteria include openings to the body from nasogastric and feeding tubes, dialysis, intravenous (IV) ports, and intubation.

Certain staphylococci are contracted through gymnasium and health club locker rooms and through close-contact sports. Generally, the staphylococcal infections may result when persons who have breaks or cuts in their skin share items such as towels, sports equipment, uniforms, and razors. Another risk factor is having direct contact with a person (a carrier) who is infected with the bacteria but does not have symptoms.

## SYMPTOMS

Staphylococcal infections may present with various symptoms depending on the point of entry. Skin symptoms include boils or furuncles that usually form around hair follicles or oil glands. A common place for boils to occur is under the arms, in the groin area, or on the buttocks. The area becomes red and swollen,

is sometimes warm to the touch, may hold pus, and can be painful. A rash may occur with blisters that ooze liquid. Swollen red bumps on the eyelids, known as sties, may be caused by staphylococcal bacteria.

Food poisoning by staphylococcal bacteria may produce gastrointestinal symptoms including nausea, stomach cramps, diarrhea, and vomiting. Symptoms occur within one to six hours after ingesting contaminated food. Foods that are most likely to contaminate are those requiring no cooking and which are prepared by hand.

Severe staphylococcal infections such as bacteremia (commonly known as blood poisoning) may present with persistent fever. A life-threatening response to a staphylococcal infection might include symptoms such as high fever, seizures, nausea and vomiting, fatigue, chest pain, tender lymph nodes, headache, muscle pain, mental confusion or disorientation, and skin rash. Additional symptoms include chills and aching joints.

## SCREENING AND DIAGNOSIS

Screening and diagnosis are based on a physical examination, on the suspected location or point of bacterial entry, and on the presenting symptoms. The health provider also can use microscopic review of a tissue sample or culture of pus from a boil or lesion to confirm a diagnosis. A rash or sores around the mouth and nose, or crusty, oozing blisters, might indicate the skin condition impetigo. When the skin becomes infected and dimples form around the hair follicles (and look like an orange peel), the health care provider may suspect cellulitis. Symptoms such as redness, fever, boils, or rashes are often indicative of staphylococcal infections. In severe cases, a blood culture may be necessary to confirm the extent of the infection.

If a patient is in the hospital or has been recently discharged from the hospital, the provider may suspect methicillin-resistant *S. aureus* (MRSA), an infection commonly acquired in hospital settings. MRSA may occur in persons who congregate in crowded areas such as health clubs, dormitories, and military barracks.

Staphylococcal infections can result from cuts or scrapes of the skin, uncomplicated food poisoning, or more serious and possibly life-threatening conditions such as osteomyelitis, toxemia, endocarditis, and bacteremia. Taking a thorough medical history of the infected person will allow the health care provider to assess risk factors when determining treatment.

## TREATMENT AND THERAPY

Generally, staphylococcal infections can be treated with oral or topical antibiotics. Because of the overuse of antibiotics, however, *S. aureus* has become increasingly resistant to antibiotics and difficult to treat. The health care provider may need to drain boils or abscesses. One should keep any open wound clean. Some providers prescribe warm, wet compresses to encourage healing. More severe cases require hospitalization with supportive therapeutic interventions. Food poisoning by staphylococcal bacteria is generally diagnosed by symptoms and allowed to run its course unless the person has a complicating chronic disease or has a compromised immune system.

## PREVENTION AND OUTCOMES

Prevention of staphylococcal infections includes good handwashing technique and using an antiseptic hand sanitizer. One should clean and apply a protective covering or bandage with antibiotic ointment to cuts and scrapes; avoid skin-to-skin contact to decrease the chance of contracting or spreading staph infections; and wash hands after shaking hands and avoid touching one's face with one's own hands. One should avoid sharing personal belongings such as toiletries, towels, and combs and brushes. Good nutrition, adequate sleep, and regular exercise can help build a strong immune system to resist infections.

*Marylane Wade Koch, M.S.N., R.N.*

## FURTHER READING

Honeyman, Allen L., Herman Friedman, and Mauro Bendinelli, eds. Staphylococcus aureus *Infection and Disease.* New York: Kluwer Academic, 2002. Articles by noteworthy scientific experts and physicians discuss infectious diseases and the bacterium *Staphylococcus aureus.*

Park, Alice. "What You Need to Know About Staph." *Time,* October 18, 2007. Provides insights and statistics about MSRA from the Centers for Disease Control and Prevention and addresses the appropriate use of antibiotics to cure this infection.

Rojo, P., et al. "Community-Associated *Staphylococcus aureus* Infections in Children." *Expert Review of Anti-infective Therapy* 8, no. 5 (May, 2010): 541-554.

Stapleton, Paul D., and Peter Taylor. "Methicillin Resistence in *Staphylococcus aureus*: Mechanisms and Modulations." *Science Progress,* March 22, 2002. A detailed look at the characteristics and impact of methicillin resistence in *S. aureus.*

Tang, Y. W., and C. W. Stratton. "*Staphylococcus aureus*: An Old Pathogen with New Weapons." *Clinics in Laboratory Medicine* 30, no. 1 (March, 2010): 179-208.

## WEB SITES OF INTEREST

*Clean Hands Coalition*
http://www.cleanhandscoalition.org

*KidsHealth*
http://kidshealth.org

*National Institutes of Health*
http://www.nlm.nih.gov/medlineplus/staphylococcalinfections.html

**See also:** Antibiotic resistance; Bacteria: Classification and types; Bacteria: Structure and growth; Bacterial infections; Contagious diseases; Drug resistance; Hospitals and infectious disease; Methicillin-resistant staph infection; Opportunistic infections; *Staphylococcus*; Wound infections.

# *Staphylococcus*

CATEGORY: Pathogen
TRANSMISSION ROUTE: Direct contact

## DEFINITION

*Staphylococcus* is a genus of gram-positive cocci, or bacteria, with a thick peptidoglycan layer in their cell walls (gram-positive) that appear under the microscope as clusters of spherical cells (cocci). The staphylococci can grow in the presence or absence of oxygen and are distinguished from bacteria in the genus *Streptococcus* in the laboratory by the production of the enzyme catalase by staph species.

## NATURAL HABITAT AND FEATURES

Staphylococci are present among the normal microbiota of human skin and the mucous membranes

## Taxonomic Classification for *Staphylococcus*

**Kingdom:** Bacteria
**Phylum:** Firmicutes
**Class:** Bacilli
**Order:** Bacillales
**Family:** Staphylococcaceae
**Genus:** *Staphylococcus*
**Species:**
*S. aureus*
*S. epidermidis*

of the respiratory and gastrointestinal tracts. Approximately 90 percent of infants become carriers of staphylococci within ten days of birth. For some staphylococcal species, the carrier rate is higher among medical personnel than among the general population.

### PATHOGENICITY AND CLINICAL SIGNIFICANCE

While *S. epidermidis* is a universal symbiotant of the human skin, it can cause opportunistic infections. Other staph species are responsible for sinusitis, various infections of the skin, food poisoning, infections of the blood and bone, and toxic shock syndrome.

*S. aureus* is responsible for most staph infections in humans. Most people carry it in their nose and spread it to the surface of the skin or clothing. *S. aureus* invades the epidermis at a site of injury, at a gland opening, or at a hair follicle. White blood cells and plasma enter the area by passing through dilated capillaries, producing the swelling and redness of boils, furuncles, and infected wounds. Pus formation results when white blood cells and dead bacteria accumulate at the site.

Usually, a fibrin clot forms around the infection site and prevents the spread of bacteria into the blood. A pus-filled blemish near the surface of the skin is called a boil. When the infection penetrates into deeper layers of the skin, it is referred to as a furuncle. Boils and furuncles are treated by drainage through a surgical incision in an effort to avoid applying pressure and pushing bacteria into uninfected tissue or the blood.

Staphylococcal infection of newborns is a serious concern. *S. aureus* is readily transmitted between carriers to newborns by direct contact. The sites infected most frequently are infants' eyes and umbilical cords. The increased prevalence of antibiotic-resistant strains has led to widespread use of commercial disinfectants in hospital settings.

Severe staphylococcal infections may occur as complications of trauma that breaks the skin, such as trauma from surgery, accident, or burn. Illnesses that leave the immune system weakened, such as cancer, acquired immunodeficiency syndrome, or cirrhosis of the liver leave people susceptible to pneumonia, bone infections (osteomyelitis), deep tissue abscesses, and infections of the surface of the heart (endocarditis) and the spinal cord and brain (meningitis).

Staphylococcal food poisoning occurs when food is left unrefrigerated. The origin of the bacteria is usually a cook or other food preparer who unknowingly carries *S. aureus* and contaminates food during its preparation. The bacteria grow in the food and produce a toxin. Dairy items such as creamed food products and custard, and bread stuffing, support the growth of *S. aureus* cells and their production of the toxin. Once the toxin contaminates food, rewarming does not make the food safe. While the bacterial cells may be killed, the toxin remains. Staphylococcal food intoxication occurs a few hours after eating contaminated food. Sudden nausea, vomiting, and diarrhea that lasts twenty-four to forty-eight hours characterize this common cause of food poisoning.

*S. aureus* and tampons are linked to the occurrence of toxic shock syndrome (TSS) in menstruating girls and women. In 1980, the public took note when there were 299 TSS cases and 25 deaths in the United States. Nearly all the women became ill during their menstrual period while using super absorbent tampons. The Centers for Disease Control and Prevention recommended that women avoid using tampons continuously during their menstrual cycle. Presumably, the super absorbent tampons injured the vaginal mucous membrane and facilitated the growth of *S. aureus*, and the uptake of bacterial toxin into the bloodstream. The symptoms of TSS include the sudden onset of high fever, nausea, vomiting, diarrhea, and muscle cramps (myalgia). A sunburn-like rash develops eight to ten days after the symptoms first appear. In severe cases, a person can go into shock.

Methicillin-resistant *S. aureus* (MRSA) and oxacillin-resistant *S. aureus* (ORSA) infections are caused by strains of bacteria resistant to several of the antibiotics commonly used to treat ordinary staph infections. These infections occur most often in people who have been in hospitals, nursing homes, and dialysis centers. When an MRSA occurs in these settings, it is known as health-care-acquired MRSA (HA-MRSA).

Since 2000, another type of MRSA infection has become more prevalent in otherwise healthy people. This form, community acquired MRSA (CA-MRSA), often begins as a skin lesion. It is spread by skin-to-skin contact. People at risk for CA-MRSA include high school wrestlers, child-care staff, and those who live in crowded conditions.

## DRUG SUSCEPTIBILITY

Antibiotics are not effective against staphylococcal infections of the skin because of the fibrin clot that walls off the infection from the normal circulation. An exception is staphylococcal impetigo, which can be treated with topical antibiotics.

After the introduction of penicillin, the strains of *S. aureus* circulating in the United States were rapidly replaced with resistant ones. Staphylococcal pneumonia, osteomyelitis, deep tissue abscesses, endocarditis, and meningitis are treated with prolonged and intensive antibiotic therapy. Nafcillin is administered for methicillin-sensitive strains, and intravenous vancomycin is used for MRSA strains. Trimethoprim-sulfamethoxazole or rifampin is used with vancomycin in severe cases and in CA-MRSA infections. Linezolid is frequently used for treating staph meningitis.

*Kimberly A. Napoli, M.S.*

## FURTHER READING

Brachman, Philip S., and Elias Abrutyn, eds. *Bacterial Infections of Humans: Epidemiology and Control.* 4th ed. New York: Springer, 2009. A college-level introduction that focuses on the mechanisms of pathogenicity.

Crossley, Kent B., Kimberly K. Jefferson, and Gordon L. Archer, eds. *Staphylococci in Human Disease.* Hoboken, N.J.: John Wiley & Sons, 2009. Informative text on the role of *Staphylococcus* in infectious disease.

"Methicillin-Resistant *Staphylococcus aureus* (MRSA)." Available at http://www.webmd.com/a-to-z-guides/methicillin-resistant-staphylococcus-aureus-mrsa-overview.

Tortora, Gerard J., Berdell R. Funke, and Christine L. Case. *Microbiology: An Introduction.* 10th ed. San Francisco: Benjamin Cummings, 2010. Text addresses infectious diseases of each major organ system.

## WEB SITES OF INTEREST

*Community and Hospital Infection Control Association*
http://www.chica.org

*PathoSystems Resource Integration Center*
http://www.patricbrc.org

**See also:** Antibiotic resistance; Bacteria: Classification and types; Food-borne illness and disease; Hospitals and infectious disease; Methicillin-resistant staph infection; Opportunistic infections; Secondary infection; Skin infections; Staphylococcal infections; *Streptococcus.*

---

STDs. *See* Sexually transmitted diseases (STDs).

---

# *Stenotrophomonas* infections

CATEGORY: Diseases and conditions
ANATOMY OR SYSTEM AFFECTED: All

## DEFINITION

*Stenotrophomonas* infections are caused by the bacterial microorganism *Stenotrophomonas maltophilia*, which is common in the environment and can be found in bodies of water, soil, and plants. It is also commonly found in hospitals, mainly in contaminated solutions and on medical equipment. *S. maltophilia*, which can be carried by humans, is not a particularly virulent organism.

## CAUSES

*S. maltophilia* is an aerobic, gram-negative bacillus. It is able to colonize body secretions without causing an infection. To cause infection, it must be introduced into the body by contaminated medical equipment, devices, or solutions; by eating contaminated food or drinks, including tap water; or by the hands of health care workers. Usually, the body's normal defenses are able to resist *S. maltophilia* infections.

## RISK FACTORS

*Stenotrophomonas* infections usually develop in persons who have existing chronic diseases or who are immunosuppressed. Chronic diseases include diabetes, heart disease, and cystic fibrosis. Immunosuppressed persons are those who are on chemotherapy or glucocorticoid drugs or who have acquired immunodeficiency syndrome.

## SYMPTOMS

*S. maltophilia* can cause sepsis, pneumonia, urinary tract infections, soft tissue infections, eye infections, endocarditis, and meningitis. Common symptoms of infection are fever; elevated heart rate; decreased blood pressure; pain, redness, and swelling at the site; and fatigue. Pneumonia causes shortness of breath, a productive cough, and wheezing. Urinary tract infection causes frequency, burning on urination, and cloudy, foul-smelling urine. Endocarditis causes decreased cardiac output, irregular heartbeat, and heart failure. Meningitis causes vomiting, lethargy, a decreased level of consciousness, neck pain, and confusion.

## SCREENING AND DIAGNOSIS

There is no routine screening for *S. maltophilia* infections. Diagnosis depends on the symptoms of infection and a culture of the organism from the affected tissue. Also, cultures can be performed on the blood, urine, spinal fluid, and sputum.

## TREATMENT AND THERAPY

*Stenotrophomonas* infections are treated with antibiotics. *S. maltophilia* is resistant to penicillin, cephalosporin, gentamycin, and tobramycin, so, usually, *S. maltophilia* infections can be treated with minocycline, meropenem, levoquin, cipro, colistin/polymyxin B, and, sometimes, trimethoprine/sulfamethoxazole.

## PREVENTION AND OUTCOMES

There is no way to prevent *Stenotrophomonas* infection in susceptible persons because *S. maltophilia* is so common. In hospital settings, persons with *S. maltophilia* infections should be isolated, and medical staff should maintain careful isolation procedures. Medical equipment, linens, furniture, and rooms should be carefully cleaned after patient treatment. Culturing of intravenous solutions, medical devices, and irrigation fluids should be performed periodically to ensure their sterility.

*Christine M. Carroll, R.N.*

## FURTHER READING

Denton, Miles, and Kevin G. Kerr. "Microbiological and Clinical Aspects of Infection Associated with *Stenotrophomonas maltophilia*." *Clinical Microbiology Reviews* 11 (1998): 57-80.

Kim, Jae-Han, et al. "Two Episodes of *Stenotrophomonas maltophilia* Endocarditis of Prosthetic Mitral Valve." *Journal of the Korean Medical Society* 17 (2002): 263-265.

Toleman, M. A., et al. "Global Emergence of Trimethoprim/Sulfamethoxazole Resistance in *Stenotrophomonas maltophilia* Mediated by Acquisition of Sul Genes." *Emerging Infectious Diseases* 13 (2007): 559-565.

## WEB SITES OF INTEREST

*Centers for Disease Control and Prevention*
http://www.cdc.gov

*Microbiology and Immunology On-line: Mycology*
http://pathmicro.med.sc.edu/book/mycol-sta.htm

**See also:** Allergic bronchopulmonary aspergillosis; Antifungal drugs: Types; Aspergillosis; *Aspergillus*; Atypical pneumonia; Blastomycosis; *Bordetella*; Chromoblastomycosis; *Coccidioides*; Coccidiosis; Cryptococcosis; Diagnosis of fungal infections; Fungal infections; Fungi: Classification and types; Histoplasmosis; Hospitals and infectious disease; Mucormycosis; Paracoccidioidomycosis; Soilborne illness and disease; Waterborne illness and disease.

---

**Stigma.** *See* Psychological effects of infectious disease; Quarantine; Social effects of infectious disease.

---

**Stomach flu.** *See* Food-borne illness and disease; Intestinal and stomach infections; Norovirus infections; Viral gastroenteritis.

# Strep throat

CATEGORY: Diseases and conditions
ANATOMY OR SYSTEM AFFECTED: Pharynx, throat, tonsils
ALSO KNOWN AS: Streptococcal pharyngitis

## DEFINITION

Strep throat is a bacterial infection in the throat and tonsils that is caused by group A *Streptococcus* bacteria. It is the most common bacterial infection affecting the throat. If the affected person has common cold symptoms accompanying the sore throat, such as coughing, sneezing, or nasal congestion, the sore throat is most likely of viral, not bacterial, origin.

## CAUSES

Strep throat is caused by streptococcal bacteria. There are many different types of strep bacteria, but the cause of strep throat is group A strep bacteria. Some group A strains can lead to a scarlet fever rash or, occasionally, to rheumatic fever and rare kidney complications. Strep throat is spread by person-to-person contact with saliva or nasal secretions.

## RISK FACTORS

Strep throat is most common in children between the age of five and fifteen years. Strep infections in children under the age of three years do not usually affect the throat. Strep throat occurs most frequently in late fall, winter, and early spring.

## SYMPTOMS

Symptoms of strep throat usually occur between two and five days after a person is exposed. Symptoms typically include a general ill feeling, difficulty swallowing, a sudden fever, loss of appetite, nausea, rash, tender and swollen lymph nodes in the neck, and a red throat, sometimes with white patches. On occasion, the infection is also accompanied by headache, muscle aches, neck pain, chills, abnormal taste, and nasal congestion. Strep throat may be quite mild, with only a few symptoms, or may be severe, with many symptoms present.

## SCREENING AND DIAGNOSIS

The person's throat is swabbed and tested for the strep bacteria. A rapid test is commonly performed. A rapid test that returns negative is often followed by a culture to see if strep grows from that culture. This culture typically takes about two days.

## TREATMENT AND THERAPY

Although strep throat usually gets better without treatment, antibiotics are often administered to prevent more serious complications, such as sinusitis, mastoiditis, ear infection, scarlet fever, or rheumatic fever. Amoxicillin or penicillin are effective and should be taken for ten days, even if the symptoms disappear in a few days. Strep throat symptoms can be relieved by drinking warm liquids, gargling with warm salt-water, sucking on throat lozenges, using a cool-mist vaporizer or humidifier, and using over-the-counter pain medications such as acetaminophen. Children should not use aspirin; doing so could lead to a condition called Reye's syndrome.

## PREVENTION AND OUTCOMES

Persons diagnosed with strep throat should avoid public gatherings until they have been on antibiotics for a minimum of twenty-four hours. One should keep family toothbrushes and utensils separate, unless they have been thoroughly washed. If strep throat continues to occur in a family, medical screening should be carried out to determine if a family member is a strep carrier. Treatment can prevent others from getting strep throat.

*Alvin K. Benson, Ph.D.*

## FURTHER READING

Frazier, Margaret Schell, and Jeanette Wist Drzymkowski. *Essentials of Human Diseases and Conditions.* 4th ed. St. Louis, Mo.: Saunders/Elsevier, 2009.

Glaser, Jason. *Strep Throat: First Facts.* Mankato, Minn.: Capstone Press, 2006.

Landau, Elaine. *Strep Throat: Head-to-Toe Health.* Tarrytown, N.Y.: Benchmark Books, 2010.

Pechère, Jean Claude, and Edward L. Kaplan, eds. *Streptococcal Pharyngitis: Optimal Management.* New York: S. Karger, 2004.

Vincent, Miriam T. "Sore Throat-Strep Throat? When to Worry." *Pediatrics for Parents* 21, no. 8 (August 1, 2004): 11-12.

## WEB SITES OF INTEREST

*Centers for Disease Control and Prevention*
http://www.cdc.gov

*Clean Hands Coalition*
http://www.cleanhandscoalition.org

*KidsHealth*
http://kidshealth.org

*National Institutes of Health*
http://www.nlm.nih.gov

**See also:** Bacterial infections; Children and infectious disease; Common cold; Contagious diseases; Fever; Group A streptococcal infection; Home remedies; Infection; Influenza; Over-the-counter (OTC) drugs; Pharyngitis and tonsillopharyngitis; Saliva and infectious disease; Streptococcal infections; *Streptococcus.*

# Streptococcal infections

CATEGORY: Diseases and conditions
ANATOMY OR SYSTEM AFFECTED: All
ALSO KNOWN AS: Strep infections, strep throat

## DEFINITION

Streptococcal infections are caused by spherical gram-positive streptococcal bacteria that reproduce in a twisted, chainlike fashion. These bacteria may be found in humans on the skin and in the respiratory, genitourinary, and gastrointestinal systems. Under certain conditions, these opportunist bacteria can cause minor to life-threatening infections.

## CAUSES

*Streptococcus* can be divided into group A *Streptococcus* (GAS) and group B *Streptococcus* (GBS). Scientists have identified more than one hundred different strains of GAS. Although the diseases caused by these bacteria are clearly defined, the mechanisms of how these pathogens act are complex and not well understood. The extent of the illness produced in the host depends on the interaction between the host and his or her immune system and the virulence of the pathogen.

The most common GAS is *S. pyogenes*, which may be part of the normal flora of the throat and skin and may be found in an asymptomatic carrier host. In infected persons, bacteria are present in the nose and mouth, and in eye secretions. This strain can produce strep throat, tonsillitis, and cellulitis, and more serious diseases such as scarlet fever, glomerulonephritis, rheumatic heart disease, toxic shock syndrome, and bacteremia.

*S. pneumoniae*, lancet-shaped cocci strep, causes community-acquired bacterial pneumonia, meningitis, sinusitis, endocarditis, and mastoiditis. *S. agalactiae*, group B strep, is found in the intestine, vagina, and rectum of up to 35 percent of all healthy women with no symptoms. This organism, however, can be passed to a fetus during delivery and can result in a life-threatening infection in the newborn.

## RISK FACTORS

The risk of streptococcal infections varies based on the strain. Generally, the risk is greater when the host has a weakened immune system or a chronic disease such as diabetes. Certain treatments such as chemotherapy or drugs such as steroids may increase the risk of infection. Teenagers are at risk for strep throat infections, and a higher incidence is seen in the early spring.

Older adults, infants, and persons with a chronic disease are more susceptible to *S. pneumoniae*. A pregnant woman can transmit *S. agalactiae* to her baby during delivery.

## SYMPTOMS

Group A strep infections present with varied symptoms, depending on the type of infection. The most common condition is strep throat with symptoms such as an inflamed red throat with white patches on the tonsils, difficulty swallowing, enlarged lymph nodes with a swollen or tender neck, headache, weakness, a loss of appetite, stomach pain, and a fever. Impetigo, a strep skin rash, develops as weepy red sores. Serious illnesses, however, such as scarlet or rheumatic fever, postpartum fever, wound infection, and pneumonia may also result from a strep infection.

A life-threatening response to group A strep that occurs when bacteria enter the blood or lungs is known as invasive GAS disease. Two uncommon but damaging diseases are toxic shock syndrome and necrotizing fasciitis, which manifests as pain, swelling, fever, and redness at the site of the infection and destroys muscles and skin. Early toxic shock syndrome may occur with dizziness, fever, flulike symptoms, and confusion, all of which could progress to shock symptoms, including a drop in blood pressure and a general failure of body organs. The host risks death in about 35 percent of cases of toxic shock syndrome.

## SCREENING AND DIAGNOSIS

Screening and diagnosis of streptococcal infections are based on physical examination, the presenting symptoms, and the results of laboratory tests. Strep throat is diagnosed with a rapid strep test of a swab of the infected person's throat mucosa. This simple test takes about twenty minutes to complete and is completed in the doctor's office. If there is a positive result, no further testing is needed. If a negative result occurs in a person who has significant symptoms, a throat culture is sent to a lab for diagnosis, which occurs within twenty-four to forty-eight hours.

Group B strep is diagnosed by a review of presenting symptoms and risk factors and a lab examination of blood or spinal fluid, or both. The diagnosis of infection with *S. pneumoniae* is confirmed through a chest X ray and a lab culture called an optochin susceptibility test.

## TREATMENT AND THERAPY

A thorough medical history will allow the health care provider to assess risk factors when determining effective therapy. Generally, streptococcal infections can be effectively treated with appropriate oral or intravenous antibiotics. The primary classes of drug treatment include penicillin, cephalosporins, and erythromycins. Because of overuse, however, some antibiotics are no longer effective against strep infections. Persons with a sore throat and confirmed strep throat should not return to work or school until a minimum of twenty-four hours have passed after starting antibiotics.

To avoid spreading the disease, one should wash the dishes and utensils of infected persons in hot, soapy water and keep them separate from other dishes and utensils. After a person has been treated with antibiotics, his or her toothbrush should be replaced to prevent contamination. Also, one should encourage infected persons to cover their mouths while coughing or sneezing to minimize the spread of the disease by droplets.

## PREVENTION AND OUTCOMES

Prevention of streptococcal infections includes frequent handwashing with soap and warm water or applying antiseptic hand sanitizer. One should minimize skin-to-skin contact with any infected person; wash hands thoroughly before preparing or eating foods and after shaking hands; keep hands away from face and mouth; and avoid sharing personal belongings such as toiletries, towels, or combs and brushes.

Adults age sixty-five years and older and those with a serious chronic disease should be encouraged to take the pneumococcal vaccine. About 30 percent of persons who contract pneumonia may get a secondary bacteremia, which can result in death. A pregnant woman who is a carrier of GBS should be tested in the ninth month of her pregnancy to ensure the fetus receives appropriate antibiotics during labor.

To avoid skin infections, one should clean and apply a protective bandage with antibiotic ointment to all cuts and scrapes. Good nutrition, adequate sleep, and regular exercise can help build a resistant immune system.

*Marylane Wade Koch, M.S.N., R.N.*

## FURTHER READING

Centers for Disease Control and Prevention. "Group A Streptococcal (GAS) Disease." Available at http://www.cdc.gov/ncidod/dbmd/diseaseinfo/groupas-treptococcal.

Gorham, Christine. "Health: Is It Strep Throat?" *Time*, April 19, 2004. Discusses the common sore throat and the need to differentiate a strep throat infection for appropriate treatment without overuse of antibiotics.

"Overdoing Antibiotics." *Harvard Health Letter*, November, 2002. Includes a detailed discussion of antibiotic resistance and the complex issues associated with this challenge to treat infections, including strep infections, with practical solutions.

Parker, James N., and Philip M. Parker, eds. *The Official Patient's Sourcebook on "Streptococcus pneumoniae" Infections.* San Diego, Calif.: Icon Health, 2002. Draws from public, academic, government, and peer-reviewed research to provide a wide-ranging handbook for patients with pneumonia infections.

Pechère, Jean Claude, and Edward L. Kaplan, eds. *Streptococcal Pharyngitis: Optimal Management.* New York: S. Karger, 2004. Provides articles written by medical experts to address the common issues of streptococcal pharyngitis (strep throat) and the evolving challenges of treatment.

Vincent, Miriam T. "Sore Throat-Strep Throat? When to Worry." *Pediatrics for Parents* 21, no. 8 (August 1,

2004): 11-12. An informative article on distinguishing between sore throat and strep throat.

## WEB SITES OF INTEREST

*Centers for Disease Control and Prevention*
http://www.cdc.gov

*Clean Hands Coalition*
http://www.cleanhandscoalition.org

*KidsHealth*
http://kidshealth.org

*National Institutes of Health*
http://www.nlm.nih.gov/medlineplus/
streptococcalinfections.html

**See also:** Bacteria: Classification and types; Bacterial infections; Cellulitis; Children and infectious disease; Contagious diseases; Group A streptococcal infection; Group B streptococcal infection; Mononucleosis; Opportunistic infections; Strep throat; *Streptococcus*; Vertical disease transmission; Wound infections.

---

# *Streptococcus*

CATEGORY: Pathogen
TRANSMISSION ROUTE: Direct contact, inhalation

## DEFINITION

*Streptococcus* is a genus of gram-positive cocci, or bacteria, with a thick peptidoglycan layer in their cell walls (gram-positive) that appear under the microscope as chains of two or more spherical cells (cocci). The streptococci can grow in low concentrations of oxygen or without oxygen and are distinguished from bacteria in the genus *Staphylococcus* in the laboratory by the production of the enzyme catalase by staph species.

The streptococci are classified in a number of ways, including by the identity of molecules on the cell surface and by the presence and variety of hemolysin, or enzyme, that lyse red blood cells. Alpha-hemolytic species lyse red blood cells and oxidize hemoglobin to leave an opaque green residue on blood agar petri dishes. Beta-hemolytic species leave a transparent halo around colonies on blood agar petri dishes. Gamma-hemolytic species exhibit neither of these traits.

---

## Taxonomic Classification for *Streptococcus*

**Kingdom:** Bacteria
**Phylum:** Firmicutes
**Class:** Bacilli
**Order:** Lactobacillales
**Family:** Streptococcaceae
**Genus:** *Streptococcus*
**Species:**
S. *agalactiae*
S. *mitis*
S. *mutans*
S. *pneumoniae*
S. *pyogenes*
S. *sanguinis*
S. *viridans*

---

## NATURAL HABITAT AND FEATURES

Streptococci are a part of the normal microbiota of humans and other mammals. Some streptococci can cause infectious diseases. The progression from latency to infectious disease is not well understood, but scientists have investigated the possibility that virus-induced genetic changes in streptococcal species are responsible for the sudden appearance of "flesh-eating" disease, or necrotizing fasciitis.

## PATHOGENICITY AND CLINICAL SIGNIFICANCE

*S. pyogenes* is a notable member of the beta-hemolytic streptococci. *Pyogenes* is an opportunistic pathogen widely distributed in humans. It causes acute bacterial pharyngitis, commonly known as strep throat, and infections of the skin and circulatory system. These bacteria are able to evade the human immune system though various means. That is, the cells are covered in hyaluronic acid, which is a component of human connective tissue and, therefore, nonimmunogenic; and a series of proteins, M proteins, prevents the engulfment of bacterial cells by immune cells. Two toxins that destroy immune cells also cause beta-hemolysis of red blood cells.

*Pyogenes* strains that produce erythrogenic exotoxins, the extracellular proteins responsible for the scarlet fever rash, may produce one of three varieties. Exposure to one variety does not induce immunity to the others, so a person may have recurring infection. These toxins are not encoded on the bacterial chromosome, but on plasmids. Prompt antibiotic therapy of strep throat has reduced the incidence of scarlet fever.

Acute rheumatic fever and acute glomerulonephritis are also consequences of untreated strep throat. The symptoms of rheumatic fever occur about three to four weeks following strep throat and include pains in the joints and long-term damage to the heart, likely because of an autoimmune response. Glomerulonephritis is swelling of the kidneys following strep throat or a streptococcal skin infection.

Streptococcal impetigo is a localized skin infection caused by *pyogenes*. Erysipelas is an acute infection of the skin with fever. Strains that express the enzyme streptokinase may dissolve a blood clot to penetrate to deeper tissue. Infection of deep muscle and fat tissue, the lungs, and blood can be life-threatening. Necrotizing fasciitis (infection of muscle and fat tissue) kills about 20 percent of infected persons, and streptococcal toxic shock syndrome (an infection causing low blood pressure and shock and injury to the kidneys, liver, and lungs) kills up to 60 percent of infected persons.

Another beta-hemolytic species, *agalactiae*, is the major cause of meningitis, pneumonia, and infections of the bloodstream in newborns. The female genital tract is the natural habitat for *agalactiae*, with 25 to 35 percent of the female population being carriers. Newborns are infected at birth or during their stay in a hospital nursery. Antibiotic therapy of pregnant women who carry *agalactiae* prevents transmission to their fetuses at birth.

Most human cases of bacterial pneumonia are caused by alpha-hemolytic *pneumoniae*. This species grows as pairs of cocci coated in a thick carbohydrate capsule. Colonies on blood agar petri dishes are surrounded by transparent agar and a mucoid appearance. *Pneumoniae* is an inhabitant of the upper respiratory tract of up to 70 percent of the population. In immunocompromised hosts, such as many elderly persons, and in those with a viral infection, this strain causes pneumonia. The infection in the lungs results in fluid retention and difficulty in breathing. Recovery follows after five to six days, even without antibiotic treatment. An increase of circulating antibodies accompanies a decrease in the severity of the symptoms. Penicillin or erythromycin hastens recovery, while a few persons with pneumococcal-pneumonia, primarily the elderly, die even though they are being treated with antibiotics.

Spinal meningitis caused by *pneumoniae* had been the second leading cause of bacterial meningitis. This changed when a glycoconjugate vaccine was added to the infant immunization schedule in the United States and other countries.

*Mutans*, *mitis*, and *sanguinis* are alpha-hemolytic streptococci that are normal inhabitants of the human mouth. *Mutans* and *mitis* are found in dental plaque. *S. mutans* produces dextran from sucrose. Dextran is the sticky component of dental plaque that allows many bacterial species to stick to tooth surfaces. When bacteria grow on the teeth, they produce acid that contributes to the creation of cavities. Non-hemolytic species, also called gamma-hemolytic streptococci, are not human pathogens.

## DRUG SUSCEPTIBILITY

Streptococcal infections are treated primarily with antibiotics. Widespread incidence of resistance has not occurred to the extent that it has in the staphylococcal species. Multiply resistant strains have been documented, though. The treatment of strep throat has become more difficult because of antibiotic resistance of non-strep bacteria in the throat. Other bacteria can destroy penicillin and other beta-lactam antibiotics and, thus, shield sensitive *pyogenes* from their effect.

*Kimberly A. Napoli, M.S.*

## FURTHER READING

Brachman, Philip S., and Elias Abrutyn, eds. *Bacterial Infections of Humans: Epidemiology and Control.* 4th ed. New York: Springer, 2009. A college-level introduction that focuses on the mechanisms of pathogenicity.

Parker, James N., and Philip M. Parker, eds. *The Official Patient's Sourcebook on "Streptococcus pneumoniae" Infections.* San Diego, Calif.: Icon Health, 2002. Draws from public, academic, government, and peer-reviewed research to provide a wide-ranging handbook for patients with pneumonia infections.

Tortora, Gerard J., Berdell R. Funke, and Christine L. Case. *Microbiology: An Introduction.* 10th ed. San Francisco: Benjamin Cummings, 2010. A great reference for those interested in exploring the microbial world. Provides readers with an appreciation of the pathogenicity and usefulness of microorganisms.

## WEB SITES OF INTEREST

*National Institutes of Health*
http://www.nlm.nih.gov/medlineplus/streptococ-calinfections.html

*PathoSystems Resource Integration Center*
http://www.patricbrc.org

**See also:** Bacteria: Classification and types; Group A streptococcal infection; *Staphylococcus*; Strep throat; Streptococcal infections.

---

# Stress and infectious disease

CATEGORY: Epidemiology

## DEFINITION

Stress is physical or psychological pressure, worry, or tension. Infectious diseases are those illnesses of the human body caused by pathogenic organisms such as bacteria and viruses. Research has linked stress to the development of infectious disease in humans.

## STRESS AND THE HUMAN BODY

In 1936, scientist Hans Selye introduced his general adaption syndrome model, which describes how the human body attempts to restore homeostasis (balance) when subjected to physical stress that threatens life. Selye, the founder of stress research, believed that human bodies react in predictable ways to external stressors, and that chronic exposure to stress could change the body chemically, resulting in disease. Selye's three-step model included stages of alarm, resistance, and exhaustion.

In the alarm stage, the body experiences hormonal changes to address the perceived threat. The body's defenses activate the hypothalamic-pituitary-adrenal axis, sympathetic nervous system, and adrenal glands to release chemicals such as cortisol, adrenaline, and noradrenalin. Catecholamines produce an emotional response, such as fear. The immune system mobilizes to respond to the threat, equipping the body with the chemical energy needed to "fight or take flight."

The second stage of stress is resistance, in which the body attempts to return to homeostasis. Metabolic changes keep the body functioning. If the threat continues, the body stays stressed without recovery, leading to stage three, exhaustion. All reserves are used up. Fatigue, burnout, and dysfunction, along with impaired thinking and damage to body cells and tissues occur, resulting in disease. In experimental animals, repeated severe stress resulted in physiological changes such as a smaller thymus gland, gastrointestinal ulcers, larger adrenal glands, and sometimes death.

## TYPES OF STRESS

The concept of stress has been studied by many scientists for decades. Stress is commonly categorized as acute or chronic. Acute stress involves an immediate threat that causes the alarm reaction. An example of acute stress is stepping on a snake or being frightened by an unknown noise at night. When the stress passes, the body recovers and relaxes.

With chronic stress, such as long-term disease or job, financial, or relationship worries, the body remains in a threatened state. This does not allow the body to recover, and it lowers the immune response, putting the body at risk for illness. Diseases that can result from long-term stress include severe headaches, high blood pressure, depression, stomach ulcers, and increased incidence of colds, the flu, and other infections.

## RESEARCH

To investigate if stress decreases host resistance to infection, Sheldon Cohen and colleagues (in 1991) studied the connection between psychological stress and the common cold resulting from respiratory viruses. They found that the incidence of common colds increased in a dose-response manner with psychological stress. These scientists from Carnegie Mellon University concluded that increased psychological stress was directly related to increased rates of infection from respiratory viruses.

In 1993, T. W. Klein of the University of South Florida, College of Medicine, found that neuroendocrine hormones can change the functioning of immune cells. His experimental studies demonstrated a connection between stress and infection, with human subjects under increased stress more likely to contract an infection with a cold virus.

Cohen and colleagues (in 1998) published a study related to life stressors and the common cold in the journal *Health Psychology*. The study's goal was to define the nature of life stressors and the biological link to disease susceptibility. The researchers looked at white blood cell activity and natural killer (NK) cell activity in the host's blood sample before the virus "challenge." The hormones epinephrine, norepinephrine, and cortisol were measured in urine the day before host exposure to the virus. The results of the study showed that the total rate of infection was 84 percent.

Scientists continue to look at ways that stress impacts infectious disease. In 2009, researchers at the University of Saskatchewan published an article in the *International Journal of General Medicine*, reviewing modern approaches to stress and infectious disease, with emphases on respiratory illnesses. The researchers claimed that stress can affect levels of specific hormones that activate or suppress the immune system. However, the focus of the study was on how stress affects disease susceptibility and on how new medical approaches can address remaining complex questions.

## IMPACT

Stress affects everyone, even though human experience, perception, and response varies. Stress can be either mental or physical, or both. Physical symptoms that plague the general population, such as headaches or insomnia, often occur with stress and result in lost days from work and school. Research on the common cold and other respiratory infections has linked infections to stress.

More than one billion people experience colds each year. The impact of the common cold on the work force can be quantified: about 23 million days of work at a cost of $25 billion in lost productivity each year. Some 26 million school days are missed by students sick with colds each year, impacting the educational system and student learning. About $2.5 billion is spent to treat colds annually, aiding the pharmaceutical industry.

Stress and resulting infections greatly affect the function and economic well-being of the general population, health and medical care, business and industry, health insurance, and government, which, in the United States, for example, assumes the costs of health care for persons on Medicare and Medicaid. Discovering the relationship of stress to costly and life-altering infections can encourage new ways to cope with day-to-day and chronic stresses for improved health and quality of life.

*Marylane Wade Koch, M.S.N., R.N.*

## FURTHER READING

Ader, Robert, ed. *Psychoneuroimmunology.* 4th ed. Boston: Academic Press/Elsevier, 2007. A classic text in the field of psychoneuroimmunology, the study of interactions between psychology and the immune and nervous systems of the human body.

Cohen, Sheldon, et al. "Types of Stressors that Increase Susceptibility to the Common Cold in Healthy Adults." *Healthy Psychology* 17, no. 3 (1998): 214-223. Details a follow-up study from Cohen's work in 1991 regarding the relationship of stress to the common cold.

Cooper, Cary L. *Handbook of Stress Medicine and Health.* 2d ed. Boca Raton, Fla.: CRC Press, 2005. Reviews stress and its direct relationship to health, long-term stress, and the immune system.

Lovallo, William R. *Stress and Health: Biological and Physiological Interactions.* Thousand Oaks, Calif.: Sage, 2005. Explains links among stress, health, and disease, with attention to the psycho-physiological responses of the body to stress.

Steptoe, Andrew, and Jane Wardle, eds. *Psychosocial Processes and Health: A Reader.* New York: Cambridge University Press, 1994. Contains research studies on various aspects of health, including life stress and psycho-physiological processes in disease.

## WEB SITES OF INTEREST

*American Institute of Stress*
http://www.stress.org

*Mayo Clinic, Stress and Health Risks*
http://www.mayoclinic.com/health/stress/sr00001

*National Institute of Mental Health*
http://www.nimh.nih.gov

**See also:** Aging and infectious disease; Centers for Disease Control and Prevention (CDC); Children and infectious disease; Contagious diseases; Epidemiology; Infection; Men and infectious disease; National Institutes of Health; Outbreaks; Psychological effects of infectious disease; Public health; Schools and infectious disease; Social effects of infectious disease; Women and infectious disease.

# Strongyloidiasis

CATEGORY: Diseases and conditions
ANATOMY OR SYSTEM AFFECTED: All

## DEFINITION

Strongyloidiasis is a disease caused by the worm *Strongyloides stercoralis*. This worm species lives in the soil of tropical and subtropical regions, the southeastern United States, and parts of Europe, Australia, and Japan. Many people from endemic areas are chronically infected.

## CAUSES

Larvae infect people who walk barefoot on fecal-contaminated soil. The larvae migrate to the small intestine, invade blood vessels, and migrate to the lungs, where they are swallowed. Adult worms attach to the small intestine and produce larvae that pass into stool.

## RISK FACTORS

Activities, both recreational and occupational, that expose people to fecal-contaminated soil in endemic areas increase the risk of strongyloidiasis. In temperate climates, strongyloidiasis is more common among alcoholics, Caucasians, males, and the poor. Cancer, impaired bowel activity, low stomach acid content, diabetes mellitus, and medications that weaken the immune system predispose persons to severe infection.

## SYMPTOMS

Most people with strongyloidiasis do not have symptoms of infection. After larvae enter the skin, a local skin reaction may develop. Cough and breathing problems occur after several days if larvae migrate to the lungs. Abdominal pain, nausea, and diarrhea occur after several weeks if larvae are swallowed. People with weakened immune systems may develop infection of the brain, lungs, heart, kidneys, or liver.

## SCREENING AND DIAGNOSIS

Larvae can be seen in stool under the microscope or by smearing stool onto culture media. People with strongyloidiasis have positive antibodies against *Strongyloides* even if the stool examination is negative. People with weakened immune systems may have noticeable changes on their chest X rays. Bronchoscopy, in which a fiber optic scope is inserted into the airways, can obtain specimens for culture that identify *Strongyloides* on special growth media.

## TREATMENT AND THERAPY

Mild *Strongyloides* infection is treated with ivermectin or thiabendazole. People with weakened immune systems and disseminated infection are also treated with antibacterial drugs. After treatment, stool should be examined for larvae to ensure eradication. Despite treatment, many people with disseminated infection die.

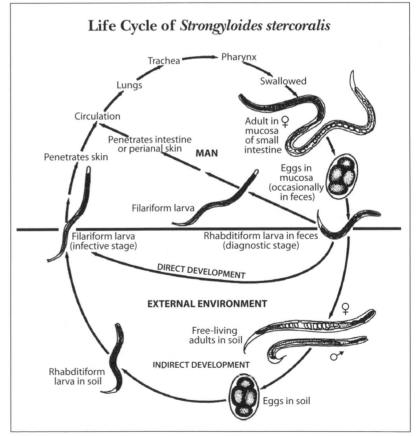

*The cycle of infection of the parasitic worm* Strongyloides stercoralis. *(CDC)*

## PREVENTION AND OUTCOMES

People who live in endemic areas should wear proper footwear when walking on fecal-contaminated soil. People with risk factors for developing strongyloidiasis should be screened with antibody testing before starting medications that weaken the immune system.

*David A. Saunders, M.D., and Steven D. Burdette, M.D.*

## FURTHER READING

Berger, Stephen A., and John S. Marr. *Human Parasitic Diseases Sourcebook*. Sudbury, Mass.: Jones and Bartlett, 2006.

Keiser, Paul, and Thomas Nutman. "*Strongyloides stercoralis* in the Immunocompromised Population." *Clinical Microbiology Reviews* 17, no. 1 (January, 2004): 208-217.

Lam, C. S. "Disseminated Strongyloidiasis: A Retrospective Study of Clinical Course and Outcome." *European Journal of Clinical Microbiology and Infectious Diseases* 25, no. 1 (January, 2006): 14-18.

Maguire, James. "Intestinal Nematodes (Roundworms)." In *Mandell, Douglas, and Bennett's Principles and Practice of Infectious Diseases*, edited by Gerald L. Mandell, John F. Bennett, and Raphael Dolin. 7th ed. New York: Churchill Livingstone/Elsevier, 2010.

Weller, P. F., and T. B. Nutman. "Intestinal Nematodes." In *Harrison's Principles of Internal Medicine*, edited by Joan Butterton. 17th ed. New York: McGraw-Hill, 2008.

## WEB SITES OF INTEREST

*American Society of Tropical Medicine and Hygiene*
http://www.astmh.org

*Centers for Disease Control and Prevention*
http://www.cdc.gov/parasites

**See also:** Amebic dysentery; Ascariasis; Cryptosporidiosis; Fecal-oral route of transmission; Giardiasis; Hookworms; Intestinal and stomach infections; Parasitic diseases; Peritonitis; Pinworms; Roundworms; Soilborne illness and disease; Travelers' diarrhea; Tropical medicine; Whipworm infection; Worm infections.

# Subacute sclerosing panencephalitis

CATEGORY: Diseases and conditions
ANATOMY OR SYSTEM AFFECTED: Brain, central nervous system, spinal cord
ALSO KNOWN AS: Dawson disease

## DEFINITION

Subacute sclerosing panencephalitis (SSPE) is a rare, chronic central nervous system (brain and spine) condition that occurs up to ten years after getting the measles. It usually results in progressive deterioration from inflammation of the brain and nerve cell death. When left untreated, SSPE almost always leads to death.

## CAUSES

SSPE is caused by an altered form of the measles virus. It occurs anywhere from two to ten years after contracting measles.

## RISK FACTORS

Two factors that are thought to increase the risk of SSPE are infection in infancy and not being vaccinated against measles. Persons at higher risk for SSPE are children age five to fifteen years, males, and persons of certain ethnic origin. Arabs and Sephardic Jews have an incidence that is six times higher than Ashkenazi Jews, and Caucasians have a four-fold higher incidence than African Americans in the United States.

## SYMPTOMS

Symptoms of SSPE include abnormal behavior, irritability, intellectual deterioration, memory loss, involuntary movements, seizures, an inability to walk, speech impairment with poor comprehension, difficulty swallowing, blindness, muteness, and coma.

## SCREENING AND DIAGNOSIS

A doctor will ask about symptoms and medical history and will perform a physical exam. Other tests may include blood tests to look for the measles antibody; an electrocardiogram (ECG, EKG) to record the heart's activity by measuring electrical currents through the heart muscle; a magnetic resonance imaging (MRI) scan (a scan that uses radio waves and a powerful magnet to produce detailed computer images), and a computed tomography (CT) scan (a detailed X-ray picture that identifies abnormalities of fine tissue structure).

## TREATMENT AND THERAPY

A doctor should be consulted about the best treatment plan. Treatment options include supportive therapy. With advanced disease, tube feedings and nursing care may be necessary. Also, anticonvulsant medications can reduce some symptoms of SSPE. There is some evidence that certain medications (such as inosine pranobex, interferon alpha, interferon beta, and ribavirin) may help stabilize the disease, delay its progression, or both.

## PREVENTION AND OUTCOMES

The best way to prevent SSPE is to avoid contracting measles. One can do this by getting the measles vaccine (usually given at twelve to fifteen months of age and again at four to six or eleven to twelve years of age). Persons who are not vaccinated should avoid contact with people who are infected with measles until all the infected person's symptoms are gone.

*Krisha McCoy, M.S.;*
*reviewed by Judy Chang, M.D., FAASM*

## FURTHER READING

Campbell, H., et al. "Review of the Effect of Measles Vaccination on the Epidemiology of SSPE." *International Journal of Epidemiology* 36 (2007): 1134-1148.

Daube, Jasper R., ed. *Clinical Neurophysiology.* 3d ed. New York: Oxford University Press, 2009.

EBSCO Publishing. *DynaMed: Subacute Sclerosing Panencephalitis* (SSPE). Available through http://www.ebscohost.com/dynamed.

_____. *Health Library: Measles.* Available through http://www.ebscohost.com.

National Institute of Neurological Disorders and Stroke. "Subacute Sclerosing Panencephalitis." Available at http://www.ninds.nih.gov.

Solomon, T., and R. Knee. "Subacute Sclerosing Panencephalitis." In *MedLink Neurology,* edited by S. Gilman. San Diego, Calif.: MedLink, 2003.

Wagner, Edward K., and Martinez J. Hewlett. *Basic Virology.* 3d ed. Malden, Mass.: Blackwell Science, 2008.

Woolsey, Thomas A., Joseph Hanaway, and Mokhtar Gado. *Brain Atlas: A Visual Guide to the Human Central Nervous System.* 2d ed. New York: John Wiley & Sons, 2002.

## WEB SITES OF INTEREST

*Canadian Neurological Sciences Federation*
http://www.ccns.org

*Centers for Disease Control and Prevention*
http://www.cdc.gov

*National Institute of Neurological Disorders and Stroke*
http://www.ninds.nih.gov

**See also:** Encephalitis; Inflammation; Measles; MMR vaccine; Postherpetic neuralgia; Progressive multifocal leukoencephalopathy; Shingles.

# Superbacteria

CATEGORY: Pathogen
ALSO KNOWN AS: Multidrug-resistant organisms, multidrug-resistant strains

## DEFINITION

Superbacteria are organisms that have developed resistance to many antibiotic drugs. Infections caused by these bacteria can be extremely difficult to treat, as some have become resistant to all antibiotics that were once effective against them. Because resistance can spread from one bacterium to another, resistant strains of many different types of bacteria have emerged.

Superbacteria have become a serious health threat worldwide; antibiotic-resistant strains are present on every continent, including Antarctica. The incidence of illness caused by drug-resistant bacteria is increasing dramatically around the world. Resistant strains of disease-causing bacteria, originally found primarily in hospitals, have now moved beyond health care facilities and into communities.

## EMERGENCE AND SPREAD OF SUPERBACTERIA

When bacteria are exposed to an antibiotic, most of them will die. However, a few bacteria may acquire changes in their DNA (deoxyribonucleic acid) that allow them to survive in the presence of the drug. These bacteria will multiply, creating a drug-resistant group. This vertical transmission (that is, the method of passing resistance genes) requires time for resistance-causing mutations to arise and stays within the same type of bacteria.

## Superbacteria: Methicillin-Resistant Staphylococci

Staphylococcal infections, especially methicillin-resistant *Staphylococcus aureus* (MRSA), occur most frequently in persons with weakened immune systems. Persons in hospitals and nursing homes, and persons on dialysis, may develop surgical wound infections, bloodstream infections, pneumonia, prosthetic joint or heart valve infections, and other types of staphylococcal infections as a result of acquiring hospital-associated MRSA (HA-MRSA) during medical treatment. These superbacteria may come from the patients themselves, from other patients, or from health care workers. Whatever the source, these infections are potentially preventable.

Persons scheduled to undergo elective surgery, such as joint replacement, are now screened for staphylococcal colonization by nasal culture, and those persons who are positive are treated with nasal mupirocin or even oral antibiotics to eradicate the staphylococci before surgery. Persons harboring staphylococci who are admitted to hospitals are being isolated to prevent transmission to both health care workers and other patients. Many U.S. states have passed legislation requiring health care institutions to report their records publicly, including records of infection rates, and this awareness is accelerating these preventive measures.

MRSA is no longer limited to patients in health care facilities. Community-associated MRSA (CA-MRSA) also is prominent. It most commonly manifests as a skin or soft tissue infection, such as a boil or abscess. Close skin-to-skin contact, cuts or abrasions, and contaminated items may lead to infection. Skin lesions have allowed CA-MRSA to cause infections in wrestlers, fencers, rugby players, football players, and other athletes. Similarly, in one case, skin abrasions in hot-tub users in Alaska resulted in CA-MRSA outbreaks. Children, some without any identified predisposing risk, have also become infected with CA-MRSA.

Typing of CA-MRSA strains using a technique called pulsed-field gel electrophoresis has identified a specific strain of CA-MRSA called USA 300 for causing nearly all infections in the United States.

Both HA-MRSA and CA-MRSA are treatable with antibiotics, but those that are effective in each type are quite different. HA-MRSA infections are treated with vancomycin, daptomycin, or linezolid. These antimicrobial agents are very expensive and usually require intravenous administration. CA-MRSA infections are treated with less expensive oral agents such as trimethoprim-sulfamethoxazole, tetracylines, fluoroquinolones, or clindamycin. Neither HA-MRSA nor CA-MRSA infections can be treated successfully with beta-lactam antibiotics, which are the antibiotics of first choice for other *S. aureus* infections.

Recognition of the persons at risk and the differences in effective antibiotic therapies are critical because the lack of appropriate initial treatment may result in the spread of the infection into the bloodstream, which leads to more severe illness.

*H. Bradford Hawley, M.D.*

The rapid spread of multiple resistance genes among species of bacteria occurs through a second method of gene transfer: horizontal transmission. Bacteria often carry their antibiotic resistance genes on bits of DNA called plasmids, which are commonly passed between bacteria. One plasmid can contain genes for resistance to numerous different antibiotics. Bacteria that receive such a plasmid will become resistant to multiple antibiotics in one rapid event. They can then spread this resistance even further when they multiply.

The widespread use of antibiotics in medicine and agriculture has led to the emergence and spread of superbacteria. Frequent exposure of bacteria to antibiotics increases the likelihood that they will develop resistance. Hospitals provide ideal conditions for bacteria to acquire resistance, because antibiotics are often used liberally and because many species of disease-causing bacteria are present.

Drug-resistant bacteria also arise on farms that produce meat and poultry, where antibiotics are routinely given to healthy animals to prevent disease and to promote growth. Incomplete treatment of pathogens with antibiotics can also promote resistance. When a person stops taking prescribed antibiotics before all bacteria are eliminated, the remaining bacteria may become resistant.

### ASSOCIATED DISEASES AND PATHOGENS

*Staph infections.* Methicillin-resistant *Staphylococcus aureus* (MRSA) causes skin and soft tissue infections, which can be invasive and life-threatening. MRSA is usually resistant to aminoglycosides, macrolides, tetracycline, chloramphenicol, lincosamides, and methicillin. MRSA infection is a major public health problem. According to the Centers for Disease Control and Prevention (CDC), MRSA infection in 2008 caused life-threatening illness in 90,000 people and 15,250 deaths in the United States alone.

*Tuberculosis.* Nearly one-third of the world's population is infected with *Mycobacterium tuberculosis*, the bacterium that causes the lung disease tuberculosis (TB). About ten percent of those infected will develop TB. The rise of antibiotic resistance now threatens the only treatment for TB, which is antibiotic therapy. Strains of *M. tuberculosis* that are resistant to a minimum of one antibiotic have been documented in every country surveyed by the World Health Organization. Multidrug-resistant TB (MDR TB) is caused by strains of *M. tuberculosis* that are resistant to both isoniazid and rifampicine, the two most effective anti-TB drugs.

*Opportunistic infections.* Persons with compromised immune systems are vulnerable to infection by organisms that are normally harmless in healthy people. Acquired in hospitals, opportunistic infections can be life-threatening without appropriate antibiotic treatment. Drug-resistant strains of the bacteria responsible for these infections pose a growing threat to hospitalized persons. The CDC estimates that annually, two million persons in the United States get some sort of infection while in the hospital; 70 percent of the bacteria that cause these infections are resistant to a minimum of one antibiotic typically used to treat them.

Strains of *Klebsiella pneumoniae* have developed resistance to carbapenems, one of the few classes of antibiotics effective against these gram-negative bacteria. *Enterobacter* variants are also carbapenem-resistant, and they are resistant to all penicillin derivatives and cephalosporins. *Enterococcus faecium* has developed strains that are resistant to both ampicillin and vancomycin. Pan-resistant strains of *Pseudomonas aeruginosa* and *Acinetobacter baumannii* are no longer treatable with any known antibiotics.

## IMPACT

Superbacteria present a serious global threat to human health. The worldwide spread of antibiotic resistance jeopardizes the usefulness of antibiotics in the treatment of bacterial diseases. Health care providers increasingly face the challenge of treating infections for which few or no effective antibiotics exist. People with resistant infections face longer hospital stays, more severe illness, and an increased chance of death from certain diseases. The resulting costs are high, both in terms of health care dollars and human lives. Solutions will require global efforts to reduce overuse and misuse of antibiotics, to prevent the spread of resistant organisms, and to develop new antibiotic agents.

*Kathryn Pierno, M.S.*

## FURTHER READING

Groopman, Jerome. "Superbugs." *The New Yorker* 84 (2008): 46-55. Recounts outbreaks of drug-resistant bacteria and discusses the causes and economic impact of multidrug resistance.

Klevens, R. M., et al. "Invasive Methicillin-Resistant *Staphylococcus aureus* Infections in the United States." *Journal of the American Medical Association* 298 (2007): 1761-1763. A study that examines the prevalence of MRSA infection in the United States.

Muto, C. A., et al. "SHEA Guideline for Preventing Nosocomial Transmission of *Staphylococcus aureus* and *Enterococcus.*" *Infection Control and Hospital Epidemiology* 24 (2003): 362-386. Presents evidence-based recommendations for preventing the spread of antibiotic-resistant bacteria in hospitals.

Nikaido, Hiroshi. "Multidrug Resistance in Bacteria." *Annual Review of Biochemistry* 78 (2009): 119-146. Review article describes the molecular mechanisms of antibiotic resistance in bacteria.

Sachs, Jessica Snyder. *Good Germs, Bad Germs: Health and Survival in a Bacterial World.* New York: Hill and Wang, 2008. Describes for general readers the nature and scope of antibiotic resistance and discusses the practices that have led to drug-resistant bacteria.

Sharma, Surendra, and Alladi Mohan. "Multidrug-Resistant Tuberculosis: A Menace that Threatens to Destabilize Tuberculosis Control." *Chest* 130 (2006): 261-272. A comprehensive review of drug-resistant tuberculosis worldwide, including its epidemiology, molecular mechanisms, diagnosis, and treatment.

## WEB SITES OF INTEREST

*Centers for Disease Control and Prevention*
http://www.cdc.gov/drugresistance

*National Institute of Allergy and Infectious Diseases*
http://www.niaid.nih.gov/topics/antimicrobialresistance

*Todar's Online Textbook of Bacteriology*
http://www.textbookofbacteriology.net

*World Health Organization*
http://www.who.int/drugresistance

**See also:** Alliance for the Prudent Use of Antibiotics; Antibiotic resistance; Antibiotics: Types; Bacteria: Classification and types; Bacteria: Structure and growth; Bacterial infections; Drug resistance; Epidemiology; Hospitals and infectious disease; Iatrogenic infections; Infection; Methicillin-resistant staph infection; Microbiology; Opportunistic infections; Reinfection; Secondary infection; Vancomycin-resistant enterococci infection; Vertical disease transmission; Wound infections.

---

Surgical wound infections. *See* Wound infections.

---

# Syphilis

CATEGORY: Diseases and conditions
ANATOMY OR SYSTEM AFFECTED: Genitalia, mouth, reproductive system, skin
ALSO KNOWN AS: Bejel, lues, pinta, yaws

## DEFINITION

Syphilis is a highly infectious sexually transmitted disease (STD) that is caused by infection by the bacterium *Treponema pallidum pallidum*. This bacterium is a wormlike spiral-shaped organism that burrows into the mucous membranes of the mouth and genitals. Syphilis can be congenital (passed to a fetus from an infected pregnant girl or woman) or acquired. The disease occurs in four stages: primary, secondary, latent (hidden), and tertiary (late).

## CAUSES

Transmission of syphilis occurs through contact with an infected person through vaginal, anal, or oral sex. The bacteria will often enter the body through mucous membranes of the urogenital area, but may also enter through chafed, scraped, or cut skin. Pregnant women with syphilis can infect their fetus through the placenta.

## RISK FACTORS

Risk factors for syphilis include unprotected sex, multiple sex partners, human immunodeficiency virus (HIV) infection, open sores or a rash, and sharing contaminated needles. Men are more vulnerable than women in contracting syphilis during sex.

## SYMPTOMS

The symptoms of syphilis, which can mimic many diseases, vary depending on the stage of the disease. In its primary stage, syphilis causes small, usually painless sores (called chancre) on the lips, mouth, genital area, or anus. In men, these sores usually develop on the penis. In women, they occur on the outer genitals or within the vagina.

In the secondary stage of syphilis, a rash forms about four to ten weeks after the appearance of the chancre sore. This rash may be over the entire body and often appears in the palms of the hands and soles of the feet.

As syphilis spreads throughout the body, additional symptoms include fever, sore throat, weakness, muscle aches, joint pain, hair loss, swollen lymph nodes, decreased appetite, and headaches. Vision, hearing, and reflex problems begin to appear as the nerves become affected. The pupils become dilated to different sizes. Irritability also develops.

During the latent stage, after the symptoms experienced in the second stage clear, the infected person does not experience any symptoms but is still infectious. This stage can last many years.

In the tertiary stage, symptoms range from mild to devastating. The symptoms vary depending on the areas affected and the complications that develop. There are three types of tertiary syphilis: benign tertiary syphilis, cardiovascular syphilis, and neurosyphilis.

In benign tertiary syphilis, a lesion, known as a gumma, forms on the skin, often just below the knee, but can also form on bone and visceral tissue and cause deep pain. These lesions grow slowly, heal slowly, and leave scars. They usually consist of a center of dead tissue surrounded by granular tissue. Cardiovascular syphilis may lead to an aneurism of the aorta or leakage of the aortic valve, which lead to chest pain, heart failure, or death. Neurosyphilis can sometimes cause no symptoms. If the brain is involved, it is called meningovascular neurosyphilis. The symptoms of meningovascular neurosyphilis include headache, dizziness, poor concentration, insomnia, neck stiffness,

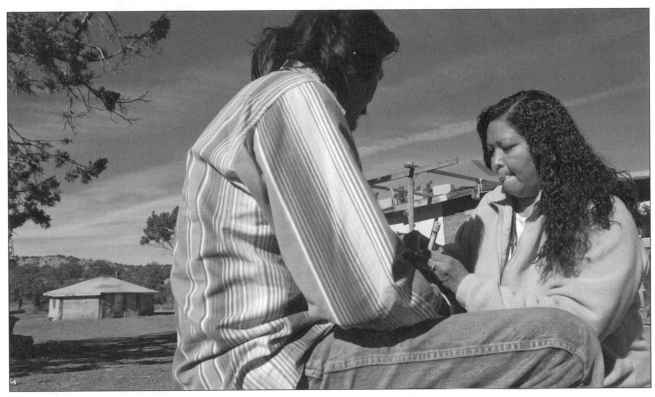

*A public health nurse draws blood from a man in New Mexico to check for syphilis.* (AP/Wide World Photos)

blurred vision, small irregular pupils, mental confusion, and seizures. When the spinal cord is infected, symptoms include weakness of the muscles of the arms and shoulders. As the disease progresses, infected persons experience loss of muscle control of arms, legs, loss of sphincter control, and bladder-related symptoms.

Congenital syphilis is passed from a woman to her fetus during pregnancy or childbirth. Symptoms of congenital syphilis include highly contagious watery discharge from the nose; painful inflammation of bone; rash of the palms of the hands and soles of the feet; anemia; an enlarged liver; swelling of the lymph nodes; an enlarged spleen; and a failure to grow. Congenital syphilis also increases the risk of fetal death.

### SCREENING AND DIAGNOSIS

Because symptoms of syphilis are similar to other conditions, an accurate diagnosis is critical. Diagnosis is made through blood testing, direct examination (when chancre are visible), and patient history. For cases in the early stages, samples taken from the chancre sore are tested for the presence of infection by *T. pallidum*. Blood is tested in a laboratory for antibodies using a test called VDRL (venereal disease research laboratory) and RPR (rapid reagin test). Definitive diagnosis is made using a fluorescent antibody absorption test. The VDRL and RPR are screening tests that are also useful for monitoring a person's response to treatment. A sample of cerebrospinal fluid may be tested to diagnose brain involvement in neurosyphilis.

### TREATMENT AND THERAPY

Antibiotics are used to treat syphilis. Penicillin is preferred, but other antibiotics, such as doxycycline or tetracycline, can be used by those with a penicillin allergy. Azithromycin has been shown to be as effective as penicillin in the early stages of syphilis.

### PREVENTION AND OUTCOMES

Syphilis is a sexually transmitted disease, therefore it can be prevented by use of condoms during sex. To prevent congenital syphilis, the Centers for Disease

Control and Prevention recommends that all pregnant girls and women be screened for syphilis. It is also important to trace and contact all the sexual partners of an infected person so they may be treated. To prevent contamination before identification of infection, health care professionals should use proper protection.

*Joan Letizia, Ph.D.*

**FURTHER READING**

Hook, E. W., et al. "A Phase III Equivalence Trial of Azithromycin Versus Benzathine Penicillin for Treatment of Early Syphilis." *Journal of Infectious Diseases* 201 (2010): 1729-1735. Discusses a study comparing azithromycin with penicillin in treating early syphilis. The results indicate that a 2-gram-dose of azithromycin was equivalent to benzathine penicillin G for the treatment of early syphilis.

Kent, Molly E., and Romanelli, Frank. "Reexamining Syphilis: An Update on Epidemiology, Clinical Manifestations, and Management." *Annals of Pharmacotherapy* 42 (2008): 226-236. This article reviews the epidemiology, clinical features, diagnosis, and treatment of syphilis.

Khare, Manjiri. "Infectious Disease in Pregnancy." *Current Obstetrics and Gynaecology* 15 (2005): 149-156. An overview of the many infectious diseases, including syphilis, that are transmissible during pregnancy.

McCutchen, J. Allen. "Sexually Transmitted Diseases." In *The Merck Manual of Diagnosis and Therapy*, edited by Mark H. Beers et al. 18th ed. Whitehouse Station, N.J.: Merck Research Laboratories, 2006. The syphilis section of this chapter gives a detailed overview of the disease, including its etiology, pathology, epidemiology, course, treatment, and surveillance.

**WEB SITES OF INTEREST**

*American Social Health Association*
http://www.ashastd.org

*Centers for Disease Control and Prevention*
http://www.cdc.gov/std/syphilis

*National Institutes of Health*
http://www.nlm.nih.gov/medlineplus/syphilis.html

**See also:** Bacterial infections; Childbirth and infectious disease; Chlamydia; Contagious diseases; Genital herpes; Genital warts; Gonorrhea; Herpesvirus infections; Human papillomavirus (HPV) infections; Men and infectious disease; Pregnancy and infectious disease; Public health; Sexually transmitted diseases (STDs); Social effects of infectious disease; Transmission routes; *Treponema*; Women and infectious disease.

Swine flu. *See* H1N1 influenza.

# T

## T lymphocytes

CATEGORY: Immune response
ALSO KNOWN AS: Helper T cells, killer T cells

### DEFINITION

T lymphocytes are specialized white blood cells that are essential components of the human immune system. Although they are produced in bone marrow, T lymphocytes migrate to the thymus gland to mature until they are needed. Normal lymphocytes and other types of white blood cells are always present in sufficient numbers to fight infection, but special T lymphocytes are released into the bloodstream by the immune system to perform as mediators of cellular immunity. As such, they help humans respond at the cellular level to different types of disease-causing organisms (pathogens), foreign cells (non-self-cells) that have entered the body, tumor cells, and abnormal self-cells that attack the body's own tissues.

### CELL ACTIVATION AND FUNCTION

T lymphocytes participate in hypersensitivity reactions, reactions to allergens or toxic substances, graft-versus-host reactions (as in transplantation), and other types of immune reactions. The immune system activates what are called helper T cells (CD4+ T cells) when it detects specific types of proteins (antigens) on the surface of non-self-cells that have invaded the body. Helper T cells secrete cytokines and lymphokines (interleukins) that signal other white cells to increase their numbers and reinforce their normal functions.

Killer T cells (CD8+ cells) are activated to attack specific tumor cells and certain viruses and parasites whose surface antigens they recognize. Regulatory T cells perform a slightly different function, protecting against self-cells that mistakenly attack certain body tissues (such as joint tissue in rheumatoid arthritis or eye tissue in thyroid eye disease) in autoimmune disease.

### ROLE IN DISEASE

The role of the immune system in protecting the body relies on layers of defense provided by different activities of the innate immune system and the adaptive immune system. Consequently, the immune response can range from general, everyday protection against invaders by a relatively nonspecific response of the innate immune system to increasingly specific responses of the adaptive immune system, whose immunologic memory allows it to recognize certain invaders. Infectious organisms, foreign cells, and tumor cells all have unique protein-based antigens on their cell surfaces that can be detected by the adaptive immune system. These antigen-presenting cells (APCs) are targeted by immune system cells, which then bind to the antigens. This process, in turn, activates other immune system components, such as macrophages, growth factors, and natural killer cells, forming an integrated defense mechanism.

As a critical component of the adaptive immune system, T lymphocytes make up the body's special reserve forces. They are called on when antigen-specific action is needed to halt the harmful activity of bacteria, viruses, parasites, tumor cells, cells from foreign tissue, or out-of-control self-cells that may be responsible for progressive disease.

*L. Lee Culvert, B.S., CLS*

### FURTHER READING

Chatilla, Talal A. "Role of Regulatory T Cells in Human Diseases." *Journal of Allergy and Clinical Immunology* 116 (2005): 949-959.

Monroe, John G., and Michael J. Lenardo. "Regulation of Activation of B and T Lymphocytes." In *Hematology: Basic Principles and Practice*, edited by Ronald Hoffman et al. 5th ed. Philadelphia: Churchill Livingstone/Elsevier, 2009.

Sompayrac, Lauren M. *How the Immune System Works.* 3d ed. Hoboken, N.J.: Wiley-Blackwell, 2008.

"T-Cell Mediated Immunity." In *Janeway's Immunobiology*, by Kenneth Murphy, Paul Travers, and Mark Walport. 7th ed. New York: Garland Science, 2008.

## WEB SITES OF INTEREST

*AIDSgov*
http://www.aids.gov

*Microbiology and Immunology On-line*
http://pathmicro.med.sc.edu/book/welcome.htm

*National Institutes of Health*
http://www.nih.gov

**See also:** AIDS; Antibodies; Autoimmune disorders; Bacterial infections; HIV; Immune response to bacterial infections; Immune response to parasitic diseases; Immune response to viral infections; Immunity; Immunoassay; Immunodeficiency; Microbiology; Neutropenia; Seroconversion; Virulence.

# Taeniasis

CATEGORY: Diseases and conditions
ANATOMY OR SYSTEM AFFECTED: Digestive system, gastrointestinal system, intestines, stomach
ALSO KNOWN AS: Beef tapeworm, cysticercosis, pork tapeworm

## DEFINITION

Taeniasis is an infestation by the tapeworm from the genus *Taenia*. Tapeworms are either of the species *T. saginata* or of the species *T. solium*, both of which can be found worldwide wherever cows and swine are raised.

## CAUSES

Humans are final hosts for these worms, which enter the human body when a person eats undercooked meat from cows (*T. saginata*) or pigs (*T. solium*). The worms are present in the meat of a formerly infected animal in the form of cysts. In the human intestine, however, the tapeworms, after being ingested by a person, develop and grow up to twelve feet long. Both types of tapeworm grow into segments called proglottids that produce thousands of eggs. Eventually, proglottids break off and are passed from the host in feces. A second route of infestation comes from directly swallowing the eggs (because of one's poor hygiene or because of contamination, including self-contamination, with the eggs of *T. solium*).

## RISK FACTORS

Eating undercooked beef or pork is the most common risk factor in acquiring taeniasis. Other risk factors are eating food that has been handled by an infected person and having direct contact with an infected person.

## SYMPTOMS

Most taeniasis infestations produce no symptoms, other than minor intestinal distress. The infestation is usually discovered by seeing proglottids in the feces, particularly if the proglottids are moving. In rarer cases, swallowed *T. solium* eggs may move through the body to lodge in other areas, particularly the eye, heart, and central nervous system, including the brain. When this happens, the larvae form cysts that may provoke an immune response. This condition is known as cysticercosis and it can be much more serious than intestinal taeniasis. Cysticercosis of the eye can cause blindness and neurocysticercosis, which affects the brain, can lead to seizures and death.

## SCREENING AND DIAGNOSIS

Because tapeworm infestation usually has no symptoms, infection is generally detected by inspecting the feces for worm eggs, or proglottids. A complete blood count differential can also be done as confirmation. To detect cysticercosis, the doctor may order magnetic resonance imaging or a computed tomography scan.

## TREATMENT AND THERAPY

The preferred drug for treating tapeworms is oral praziquantel. The drugs niclosamide and albendazole may also be used. With treatment, intestinal tapeworm infestations can be eliminated. If the larvae have moved into body tissues, however, treatment can be very difficult. In some severe cases, surgery may be needed to remove the cysts.

## PREVENTION AND OUTCOMES

Taeniasis infestations are best avoided through hygiene measures, including meat inspection, and beef and pork should be cooked at high enough temperatures to kill any potential eggs. Also, careful personal hygiene, including handwashing after bowel movements, can help to avoid spreading the disease.

*David Hutto, Ph.D.*

## FURTHER READING

Centers for Disease Control and Prevention. "Taeniasis." Available at http://www.dpd.cdc.gov/dpdx/html/taeniasis.htm.

Icon Health. *Tapeworms: A Medical Dictionary, Bibliography, and Annotated Research Guide to Internet References.* San Diego, Calif.: Author, 2004.

The Merck Manuals, Online Medical Library. "*Taeniasis solium* and Cysticercosis."
Available at http://www.merck.com/mmhe.

Roberts, Larry S., and John Janovy, Jr. *Gerald D. Schmidt and Larry S. Roberts' Foundations of Parasitology.* 8th ed. Boston: McGraw-Hill, 2009.

"Tapeworm Infestation." In *The American Medical Association Encyclopedia of Medicine,* edited by Charles B. Clayman. New York: Random House, 1994.

World Health Organization. "Taeniasis/Cysticercosis." Available at http://www.who.int/zoonoses/diseases/taeniasis.

## WEB SITES OF INTEREST

*National Center for Emerging and Zoonotic Infectious Diseases*
http://www.cdc.gov/ncezid

*U.S. Department of Agriculture, Food Safety Information Center*
http://foodsafety.nal.usda.gov

*World Health Organization*
http://www.who.int/zoonoses

**See also:** Ascariasis; Capillariasis; Cysticercosis; Developing countries and infectious disease; Filariasis; Flukes; Food-borne illness and disease; Hookworms; Immune response to parasitic diseases; Intestinal and stomach infections; Parasitic diseases; Pigs and infectious disease; Pinworms; Tapeworms; Tropical medicine; Whipworm infection; Worm infections; Zoonotic diseases.

# Tapeworms

CATEGORY: Pathogen
TRANSMISSION ROUTE: Ingestion

## DEFINITION

Tapeworms are flatworm members of the class Cestoda, with seven species known to infect humans with intestinal worms. Other species can create diseases in humans by forming cysts in body tissues.

## NATURAL HABITAT AND FEATURES

Tapeworms are parasitic flatworms (also known as cestodes), with more than one thousand known species in worldwide distribution. The worms are located in the intestinal tract of the final host, although a larval-stage disease is also encountered in other body tissues. Tapeworms have a complicated life cycle of intermediate and final hosts. In intermediate hosts the cestode travels through the circulation system and forms a larval cyst within body tissues of the host. When the final host eats the intermediate host, the cestode develops into the mature worm in the intestine, where it absorbs nutrients through its skin as it passes through the host's intestine. Depending on the

---

**Taxonomic Classification
for Tapeworms**

**Kingdom:** Animalia
**Phylum:** Platyhelminthes
**Class:** Cestoda
**Order:** Cyclophyllidea
**Family:** Taeniidae
**Genus:** *Taenia*
**Species:**
*T. solium*
*T. saginata*
*T. asiatica*
**Order:** Cyclophyllidea
**Family:** Hymenolepididae
**Genus:** *Hymenolepsis*
**Species:**
*H. nana*
*H. diminuta*
**Order:** Cyclophyllidea
**Family:** Dipylidiidae
**Genus:** *Dipylidium*
**Species:** *D. caninum*
**Order:** Pseudophyllidea
**Family:** Diphyllobothriidae
**Genus:** *Diphyllobothrium*
**Species:** *D. latum*

## Flatworm (Tapeworm) Facts

**Geographical location:** Worldwide
**Habitat:** Cestoda (tapeworms) may be found in streams, but adults live within the body of a host
**Gestational period:** Varies among flatworm species. Most species lay eggs within a few days after fertilization; eggs usually hatch within a few days to a few weeks after being deposited
**Life span:** Varies among flatworm species
**Special anatomy:** Elongated, bilateral invertebrates without appendages, have neither a true body cavity nor a circulatory system; parasitic species have specially adapted mouth parts for attaching to the tissues of the host

species, the worms can range in size from less than one inch to more than 50 feet long.

The head of a tapeworm is called a scolex, and it usually has suckers that enable the worm to attach to the intestine; some species also have hooks. The body of the worm is referred to as the strobila, which is made up of segments called proglottids. Proglottids can produce thousands of eggs, which are released to pass from the host in the feces. Most tapeworms are hermaphroditic, and a single tapeworm can produce many thousands of viable eggs. Eventually, proglottids break off from the body of the tapeworm and also pass in the feces. Some tapeworms, such as the *Taenia* species, may live for as long as twenty years, while *Hymenolepsis nana* (dwarf tapeworm) lives for one year only.

Tapeworms causing intestinal infestation in humans are usually known by the name of the intermediate host. The worms that infest humans are *T. saginata* (beef tapeworm), *T. solium* (pork tapeworm), *T. asiatica* (earlier confused with *T. saginata*), *Diphyllobothrium latum* (fish tapeworm), *Dipylidium caninum* (dog tapeworm), *H. diminuta* (rat tapeworm), and *H. nana* (dwarf tapeworm). The dwarf tapeworm is so named not only because of its small size but also because the worm was thought to lack an intermediate host.

### Pathogenicity and Clinical Significance

Most tapeworm infestations in humans involve mature worms in the intestines and involve few symptoms, if any. When symptoms are noticed, they usually manifest as intestinal distress, such as nausea, loss of appetite, abdominal pain, weight loss, or diarrhea. Because of a lack of symptoms, the host can carry the tapeworm for many years without being aware he or she is doing so. Although most tapeworm infestation does not cause a visible problem for the host, a worm that grows very large may block the bile duct, the pancreatic duct, or the intestine.

Tapeworms are generally acquired from intermediate hosts by eating poorly cooked or raw beef, pork, or fish containing encysted larvae. A second route of transmission also involves intermediate hosts, whereby a person accidentally ingests the host through eating insects in dried foods such as grains and cereals (*H. diminuta*). Another route is more direct: children accidentally ingesting fleas or lice from dogs (*D. caninum*). Children also are most susceptible to acquiring *H. nana*.

A larval-stage infestation, which can be a much more serious disease, comes from directly ingesting tapeworm eggs, either from contaminated food and water or from self-infection with *T. solium* eggs by hosts who already carry pork tapeworm. In addition to *T. solium*, such larval-stage disease is caused by *Spirometra* species, *T. multiceps*, and *Echinoccocus granulosus*, *E. multilocularis*, and *E. vogeli*.

When eggs from these species are swallowed, they form larvae that move through the blood to body tissues and then form cysts, using the human as an intermediate host. This form of infestation has various names, depending on the species and type of cyst involved. When the larvae come from *T. solium*, the disease is known as cysticercosis. Such larval-stage diseases can have serious health consequences, particularly if the cysts lodge in the heart, eye, or central nervous system, including the brain. If the cysts migrate to other organs within the body, they can disrupt the functioning of the organ; in the eye they may lead to blindness. When cysts form in the central nervous system, including the brain (neurocysticercosis), they can result in headaches, seizures, meningitis, hydrocephalus, dementia, and death.

### Drug Susceptibility

Most intestinal infestations are treated with praziquantel in a single oral dose. With treatment, there is a good chance of ridding the body of the parasite altogether. After treatment, it is possible that only part of the worm will be seen in the feces, as the host may begin to break the worm down by digestion before it is excreted. Other possible anthelmintic drugs include albendazole and niclosamide.

Cysticercosis and other larval-stage infestations are not necessarily treated unless they involve the brain. When they are treated, praziquantel may also be used, though in persons with neurocysticercosis, side effects may require administration of corticosteroids and praziquantel. In some cases, surgery is necessary to remove the cysts of larval disease.

*David Hutto, Ph.D.*

## FURTHER READING

Ash, Lawrence R., and Thomas C. Orihel. *Atlas of Human Parasitology.* 3d ed. Chicago: American Society of Clinical Pathologists, 1990. Short articles with very good photographs of both adult worms and eggs of all common cestode diseases.

Grove, David I. *A History of Human Helminthology.* Wallingford, England: CAB International, 1990. Contains chapters on a variety of helminthic diseases, with detailed chapters on the most common cestode diseases.

Icon Health. *Tapeworms: A Medical Dictionary, Bibliography, and Annotated Research Guide to Internet References.* San Diego, Calif.: Author, 2004. A helpful reference guide to tapeworms and tapeworm infection.

Roberts, Larry S., and John Janovy, Jr. *Gerald D. Schmidt and Larry S. Roberts' Foundations of Parasitology.* 8th ed. Boston: McGraw-Hill, 2009. A graduate-level textbook covering all aspects of parasitology. The text is highly technical and intended for the informed reader. The book is well illustrated.

"Tapeworm." In *Johns Hopkins Family Health Book,* edited by Michael Klag. New York: HarperCollins, 1999. Describes six types of tapeworm that infest humans as adult worms. Includes advice to patients on what to look for and when to call a doctor.

"Tapeworm Infestation." In *The American Medical Association Encyclopedia of Medicine,* edited by Charles B. Clayman. New York: Random House, 1994. A discussion of the basic life cycle and clinical effects of pork, beef, fish, and dwarf tapeworms.

## WEB SITES OF INTEREST

*National Center for Emerging and Zoonotic Infectious Diseases*
http://www.cdc.gov/ncezid

*U.S. Department of Agriculture, Food Safety Information Center*
http://foodsafety.nal.usda.gov

*World Health Organization*
http://www.who.int/zoonoses

**See also:** Ascariasis; Capillariasis; Cysticercosis; Developing countries and infectious disease; Filariasis; Flukes; Food-borne illness and disease; Hookworms; Immune response to parasitic diseases; Intestinal and stomach infections; Parasitic diseases; Pigs and infectious disease; Pinworms; Taeniasis; Tropical medicine; Whipworm infection; Worm infections; Zoonotic diseases.

---

TB. *See* Tuberculosis (TB).

---

Terrorism. *See* Biological weapons; Bioterrorism.

---

# Tetanus

CATEGORY: Diseases and conditions
ANATOMY OR SYSTEM AFFECTED: Jaw, mouth, musculoskeletal system, nervous system
ALSO KNOWN AS: Lockjaw

## DEFINITION

Tetanus is a bacterial infection that affects the nervous system. Tetanus bacteria from soil, dust, or manure enter the body through a break in the skin. The infection may result in severe muscle spasms. Such spasms lead to lockjaw, which prevents opening or closing of the mouth. Tetanus can be fatal.

## CAUSES

Tetanus is caused by a toxin produced by the spores of the bacterium *Clostridium tetani.*

## RISK FACTORS

The risk for tetanus is increased for persons who are not immunized against tetanus or who are not updating tetanus shots regularly, are intravenous-drug users, are age fifty years and older, have skin sores or wounds, have had burns, and have had exposure of open wounds to soil or to animal feces.

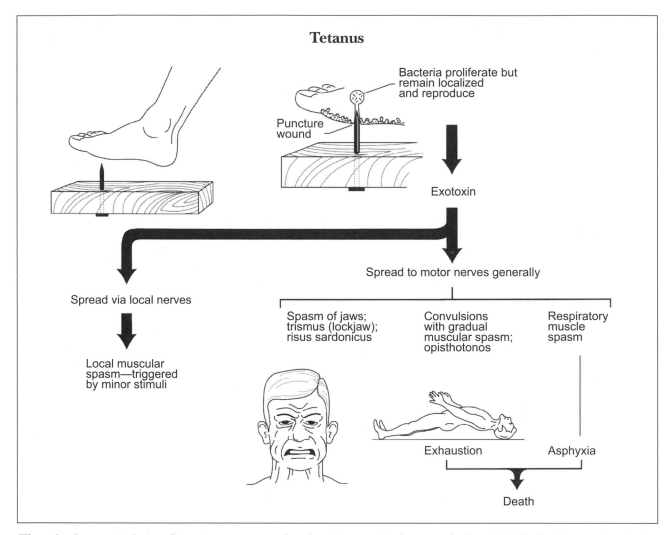

**Tetanus**

Bacteria proliferate but remain localized and reproduce

Puncture wound

Exotoxin

Spread via local nerves

Local muscular spasm—triggered by minor stimuli

Spread to motor nerves generally

Spasm of jaws; trismus (lockjaw); risus sardonicus

Convulsions with gradual muscular spasm; opisthotonos

Respiratory muscle spasm

Exhaustion

Asphyxia

Death

*The cycle of tetanus infection: Bacteria enter a wound and produce a toxin that spreads through the body, often causing death.*

## SYMPTOMS

Symptoms of tetanus may include headache; stiff jaw muscles (lockjaw) or neck muscles; drooling or trouble swallowing; muscle spasticity or rigidity; sweating; fever; irritability; pain or tingling at the wound site; high or low blood pressure; seizures; difficult breathing; heart beat that is irregular, too fast or too slow; cardiac arrest; dehydration; and pneumonia (a complication of the infection).

## SCREENING AND DIAGNOSIS

A doctor will ask about symptoms and medical history and will perform a physical exam. The diagnosis is based mainly on the patient's medical history but may include a culture of the wound; culture results, however, are not always accurate.

## TREATMENT AND THERAPY

Treatment may include hospitalization to manage complications of the infection; opening and cleaning of the wound, or sometimes surgical removal of the entire wounded area; antibiotics; a tetanus immunoglobulin (antibodies against tetanus that help neutralize the tetanus toxin); and a tetanus shot, if the patient's tetanus vaccine is not up to date.

For cases in which the patient has trouble breathing or swallowing, a breathing tube may be inserted into the throat to help keep the airway open. In certain situations, a surgical procedure called a tracheotomy may be done to provide an open airway.

## Prevention and Outcomes

The best means of prevention is immunization. All children (with a few exceptions) should receive the DTaP vaccine, which protects against diphtheria, tetanus, and pertussis. This is a series of five shots and a booster shot. The regular immunization schedule (for children and adults) is as follows: DTaP vaccines at two, four, and six months of age; at fifteen to eighteen months of age; and at four to six years of age; and a booster dose of Tdap given at eleven or twelve years of age (for children who have not already had the Td booster).

Children age thirteen to eighteen years who missed the booster dose or received Td only can receive one dose of Tdap five years after the last dose and can receive a booster of Tdap (a onetime dose for persons age nineteen to sixty-four years) or Td (every ten years) to provide continued protection.

For children ages four months to six years who have not yet received the vaccination, the Centers for Disease Control and Prevention recommends the following "catch-up" schedule: first and second dose (with a minimum four-week interval between doses); second and third dose (with a minimum four-week interval between doses); third and fourth dose (with a minimum six-month interval between doses); and fourth and fifth dose (with a minimum six-month interval between doses). The fifth dose is not necessary if the fourth dose was administered at age four years or older.

DTaP is not indicated for persons age seven years or older. Children age seven years and older and adults who have not been vaccinated should also be vaccinated. The choice and timing will vary based on age and prior vaccine exposure.

In addition to the vaccine, one can prevent tetanus by taking proper care of wounds, including promptly cleaning all wounds and consulting a doctor for medical care. One should consult a doctor especially if the patient has not had a tetanus vaccination in the ten years before injury.

*Jenna Hollenstein, M.S., RD;*
*reviewed by David L. Horn, M.D., FACP*

## Further Reading

Brachman, Philip S., and Elias Abrutyn, eds. *Bacterial Infections of Humans: Epidemiology and Control.* 4th ed. New York: Springer Science, 2009.

Brown, Pamela. *Quick Reference to Wound Care.* Sudbury, Mass.: Jones and Bartlett, 2009.

"Centers for Disease Control and Prevention Report Finds Tetanus Reaching Younger Adults." *Vaccine Weekly,* July 16, 2003, 21-22.

Centers for Disease Control and Prevention. "Recommended Immunization Schedules for Persons Aged 0-18 Years—United States, 2008." *Morbidity and Mortality Weekly Report* 57 (2008): Q1-Q4. Available at http://www.cdc.gov/mmwr/preview/mmwrhtml/mm5701a8.htm.

_____. "Tetanus (Lockjaw) Vaccination." Available at http://www.cdc.gov/vaccines/vpd-vac/tetanus.

Gremillion, Henry A., ed. *Temporomandibular Disorders and Orofacial Pain.* Philadelphia: Saunders/Elsevier, 2007.

Pan American Health Organization. World Health Organization. *Control of Diphtheria, Pertussis, Tetanus, "Haemophilus influenzae" Type B, and Hepatitis B Field Guide.* Washington, D.C.: Author, 2005.

## Web Sites of Interest

*American Academy of Pediatrics*
http://www.healthychildren.org

*Caring for Kids*
http://www.caringforkids.cps.ca

*Centers for Disease Control and Prevention*
http://www.cdc.gov/vaccines

*College of Family Physicians of Canada*
http://www.cfpc.ca

*National Foundation for Infectious Diseases*
http://www.nfid.org

*National Institute of Allergy and Infectious Diseases*
http://www.niaid.nih.gov

**See also:** Airborne illness and disease; Bacterial infections; Botulism; Children and infectious disease; *Clostridium*; Diphtheria; DTaP vaccine; Melioidosis; Soilborne illness and disease; Vaccines: History; Vaccines: Types; Wound infections.

# Tetracycline antibiotics

CATEGORY: Treatment

## DEFINITION

Tetracycline, which is produced by *Streptomyces* spp., is a broad-spectrum antibiotic that is useful against a wide range of gram-positive and gram-negative bacteria. Tetracyclines are not generally first-line agents but are still often prescribed. Activity is similar to the macrolide antibiotics, such as erythromycin. Tetracyclines are commonly used as topical or oral agents for acne. They are also among the drugs of choice for Lyme disease and anthrax infection and remain somewhat commonly used against rickettsial infections and sexually transmitted diseases, especially chlamydia.

## MECHANISM OF ACTION

Tetracyclines are bacteriostatic agents that work by inhibiting protein synthesis at the ribosomal level. They bind to ribonucleic acid (RNA) at the 30S site and then inhibit subsequent binding of the aminoacyl-transfer-RNA to the ribosome. This action terminates peptide chain growth. More lipophilic agents in this class, such as minocycline, also disrupt cytoplasmic membrane function and cause key cellular components to leak from the cell, leading to cell death.

## DRUGS IN THIS CLASS

The common drugs in this class are tetracycline, doxycycline, demeclocycline, and minocycline. They are well absorbed and can be taken by mouth. They should not, however, be taken within two hours of ingesting dairy products, antacids, or other foods or multivitamin and mineral preparations that contain calcium, iron, aluminum, or magnesium; chelation of the drug with the metal ion will result. The drug will then become insoluble and the drug will not be properly absorbed.

Drugs in this class are associated with nausea,

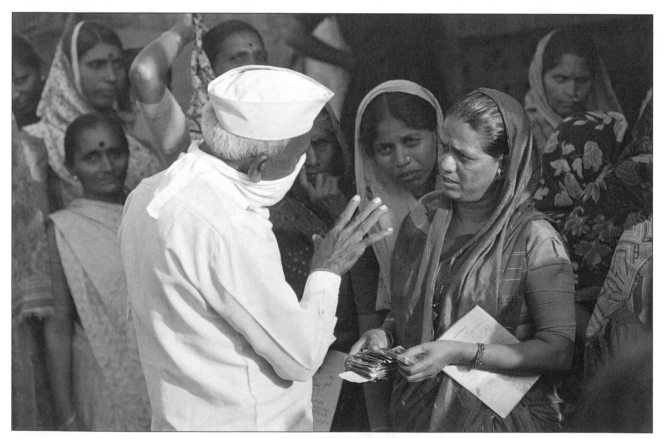

*Tetracycline antibiotics are distributed during the 1994 pneumonic plague outbreak in India.* (AP/Wide World Photos)

vomiting, diarrhea, dizziness, and vertigo. Like other broad-spectrum antibiotics, they frequently lead to superinfection, particularly of *Candida albicans.* They should not be prescribed to children under the age of twelve years because they are highly associated with a progressive and permanent discoloration of teeth, particularly during the years in which the permanent set is developing. They also are not advised for pregnant women because of the potential of liver toxicity.

All agents in this class can lead to photosensitivity, so persons should be advised to limit sun exposure to avoid serious sunburn, particularly when first beginning the medication. This reaction is most common with demeclocycline.

Another unique issue related to tetracyclines is the presence of a Fanconi-like syndrome caused by anhydro-4-epitetracycline, a degradation product that can form over time; it is toxic to the kidneys and can be fatal. For this reason, outdated or expired tetracycline and demeclocycline should never be taken. Because the degradation product is formed by a dehydration reaction at C-6, only tetracyclines that have a C-6 hydroxyl group are at risk for this problem. Minocycline and doxycycline do not have this group and are free of this toxicity.

### IMPACT

Tetracycline products are most often used for acne and for Lyme disease prophylaxis. Minocycline and doxycycline are most commonly used. Doxycycline, which received widespread attention in the wake of the October, 2001, anthrax bioterrorism scare in the United States, is one of the primary agents used for anthrax, including inhalation anthrax. Tetracyclines also are commonly included in animal feed.

*Karen M. Nagel, Ph.D.*

### FURTHER READING

"Antibiotics and Antimicrobial Agents." In *Foye's Principles of Medicinal Chemistry*, edited by Thomas L. Lemke et al. 6th ed. Philadelphia: Lippincott Williams & Wilkins, 2008.

Murray, Patrick R., Ken S. Rosenthal, and Michael A. Pfaller. *Medical Microbiology.* 6th ed. Philadelphia: Mosby/Elsevier, 2009.

Sanford, Jay P., et al. *The Sanford Guide to Antimicrobial Therapy.* 18th ed. Sperryville, Va.: Antimicrobial Therapy, 2010.

Tortora, Gerard J., Berdell R. Funke, and Christine L.
Case. "Antimicrobial Drugs." In *Microbiology: An Introduction.* 10th ed. San Francisco: Benjamin Cummings, 2010.

### WEB SITES OF INTEREST

*Alliance for the Prudent Use of Antibiotics*
http://www.tufts.edu/med/apua

*eMedicineHealth: Antibiotics*
http://www.emedicinehealth.com/antibiotics

**See also:** Alliance for the Prudent Use of Antibiotics; Aminoglycoside antibiotics; Antibiotics: Types; Bacteria: Classification and types; Cephalosporin antibiotics; Glycopeptide antibiotics; Ketolide antibiotics; Lipopeptide antibiotics; Macrolide antibiotics; Oxazolidinone antibiotics; Penicillin antibiotics; Prevention of bacterial infections; Quinolone antibiotics; Reinfection; Secondary infection; Superbacteria; Treatment of bacterial infections.

---

# Thiazole antifungals

CATEGORY: Treatment

### DEFINITION

Thiazole antifungals belong to the azole family, which includes imidazole and triazole. These three can be differentiated from the other members in this family by the presence of a thiazole functional group, a five-membered ring containing one nitrogen and one sulfur. Imidazole groups are similar rings with two nitrogens, whereas triazoles contain three nitrogens.

### MECHANISM OF ACTION

Thiazole antifungals act in a similar fashion to imidazole and triazole antifungals. All drugs in this family work by inhibiting cytochrome P450 demethylase, an enzyme responsible for converting lanosterol to ergosterol. Blocking this conversion leads to buildup of lanosterol, which is not typically present in fungal cell walls to the extent it is in ergosterol. Lanosterol contains a 14 alpha-methyl group not present in ergosterol; this chemical substitution results in a different shape and different physical properties of this sterol. The fungal cell membrane thereby exhibits permeability changes and becomes leaky, allowing key cellular components to exit the cell. This leads to cell death.

## DRUGS IN THIS CLASS

No drugs containing these groups are approved to treat fungal infections in humans, but several tri-substituted thiazole derivatives are being investigated. Researchers in Saudi Arabia report that four compounds in a series of thiazole derivatives showed significant activity against *Candida albicans*, and thirteen were somewhat active against gram-positive bacteria, including *Staphylococcus aureus* and *Bacillus subtilis*. A research group from Greece also reported significant antifungal and antibacterial activity with a series of thirteen thiadiazole derivatives.

Other researchers have had promising results against *Cryptococcus neoformans* with a thiazol-4-one derivative. The agent showed fungicidal activity and could be useful in the development of new agents against cryptococcosis, a fungal infection that can be life-threatening in persons with impaired immune systems.

None of the foregoing derivatives have undergone clinical testing, but all have shown some promise in the development of new antifungal agents.

## THIAZOLE-BASED FUNGICIDES AND ANTIPARASITIC AGENTS

A number of fungicides containing thiazole groups are in common use worldwide in the agricultural industry to improve yield and plant quality. Thiabendazole is one common agent used to control mold, blight, and other fungal diseases in fruits and vegetables and parasitic infections in livestock. It had been available as an oral suspension or tablet for human use against parasites, but, by order of the U.S. Food and Drug Administration, distribution has been discontinued in the United States. A topical product is available in other countries. Mebendazole (Vermox) is available as a tablet for the treatment of parasitic infections such as ringworm and hookworm, but it does not appear to have any antifungal activity.

## IMPACT

Immunocompromised persons are susceptible to a number of fungal infections that healthy persons can easily fight. The infections include *C. albicans* and *C. neoformans*, which often become resistant to broad-spectrum antifungal agents. Newer agents must constantly be developed, particularly for those persons with impaired immune systems because of human immunodeficiency virus (HIV) infection, chemotherapy, or organ transplantation.

*Karen M. Nagel, Ph.D.*

## FURTHER READING

Al-Saadi, M. S., H. M. Faidallah, and S. A. Rostom. "Synthesis and Biological Evaluation of Some 2,4,5-Trisubstituted Thiazole Derivatives as Potential Antimicrobial and Anticancer Agents." *Archiv der Pharmazie—Chemistry in Life Sciences* 341 (2008): 424-434.

Camoutsis, C., et al. "Sulfonamide-1,2,4-Thiadiazole Derivatives as Antifungal and Antibacterial Agents: Synthesis, Biological Evaluation, Lipophilicity, and Conformational Studies." *Chemical and Pharmaceutical Bulletin* 58 (2010): 160-167.

Griffith, R. K. "Antifungal Drugs." In *Foye's Principles of Medicinal Chemistry*, edited by Thomas L. Lemke and William O. Foye. 6th ed. Philadelphia: Wolters Kluwer, 2008.

Gullo, Antonio. "Invasive Fungal Infections." *Drugs* 69 (2009): 65-73.

Insuasty, B., et al. "Fungicide Activity of 5-(4-Chlorobenzylidene)-(Z)-2-Dimethylamino-1,3-Thiazol-4-One Against *Cryptococcus neoformans*." *Archiv der Pharmazie—Chemistry in Life Sciences* 343 (2010): 48-53.

Murray, Patrick R., Ken S. Rosenthal, and Michael A. Pfaller. *Medical Microbiology*. 6th ed. Philadelphia: Mosby/Elsevier, 2009.

Ryan, Kenneth J. "Pathogenesis of Fungal Infection." In *Sherris Medical Microbiology*, edited by Kenneth J. Ryan and C. George Ray. 5th ed. New York: McGraw-Hill, 2010.

## WEB SITES OF INTEREST

*Centers for Disease Control and Prevention, Division of Foodborne, Bacterial, and Mycotic Diseases*
http://www.cdc.gov/nczved/divisions/dfbmd

*DoctorFungus*
http://doctorfungus.org

*Microbiology and Immunology On-line: Mycology*
http://pathmicro.med.sc.edu/book/mycol-sta.htm

**See also** Antifungal drugs: Mechanisms of action; Antifungal drugs: Types; Diagnosis of fungal infections; Echinocandin antifungals; Fungal infections; Fungi: Classification and types; Imidazole antifungals; Immune response to fungal infections; Infection; Mycoses; Polyene antifungals; Prevention of fungal infections; Treatment of fungal infections; Triazole antifungals.

---

Third World. *See* Developing countries and infectious disease; Tropical medicine.

---

# Thrush

CATEGORY: Diseases and conditions
ANATOMY OR SYSTEM AFFECTED: Larynx, mouth, respiratory system, skin, throat, tongue
ALSO KNOWN AS: Oropharyngeal candidiasis

## DEFINITION

Thrush is a fungal infection of the mouth caused by an overgrowth of the yeast organism *Candida albicans.* Thrush usually begins on the tongue and inside the cheeks and may spread to the palate, gums, tonsils, and throat. In severe cases, the infection may spread to the larynx (voice box), digestive tract, respiratory system, and skin.

## CAUSES

Many microorganisms, including yeast and bacteria, live in the mouth. Thrush occurs when the normal balance of these organisms is upset. This allows an overgrowth of *Candida* to occur.

## RISK FACTORS

Risk factors for developing thrush include age (infants, toddlers, and the elderly); a weakened immune system from human immunodeficiency (HIV) virus infection, acquired immunodeficiency syndrome (AIDS), cancer, or medical treatments for cancer, such as chemotherapy; stress; prolonged illness; use of antibiotics; use of oral or inhaled corticosteroids; diabetes; hormonal changes, such as those associated with pregnancy or the use of birth control pills; wearing dentures; conditions that cause a dry mouth; and smoking.

## SYMPTOMS

The symptoms of thrush, which occur in the mouth, include white, raised patches; red, slightly raised patches; discharge with a curdlike appearance (like cottage cheese); thick, dark brownish coating in the mouth; dry mouth; and fissures or cracks in the mouth. If the infection spreads into the esophagus, one may also experience difficulty or pain with swallowing or a sensation of something "stuck" in the throat. If thrush spreads systemically, one may develop a fever.

## SCREENING AND DIAGNOSIS

A doctor will ask about symptoms and medical history and will examine the patient's mouth. A sample of cells from the affected area may be scraped off and examined under a microscope.

## TREATMENT AND THERAPY

The goal of treatment is to restore the normal balance of bacteria and yeast in the mouth. Treatments may include antifungal medications such as lozenges, troches (a type of lozenge that dissolves in the mouth), tablets, or oral rinses; medications that are active against yeast, such as nystatin (Bio-Statin and Nilstat), clotrimazole (Lotrimin and Mycelex), miconazole, and gentian violet; and, for breast-feeding mothers of infants with thrush, a topical antifungal medication placed on the woman's nipples to reduce the infant's infection.

Oral hygiene practices that may aid in healing include rinsing one's mouth with warm salt-water and gently scraping off patches with a toothbrush. Finally, underlying conditions that may contribute to thrush can be identified and treated.

## PREVENTION AND OUTCOMES

Preventive measures can be taken to reduce the risk of thrush. Thrush in adults is often associated with AIDS, so persons with thrush should obtain a blood test for HIV and follow recommended prevention guidelines, such as using condoms and other protection and avoiding needles except under sterile conditions.

Persons who are at high risk for or who are prone to thrush may be given an antifungal medication as a preventive measure. If prone to thrush, one should avoid overuse of mouthwashes and mouth sprays, which can upset the normal balance of yeast and bacteria in the mouth. If a baby is prone to thrush and if that baby drinks from a bottle, the baby should drink from the bottle with disposable nipples.

One should avoid unnecessary use of antibiotics; if avoiding antibiotics is not an option, one should consider eating yogurt or using acidophilus tablets (probiotics) during antibiotic treatment and for several weeks thereafter. One should decrease his or her intake of sugar and yeast-containing foods and beverages, such as bread, wine, and beer, and, if using a cortisone inhaler, should rinse the mouth thoroughly after each use.

*Jennifer Hellwig, M.S., RD;*
*reviewed by Elie Edmond Rebeiz, M.D., FACS*

## FURTHER READING

Greenspan, Deborah, and John S. Greenspan. "HIV-related Oral Disease." *The Lancet* 348 (September, 1996): 729-733.

Langlais, Robert P., and Craig S. Miller. *Color Atlas of Common Oral Diseases.* 4th ed. Philadelphia: Lippincott Williams & Wilkins, 2009.

Mandell, Gerald L., John E. Bennett, and Raphael Dolin, eds. *Mandell, Douglas, and Bennett's Principles and Practice of Infectious Diseases.* 7th ed. New York: Churchill Livingstone/Elsevier, 2010.

Martin, Jeanne Marie. *Complete "Candida" Yeast Guidebook: Everything You Need to Know About Prevention, Treatment, and Diet.* Rev. ed. New York: Three Rivers Press, 2000.

Ohnmacht, Galen A., et al. "A Prospective, Randomized, Double-Blind, Placebo-Controlled Trial Evaluating the Effect of Nystatin on the Development of Oral Irritation in Patients Receiving High-Dose Intravenous Interleukin-2." *Journal of Immunotherapy* 24, no. 2 (March/April, 2001): 188-192.

Winn, Washington C., Jr., et al. *Koneman's Color Atlas and Textbook of Diagnostic Microbiology.* 6th ed. Philadelphia: Lippincott Williams & Wilkins, 2006.

## WEB SITES OF INTEREST

*AIDSgov*
http://www.aids.gov

*AIDSinfo*
http://aidsinfo.nih.gov

*Canadian AIDS Treatment Information Exchange*
http://www.catie.ca

*Canadian Dental Association*
http://www.cda-adc.ca

*Centers for Disease Control and Prevention*
http://www.cdc.gov

*National Foundation for Infectious Diseases*
http://www.nfid.org

**See also:** AIDS; Antifungal drugs: Types; *Candida*; Candidiasis; *Capnocytophaga* infections; Children and infectious disease; Diagnosis of fungal infections; Epiglottitis; Fungal infections; HIV; Laryngitis; Mononucleosis; Mouth infections; Nasopharyngeal infections; Pharyngitis and tonsillopharyngitis; Treatment of fungal infections; Women and infectious disease.

# Ticks and infectious disease

**CATEGORY:** Transmission

## DEFINITION

Ticks are members of the Arthropod phylum of the animal kingdom, and they serve as the vectors for a wide variety of human pathogens. Ticks are not insects; they are arachnids like scorpions, spiders, and mites. Ticks are divided into four families, but only two families, the Argasidae and the Ixodidae, are associated with human disease. Of the 878 known species, about 222 have been reported to feed on people; however, only 33 species commonly do so.

## ANATOMY

The body of the tick comprises two fused parts, the capitulum (a "false" head) and the idiosome (the main body) to which the legs are attached. Larvae have six legs, and the nymphs and adults have eight legs. The body of the ixodid, or hard tick, bears a dorsal shield called the scutum. In males, the scutum covers the entire body, but in females, the hard cuticle is smaller and makes up only the anterior portion of the body. Unfed hard ticks are flattened and seed-like in appearance. In contrast, the argasid, or soft tick, has a nearly absent hard cuticle and is shaped like a raisin. There is little difference in the appearance of males and females.

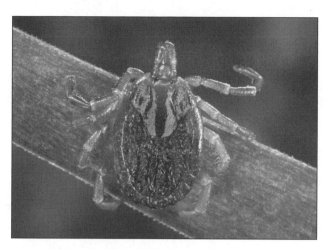

*A female Ixodides tick.* (CDC)

## LIFE CYCLE AND FEEDING

Ticks have four life stages: egg, larvae, nymph, and adult. They are ectoparasites that require a blood meal to survive and to develop or move to the next stage and reproduce. Ticks feed upon a variety of vertebrate hosts, with mammals and birds predominating. After the larvae hatches from the egg, the first meal is taken, which enables movement to the next stage of development, the nymph. Nymphs may progress through several stages (instars) before advancing to the final adult stages. Blood meals are taken between stages. Adults, both male and female, take blood meals for survival and reproductive development.

Soft ticks are found mostly in tropical and subtropical regions, and they tend to live in narrow ranges of temperature and humidity. They are nest-dwelling and live up to twenty years. Nymphs may have as many as seven instars, each preceded by a blood meal.

Hard ticks are much more significant in disease transmission (in the United States). Hard ticks, which can live from one to six years, may have from one to three hosts during their life cycles. Female hard ticks die after laying one batch of eggs; the male dies after mating. Hard-tick habitats vary according to species, but they live in environments, such as open fields and wooded areas, that are less sheltered than those of soft ticks.

Ticks employ a variety of methods to find their hosts. Soft ticks leave their nests and crawl to their hosts for a quick meal before returning to their nests. Hard ticks quest by crawling to the tips of vegetation and waiting for a passing host, which the tick detects through the host's vibration, heat, shadow, odor, or carbon dioxide output. When the tick detects a host, it releases from the vegetative perch and quickly clings to the host.

A host can carry a tick to an entirely new place. In the case of a migrating bird host, the tick may even be carried to a new continent. The body weight of a soft tick may increase five to twelve times following a blood meal, but the female hard tick may weigh 125 to 150 times more after feeding. Hard ticks feed slowly and for several days before dropping from their hosts.

Ticks spend only a small portion of their lives on hosts taking blood meals. Ticks spend most of their time struggling to stay alive in a fasting state and often in a less than ideal environment. An ideal environment for a tick is one with 85 percent or greater humidity and with a temperature between 43° and 45° Fahrenheit (6° and 7° Celsius). Humidity is paramount, and rain is welcomed by ticks. Ticks can prevent desiccation while fasting, and they respond to over-hydration during feeding.

## TICKBORNE DISEASES

Ticks transmit several bacterial infections, but humans are only rarely infected; for humans, the usual method of acquisition is by inhaling spores or bacteria associated with infected animals, such as sheep and goats. Spirochetal infections caused by ticks fall into three categories: Lyme disease, southern tick-associated rash illness, and the tickborne relapsing fevers.

Lyme disease is now the most common arthropod-borne infectious disease in the United States and in Europe. This disease is caused by a spirochete, *Borrelia burgdorferi*, and is transmitted by several species of hard ticks. A less common bacterial infection is tularemia, which is caused by the gram-negative coccobacillus *Francisella tularensis*. The disease may be transmitted by the bite of the deer fly or hard tick or by direct contact with an infected animal, such as a rabbit or muskrat. The American dog tick, *Dermacentor variabilis*, is the usual vector. The newest bacteria to be added to the list are the *Ehrlichia* and *Anaplasma*. Human ehrlichiosis and anaplasmosis are transmitted by hard ticks and are now endemic to many regions of the United States. Q fever is caused by a gram-negative, intracellular bacterium, *Coxiella burnetti*, that is related to *Legionella pneumophila*.

The tickborne rickettsial diseases are in the spotted

fever group. In the United States, the most significant of these fevers is Rocky Mountain spotted fever, caused by *Rickettsia rickettsii* and transmitted by hard ticks. The illness, which was first described in the Snake River Valley of Idaho, is now more commonly found in the American South.

Protozoa also can be transmitted to humans by ticks. Texas cattle fever, the first infectious disease attributed to tick bites, was described in 1893 by Theobald Smith. This illness is caused by *Babesia bigemina* and does not affect humans. Two other species, *B. divergens* and *B. microti*, cause disease in humans. The most common form of babesiosis (which is similar to malaria) in the United States is caused by *B. microti* and is transmitted by the same hard tick that carries the pathogen for Lyme disease.

The viral pathogens transmitted by ticks fall into three groups: encephalitide, hemorrhagic fever, and coltivirus. Powassan and West Nile are the two encephalitis viruses seen in the United States. Colorado tick fever and Salmon River viruses are coltiviruses that occasionally cause disease in Western states. The hemorrhagic fever viruses are not endemic to the Americas.

Tick paralysis is a rare disease associated with the bite of a hard tick. Acute ataxia and ascending paralysis occur four to seven days after the bite of a female tick. The exact mechanism of disease is unknown, but the disease is cured by removal of the tick. No infectious agent is involved.

## PREVENTION AND TREATMENT

Tick bites can be prevented by avoiding infested areas and by wearing protective, light-colored, clothing. A chemical that can be used on clothes to kill and repel ticks is permethrin. For skin protection, one can use an insect repellant containing NN-diethyl metatoluamide (DEET). Ticks should be carefully removed from the skin by using tweezers or forceps to avoid handling or crushing the ticks, as the infected blood of the engorged tick can cause infection if it comes into contact with the eyes, with other mucous membranes, or with broken skin. Specific antibiotic treatment is available for all of the infectious diseases transmitted by ticks, except for the viral diseases.

## IMPACT

Tickborne diseases are varied and many. The exact number of cases occurring annually worldwide is un-known, but it certainly numbers in the hundreds of thousands. Many of these diseases, such as Lyme disease and tickborne encephalitis, appear to be increasing. The climate changes associated with global warming have resulted in large areas of ideal tick habitat, providing both warmth and moisture. A direct connection among climate change, tick populations, and tickborne diseases has been scientifically documented.

*H. Bradford Hawley, M.D.*

## FURTHER READING

Anderson, John F. "The Natural History of Ticks." *Medical Clinics of North America* 86 (2002): 205-218. A good review of tick biology and taxonomy.

_____, and Louis A. Magnarelli. "Biology of Ticks." *Infectious Disease Clinics of North America* 22 (2008): 195-215. A complete article on the anatomy, feeding, and life cycles of ticks.

Atkinson, P. W., ed. *Vector Biology, Ecology, and Control.* New York: Springer Science, 2010. This book is a good source for the reader needing a detailed study of vectors and the latest methods for effective vector control.

Diaz, James H. "Ticks, Including Tick Paralysis." In *Mandell, Douglas, and Bennett's Principles and Practice of Infectious Diseases,* edited by Gerald L. Mandell, John F. Bennett, and Raphael Dolin. 7th ed. New York: Churchill Livingstone/Elsevier, 2010. A summary of ticks and their associated illnesses. Includes color illustrations.

Suss, Jochen, et al. "What Makes Ticks Tick? Climate Change, Ticks, and Tick-Borne Diseases." *Journal of Travel Medicine* 15 (2008): 39-45. This article reviews studies of climate change, tick populations, and tickborne diseases in Europe.

## WEB SITES OF INTEREST

*Centers for Disease Control and Prevention*
http://www.cdc.gov/ticks

*National Institute of Allergy and Infectious Diseases*
http://www.niaid.nih.gov/topics/vector

**See also:** Acariasis; Anaplasmosis; Arthropod-borne illness and disease; Blood-borne illness and disease; *Borrelia*; Colorado tick fever; Ehrlichiosis; Encephalitis; Hemorrhagic fever viral infections; Insect-borne illness and disease; Lyme disease; Mediterranean spotted fever; Mites and chiggers and infectious disease; Mosquitoes and infectious disease; Parasites: Classification and types; Parasitic diseases; Plague; Reoviridae; *Rickettsia*; Rocky Mountain spotted fever; Transmission routes; Tularemia; Vectors and vector control.

# Tinea capitis

CATEGORY: Diseases and conditions
ANATOMY OR SYSTEM AFFECTED: Head, scalp, skin
ALSO KNOWN AS: Fungal infection of the scalp, ringworm of the scalp

## DEFINITION

Tinea capitis is a fungal infection of the scalp. It is caused by a type of fungus called a dermatophyte. It occurs most often in children and is rare in adults.

## CAUSES

The fungi thrive in warm, humid environments. Factors that may contribute to tinea capitis include living in a hot, humid climate, and excessive sweating.

## RISK FACTORS

Factors that increase the chance for tinea capitis include age (ten years of age and younger); race (African); attending or working in a day-care center; exposure to pets with the infection; poor hygiene; sharing combs, brushes, or hats; having diabetes; and having an immune system disorder, such as human immunodeficiency virus (HIV) infection.

## SYMPTOMS

Symptoms of tinea capitis include itching of the scalp, bald patches, and areas with swelling, sores, or irritated skin. If not properly treated, the infection may cause permanent hair loss and scarring.

## SCREENING AND DIAGNOSIS

A doctor will ask about symptoms and medical history and will perform a physical exam. Infected children may need to be referred to a specialist, such as a dermatologist, whose work is focused on skin conditions. Diagnosis is often made by a close inspection of the scalp. If the diagnosis is uncertain, the doctor may scrape the child's scalp or clip a few hairs for testing.

Tests on the sample may include a microscopic examination and a fungal culture.

## TREATMENT AND THERAPY

The main treatment for tinea capitis is prescription antifungal medications. It is taken by mouth. Medicated shampoos are not effective, but they can help prevent the spread of infection to other people. Tinea capitis may be difficult to treat, and it may return after treatment. It sometimes goes away on its own at puberty.

## PREVENTION AND OUTCOMES

To help reduce the chance of getting tinea capitis, one should shampoo the infected child's hair regularly; should ensure the child does not share headgear, brushes, or combs; and should wash towels, clothes, and any shared items used by an infected person to prevent spreading it to others in the household. One should also take pets to a veterinarian for treatment if they develop skin rashes.

*Diane W. Shannon, M.D., M.P.H.;*
*reviewed by Ross Zeltser, M.D., FAAD*

## FURTHER READING

American Academy of Dermatology. "Tinea (Dermatophyte) Infections." Available at http://www.aad.org.

American Academy of Family Physicians. "Diagnosis and Management of Common Tinea Infections." Available at http://www.aafp.org/afp/980700ap/noble.html.

_____. "Tinea Infections: Athlete's Foot, Jock Itch, and Ringworm." Available at http://www.aafp.org/afp/980700ap/980700b.html.

Berger, T. G. "Dermatologic Disorders." In *Current Medical Diagnosis and Treatment 2011*, edited by Stephen J. McPhee and Maxine A. Papadakis. 50th ed. New York: McGraw-Hill Medical, 2011.

National Library of Medicine. "Tinea Capitis." Available at http://www.nlm.nih.gov/medlineplus/ency/article/000878.htm.

Richardson, Malcolm D., and Elizabeth M. Johnson. *The Pocket Guide to Fungal Infection.* 2d ed. Malden, Mass.: Blackwell, 2006.

## WEB SITES OF INTEREST

*American Academy of Dermatology*
http://www.aad.org

*Canadian Dermatology Association*
http://www.dermatology.ca

**See also:** Antifungal drugs: Types; Athlete's foot; Children and infectious disease; Chromoblastomycosis; Dermatomycosis; Diagnosis of fungal infections; Fungal infections; Jock itch; Onychomycosis; Plantar warts; Reinfection; Ringworm; Scabies; Skin infections; Tinea corporis; Tinea versicolor; Treatment of fungal infections.

# Tinea corporis

CATEGORY: Diseases and conditions
ANATOMY OR SYSTEM AFFECTED: Skin
ALSO KNOWN AS: Ringworm, tinea circinata, tinea glabrosa

## DEFINITION

Tinea corporis, commonly called ringworm, is a superficial dermatophyte infection that is characterized by lesions typically appearing on the arms, legs, or trunk of the body. It is a common infection that is seen more often in hot, humid climates. It may occur in people of all ages, but is most often found in children. The infection can be produced by the following fungal genera: *Trichophyton*, *Microsporum*, or *Epidermophyton*.

## CAUSES

Tinea corporis is caused by dermatophyte fungi. Almost one-half of the reported cases are caused by the *T. rubrum* fungus. Tinea corporis is a contagious disease that can be spread by person-to-person contact. It is also transmitted by animal-to-human contact and by touching contaminated, inanimate objects (fomites) such as combs, hair brushes, bedding, personal care products, shower floors and walls, and soils.

## RISK FACTORS

The risk for contracting tinea corporis is increased by long-term wetness of the skin, minor skin and nail injuries, poor hygiene, excessive sweating, and contact with infected people, pets, and objects. Because fungi thrive in warm, moist areas, living in such areas increases the risk of contracting tinea corporis.

## SYMPTOMS

Tinea corporis manifests as a lesion that starts as a flat, scaly spot that develops into a red-colored, elevated border that advances outward in a circular shape. As the rash develops, it may become dry, flaky, and itchy. Almost invariably, there is hair loss in areas where the infection occurs.

## SCREENING AND DIAGNOSIS

The primary diagnosis is based on examination of the skin. Skin scrapings are taken and examined underneath a microscope to reveal the presence of tinea corporis fungi. If the scrapings are negative, they may be sent for culture, which may take several days for development. In some cases, potassium hydroxide tests may reveal the culprit.

## TREATMENT AND THERAPY

The skin of an infected person should be kept clean and dry. Ringworm typically responds well to topical treatment. Topical antifungal creams containing miconazole or clotrimazole are effective in controlling and eliminating the infection. Oral antifungal medications, such as ketoconazole or terbinafine, are sometimes used in cases of severe, widespread fungal infection. Antibiotics are often used to treat secondary bacterial infections.

## PREVENTION AND OUTCOMES

Practicing good hygiene is the best safeguard against ringworm infections. One should keep skin dry; avoid contact with contaminated material; wear loose-fitting clothing; keep combs, bathroom surfaces, bedding, and clothing clean and dry; and thoroughly wash hands after handling animals and plants or coming into contact with the infection. If a person becomes infected, one should take proper measures to prevent the infection from spreading to others.

*Alvin K. Benson, Ph.D.*

## FURTHER READING

Andrews, M. D., and M. Burns. "Common Tinea Infections in Children." *American Family Physician* 77 (2008): 1415-1420.

Beers, Mark H., et al., eds. *The Merck Manual of Diagnosis and Therapy*. 18th ed. Whitehouse Station, N.J.: Merck Research Laboratories, 2006.

Berger, T. G. "Dermatologic Disorders." In *Current Medical Diagnosis and Treatment 2011*, edited by Stephen J. McPhee and Maxine A. Papadakis. 50th ed. New York: McGraw-Hill Medical, 2011.

Burns, Tony, et al., eds. *Rook's Textbook of Dermatology.* 8th ed. 4 vols. Hoboken, N.J.: Wiley-Blackwell, 2010.

Jackson, Scott, and Lee T. Nesbitt. *Differential Diagnosis for the Dermatologist.* New York: Springer, 2008.

Lanigan, S. W., and Zohra Zaidi. *Dermatology in Clinical Practice.* New York: Springer, 2010.

### Web Sites of Interest

*British Mycological Society*
http://fungionline.org.uk

*DoctorFungus.org*
http://doctorfungus.org

**See also:** Antifungal drugs: Types; Athlete's foot; Chromoblastomycosis; Dermatomycosis; *Epidermophyton*; Fungal infections; Jock itch; *Microsporum*; Onychomycosis; Skin infections; Tinea capitis; Tinea versicolor; *Trichophyton.*

# Tinea versicolor

Category: Diseases and conditions
Anatomy or system affected: Skin
Also known as: Pityriasis versicolor

### Definition

Tinea versicolor is a type of dermatomycosis that is caused by a yeast that interferes with normal tanning. Dermatomycosis includes a variety of superficial skin infections caused by fungi or yeast. These types of infections almost always only affect skin, hair, and nails. In people with severe immune problems, these infections can become more serious and invasive.

Tinea versicolor can result in uneven skin color and usually affects the back, upper arms, underarms, chest, and neck. It rarely affects the face.

### Causes

The fungus that causes tinea versicolor, *Malassezia furfur*, is normally present in small numbers on the skin and scalp. Overgrowth of the yeast leads to infection.

### Risk Factors

Risk factors for tinea versicolor include age (more common in adolescents and young adults), gender (more common in boys and men), skin condition (more common in people with naturally oily or excessively sweaty skin), and climate (more common in warm and humid climates).

### Symptoms

Symptoms include uneven skin color, with either white or light brown patches; light scaling on affected areas; slight itching that is worse when the person is hot; and patches that are most noticeable in summer months.

### Screening and Diagnosis

A doctor will ask about symptoms and medical history and will perform a physical exam. The patient may be referred to a dermatologist, a specialist in skin disorders and conditions. The doctor may use an ultraviolet light to see the patches more clearly and may scrape the patch for testing.

### Treatment and Therapy

Treatment options for tinea versicolor include topical medications such as selenium sulfide lotion (2.5 percent) or shampoo (1 percent; such as Dandrex, Exsel, and Selsun Blue), applied daily for one week and then monthly for several months to prevent recurrences. Another option is oral medication, such as prescription antifungal drugs. Oral medications make treatment shorter, but they are more expensive and associated with more adverse side effects.

Once the infection is successfully treated, the patient's skin will naturally return to its normal color. However, this process usually takes several months. Also, the condition may improve in the winter only to return again in the summer months.

### Prevention and Outcomes

One should avoid excessive heat and sweating to reduce the risk of tinea versicolor.

*Diane W. Shannon, M.D., M.P.H.;
reviewed by Ross Zeltser, M.D., FAAD*

### Further Reading

American Academy of Dermatology. "Tinea Versicolor." Available at http://www.aad.org.

Berger, T. G. "Dermatologic Disorders." In *Current*

*Medical Diagnosis and Treatment 2011*, edited by Stephen J. McPhee and Maxine A. Papadakis. 50th ed. New York: McGraw-Hill Medical, 2011.

National Library of Medicine. "Tinea Versicolor." Available at http://www.nlm.nih.gov/medlineplus/ency/article/001465.htm.

Richardson, Malcolm D., and Elizabeth M. Johnson. *The Pocket Guide to Fungal Infection.* 2d ed. Malden, Mass.: Blackwell, 2006.

## WEB SITES OF INTEREST

*American Academy of Dermatology*
http://www.aad.org

*Canadian Dermatology Association*
http://www.dermatology.ca

*Microbiology and Immunology On-line: Mycology*
http://pathmicro.med.sc.edu/book/mycol-sta.htm

**See also:** Antifungal drugs: Types; Athlete's foot; Chromoblastomycosis; Dandruff; Dermatomycosis; Diagnosis of fungal infections; Fungal infections; Jock itch; *Malassezia*; Onychomycosis; Plantar warts; Reinfection; Ringworm; Scabies; Skin infections; Tinea capitis; Tinea corporis.

---

Tissue death. *See* Gangrene; Necrotizing fasciitis.

---

# Tooth abscess

CATEGORY: Diseases and conditions
ANATOMY OR SYSTEM AFFECTED: Mouth, teeth, tissue
ALSO KNOWN AS: Dental abscess

## DEFINITION

A tooth abscess is a sac of pus (infected material) in a tooth or the gums. There are two types of tooth abscesses: abscess of the pulp (the blood and nerve supply inside the tooth) and abscess between the tooth and gum.

## CAUSES

A tooth abscess is caused by bacteria. It begins when bacteria invade and infect a tooth, resulting in pus buildup. When the pus is unable to drain, an abscess results. Conditions that allow bacteria to invade a tooth include severe tooth decay and a break or crack in a tooth that lets bacteria invade the pulp. Food or other foreign matter that becomes trapped between the tooth and gum may lead to a bacterial infection in the area around the tooth.

## RISK FACTORS

Factors that increase the chance of developing a tooth abscess include the buildup of tartar or calculus beneath the gum line; poor fluoride application to teeth through fluoridated water, toothpaste, or mouthwash; poor dental hygiene (leading to cavities and periodontal diseases); and malnutrition, including severe vitamin and mineral deficiencies.

## SYMPTOMS

A person with the following symptoms should not assume he or she has a tooth abscess. These symptoms may be caused by other conditions: throbbing or lingering pain in a tooth or gum area; pain when biting on a tooth; spontaneous tooth pain; redness, tenderness, or swelling of the gums; fever; swollen neck glands; tooth discoloration; bad breath or foul taste in mouth; and an open, draining sore on the gums. If left untreated, complications of tooth abscess include the loss of the tooth and surrounding tissue or bone and the spread of the infection to surrounding tissue or bone.

## SCREENING AND DIAGNOSIS

A dentist will ask about symptoms and medical history and will perform a detailed examination of the patient's teeth and gums. The dentist will test for pain and sensitivity by lightly tapping on the tooth, stimulating the tooth nerve with heat or cold, stimulating the tooth nerve with a low electrical current, and sliding a probe between the tooth and gum to measure gaps or tissue loss. The dentist will also take an X ray of the tooth and surrounding bone.

## TREATMENT AND THERAPY

Treatment for a tooth abscess includes the following:

*Removal of the abscess with a root canal.* If an abscess results from tooth decay or a break or crack in the tooth, the tooth and surrounding tissue are numbed and a hole is drilled through the top of the tooth. Pus and dead tissue are removed from the center of the tooth, and the interior of the tooth and the root (nerve) canals are cleaned and filled with a permanent filling. A crown is then placed on the tooth to protect it. If an abscess results from infection between the tooth and gum, then the abscess is drained and thoroughly cleaned. The root surface of tooth is cleaned and smoothed. In some cases, surgery to reshape the gum is done to prevent recurrence of infection.

*Tooth extraction.* Removal of the tooth may be required if tooth decay or tooth infection are too extensive for filling or root canal treatment; if the break or crack in the tooth is too severe to be repaired; or if the infection or loss of tissue or bone between the tooth and gum is severe. If the tooth is extracted, it will be replaced with a partial bridge, denture, or tooth implant.

*Medication.* Antibiotics are prescribed to fight residual infection of the tooth or gums. Also, the dentist could recommend nonprescription pain relief drugs (such as ibuprofen or acetaminophen) and warm saltwater rinses.

## PREVENTION AND OUTCOMES

To help reduce the chance of getting a tooth abscess, one should practice proper dental hygiene that includes brushing teeth with fluoride toothpaste after meals (or a minimum of twice per day), daily flossing between teeth and gums, getting regular dental checkups (every six months), and getting regular professional teeth and gum cleaning (every six months).

*Rick Alan; reviewed by Laura Morris-Olson, D.M.D.*

## FURTHER READING

Langlais, Robert P., and Craig S. Miller. *Color Atlas of Common Oral Diseases.* 4th ed. Philadelphia: Lippincott Williams & Wilkins, 2009.

Porter, Robert S., et al., eds. *The Merck Manual Home Health Handbook.* 3d ed. Whitehouse Station, N.J.: Merck Research Laboratories, 2009.

Sutton, Amy L., ed. *Dental Care and Oral Health Sourcebook.* 3d ed. Detroit: Omnigraphics, 2008.

Whitworth, John M. *Rational Root Canal Treatment in Practice.* Chicago: Quintessence, 2002.

## WEB SITES OF INTEREST

*Academy of General Dentistry*
http://www.agd.org

*American Dental Association*
http://www.ada.org

*Canadian Dental Association*
http://www.cda-adc.ca

*Canadian Dental Hygienists Association*
http://www.cdha.ca

**See also:** Abscesses; Actinomycosis; Acute necrotizing ulcerative gingivitis; Bacterial infections; Gingivitis; Mouth infections; Vincent's angina.

# Toxocariasis

CATEGORY: Diseases and conditions
ANATOMY OR SYSTEM AFFECTED: Eyes, gastrointestinal system, liver, lungs, respiratory system, vision
ALSO KNOWN AS: Visceral larva migrans

## DEFINITION

Toxocariasis is an infection caused by ingesting the eggs of nematode worms that are normally found in dogs (as *Toxocara canis*) and cats (as *T. cati*). Once the eggs have entered the human body, they hatch into larvae that are less than 0.5 millimeters (mm) long and 0.02 mm wide. The larvae then penetrate the walls of the digestive tract and commonly migrate to the liver, lungs, eyes, or anywhere the blood vessels are large enough to accommodate them. The presence of the worms may lead to serious infections such as myocarditis, encephalitis, or enophthalmitis. In the United States, more than ten thousand toxocariasis infections are diagnosed annually. Almost 14 percent of the U.S. population is infected with the *Toxocara* parasite at any given time.

## CAUSES

Commonly occurring worms in dogs and cats lay eggs that are excreted in the feces of the animal. These eggs can survive in the environment for many years, so it is likely, for example, that the soil in many public parks and playgrounds is highly contaminated. Humans can ingest the eggs from touching their mouths with contaminated hands. Once ingested, the eggs release larvae that penetrate through the bowel and migrate throughout the body, including the liver, lungs, eyes, and brain.

## RISK FACTORS

The risk of ingesting *Toxocara* eggs increases for people who live with or work with dogs or cats or for those who eat without thoroughly washing their hands after touching potentially contaminated soil or sand in a park, yard, or playground. Young children have a higher prevalence of infection because they tend to frequently put their hands or other objects, such as toys, in their mouths.

## SYMPTOMS

Toxocariasis is often asymptomatic, but some persons do experience fever, cough, abdominal pain, rash, or enlarged lymph nodes. Worm migration to the eyes can lead to vision disturbances, swelling around the eyes, or the appearance of a crossed eye.

## SCREENING AND DIAGNOSIS

Most cases of toxocariasis go undiagnosed and do not cause problems or symptoms; however, cases are occasionally diagnosed during routine eye exams or through X rays taken to diagnose other issues. Diagnosis of toxocariasis can be made by immunological testing and can be confirmed by the presence of larvae in tissue acquired during a tissue biopsy.

## TREATMENT AND THERAPY

Toxocariasis is commonly treated with a five-day-course of albendazole, a broad-spectrum anthelmintic, inhibiting the worms' ability to eat glucose and thus causing the death of the worms. Corticosteroids may be used to treat the symptomatic reactions of infestation. More serious complications, such as eye or organ involvement, may require surgery or chemotherapy.

## PREVENTION AND OUTCOMES

Toxocariasis can be prevented by keeping *Toxocara* eggs from entering the body by practicing good hand-washing technique and by avoiding touching one's face and mouth area with contaminated hands. Children should be prevented from touching their mouths, especially while at parks or playgrounds, and from ingesting dirt. Many playgrounds and urban areas have posted signs that restrict dogs from areas where children play.

*April Ingram, B.S.*

## FURTHER READING

Despommier, Dickson. "Toxocariasis: Clinical Aspects, Epidemiology, Medical Ecology, and Molecular Aspects." *Clinical Microbiology Reviews* 16 (2003): 265-272.

_____, et al. *Parasitic Diseases.* 5th ed. New York: Apple Tree, 2006.

Smith, Hazel, et al. "How Common Is Human Toxocariasis? Towards Standardizing Our Knowledge." *Trends in Parasitology* 25 (2009): 182-188.

## WEB SITES OF INTEREST

*About Kids Health*
http://www.aboutkidshealth.ca

*Centers for Disease Control and Prevention*
http://www.cdc.gov/parasites

*Clean Hands Coalition*
http://www.cleanhandscoalition.org

*Companion Animal Parasite Council*
http://www.capcvet.org

*Microbiology and Immunology On-line: Parasitology*
http://pathmicro.med.sc.edu/book/parasit-sta.htm

**See also:** Cats and infectious disease; Children and infectious disease; Dogs and infectious disease; Fecal-oral route of transmission; Hygiene; Intestinal and stomach infections; Oral transmission; Parasites: Classification and types; Parasitic diseases; Roundworms; Soilborne illness and disease; Toxoplasmosis; Treatment of parasitic diseases; Worm infections; Zoonotic diseases.

---

# Toxoplasmosis

CATEGORY: Diseases and conditions
ANATOMY OR SYSTEM AFFECTED: All

## DEFINITION

Toxoplasmosis is an infection caused by a tiny organism called a protozoan. Many people are infected with this protozoan, but few people have any related symptoms or problems.

## CAUSES

Toxoplasmosis is passed from animals to humans. People can contract it by touching contaminated cat feces or something that has had contact with cat feces, such as soil or insects; by eating undercooked, infected meat; and by touching one's mouth after touching contaminated meat. In rare cases, receiving a blood transfusion or an organ transplant can lead to the infection.

A pregnant woman who gets toxoplasmosis for the first time has a 15 to 60 percent chance of passing it to her fetus. Active infection usually occurs only once in a person's life, although the protozoan remains inactive in the body. If a woman has become immune to the infection before getting pregnant, she will not pass the condition to her fetus.

## RISK FACTORS

People at risk for having symptoms from toxoplasmosis are infants born to women who are first exposed to toxoplasmosis just before becoming pregnant or during pregnancy; people with weakened immune systems from conditions such as human immunodeficiency virus infection, acquired immunodeficiency syndrome, and cancer; and those who have had an organ transplant.

## SYMPTOMS

Most people do not have symptoms, but those who do may experience swollen lymph nodes, a fever, fatigue, a sore throat, muscle aches and pains, and a rash. People with weakened immune systems may develop toxoplasmosis infections in multiple organs. Infection is most common in the brain (encephalitis), eye (chorioretinitis), and lung (pneumonitis). Symptoms may include a fever; seizures; a headache; visual defects; problems with speech, movement, or thinking; mental illness; and shortness of breath.

In infants, the severity of symptoms depends on when during preg-

nancy the mother became infected. If infection occurs during the first three months of pregnancy, the fetus is less likely to become infected, but if the fetus does becoming infected, symptoms will be much more severe. The fetus is more likely to become infected during the last six months of pregnancy, but symptoms will be less serious. Toxoplasmosis can also cause miscarriage or stillbirth.

About one in ten infants born with toxoplasmosis has severe symptoms, including visual defects because of eye infections (chorioretinitis), enlarged liver and spleen, jaundice (yellow skin and eyes), pneumonitis, myocarditis (inflammation of the heart), brain malfor-

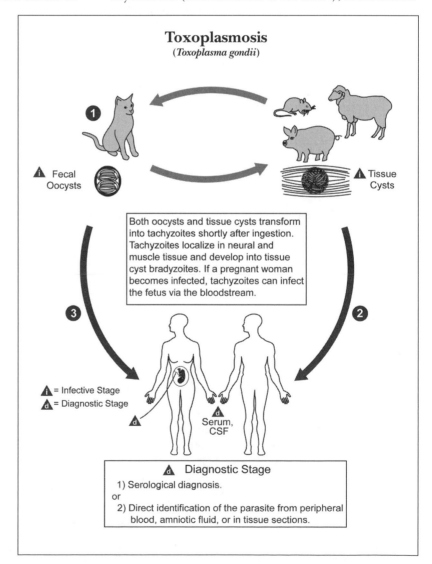

*The cycle of infection of the protozoan parasite* Toxoplasma gondii. *(CDC)*

mations, mental retardation, cerebral palsy, and seizures. Many infants infected with toxoplasmosis who seem healthy at birth may develop problems months or years later. These include visual defects, hearing loss, learning disabilities, and seizures.

### SCREENING AND DIAGNOSIS

A doctor will ask about symptoms and medical history and will perform a physical exam. Blood tests are done to look for antibodies produced by the body to fight the toxoplasmosis. Other lab tests are done to look for the protozoan itself. Pregnant women who are infected will undergo prenatal tests, including ultrasound and amniocentesis, to determine if the fetus is infected.

### TREATMENT AND THERAPY

People who are healthy and not pregnant do not need treatment. Symptoms usually disappear within a few weeks or months. People with a weakened immune system are treated with antitoxoplasmosis medicines for several months. If a pregnant woman is infected but the fetus is not, the woman is usually given the antibiotic spiramycin. This medicine can decrease the chance of the fetus becoming infected by about 60 percent.

Fetuses with confirmed toxoplasmosis infections are treated by giving the pregnant woman a combination of the following medications: spiramycin, pyrimethamine, sulfadiazine, and folinic acid. These drugs can reduce the severity of, but not eliminate, a newborn's symptoms. Once born, the infant will be given different combinations of medicines.

### PREVENTION AND OUTCOMES

Women who are pregnant or considering becoming pregnant should consult a physician about having a blood test to determine if they are immune to toxoplasmosis (which would indicate a previous exposure). If not immune, women should take the following steps to avoid sources of toxoplasmosis: Avoid eating raw or undercooked meat (if one touches raw meat, avoid touching one's eyes, mouth, or nose); wash one's hands and cutting boards, knives, and sink with soap and warm water; and wash all raw vegetables and fruits.

One should also avoid emptying a cat's litter box; avoid children's sand boxes because they are often used by cats as a litter box; avoid feeding a cat raw or undercooked meat; and keep one's cat indoors to pre-

vent it from hunting rodents or birds that could be infected. Also, when gardening, one should wear gloves; keep one's hands away from one's eyes, mouth, and nose; and wash one's hands when finished. These steps also apply to persons with weakened immune systems.

*Laurie Rosenblum, M.P.H.;*
*reviewed by Jeff Andrews, M.D., FRCSC, FACOG*

### FURTHER READING

Ambroise-Thomas, Pierre, and Eskild Petersen, eds. *Congenital Toxoplasmosis: Scientific Background, Clinical Management, and Control.* New York: Springer, 2000.

American Congress of Obstetricians and Gynecologists. "Perinatal Viral and Parasitic Infections." *ACOG Practice Bulletin,* no. 20 (2000). Available at http://www.acog.org.

Despommier, Dickson D., et al. *Parasitic Diseases.* 5th ed. New York: Apple Tree, 2006.

Joynson, David H. M., and Tim G. Wreghitt, eds. *Toxoplasmosis: A Comprehensive Clinical Guide.* Rev. ed. New York: Cambridge University Press, 2005.

Martin, Richard J., Avroy A. Fanaroff, and Michele C. Walsh, eds. *Fanaroff and Martin's Neonatal-Perinatal Medicine: Diseases of the Fetus and Infant.* 2 vols. 8th ed. Philadelphia: Mosby/Elsevier, 2006.

Parker, James N., and Philip M. Parker, eds. *The Official Patient's Sourcebook on Toxoplasmosis.* San Diego, Calif.: Icon Health, 2002.

### WEB SITES OF INTEREST

*Center for the Evaluation of Risks to Human Reproduction*
http://cerhr.niehs.nih.gov

*Centers for Disease Control and Prevention*
http://www.cdc.gov/parasites

*Companion Animal Parasite Council*
http://www.capcvet.org

*March of Dimes*
http://www.modimes.org

*National Center for Emerging and Zoonotic Infectious Diseases*
http://www.cdc.gov/ncezid

*Women's Health Matters*
http://www.womenshealthmatters.ca

**See also:** AIDS; Antibiotics: Types; Cats and infectious disease; Childbirth and infectious disease; Diagnosis of protozoan diseases; Encephalitis; Fecal-oral route of transmission; Fever; Food-borne illness and disease; HIV; Parasitic diseases; Parasitology; Pregnancy and infectious disease; Prevention of protozoan diseases; Protozoa: Structure and growth; Protozoan diseases; Toxocariasis; Treatment of protozoan diseases; Zoonotic diseases.

# Trachoma

CATEGORY: Diseases and conditions
ANATOMY OR SYSTEM AFFECTED: Eyes, vision
ALSO KNOWN AS: Egyptian ophthalmia, granular conjunctivitis

## DEFINITION

Trachoma is a chronic and extremely contagious infection of the conjunctiva of the eye that is caused by the microorganism *Chlamydia trachomatis*. It is a leading cause of blindness around the world and is most prevalent in developing countries and in disadvantaged populations. If the inflammation persists and is left untreated, the eyelid may turn inward, causing the eyelashes to rub on the surface of the eye and leading to the formation of painful scar tissue; this results in irreversible blindness.

## CAUSES

Trachoma infection is caused by the bacterium *C. trachomatis* and can easily be spread from person to person by direct contact with contaminated secretions or by contact with secretions on towels, wash cloths, or clothing. Flies also act as vectors by transmitting the microorganism from secretions. This occurs often in young children, who are unable to brush flies from their faces.

## RISK FACTORS

Poor hygiene, especially a lack of facial cleanliness, and the absence of clean water sources have been linked to high rates of trachoma infection. Also, proximity to livestock and a lack of proper latrines or waste disposal increase the number of flies in an area. This increases disease transmission throughout a community.

## SYMPTOMS

Symptoms of trachoma are usually red, sticky looking eyes, similar in appearance to other eye infections. Other symptoms may include swollen eye lids, a runny nose, swollen or tender lymph nodes, and discharge from the eyes. Clinical examination may reveal small white follicles on the undersurface of the upper eyelid.

## SCREENING AND DIAGNOSIS

In trachoma-endemic areas, attempts are made to provide annual screening programs in communities. Laboratory testing is normally not available for trachoma screening, so clinical examinations by trained personnel are performed in the community. During the screening, the eyelid is inverted. Further examination of the conjunctiva will reveal a presence or absence of round, whitish swellings called follicles. These follicles can be mild or rough and thickened, causing deformities of the conjunctiva and eyelid. A grading classification system has been established to describe the findings of examination. This system includes the following: TF (trachomatous inflammation, follicular), TI (trachomatous inflammation, intense), TS (trachomatous scarring), TT (trachomatous trichiasis), and CO (corneal opacity).

## TREATMENT AND THERAPY

Trachoma can be treated with oral antibiotics for three to six weeks. Because reinfection is common in endemic areas, one should take preventive precautions. If lid deformities occur because of recurring infection, causing the eyelashes to turn inward (trichiasis), then surgery may be necessary to attempt to correct the deformities.

## PREVENTION AND OUTCOMES

The World Health Organization has initiated a Global Alliance for the Elimination of Trachoma by 2020. This alliance has implemented a "SAFE" strategy to apply medical, behavioral, and environmental approaches to trachoma control around the world. The SAFE strategy comprises the following directives: "Surgery for trichiasis," "Antibiotics to treat *Chlamydia trachomatis* infection," and "Facial cleanliness and Environmental improvement to reduce transmission of *C. trachomatis* from one person to another."

*April Ingram, B.S.*

## FURTHER READING

Miller, K. E. "Diagnosis and Treatment of *Chlamydia trachomatis* Infection." *American Family Physician* 73 (2006): 1411-1416.

Olitzky, S. E., et al. "Disorders of the Conjunctiva." In *Nelson Textbook of Pediatrics*, edited by Richard E. Behrman, Robert M. Kliegman, and Hal B. Jenson. 18th ed. Philadelphia: Saunders/Elsevier, 2007.

Solomon, Anthony W., et al. "Trachoma Control: A Guide for Programme Managers." Geneva: World Health Organization, 2006.

Taylor, Hugh R. *Trachoma: A Blinding Scourge from the Bronze Age to the Twenty-first Century.* East Melbourne, Vic.: Centre for Eye Research Australia/Haddington Press, 2008.

World Health Organization. "Trachoma." Available at http://www.who.int/blindness/causes/priority.

Wright, Heathcote, Angus Turner, and Hugh Taylor. "Trachoma." *The Lancet* 371 (2008): 1945-1954.

## WEB SITES OF INTEREST

*American Academy of Ophthalmology*
http://www.aao.org

*Centers for Disease Control and Prevention*
http://www.cdc.gov

*International Trachoma Initiative*
http://www.trachoma.org

**See also:** Acanthamoeba infection; Bacteria: Classification and types; Bacterial infections; *Chlamydia*; Conjunctivitis; Developing countries and infectious disease; Eye infections; Flies and infectious disease; Hordeola; Inflammation; Keratitis; Ophthalmia neonatorum.

# Transmission routes

CATEGORY: Transmission

## DEFINITION

Epidemiology, the study of disease transmission, identifies the organisms responsible for disease, the hosts that transmit the disease, and the possible routes of disease transmission. Infections and pathogens (disease-causing agents such as bacteria, viruses, and protozoa) may be spread from animal to animal, animal to human (zoonotic transmission), or human to human through several means. Pathogens are not limited to one transmission route; some have many. Properly classifying how pathogens are transmitted is critical to the effective treatment of an infected person and to controlling the spread of disease.

## TYPES OF TRANSMISSION

*Vertical.* Vertical transmission is the passing of a disease-causing agent from one generation to another, as when a parent transmits a pathogen to potential offspring at conception, during the perinatal period (pregnancy), at labor and delivery, or shortly after birth. The pathogen may be transferred either in sperm, by crossing the placenta, by fetal or newborn exposure to secretions or blood, or through breast-feeding.

Common examples of vertically transmitted diseases include human immunodeficiency virus (HIV) infection, hepatitis, cytomegalovirus, and toxoplasmosis. Pregnant women may be asymptomatic, but affected fetuses can have severe disease presentation after birth depending on the timing of exposure. Infections can lead to multiple medical and developmental concerns or to fetal or neonatal death.

Women (both pregnant and those planning to become pregnant) are screened on routine blood work for many of the diseases that show vertical transmission. Treatments, although specifically tailored to the individual disease, include maternal or neonatal medication (or both), changing delivery route from a vaginal delivery to a cesarean section to avoid maternal-fetal contact in the birth canal, and avoiding breast-feeding. Vaccines for certain diseases, such as hepatitis B, are administered in the newborn period to prevent disease development and transmission to future generations.

*Horizontal.* Horizontal transmission refers to the passing of a disease or pathogen from one person to another in the same generation. The disease is not passed from woman to fetus in the perinatal period. Symptoms depend on the specific type of acquired infection. Horizontal disease transmission occurs by direct or indirect pathogenic contact.

Direct contact occurs when a susceptible person touches or otherwise physically comes into contact with the pathogenic source or an infected person. Therefore, for transmission to occur, the source of disease and the potential recipient must be close to one another. This transmission can occur when touching an open wound, a mucous membrane, blood, or saliva. Sexually transmitted diseases occur by reproductive transmission, a form of direct contact. The respiratory route is also considered a pathway for direct transmission of disease.

Indirect transmission occurs when a person has contact with an object or host that carries the pathogen, allowing transmission of disease without physical contact between persons. This may occur through vector transmission (that is, through an insect or animal) or through fomite transmission (that is, through contaminated, inanimate objects).

*Sexual and reproductive.* Sexually transmitted diseases (STDs) are transmitted by direct contact through touching or sharing of saliva or body secretions. One sexual partner's infection may be transmitted to the other partner through genital, anal, or oral contact. Risk factors include unprotected sexual intercourse.

More than twenty-five STDs exist, including HIV infection, chlamydia, gonorrhea, and herpes. STDs are very common; one study estimated 333 million new cases in one year of syphilis, gonorrhea, trichomoniasis, and chlamydia.

Laboratory blood work and a physical exam will diagnose STDs. Antibiotics, antiviral medications, and vaccinations are available for some STDs. Abstinence or condom use are recommended measures to prevent future transmission of disease.

*Respiratory.* The respiratory system is a common pathway for direct contact, whereby an ill person coughs, spits, or sneezes contaminated respiratory droplets of saliva onto a susceptible person. The pathogen enters the body through the nose, mouth, or eye and causes infections such as influenza, chickenpox, the common cold, and strep throat. Airborne transmission of pathogens occurs when droplets become smaller in size and when the liquid in those droplets evaporates to a significant degree.

Precautions to avoid contracting an illness by droplet contact include good hygiene practices, such as handwashing and the avoidance of sneezing directly into the hand. Infected persons should minimize direct contact with others. Antibiotic and antiviral medications are prescribed to treat certain infections.

*Airborne.* An airborne (aerosol) route differs from the respiratory route when infective droplets become smaller in size and when they become more evapora-

tive, making it possible for the pathogen to travel farther distances. Most pathogenic droplets cannot survive when airborne, and their survival is affected by factors such as temperature and the general environment. A pathogen that replicates in the respiratory tract has the potential to be transmitted through airborne contact. Additionally, pathogens that replicate in water may also become airborne by means of shower heads or water fountains.

Airborne transmission is divided into two categories: long range and short range. Short-range transmission involves pathogenic droplets traveling less than three feet (one meter) from the person who sneezes or coughs. Therefore, for infection to be transmitted by air-flow exchange, the infected person and a susceptible person must be close to one another.

Long-range transmission occurs when droplets travel more than one meter, generally because of pressure differences in air flow from ventilation systems, open windows, a person's movement, or temperature. Dust particles containing bacteria or viruses containing the infectious agent may be carried by air currents before being inhaled or before landing on other surfaces. In general, when an infectious agent has the capacity for long-range transmission, it is also pathogenic in the short-distance range.

The symptoms of disease from airborne transmission ultimately depend on the type of pathogen, the inhaled dose, and the immune response. Common diseases include tuberculosis, measles, the common cold, and chickenpox. It remains debatable if influenza is spread mostly by direct contact or by airborne transmission. The international 2003 outbreak of severe acute respiratory syndrome (SARS), thought to originate through water aerosols, demonstrates the long-range capacity of airborne illness and the possibility that it may cause a global pandemic if not adequately controlled. Although most airborne transmission occurs through human illness, pathogens can be disseminated through biological warfare and bioterrorism.

Inadequate ventilation is a significant risk factor for airborne transmission. Precautionary measures include using proper ventilation systems when working with known pathogenic agents, isolating or quarantining infected persons, and improving door and window seals.

*Fecal-oral.* The fecal-oral route of transmission typically involves food, water, or objects contaminated with either animal or human feces or urine that are ingested, leading to the oral transmission of disease. Transmission of disease by contaminated food or water is extremely common and remains a public health burden worldwide. The Centers for Disease Control and Prevention estimates that, annually, 325,000 hospitalizations and 5,000 deaths are related to this disease route. Populations at greatest risk include young children, the elderly, pregnant women, and immunocompromised persons, such as those with human immunodeficiency virus infection or acquired immunodeficiency syndrome.

Food-borne transmission, commonly known as food poisoning, occurs as part of the fecal-oral pathway. Food-borne illness is defined as disease resulting from the consumption of food or beverages contaminated either by a microbial pathogen or by a toxic substance. Infections typically have an incubation period before they lead to illness. A common area affected is the gastrointestinal tract, with diarrhea, nausea, and vomiting. Exact symptoms pertain to the type of substance and dose ingested.

There are more than 250 food-borne diseases and illnesses, such as those caused by the bacterium *Escherichia coli* and the bacterium *Salmonella*. Laboratory analysis on stool samples can be performed to identify some of the causative agents. Because symptomatic persons are often dehydrated, rehydration with oral fluids containing electrolytes is often recommended. Some bacteria respond to antibiotics, but normally the clinical course self-resolves within a few days.

Causes of food-borne illness include improper handling of food items; improper cooking, so that food remains raw or undercooked; drinking unpasteurized milk; eating contaminated produce; and having direct contact with animals, such as at petting farms or zoos.

One should use proper handwashing technique and should use gloves when commercially preparing food. Other food preparation recommendations include thoroughly cooking all food, separating food to prevent cross-contamination, refrigerating food when not in use, and washing all produce. Any symptomatic person who prepares food for consumption is advised to discontinue work and remain home to prevent the spread of infection.

A specific category of food-borne illness is waterborne disease. Water provides an excellent breeding ground for many infectious agents. Pathogens that are excreted in fecal matter may contaminate water, leading to indirect fetal-oral waterborne transmission. Contaminated water is often used for drinking, bathing, or swimming. Measures to prevent waterborne illness include chlorinating swimming pools, avoiding water with hazardous wastes, regularly sterilizing bathtubs and sinks, and drinking treated water only.

*Vector.* Vector-borne transmission requires the use of a "vehicle" (or vector), such as an insect or arachnid, to disseminate the infection to humans. By definition, a vector can carry a disease agent but will not develop symptoms.

Vector-borne transmission occurs either mechanically or biologically. With mechanical transmission, the pathogen "uses" the vector only as a means to deposit itself, involving no replication or change in the pathogen. The infectivity of the vector is greatest within the first day of pathogen exposure, but even if the mechanical vector were to be eliminated, the pathogen would remain because it would be able to find another route for infection.

With biological transmission, also known as cyclical transmission, the pathogen uses the vector as a host to replicate and develop. For example, the pathogen "uses" a mosquito's bite, which is infected with the pathogen, to cause malaria. After the initial vector infection, the vector (the mosquito) will remain infected forever, and the host (the person bitten) will remain infectious for some time only. Unlike with mechanical transmission, eliminating biological transmission reduces, or eliminates, the disease incidence.

Nearly one-half of the world's population has a vector-borne disease. At greatest risk are persons living or traveling in tropical and subtropical climates. These climates are hot and humid, making conditions ideal for disease transmission. Many vector-borne illnesses were once thought to be controlled, but because of vector drug resistance, airline travel, and mass migrations, for example, these diseases are on the rise.

Preventive measures against infections from vector transmission include pest control in the home, in food stores, in food preparation areas, and in health care settings. Health care settings and homes are especially at risk for diseases related to mice, rats, and cockroaches.

*Nosocomial.* A nosocomial infection is an infection that is acquired in a medical setting, typically a hospital, during a person's care. Organisms of greatest concern for nosocomial infection include *Escherichia coli*, *Enterococcus*, *Staphylococcus aureus*, and *Pseudomonas*. It is estimated that annually, two million persons acquire these infections in the United States, and approximately twenty thousand persons die from resulting complications.

Nosocomial infections are caused by either direct or indirect contact with endogenous or exogenous agents. An endogenous agent is a pathogen that comes from a previously infected or colonized site in the patient's own body. An exogenous agent is a pathogen that comes from outside the patient's body. Many of the exogenous pathogens are found on inanimate objects that carry disease, such as medical equipment, supplies, and clothing. The pathogens may also come from staff members, other infected patients, and visitors. Transmission caused by a medical procedure is termed "iatrogenic" and may confer a risk for infections such as methicillin-resistant *Staphylococcus aureus* or Creutzfeldt-Jakob disease.

## IMPACT

Understanding the route of disease transmission is of utmost importance for treating an infected person and for ensuring public health. However, because significant overlap exists among the transmission routes for some illnesses, it is a challenge to determine the actual route of transmission that led to illness and, therefore, to treat and control disease.

While many forms of disease transmission can be controlled, data show that on an individual level, care is not always taken to prevent illness. Also, threats of global pandemic still exist. Continued efforts from governmental and public health agencies are needed to educate the public on disease transmission so that illness and its associated health care costs can be reduced or eliminated.

*Janet Ober Berman, M.S., CGC*

## FURTHER READING

Aitken, Celia, and Donald J. Jeffries. "Nosocomial Spread of Viral Disease." *Clinical Microbiology Reviews* 14 (2001): 528-546. Review of literature detailing the risks of specific viruses for transmission in the medical setting. Includes discussion of respective hygienic precautions.

Brower, Vicki. "Vector-Borne Diseases and Global Warming: Are Both on an Upward Swing?" *EMBO Reports* 2 (2001): 755-757. Examines the medical and political controversy about whether or not warmer global temperatures are increasing the incidence of vector-borne illnesses.

Martinson, Francis E., et al. "Risk Factors for Horizontal Transmission of Hepatitis B Virus in a Rural District in Ghana." *American Journal of Epidemiology* 147 (1997): 478-487. A case study discussing risk factors and suggestions for reducing horizontal transmission of disease.

Morrison, Leanne G., and Lucy Yardley. "What Infection Control Measures Will People Carry Out to Reduce Transmission of Pandemic Influenza?" *BMC Public Health* 9 (2009): 1-11. A pilot study assessing public knowledge and willingness to comply with infection control recommendations to reduce disease transmission.

Tang, J. W., et al. "Factors Involved in the Aerosol Transmission of Infection and Control of Ventilation in Healthcare Premises." *Journal of Hospital Infection* 64 (2006): 100-114. Discusses common and less recognized diseases that may be a risk for airborne transmission. Also illustrates common mechanisms for spreading airborne illness.

## WEB SITES OF INTEREST

*Centers for Disease Control and Prevention*
http://www.cdc.gov/ncidod/dvbid

*Community and Hospital Infection Control Association*
http://www.chica.org

*Infectious Diseases Society of America*
http://www.idsociety.org

*National Institute of Allergy and Infectious Diseases*
http://www.niaid.nih.gov/topics/vector

*National Institutes of Health*
http://www.nlm.nih.gov/medlineplus/infectionsandpregnancy

**See also:** Airborne illness and disease; Arthropod-borne illness and disease; Biological weapons; Blood-borne illness and disease; Epidemiology; Fecal-oral route of transmission; Food-borne illness and disease; Horizontal disease transmission; Hospitals and infectious disease; Iatrogenic infections; Insect-borne illness and disease; Oral transmission; Pathogens; Respiratory route of transmission; Saliva and infectious disease; Sexually transmitted diseases (STDs); Soilborne illness and disease; Vectors and vector control; Vertical disease transmission; Waterborne illness and disease.

# Travelers' diarrhea

CATEGORY: Diseases and conditions
ANATOMY OR SYSTEM AFFECTED: Abdomen, gastrointestinal system, stomach
ALSO KNOWN AS: Montezuma's revenge, turista

## DEFINITION

In persons traveling to international destinations, particularly in less developed countries, watery, loose stools (diarrhea) are most often caused by bacterial or viral infection. Most cases of travelers' diarrhea resolve within one to two days without treatment and 90 percent resolve within one week. To ease symptoms, one can take over-the-counter medications. If travelers' diarrhea does not resolve on its own in about one week, one should consult a doctor.

## CAUSES

The primary cause of travelers' diarrhea is ingestion of food or water contaminated with fecal matter. The common pathogens include bacteria (such as *Escherichia coli*, *Campylobacter*, *Shigella*, *Salmonella*, and *Yersinia*) and viruses such as rotavirus, norovirus, and enterovirus.

## RISK FACTORS

The most important risk factor for contracting travelers' diarrhea is destination. Underdeveloped countries with contaminated water supplies pose the highest risk. The following factors increase the chance of developing travelers' diarrhea: age (children two years of age or younger), people with weak immune systems, people with diabetes or inflammatory bowel disease, and those taking acid blockers or antacids (such as those for heartburn).

## SYMPTOMS

Symptoms of travelers' diarrhea include increased frequency and volume of stool, frequent loose stools (four to five watery bowel movements a day), abdominal cramping, nausea, vomiting, fever, and bloating.

## SCREENING AND DIAGNOSIS

A doctor will ask about symptoms and medical history, will perform a physical exam, and will take a stool sample from the patient to identify the pathogen.

## TREATMENT AND THERAPY

Treatment for travelers' diarrhea includes the use of antimotility agents such as loperamide (Imodium), diphenoxylate (Lomotil), and opiates, all of which reduce muscle spasms in the gastrointestinal tract, slow transit time, and thus increase absorption. Infants and those with bloody diarrhea cannot use antimotility agents. Another treatment is bismuth subsalicylate (Pepto-Bismol), an over-the-counter medication that decreases the frequency of stools. This medication should not be used by children, pregnant women, or people who have allergies to aspirin or salicylates. In addition, this medication should not be used by persons currently taking aspirin or similar drugs (such as salicylates).

Another treatment is antibiotics, such as ciprofloxacin, norfloxacin, ofloxacin, doxycycline, and trimethoprim-sulfamethoxazole, which are the most common antibiotics for treating travelers' diarrhea. Antibiotics are effective only in treating a bacterial infection.

## PREVENTION AND OUTCOMES

To help reduce the chance of getting travelers' diarrhea, one should avoid eating foods from street vendors or from unclean eating establishments, avoid raw or undercooked meat or seafood, eat foods that are fully cooked and served hot, avoid salads or unpeeled fruits, and eat only fruits and vegetables (such as bananas or oranges) that one has peeled oneself.

One should also avoid drinking tap water or using ice cubes; should drink only bottled water or, if necessary, local water that one boils for ten minutes or treats with iodine or chlorine; and should drink, as an alternative to tap water, bottled carbonated beverages, steaming hot tea or coffee, wine, or beer.

*Shara Aaron, M.S., RD;*
*reviewed by David L. Horn, M.D., FACP*

## FURTHER READING

DuPont, Herbert L., and Charles D. Ericsson. "Drug Therapy: Prevention and Treatment of Travelers' Diarrhea." *New England Journal of Medicine* 328 (June 24, 1993): 1821-1826.

Guerrant, R. L., et al. "Practice Guidelines for the Management of Infectious Diarrhea." *Clinical Infectious Diseases* 32 (2001): 331-350.

"Infectious Diarrheal Diseases and Bacterial Food Poisoning." In *Harrison's Principles of Internal Medicine*, edited by Joan Butterton. 17th ed. New York: McGraw-Hill, 2008.

Johnson, Leonard R., ed. *Gastrointestinal Physiology.* 7th ed. Philadelphia: Mosby/Elsevier, 2007.

Juckett, G. "Prevention and Treatment of Travelers' Diarrhea." *American Family Physician* 60 (1999): 119-136.

Yates, J. "Travelers' Diarrhea." *American Family Physician* 71 (2005): 2095-2100, 2107-2108.

## WEB SITES OF INTEREST

*American Gastroenterological Association*
http://www.gastro.org

*Canadian Partnership for Consumer Food Safety Education*
http://www.canfightbac.org

*Centers for Disease Control and Prevention*
http://www.cdc.gov/nczved/divisions/dfbmd/
diseases/travelers_diarrhea

**See also:** Amebic dysentery; Antibiotic-associated colitis; Antiparasitic drugs: Types; Ascariasis; Bacterial infections; *Campylobacter*; Cholera; Cryptosporidiosis; Developing countries and infectious disease; Enterovirus infections; *Escherichia coli* infection; Fecal-oral route of transmission; Food-borne illness and disease; Giardiasis; Hookworms; Intestinal and stomach infections; Norovirus infection; Parasitic diseases; Rotavirus infection; *Salmonella*; *Shigella*; Tropical medicine; Typhoid fever; Viral gastroenteritis; Viral infections; Water treatment; Waterborne illness and disease; Worm infections; *Yersinia*.

# Treatment of bacterial infections

CATEGORY: Treatment

## DEFINITION

Treatment for bacterial infections involves relieving the symptoms of disease caused by harmful (pathogenic) bacteria and curing a diseased person. Bacterial infections can be mild, leading to discomfort and inconvenience, or severe, leading to permanent disability or to death.

Common bacterial infections include bronchitis, pneumonia, tuberculosis, salmonella, strep throat, acne, and boils. The treatment for a bacterial infection depends on the type of bacterium causing the disease, the severity of the disease, the infected person's overall health, the body's response to medicines used for treatment, the bacterium's resistance to medicines, and the availability of medicines.

## TREATMENT WITHOUT DRUGS

As bacteria infect the human body, the immune system fights the invading pathogens. Symptoms such as fever, cough, swelling, fatigue, and discharge of fluids signal a bacterial infection. If the symptoms are mild, bacterial infections can be treated at home without a doctor's prescription. An increase in fluids, proper nutrition, and bed rest can relieve symptoms and allow the body's natural defenses to fight the infection.

Many plants worldwide have been used to treat bacterial infections, including certain mushrooms, tea leaves, various herbs, and the seeds and oil of the Chia plant. Honey has been promoted as an infection fighter too. However, rigorous clinical trials have not proven the effectiveness of these alternative treatments.

Though not technically a treatment, prevention is a proven method for battling bacterial infections. Common methods to prevent the spread of bacterial infections include covering the mouth when coughing or sneezing, washing the hands often, washing raw fruits and vegetables before preparing them, cooking fruits and vegetables properly, cleaning and covering cuts on the skin, and disinfecting surfaces in the room or rooms where the sick person rests.

## TREATMENT WITH DRUGS

The most common and proven drugs for treating bacterial infections are antibiotics, sometimes called antibacterials. Antibiotics are chemical substances derived from bacteria, molds, and other microorganisms. Each antibiotic works against a specific bacteria species. Antibiotics, however, do no work against viruses, fungi, and parasites.

Antibiotics either kill the targeted bacteria or prevent them from reproducing, allowing the body's immune system to destroy the pathogens. Antibiotic medicines take the form of pills that are swallowed or liquids that are swallowed or injected into the muscles or veins.

Penicillin, a chemical produced by a mold, was the first substance recognized as an antibiotic. It was identified in 1929 by Scottish bacteriologist Arthur Fleming, but it was not refined and manufactured in quantity until World War II, which saw an increased need for antibacterial medicines.

Antibiotics are variously classified according to the microorganisms they are obtained from, by their chemical structure, by the way they interact with bacteria, and by the types of bacteria they fight. Under the latter classification, antibiotics are classified into two broad groups: broad-spectrum antibiotics and narrow-spectrum antibiotics. Broad-spectrum antibiotics fight both gram-positive and gram-negative bacteria (the two major types of bacteria, classified by the thickness of the cell wall surrounding them). Tetracycline is a well-known broad-spectrum antibiotic that prevents the growth and spread of bacteria. Narrow-spectrum antibiotics target only gram-positive bacteria. The penicillins (such as amoxicillin, ampicillin, and oxacillin) are the best-known antibiotics in this group. They interfere with the growth of the bacteria's cell wall and eventually kill the bacteria.

## RESPONSES TO TREATMENT

Although antibiotics are effective in curing bacterial infections, some present side effects or cause allergic reactions. A side effect is an undesirable effect on the body caused by a drug; an allergic reaction is the immune system's uncontrolled response to a foreign substance, such as a drug. Some antibiotics interact with other drugs (therapeutic and recreational) and reduce the effectiveness of or increase the side effects of the other drugs or the antibiotic. Alcohol and most antibiotics, for example, do not mix.

Most common side effects of antibiotics are seldom serious or long lasting. They include nausea, vomiting, diarrhea, sensitivity to sunlight, and vaginal yeast infection. In some rare cases, however, antibiotics have severe effects on the function of the kidneys, liver, or other organs.

Mild allergic reactions include an itchy rash, wheezing, shortness of breath, and swelling of the lips and tongue. A more severe and life-threatening reaction is anaphylaxis, which involves a drop in blood pressure, swelling of the throat, and inability to swallow or breathe.

Not everyone experiences side effects or allergic reactions when taking antibiotics, and among those who do, not all respond the same way. The body's reaction to any foreign matter is highly individualized.

## IMPACT

Although antibiotics are effective against bacterial infections, their use has not yet eradicated bacteria-causing diseases. Furthermore, after more than sixty years of exposure to antibiotics, many bacteria have developed a resistance, chiefly because of the overuse and misuse of these drugs. Many species of harmful bacteria have acquired antibiotic-resistant genes by swapping genetic material with each other. This has led to the growth of superbugs or superbacteria, some of which are resistant to all known antibiotics. Antibiotic resistance makes it more difficult to treat bacterial infections and can lead to serious complications such as bacteria escaping into the bloodstream, coma, and even death.

The development of antibiotics in medical laboratories is a long, complex, and costly process. Commercial production is costly too. Only three new classes of antibiotics have been developed since the 1950's, and few new antibiotics have been brought to the market in recent years. Research indicates that the battle between medical science and disease-causing bacteria will continue indefinitely.

*Wendell Anderson, B.A.*

## FURTHER READING

Brachman, Philip S., and Elias Abrutyn, eds. *Bacterial Infections of Humans: Epidemiology and Control.* 4th ed. New York: Springer, 2009. A college-level introduction that focuses on the mechanisms of pathogenicity.

Furtado, G. H., and D. P. Nicolau. "Overview Perspective of Bacterial Resistance." *Expert Opinion on Therapeutic Patents* 20 (2010): 1273-1276. An overview of bacterial resistance that focuses on the most common pathogens. Also discusses strategies to curb antimicrobial resistance worldwide.

McPhee, Stephen J., and Maxine A. Papadakis, eds. *Current Medical Diagnosis and Treatment 2011.* 50th ed. New York: McGraw-Hill, 2011. Chapter 33 of this classic reference text gives a complete review of bacterial infections and their treatment.

Nikaido, Hiroshi. "Multidrug Resistance in Bacteria." *Annual Review of Biochemistry* 78 (2009): 119-146. A review article describing the molecular mechanisms of antibiotic resistance in bacteria.

Sachs, Jessica Snyder. *Good Germs, Bad Germs: Health and Survival in a Bacterial World.* New York: Hill and Wang, 2008. Describes for general readers the nature and scope of antibiotic resistance and discusses the medical and other practices that have led to drug-resistant bacteria.

## Web Sites of Interest

*Alliance for the Prudent Use of Antibiotics*
http://www.tufts.edu/med/apua

*Centers for Disease Control and Prevention*
http://www.cdc.gov/drugresistance

*Todar's Online Textbook of Bacteriology*
http://www.textbookofbacteriology.net

**See also:** Alliance for the Prudent Use of Antibiotics; Antibiotic resistance; Antibiotics: Types; Bacteria: Classification and types; Bacteria: Structure and growth; Bacterial infections; Diagnosis of bacterial infections; Drug resistance; Epidemiology; Home remedies; Infection; Microbiology; Over-the-counter (OTC) drugs; Prevention of bacterial infections.

# Treatment of fungal infections

Category: Treatment

## Definition

Fungi are single-celled or multicelled organisms that include yeasts and molds. Fungal infections are classified three ways: as noninvasive, which are those infections that appear on skin, hair, or nails; as systemic, those infections that develop deep within the tissue and often circulate through the blood; and as subcutaneous, which occur below the skin but do not spread. The most appropriate approach to treating an antifungal infection balances efficacy and toxicity. Other considerations include the infected person's health and the convenience and costs of treatment.

## Infection Types

*Noninvasive.* Many superficial fungal infections, such as athlete's foot (tinea pedis) and jock itch (tinea cruris), resolve spontaneously or with the use of a nonprescription or over-the-counter antifungal. Hygienic measures help in preventing initial spread and recurrence.

The first choice of a prescription drug to treat a superficial infection is nystatin or an azole. Nystatin has broad-spectrum activity and is available in cream, ointment, and powder formulations. Azoles are synthetic antifungals. Topical formulations of miconazole, clotrimazole, econazole, sulconazole, and oxiconazole are used for treating a wide spectrum of noninvasive fungal infections. The use of butoconazole, terconazole, and ticonazole is limited to vaginal candidiasis.

Allylamines (amorolfine, butenafine, naftifine, and terbinafine) are broad-spectrum synthetic antifungals prescribed as topical agents, mainly to treat skin and nail infections. Amorolfine is available only as a lacquer for treating nail infections. The allylamines are not effective against infections caused by *Candida* species.

Nystatin vaginal suppositories and clotrimazole vaginal tablets are used to treat vaginal candidiasis. Cutaneous infections with surface manifestations, such as some forms of candidiasis, including paronchia (nail infection), can also be treated with topical antifungals. Other cutaneous infections, such as thrush, are managed with oral agents such as nystatin lozenges and griseofulvin tablets, capsules, or suspension.

The duration of treatment for fungal infections varies according to the type, location, and persistence of infection. For example, among noninvasive infections, vaginal candidiasis may require seven to ten days of treatment. In contrast, other infections may require several months of treatment before they resolve. Difficult cases of thrush, for example, that are treated with griseofulvin, may require six months of ongoing treatment. Neither superficial nor cutaneous infections elicit a lasting immune response, so recurring infection that requires retreatment is not uncommon.

*Subcutaneous.* Subcutaneous fungal infections, which affect skin and muscle tissue, are uncommon in temperate climates. Chromoblastomycosis and maduromycosis are caused by soil fungi that enter the body through open wounds. They produce local tumors, especially of the feet. Sporotrichosis occurs when thorns or sphagnum moss penetrate the skin and introduce pathogenic spores into the lymphatic system. Ulcers associated with lymph nodes then develop, often followed by systemic manifestations. All three infections can be treated with amphotericin B administered by intravenous infusion.

Amphotericin B is highly toxic and can lead to renal dysfunction. Cutaneous and lymphocutaneous sporotrichosis can be treated with oral itraconazole or potassium iodide. Localized tumors associated with chromoblastomycosis and maduromycosis can be removed surgically.

*Systemic.* The main systemic fungal infections seen in the Unites States are histoplasmosis, coccidioidomycosis, blastomycosis, and cryptococcosis. All are difficult to manage and may require long-term, even lifelong, treatment. Some of these agents can become toxic at high doses or resistant after prolonged use.

Persons with symptomatic, mild-to-moderate, acute pulmonary histoplasmosis lasting more than four weeks should be treated with itraconazole for six to twelve weeks. Mild or moderate chronic or disseminated pulmonary histoplasmosis requires from six to twenty-four months of therapy with itraconazole in otherwise healthy persons and lifetime therapy in persons with acquired immunodeficiency syndrome (AIDS). Amphotericin B, administered for up to twelve weeks, is the drug of first choice for all cases of severe or systemic histoplasmosis. Once stabilized, an infected person can be switched to itraconazole on a schedule similar to that for less severe cases.

Coccidioidomycosis can be treated with itraconazole (200 milligrams [mg], twice daily) or fluconazole (400 to 600 mg per day) for three to six months. Fluconazole has fewer drug interactions than does itraconazole and is more easily absorbed, but it has a higher relapse rate. If the disease fails to improve or if it worsens, treatment should be switched to amphotericin B, starting at 1 to 1.5 mg per kilogram (mg/kg) of body weight per day. The dose of amphotericin B and its frequency should be reduced as improvement occurs. In coccidioidal meningitis, amphotericin can be infused directly into the cerebrospinal fluid. Even with aggressive therapy, regardless of the drug used, the risk of relapse is high. Therapy may need to be continued on a long-term basis.

Acute or chronic blastomycosis can be treated with itraconazole (400 mg per day) for six months, unless the condition is life-threatening. In this situation,

therapy should start with amphotericin B (1.5 to 2.5 mg/kg per day), followed by itraconazole for up to six months once the infected person has stabilized.

Cryptococcosis is seen mainly in persons with compromised immunity. Aggressive therapy is always recommended, starting with amphotericin B at 0.7 mg/kg per day. Flucystatin 100 mg/kg may be added to this regimen. The two agents appear to work synergistically, allowing an early discontinuation of the amphotericin B. Flucytosine should not be used alone as *Cryptococcus* species quickly develop resistance to it.

## IMPACT

Untreated or under-treated invasive and systemic fungal infections can lead to serious complications and even death. The management of invasive and systemic fungal infections, especially in immunocompromised persons, requires close clinical supervision with periodic monitoring of dosage and periodic adjustment of dosage, if necessary.

*Ernest Kohlmetz, M.A.*

## FURTHER READING

Baran, Robert, Rod Hay, and Javier Garduno. "Review of Antifungal Therapy, Part II: Treatment Rationale, Including Specific Patient Populations." *Journal of Dermatological Treatment* 19 (2008): 168-175.

Gladwin, Mark, and Bill Trattler. *Clinical Microbiology Made Ridiculously Simple.* 4th ed. Miami: MedMaster, 2007.

Richardson, Malcolm D., and Elizabeth M. Johnson. *The Pocket Guide to Fungal Infection.* 2d ed. Malden, Mass.: Blackwell, 2006.

Ryan, Kenneth J., and George Ray. *Sherris Medical Microbiology: An Introduction to Infectious Diseases.* 5th ed. New York: McGraw-Hill Medical, 2010.

Webster, John, and Roland Weber. *Introduction to Fungi.* New York: Cambridge University Press, 2007.

## WEB SITES OF INTEREST

*Centers for Disease Control and Prevention, Division of Foodborne, Bacterial, and Mycotic Diseases*
http://www.cdc.gov/nczved/divisions/dfbmd

*Medical Pharmacology Online: Antifungal Drugs*
http://www.pharmacology2000.com/antifungal/antif1.htm

*Microbiology and Immunology On-line: Mycology*
http://pathmicro.med.sc.edu/book/mycol-sta.htm

**See also:** Antifungal drugs: Mechanisms of action; Antifungal drugs: Types; Diagnosis of fungal infections; Fungal infections; Fungi: Classification and types; Fungi: Structure and growth; Mold infections; Mycoses; Opportunistic infections; Prevention of fungal infections; Skin infections.

# Treatment of parasitic diseases

CATEGORY: Treatment

## DEFINITION

Parasites are organisms that depend on hosts, including humans, for their food source and survival. Treatment for parasitic disease involves drugs and other therapies to manage the three types of parasite: protozoan, helminthic, and ectoparasitic.

## PROTOZOA

Protozoa (living, single-cell, parasitic, eukaryotic organisms) may or may not produce disease in a host. Some of these diseases are asymptomatic. However, some protozoa can prove uncomfortable and even deadly for the host. Common protozoan diseases include malaria, amebiasis, toxoplasmosis, and trichomoniasis.

Malaria is a global disease that kills more than one million people each year. Spread by the female *Anopheles* mosquito, malaria has a triad of antimalarial treatment options. The first option is chemoprophylaxis. Using the principle of prevention, persons who travel to highly infested, at-risk areas are prescribed medications to decrease the chance of contracting the disease. Chemoprophylaxis medications are given for one week before the person travels, during the trip, and for one to four weeks after return home. Chloroquine is most commonly prescribed for chemoprophylaxis. However, if the traveler cannot take this drug for some reason, other drugs, such as atovaquone-proguanil, primaquine, doxycycline, and mefloquine (for use in pregnant women), may be combined for preventive therapy.

The second treatment option for malaria is for an acute attack. The drug of choice is chloroquine, which works by interrupting the erthocyctic stage of the infection and by limiting the life cycle of malaria protozoa. If the infected person is resistant to chloroquine, then he or she can use primiquine, quine sulfate, mefloquine, or atovaquone-proguanil. Sometimes, combination antibiotics are prescribed, including doxycycline, clindamycin, and tetracycline (not used in pregnant women). Certain side effects occur, so caution should be observed with the use of these antimalarial drugs.

Amebiasis is a protozoan disease that results from ingesting *Entamoeba histolytica*. Amebiasis is usually treated with metronidazole and an opioid to control diarrhea. Antibiotics such as chloroquine and tetracycline are sometimes used with paromomycin and iodoquinol for intestinal infections.

Toxoplasmosis, caused by *Toxoplasma gondii*, transfers to humans through feces (such as feces in the litter boxes of cats), soil, or contaminated vegetables. Treatment includes four or five weeks of pyrimethamine in combination with sulfadiazine.

Trichomoniasis, commonly known as trich, is a sexually transmitted disease caused by *T. vaginalis*. A single dose of metronidazole (Flagyl) is prescribed to both the infected person and his or her sexual partner or partners.

## HELMINTHS

Helminths (multicelled parasitic worms) can often be seen with the naked eye. They usually enter humans through the skin or through the digestive tract and attach to the intestines. The most common helminths are roundworms (nematodes), tapeworms (cestodes), and flukes (trematodes). Medications used to treat helminth disease are known as anthelmintics.

The most common roundworm, *Ascaris lumbricoides*, causes ascariasis in Latin America and Asia, usually in children. To treat ascariasis, oral mebendazole (Vermox) is prescribed for three days. If the infected person is unable to take mebendazole, they can be treated with albendazole or pyrantel pamoate.

A common helminth found in the Unites States is the pinworm, a roundworm caused by *Enterobius vermicularis*. Treatment for this helminth, a single dose of mebendazole, albendazole, or pyrantel, usually provides relief, but the dose may be repeated if needed. Pinworms can cause anal itching, so antipruritic creams may be prescribed for local irritation. Hookworms are often acquired by walking barefoot on contaminated dirt. Treatment for hookworms includes albendazole and mebendazole, given for three days.

Tapeworms are usually contracted by humans by eating raw or undercooked meat contaminated with tapeworm cysts or larvae. Tapeworms can grow quite large, some as long as two to six feet (seven to twenty-five meters). Tapeworm infection is treated with a single dose of praziquantel with a laxative, given to excrete the worm and any eggs.

Flukes are flat worms that may infect the intestine. Some forty to fifty million people worldwide are infected with one of about seventy varieties of flukes. Praziquantel (Biltricide) is the treatment of choice.

## ECTOPARASITES

Ectoparasites attach themselves to skin or to the hair follicles of the host. Ticks, lice, leeches, bedbugs, and mites are all ectoparasites. Treatment is based on the type of ectoparasite involved. Ticks must be carefully removed from the host skin, and the area must be treated with alcohol. Head lice can be removed by using a shampoo medication, such as Nix, that contains permethrin. After shampooing, the nits, or lice eggs, should be removed using a small-tooth comb. A second shampoo treatment is usually recommended for use seven days after the first shampoo treatment.

## IMPACT

Parasitic disease causes devastating illness and even death. Protozoan diseases, such as malaria, kill more than one million people annually, primarily in Africa. Globally, some fifty million people each year are afflicted with amebiasis alone, resulting in forty thousand or more deaths. Trichomoniasis infects about 15 percent of women in the United States, with some 2.5 to 3 million cases seen in clinics treating sexually transmitted diseases. Each year, an estimated four hundred to four thousand cases of congenital toxoplasmosis are reported in the United States, resulting in mental retardation, blindness, epilepsy, and, occasionally, stillbirth and abortion. Helminths infect more than two billion people each year worldwide. Ascariasis, which is found in Latin America and Asia, affects some four million people and causes about sixty thousand deaths annually, primarily in children. In the United States, about forty million people, mostly children, have pinworms, while hookworms infect almost one billion people each year.

Parasitic diseases are expensive to diagnosis and treat, and they lead to reduced economic growth. Infected workers experience lost productivity and increased use of limited health care resources. Prevention and treatment of parasitic disease is a primary goal for the improvement of global health.

*Marylane Wade Koch, M.S.N., R.N.*

## FURTHER READING

Adams, Michael P., and Robert W. Koch. "Pharmacotherapy of Protozoan and Helminthic Infections." In *Pharmacology: Connections to Nursing Practice.* Upper Saddle River, N.J.: Pearson Prentice Hall, 2010. Discusses various types of parasitic diseases and their modes of transmission, symptoms, and pharmacologic treatment options.

Molyneux, David, ed. *Control of Human Parasitic Disease.* Vol. 61 in *Advances in Parasitology*, edited by J. R. Baker, R. Muller, and D. Rollinson. London: Academic Press, 2006. Describes the epidemiology and pathogenesis of parasitic disease and the low-cost but effective strategies to improve global health.

## WEB SITES OF INTEREST

*Centers for Disease Control and Prevention*
http://www.cdc.gov/parasites

*Partners for Parasite Control*
http://www.who.int/wormcontrol

**See also:** Flukes; Malaria; Parasites: Classification and types; Parasitic diseases; Pathogens; Pinworms; Protozoan diseases; Roundworms; Tapeworms; Worm infections.

# Treatment of prion diseases

CATEGORY: Treatment

## DEFINITION

Prion diseases are rare and fatal degenerative brain disorders that are caused by mutated proteins in the brain that aggregate and form visible "holes." These holes show a spongy appearance seen through a microscope, hence the name "spongiform encephalopathies." Because these diseases are terminal, treatment is meant to control symptoms that may cause discomfort; there is no cure for the disease state. Certain diseases, such as scrapie (a disease of sheep and goats), and two human diseases, Creutzfeldt-Jacob disease (CJD) and kuru, are transmitted by an infectious agent, namely a prion. Variant Creutzfeldt-Jacob disease (vCJD) and Gerstmann-Sträussler-Scheinker syndrome are two familial forms of prion disease and are considered inherited neurodegenerative disorders.

## GENERAL CONSIDERATIONS

There are no known ways to cure prion diseases; however, scientists around the world are working to develop methods to treat symptoms. Using infectious tissues from cultured cells, researchers have identified hundreds of molecules that inhibit the formation of the abnormal form of prion proteins. Groups of scientists are studying these infectious agents in animals, while other scientists are testing two molecular compounds in CJD patients. Researchers have identified antibodies and fragments of prion protein (short synthetic protein molecules) that can block the conversion of normal prion protein to the abnormal form. If successful, these studies may lead to effective methods to prevent prion infections and to the development of therapies that work either in affected patients or in the presymptomatic phases of disease.

One clinical trial, sponsored by the National Institute for Aging, assessed the potential benefits of the drug quinacrine for human sporadic CJD in the United States. Quinacrine has been used extensively as an antimalarial medication, and it is known to pass the blood-brain barrier. Because the main site of treatment for prion diseases is in the brain, where much of the neuronal damage is caused, drugs administered intravenously need to cross the blood-brain barrier to be effective. However, there is controversial evidence of the success of quinacrine for persons with CJD, as one person reported neurologic improvement. In another study, no benefit was seen in the animals being examined.

Pentosan polysulphate (PPS) is a component found in beech wood and is used generally as an anti-thrombotic and anti-inflammatory drug. It has helped persons who have thrombotic (blood clotting) disorders and interstitial cystitis (inflammation of the urinary bladder). In vitro experiments (performed in the laboratory on cultured cells) showed that PPS affected the production of prion proteins, their replication, and their cell toxicity. However, the laboratory experiments did not show any affect when used as treatment for humans with prion diseases. Because little is known about how neurons die in persons with prion diseases, it is difficult to understand the mechanism by which this drug may work. In vivo work using PPS on animals has shown that when PPS is given to animals at or near the time of experimental infection, a prolonged time exists between inoculation of infection and the appearance of disease. Some animals have shown complete protection against the development of disease. However, these experiments do not give clear evidence that PPS will have any positive effect on people with prion diseases.

Only a few people have received PPS as treatment for vCJD. These treatments were administered in the United Kingdom. PPS was given through the intra-cerebroventricular route, because PPS does not cross the blood-brain barrier. One patient had suggestions of improved neurological condition, but judgment is difficult to ascertain, and another patient showed no successful response to the drug. Other scientific papers using this treatment on a few patients have been published, with inconclusive results; however, the research has led to further investigation, though caution is emphasized because of possible side effects and the risk of administering the drug.

Another potential drug is the analgesic flupirtine, which may slow down the cognitive deterioration seen in persons with CJD; however, this drug has not shown to be significantly effective in increasing the survival rates of persons with CJD.

Much remains to be learned and understood about the use of flupirtine and other drugs for prion diseases after infection has occurred. More needs to be known about the dose and administration of the drug and about what specific diseases may react to the drugs in ways similar to the reactions in in vivo experiments.

Another form of treatment is the use of permanent feeding tubes. To help with symptoms, persons with dysphagia or swallowing difficulties, for example, may need the feeding tubes.

## IMPACT

One major dilemma in attempts to treat prion diseases is that persons with the disease are identified long after the disease has advanced. Therefore, treatments are less likely to help with symptoms or to improve the disease state. One approach for future treatment is to intercept the disease well before it deteriorates the brain and to diagnose the disease earlier in the disease state.

*Susan M. Zneimer, Ph.D., FACMG*

## FURTHER READING

Barrett, A., et al. "Evaluation of Qunicarine Treatment for Prion Diseases." *Journal of Virology* 77 (2003): 8462-8469. Discusses the use of the drug quinacrine for clinical use in human prion diseases.

Doh-ura, K., et al. "Treatment of Transmissible Spongiform Encephalopathy by Intraventricular Drug Infusion in Animal Models." *Journal of Virology* 78, no. 10 (2004): 4999-5006. Explains how PPS is being studied as a potential drug for persons with prion diseases.

Rainov, N. G., et al. "Treatment Options in Patients with Prion Disease: The Role of Long Term Cerebroventricular Infusion of Pentosan Polysulfate." In *Prions: Food and Drug Safety*, edited by T. Kitamoto. New York: Springer, 2005. Gives a comprehensive approach to the pros and cons of PPS as a drug to treat human prion diseases.

Todd, N. V., et al. "Cerebroventricular Infusion of Pentosan Polysulphate in Human Variant CJD Disease." *Journal of Infection* 50 (2005): 394-396. Describes the potential benefits of and problems with the use of PPS in humans.

## WEB SITES OF INTEREST

*Centers for Disease Control and Prevention*
http://www.cdc.gov/ncidod/dvrd/prions

*Creutzfeldt-Jakob Disease Foundation*
http://www.cjdfoundation.org

*Genetic and Rare Diseases Information Center*
http://rarediseases.info.nih.gov/gard

*National Institute of Allergy and Infectious Diseases*
http://www.niaid.nih.gov/topics/prion

*National Institute of Neurological Disorders and Stroke, Transmissible Spongiform Encephalopathies Information Page*
http://www.ninds.nih.gov/disorders/tse

*National Organization for Rare Disorders*
http://www.rarediseases.org

*National Prion Disease Pathology Surveillance Center*
http://www.cjdsurveillance.com

**See also:** Creutzfeldt-Jakob disease; Encephalitis; Fatal familial insomnia; Gerstmann-Sträussler-Scheinker syndrome; Kuru; Prions; Variant Creutzfeldt-Jakob disease.

# Treatment of protozoan diseases

CATEGORY: Treatment

## DEFINITION

Treatment for protozoan diseases involves therapy to manage infections caused by living, single-cell, parasitic, and eukaryotic organisms known as protozoa.

## COMMON PROTOZOAN DISEASES

Common protozoan diseases are malaria, amebiasis, toxoplasmosis, and trichomoniasis, which, along with their treatment protocols, are discussed here.

*Malaria.* Malaria is a deadly disease resulting from human contact with protozoa passed by the female *Anopheles* mosquito. The four infective species of protozoan *Plasmodium* that can result in malaria include *P. vivax*, the most common and debilitating; *P. falciparum*, which has the most severe symptoms and has a 10 percent fatality rate; and *P. malariae* and *P. ovale*, which are confined to Africa and are least common. In addition, *P. vivax* and *P. ovale* can hide in the liver for months or years and can produce relapses.

The pharmacological treatment of malaria can include chemoprophylaxis, or antimalarial medications, taken before a person travels to a geographic area at high risk for malaria; drugs administered during an acute attack; and drug therapy taken to prevent a relapse of illness. Chemoprophylaxis drugs are taken one week before travel to an infested (or endemic) area, during the stay there, and for one to four weeks after return from travel. The primary medication prescribed for chemoprophylaxis is chloroquine (Aralen). If the infected person cannot take this drug, combinations of drugs such as atovaquone-proguanil (Malarone); mefloquine (Lariam), which is used by pregnant women; doxycycline; and primaquine may be prescribed.

The treatment of a person with acute malaria is based on the extent of infection. The earlier the treatment occurs in the course of the infection, the more likely therapy is to be successful. Because malarial symptoms can mimic a common cold, infected persons often delay seeing a health care provider for treatment or are often misdiagnosed.

The first choice of pharmacological treatment for acute malaria is chloroquine, which interrupts the erythocytic stage of the infection and breaks the life cycle of the protozoan. If there is resistance to this drug, alternates are primaquine, mefloquine, quine sulfate, and atovaquone-proguanil. Antibiotics such as doxycyclin, clindamycin, and tetracycline (except in pregnant women) may also be administered. If infected persons have illnesses that are more progressed, they can be administered quinidine gluconate intravenously in combination with the foregoing antibiotics.

Chloroquine, the primary medication used to treat malaria, is contraindicated in persons with retinal problems because it can cause irreversible damage to the retina when given in high doses. Intermittent visual screening is indicated. Because the drug is metabolized in the liver, persons with compromised liver function, such as in alcoholism, should use this drug with caution. People with a history of hematologic disease should consider an alternate drug choice, because chloroquine can cause blood dyscrasias. As with all medications, drug interactions should be considered before therapy begins.

*Amebiasis.* Amebiasis, a protozoan disease caused by the ingestion of *Entamoeba histolytica,* usually occurs in the human digestive system. However, amebiasis can spread through colon ulcers to other parts of the body, including the liver. People living in countries outside the United States where drinking water is contaminated by poor sanitation are most likely to be infected.

Pharmacological treatment for amebiasis includes combination therapies of two or more drugs to ensure effective treatment. Metronidazole is the drug of choice, taken with an opioid to control diarrhea. Antibiotics such as chloroquine and tetracycline may be given. Paromomycin and iodoquinol can be used when the infection is limited to the intestine. Therapy is continued until consecutive stools test negative for the protozoa.

*Toxoplasmosis.* Toxoplasmosis is caused by *Toxoplasma gondii.* Cats host this parasitic organism, which can transfer to humans through feces in litter boxes or soil or on vegetables. Pregnant women are at highest risk for toxoplasmosis during the first two trimesters of pregnancy.

The pharmacological treatment of choice for toxoplasmosis includes four to five weeks of pyrimethamine, given in combination with sulfadiazine. Caution should be used with persons who have megaloblastic anemia because these drugs are folic-acid inhibitors.

*Trichomoniasis.* Trichomoniasis, or trich, is a protozoan disease that is transmitted sexually by *T. vaginalis.* As many as 50 percent of infected persons are asymptomatic.

A single dose of metronidazole (Flagyl) is an effective treatment. If the person experiences gastrointestinal upset, a lower dose of metronidazole can be used for seven days. Pharmacological treatment should also be given to any sexual partners of the infected person.

## Impact

Although some protozoa cause minimal disease and are asymptomatic, others result in devastating illness and even death. Malaria kills more than one million people around the world annually, mostly in Africa. Amebiasis affects some fifty million people each year, with forty thousand or more deaths. Trichomoniasis affects about 15 percent of women in the United States, of which nearly three million are seen in sexually transmitted disease clinics. An estimated four hundred to four thousand cases of congenital toxoplasmosis are reported annually in the United States.

Though rare, stillbirth and abortion can occur if a pregnant woman becomes infected; mental retardation, blindness, and epilepsy may result in newborns. Some protozoan diseases affect the health of both unborn fetuses and newborn infants; toxoplasmosis can cause still birth.

*Marylane Wade Koch, M.S.N., R.N.*

## Further Reading

Adams, Michael P., and Robert W. Koch. "Pharmacotherapy of Protozoan and Helminthic Infections." In *Pharmacology: Connections to Nursing Practice.* Upper Saddle River, N.J.: Pearson Prentice Hall, 2010. Discusses various types of parasitic diseases and their modes of transmission, symptoms, and pharmacologic treatment options.

Centers for Disease Control and Prevention. "Guidelines for Treatment of Malaria in the United States." Provides treatment guidelines for malaria. Available at http://www.cdc.gov/malaria/resources/pdf/treatmenttable73109.pdf.

_____. "Rapid Diagnostic Tests for Malaria: Haiti—2010." *Morbidity and Mortality Weekly Report* 59 (October 29, 2010): 1372-1373. Describes data-driven government policy change that supports rapid diagnostic testing of *Plasmodium falciparum* malaria, endemic to Haiti. This test allows more accurate testing, resulting in better diagnosis and treatment.

Sheorey, Harsha, John Walker, and Beverley-Ann Biggs. *Clinical Parasitology*. Carlton South, Vic.: Melbourne University Press, 2000. Reviews global parasitic diseases and includes information regarding classification and geographical distribution of parasites, details of diagnostic tests, availability and treatment regimens of drugs, and means of obtaining uncommon drugs.

## Web Sites of Interest

*Centers for Disease Control and Prevention*
http://www.cdc.gov/parasites

*Microbiology and Immunology On-line: Parasitology*
http://pathmicro.med.sc.edu/book/parasit-sta.htm

**See also:** Amebic dysentery; Developing countries and infectious disease; Diagnosis of protozoan diseases; Malaria; Parasitic diseases; Parasitology; Prevention of protozoan diseases; Protozoa: Structure and growth; Toxoplasmosis; Trichomonas; Tropical medicine.

# Treatment of viral infections

CATEGORY: Treatment

## Definition

Treatment for viral infections involves therapy to manage infections caused by a virus, an intracellular parasitic microorganism that is smaller than bacteria. Some common viral infections that affect humans worldwide are infectious caused by herpesvirus, influenza virus, and hepatitis virus.

## Viral Infections

The goal of a virus is to replicate itself. To do so, a virus must invade a living cell and use that cell's chemical mechanisms to replicate. The existence of a virus is dependent on the metabolic functioning of the host cell it attacks.

Some viral infections are self-limiting and will run their course without treatment. An example of this is the common cold, which has a seven- to ten-day course of illness. However, other viruses cause illness with severe symptoms and require pharmacological treatment. An example of a viral infection that requires treatment is human immunodeficiency virus (HIV) infection. Without pharmacological treatment, HIV can lead to acquired immunodeficiency syndrome (AIDS). In general, antiviral medications are designed to interfere with the functioning of a virus or with its ability to replicate. Antiviral drugs may interact with the enzymes or protein in the virus to break the viral replication cycle. The use of vaccines, when available, is one way to treat viral infections through prevention.

*Herpesvirus.* Herpes simplex viruses (HSV) belong to the family of DNA (deoxyribonucleic acid) viruses that cause blisters on a person's skin, mucous membranes, or genitals. This family of viruses includes HSV-1, HSV-2, cytomegalovirus, varicella zoster virus (chickenpox and shingles), Epstein-Barr virus, and herpesvirus type-6.

The pharmacologic treatment for herpesviruses is aimed at relieving the acute symptoms and preventing recurrences. No cure exists for herpesviruses, but medications can be employed to treat and lessen the severity of these diseases. Drug therapy can also increase the time the virus is in its latent state and can minimize symptoms.

Drug therapy for HSV-1 and HSV-2 requires five to ten days of oral antiviral medications. The most common antivirals for these infections are acyclovir (Zovirax), famciclovir (Famivir), and valacycloir (Valtrex). If blisters are present, topical medications may be used. In severely immunosuppressed persons, antiviral drugs can be given intravenously. Ocular herpes is treated with latanoprost, an antiglaucoma medication, to avoid corneal blindness. Ocular herpes can also be managed with medicated ophthalmic drops. Although recurrences may happen, antiviral prophylaxis medications are rarely used because of their high cost.

*Influenza.* The influenza virus, or flu, is labeled as

A, B, or C type. The treatment of influenza depends on the type flu a person contracts. The best treatment for influenza is to prevent infection through annual vaccination. The treatment for influenza once it is acquired is limited. Amantadine (Symmetrel) is the drug of choice; it has been available since 1966. Neuraminidase inhibitors treat active viral diseases. Oseltamivir (Tamiflu) and zanamivir (Relenza) can be given by mouth to shorten the course of the illness from seven to five days. Antivirals are ineffective in the treatment of the common cold.

*Hepatitis.* Hepatitis, or inflammation of the liver, can occur with alcoholism, drug use, autoimmune disease, metabolic disease, and diverse infections. Hepatitis, caused by numerous viruses, can be an acute infection or a chronic one. Sometimes, persons with hepatitis are asymptomatic.

Hepatitis A is spread mostly through contaminated food or tap water and will usually resolve with no treatment within a few weeks. The best treatment for hepatitis A is prevention with vaccines.

Hepatitis B is contracted through infected blood, sexual activity with an infected person, or childbirth. Acute hepatitis B usually resolves without treatment, but if treatment is needed, the drug lamivudine is available. Chronic hepatitis B can be treated with alpha interferon, lamivudine, peginterferon, or adefovir dipivoxil.

Hepatitis C is spread most often by contaminated blood. The drug of choice for treating chronic hepatitis C is peginterferon, sometimes in combination with ribavirin. Hepatitis D comes from infected blood and is treated with alpha interferon. Hepatitis E, uncommon in the United States, is contracted from contaminated food and water. Treatment is usually not needed because it will resolve on its own.

## IMPACT

Viral infections can be minor and come with few symptoms, or they can be severe and life-threatening. Global viral infections include relatively minor diseases such as the common cold, influenza, and chickenpox, but also serious diseases such as Ebola, AIDS, severe acute respiratory syndrome (SARS), and avian influenza. Other diseases are under investigation as viral and include multiple sclerosis and chronic fatigue syndrome. Virology, the study of viruses, is a critical component of modern biology and genetics.

Most persons will encounter one or more virus in-

fections during their lifetime. Of the 250,000 to 500,000 people who get influenza each year, about 20,000 of them will die. Indeed, in 1919, a worldwide flu epidemic resulted in about 20 million deaths. One in five Americans, or about 60 million people, is infected with genital herpes. Neonatal herpes has a 50 percent mortality rate. In 2008, 29 to 35 percent of the United States population was infected with viral hepatitis A. Persons living with chronic viral hepatitis B numbered up to 1.4 million, while those living with chronic infection of viral hepatitis C was 2.7 to 3.9 million persons. Influenza in a pregnant woman can damage a fetus and can kill an adult. Treating viral disease remains a key goal of global population health.

*Marylane Wade Koch, M.S.N., R.N.*

### FURTHER READING

Adams, Michael P., and Robert W. Koch. *Pharmacology: Connections to Nursing Practice.* Upper Saddle River, N.J.: Pearson Prentice Hall, 2010. Discusses various types of viral diseases, their modes of transmission, symptoms, and treatment options.

Driscoll, John S. *Antiviral Drugs.* Hoboken, N.J.: John Wiley & Sons, 2006. Presents the most commonly used antiviral drugs and discusses the mechanisms by which the drugs exert their therapeutic effects.

Knobler, Stacey, Joshua Lederberg, and Leslie A. Pray. *Considerations for Viral Disease Eradication: Lessons Learned and Future Strategies.* Washington, D.C.: National Academies Press, 2002. Summary of the proceedings of a workshop, Forum for Emerging Infections, that discusses a national initiative to eradicate viral disease with immunization.

Wagner, Edward K., and Martinez J. Hewlett. *Basic Virology.* 3d ed. Malden, Mass.: Blackwell Science, 2008. Introductory text for students and researchers about the relationship of virology to modern biology and the future of human and animal health.

### WEB SITES OF INTEREST

*Centers for Disease Control and Prevention, Division of High-Consequence Pathogens and Pathology*
http://www.cdc.gov/ncezid/dhcpp

*Flu.gov*
http://flu.gov

*Hepatitis Foundation International*
http://www.hepfi.org

*International Herpes Alliance*
http://www.herpesalliance.org

**See also:** Antiviral drugs: Mechanisms of action; Antiviral drugs: Types; Hepatitis A; Hepatitis B; Hepatitis C; Hepatitis D; Hepatitis E; Herpesvirus infections; Influenza; Parasitic diseases; Pregnancy and infectious disease; Sexually transmitted diseases (STDs); Viral infections; Viruses: Structure and life cycle; Viruses: Types.

---

# *Treponema*

CATEGORY: Pathogen
TRANSMISSION ROUTE: Direct contact

## DEFINITION

*Treponema* are gram-negative, motile, spirochete with many nutritional requirements that can be anaerobes or microaerophiles. All are commensals or parasites in humans and other animals.

## NATURAL HABITAT AND FEATURES

The name *Treponema* was derived from the Greek words *trepein* and *nema*, meaning "turning thread." Like other spirochetes, treponemes have two or more periplasmic flagella, each attached to opposite ends of the protoplasmic cylinder and unattached at the other end. They extend about two-thirds of the way along the cylinder. The membrane cell wall of the cylinder is rigid, while the complex outer sheath is flexible. When the flagella rotate in the space between the sheath and the cylinder, the entire organism rotates in the opposite direction, allowing for motility.

Because the diameters of these bacteria are usually less than 0.3 micrometers (μm), they are difficult to visualize with a Gram's stain. However, most can be visualized using dark-field or phase-contrast microscopy. They grow best at pH 7.2 to 7.4 and at temperatures between 86° and 99° Fahrenheit (30° and 37° Celsius). Treponemes have very small genomes, with approximately 1.14 million base pairs and fewer than 1,100 genes. Because of their small genomes, they have limited metabolism and depend on their hosts

---

**Taxonomic Classification for *Treponema***

**Kingdom:** Bacteria
**Phylum:** Spirochaetes
**Class:** Spirochaetes
**Order:** Spirochaetales
**Family:** Spirochchaetaceae
**Genus:** *Treponema*
**Species:**
*T. azotonutricium*
*T. bryantii*
*T. carateum*
*T. denticola*
*T. hyodysenteriae*
*T. minutum*
*T. mucosum*
*T. pallidum*
*T. paraluiscuniculi*
*T. primitia*
*T. refringens*
*T. saccharophilum*
*T. vincentii*

---

for many necessary compounds, including fatty acids and most amino acids that treponemes are unable to make. They are difficult to grow in culture because of their extensive nutritional requirements. Some, like *pallidum*, have never been successfully grown in culture; others can be co-cultured only in the presence of other cultured cells; and some, whose complex nutritional requirements have been determined, can be grown in normal culture.

Although immunity does develop after some treponemal infections, that immunity is strain specific; no *Treponema* vaccine has been developed.

The taxonomy of the genus has changed in the twenty-first century. The four main human pathogens, *pallidum*, *carateum*, *endemicum*, and *pertenue*, have all been reclassified as subspecies of *pallidum*, although the original designations, especially *carateum*, still appear in the literature. These pathogens were combined because, morphologically and genetically, almost no difference exists among these organisms. All are flattened spirochetes that cause a three-phase infection in humans. Stage one shows a small sore or chancre at the site of infection. It usually appears days or weeks after initial contact; during this stage the spirochetes are multiplying. Stage two occurs a few weeks to several months later; during this stage the bacteria disseminate and lesions appear on various parts of the body. Stage three occurs after the bacteria have become fully disseminated, which may take many years, and is the most serious; many lesions present both internally and externally.

The treatment of choice is penicillin and a single dose is usually enough to wipe out the organisms in stages one and two. Other antibiotics, such as tetracycline, chloramphenicol, erythromycin, and azithromycin, have been used, but none seem as effective as penicillin in treating human primary and secondary infections. The tertiary stage requires prolonged and sometimes more diverse antibiotic therapy.

*Pallidum* naturally infects only humans, and humans serve as the only living reservoir for the bacteria. *Pallidum,* a thin spirochete with a diameter of less than 1.5 μm, is so sensitive to environmental stress that it rarely survives more than a few seconds away from its human host. *Pallidum pallidum* causes syphilis, the most severe of the treponemal infections. Infections are usually contracted through sexual contact with an infected partner. Congenital syphilis can occur when the bacterium crosses the placental barrier or infects the fetus as it passes through the birth canal of an infected woman. The tertiary stage of syphilis occurs in about one-half of all untreated cases. Lesions can occur on the central nervous system and the circulatory system, leading to paralysis and death.

*Pallidum pertenue* causes yaws and *pallidum carateum* causes pinta. Both are transmitted through skin-to-skin contact and are most common in children in tropical and subtropical countries. Yaws is found in tropical regions worldwide and, in its tertiary stage, can lead to disfiguring lesions on the bones. Pinta is more common in Central America and South America and, even in its tertiary stages, involves only the skin.

*Pallidum endemicum* is the cause of bejel. This disease is most common in the Mediterranean region and Saharan Africa. The bacterium is usually transmitted through mouth-to-mouth contact but is sturdy enough to remain viable on eating utensils and can be transmitted by sharing utensils with an infected person. The primary and secondary stages are usually found in the mouth, while the disseminated tertiary stage leads to bone lesions.

*Denticola, mucosum,* and *vincentii* are three of the many treponemes that cause periodontal disease. Other *Treponema* spp. seem to be commensal in human oral and genital tissue without being pathogenic, unless the host is debilitated. Some *Treponema* spp. are pathogenic in other animals (for example, *hyodysenteriae* in pigs and *paraluiscuniculi* in rabbits). *Bryantii* and *saccharophilum,* found in the rumen of cows, are important in the complete breakdown of cellulose, although neither is cellulolytic itself. In termite guts, both *primitia* and *azotonutricium* are needed for the utilization of wood as food. *Azotonutricium* is the only known *Treponema* spp. that can fix atmospheric nitrogen.

*Richard W. Cheney, Jr., Ph.D.*

**FURTHER READING**

Antal, George M., Sheila A. Lukehart, and Andre Z. Meheus. "The Endemic Treponematoses." *Microbes and Infection* 4 (2002): 83-94. This article describes the main endemic treponeme infections in humans: yaws, pinta, and bejel.

Krieg, Noel R., et al., eds. *Bergey's Manual of Systematic Bacteriology.* 2d ed. New York: Springer, 2010. Volume 4 of this multivolume work describes the Spirochaetes in detail.

Madigan, Michael T., and John M. Martinko. *Brock Biology of Microorganisms.* 12th ed. Upper Saddle River, N.J.: Pearson/Prentice Hall, 2010. This text outlines many common bacteria and describes their natural history, pathogenicity, and other characteristics.

**WEB SITES OF INTEREST**

*Centers for Disease Control and Prevention*
http://www.cdc.gov

*Virtual Museum of Bacteria*
http://www.bacteriamuseum.org

**See also:** Bacteria: Classification and types; Microbiology; Pathogens; Pinta; Syphilis; Yaws.

# Triazole antifungals

CATEGORY: Treatment

**DEFINITION**

Triazole is a class of antifungal drugs that consists of five-membered rings with three nitrogen substitution molecules. These molecules interfere with the activity of fungal organic compounds that cause infections.

## DISEASES TREATED

First-generation triazoles, such as itraconazole and fluconazole, provide broad-spectrum action against superficial and deep fungal infections. Extra nitrogens present on the triazole antifungal drugs result in increased specificity and potency compared with the older imidazole antifungals, such as miconazole. Candidiasis infections, which cause oral thrush and vaginal yeast infections, and onychomycosis, a fungal nail infection, are two common examples of diseases treated with triazole antifungal agents. Aspergillosis, blastomycosis, histoplasmosis, and, in particular, cryptococcus meningitis, which are also treated with triazole antifungals, are more often observed in immune-compromised persons, such as those with human immunodeficiency virus (HIV) infection and acquired immunodeficiency syndrome (AIDS). Fluconazole may be used lifelong in persons with AIDS because of the increased risk of candidiasis relapse; however, prophylaxis for initial candidiasis in persons with HIV is not recommended.

## MECHANISM OF ACTION

Triazole antifungals disrupt sterols in fungal cytoplasmic membranes that are essential to fungal cell functioning. These drugs bind to cytochrome P450 (CYP450) liver metabolism enzymes in the body to increase the amount of C14-alpha-methylsterol and decrease the amount of ergosterol needed by the fungal cells. Triazole effects appear proportional to drug exposure as measured by the area under the curve, and they are often longer with triazoles than with older imidazole compounds. Triazoles, when used topically, may provide, in addition to their sterol effects, direct damage to fungal cell membranes.

## ADVERSE DRUG EFFECTS AND INTERACTIONS

The most common side effects of drugs in the triazole class, when taken by mouth, are gastric discomfort, such as nausea and vomiting, and hepatotoxicity. Suppression of the body's sterol and hormonal levels may occur as well. The interaction of the CYP liver-enzyme system with triazoles for the drug's effect can cause increases in other drug concentrations when the drugs are taken concomitantly with triazole antifungals. All CYP3A4 enzymes are affected by triazole antifungals to cause inhibition of other drug metabolism. Fluconazole and voriconazole, additionally, interact with CYP2C9 and CYP2C19 enzymes in the same manner. Drugs that are adversely increased by inhibited CYP metabolism include rifampin, midazolam, warfarin, and phenytoin; however, CYP drug interactions are specific to each triazole antifungal.

## IMPACT

From their early development, which resulted from natural discovery in the 1940's, through the development of second- and third-generation agents in the early twenty-first century, triazole antifungals have expanded as a class. They now include improved action in the body and widespread administration forms, from oral to topical and nonprescription to prescription.

From the early use of itraconazole and fluconazole, however, resistant fungi, especially candidiasis, have developed because of drug efflux and increased C14-alpha-demethylase changes; this resistance has led to research and development of newer agents in the triazole class.

Posaconazole, a unique late-generation triazole, is uniquely active against molds and zygomycetes in addition to typical fungal targets. Other late-generations examples, such as isavuconazole, voriconazole, ravuconazole, and albuconazole, provide longer half-lives and improved body distribution, which improve dosing regimens also.

*Nicole M. Van Hoey, Pharm.D.*

## FURTHER READING

Greer, Nickie D. "Posaconazole (Noxafil): A New Triazole Antifungal Agent." *Proceedings* (Baylor University Medical Center) 20, no. 2 (2007): 188-196. Also available at http://www.ncbi.nlm.nih.gov/pmc/articles/pmc1849883.

Griffith, R. K. "Antifungal Drugs." In *Foye's Principles of Medicinal Chemistry*, edited by Thomas L. Lemke and William O. Foye. 6th ed. Philadelphia: Wolters Kluwer, 2008.

Rex, John H., and David A. Stevens. "Systemic Antifungal Agents." In *Mandell, Douglas, and Bennett's Principles and Practice of Infectious Diseases*, edited by Gerald L. Mandell, John F. Bennett, and Raphael Dolin. 7th ed. New York: Churchill Livingstone/Elsevier, 2010.

Ryan, Kenneth J. "Pathogenesis of Fungal Infection."

In *Sherris Medical Microbiology*, edited by Kenneth J. Ryan and C. George Ray. 5th ed. New York: McGraw-Hill, 2010.

Torres, Harry A., et al. "Posaconazole: A Broad-Spectrum Triazole Antifungal." *Lancet Infectious Disease* 5 (2005): 775-785.

**WEB SITES OF INTEREST**

*DoctorFungus*
http://doctorfungus.org

*Family Practice Notebook: Pharmacology*
http://www.fpnotebook.com/der/pharm

*Medical Pharmacology Online: Antifungal Drugs*
http://www.pharmacology2000.com/antifungal/antif1.htm

*Microbiology and Immunology On-line: Mycology*
http://pathmicro.med.sc.edu/book/mycol-sta.htm

**See also:** Antifungal drugs: Mechanisms of action; Antifungal drugs: Types; Diagnosis of fungal infections; Echinocandin antifungals; Fungal infections; Histoplasmosis; Imidazole antifungals; Immune response to fungal infections; Infection; Mycoses; Onychomycosis; Polyene antifungals; Prevention of fungal infections; Thiazole antifungals; Thrush; Treatment of fungal infections.

# Trichinosis

CATEGORY: Diseases and conditions
ANATOMY OR SYSTEM AFFECTED: Gastrointestinal system, intestines, muscles, stomach, tissue
ALSO KNOWN AS: Trichinellosis, trichiniasis

## DEFINITION

Trichinosis is a parasitic disease caused by infection with the larvae of a roundworm (*Trichinella*) that is found in raw or undercooked pork, pork products, wild game, and some marine mammals.

## CAUSES

Trichinosis is caused by the ingestion of raw or undercooked meat contaminated with the encapsulated larvae of the roundworm *Trichinella*. There are six species of *Trichinella* that are known to infect humans. These are *T. spiralis*, which is found in animals worldwide; *T. britovi*, found in Europe and Asia; *T. pseudospiralis*, found in birds; *T. nativa*, found in the Arctic; *T. nelson*, found in Africa; and *T. murrelli*, found in wild animals in the United States. Most human infections are caused by *T. spiralis*.

The most important source of human infection worldwide is the domestic pig, but in countries other than the United States, the consumption of horses and wild boars has played a significant role during outbreaks. Some marine mammals (walruses and seals of the Arctic) also carry the parasitic infection.

Once consumed, the gastric juices of the stomach digest the wall surrounding the larvae, which are then released into the small intestine. The larvae penetrate the wall of the intestines, where they mature and mate. Females burrow into the intestinal wall and produce more larvae (more than one thousand). This process continues as the infection moves down the gastrointestinal tract and the worms are eliminated through feces. Larvae can also be carried through the blood and lymph system to other parts of the body. The larvae that reach muscle tissue are the only ones that survive. They burrow into the muscle fiber and cause the muscle to become inflamed. Some muscle cells become "nurse" cells that protect the larvae from the infected person's immune system.

## RISK FACTORS

Risk factors include eating pork and pork products (such as sausage), wild game, and some marine mammals that are eaten raw or undercooked. Domestic pigs that are fed garbage pose a higher risk of carrying the larvae than are pigs fed on a root vegetable diet (such as in France, where trichinosis is rare).

## SYMPTOMS

Symptoms of trichinosis vary depending on the part of the body that is infected by the parasite. If the infection is in the intestine, symptoms include nausea, diarrhea, vomiting, fatigue, fever, and stomach pain. Symptoms experienced as the parasite reaches other parts of the body include headaches, chills, cough, painful joints, muscle aches and inflammation, and swelling of the eyes. Larvae that reach nerve tissue or cardiac tissue do not survive but still cause symptoms. Infections at these areas may cause difficulty in muscle

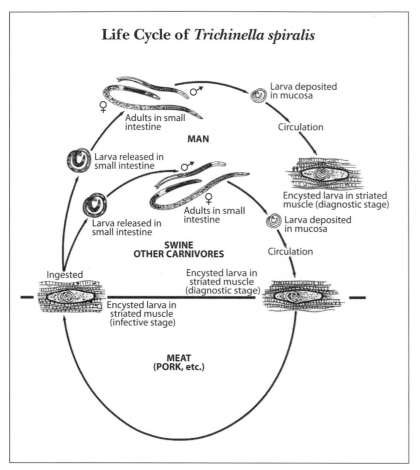

## Life Cycle of *Trichinella spiralis*

The cycle of infection of the worm Trichenella spiralis, *which causes trichinosis.* (CDC)

coordination, respiratory paralysis, and (in severe cases) death.

### SCREENING AND DIAGNOSIS

There is no test to diagnose the early (intestinal) stages of *Trichinella* infection. Having a history of consumption of raw or undercooked meat is the only indication. During later infections, as the parasite invades muscle tissue, elevated white blood cells are present. Increased levels of creatine kinase and lactate dehydrogenase (which indicate muscle cell damage) are seen in blood tests, but these are not specific to trichinosis.

Specific tests are available that measure antibodies to the parasite. These are indirect immunofluorescence, latex agglutination, and enzyme-linked immunosorbent assays; but these are not useful until a min-

imum of three weeks after infection and may give false-positive results in persons with other infections or with autoimmune diseases. Biopsy of the muscle to look for the presence of the parasite is the best diagnostic tool.

### TREATMENT AND THERAPY

Minor cases of trichinosis do not require treatment. Adult worms in the gastrointestinal tract can be eliminated with the use of thiabendazole, mebendazole, or albendazole. These are effective within one week of infection and are used to prevent further infection by the parasite. Once the parasite has invaded tissues, inflammation at infection sites is treated with prednisone.

### PREVENTION AND OUTCOMES

Trichinosis is prevented by thoroughly cooking pork and pork products. The U.S. Department of Agriculture's food safety recommendations are to cook meat to 160° Fahrenheit to avoid all food-borne diseases. *Trichinella* can be killed by cooking meats to 140°. Freezing meat is also effective in killing most *Trichinella* species. Recommended temperatures for freezing are 5° for twenty days, minus 10° for ten days, or minus 20° for six days (for a six-inch piece of meat). Salting, smoking, and drying the meat will not kill *Trichinella*.

*Joan Letizia, Ph.D.*

### FURTHER READING

Despommier, Dickson D., et al. "Trichinosis." In *Parasitic Diseases.* 5th ed. New York: Apple Trees, 2006. This chapter summarizes the basic science of *Trichinella* infection and provides clinical information on trichinosis.

Gottstein, B., et al. "Epidemiology, Diagnosis, Treatment, and Control of Trichinellosis." *Clinical Microbiology Review* 22 (2009): 127-145. This article examines trichinosis and discusses the economic importance of eliminating the parasite from the food chain.

Michelson, Marco K. "Parasitic Infections." In *The Merck Manual of Diagnosis and Therapy*, edited by Mark H. Beers et al. 18th ed. Whitehouse Station, N.J.: Merck Research Laboratories, 2006. The tissue nematodes section of this chapter includes discussion of trichinosis, which also includes its etiology, pathogenesis, and epidemiology.

Morris, J. Glenn, Jr. "How Safe Is Our Food?" *Emerging Infectious Diseases* 17 (2011). Available at http://www.cdc.gov/eid/content/17/1/126.htm.

Murray, Clinton. "Trichinosis." Available at http://emedicine.medscape.com/article/230490-overview. In addition to an overview of the disease, this article discusses the *Trichinella* species, including its life cycle.

### WEB SITES OF INTEREST

*Centers for Disease Control and Prevention*
http://www.cdc.gov/parasites/trichinellosis

*National Center for Emerging and Zoonotic Infectious Diseases*
http://www.cdc.gov/ncezid

*National Institutes of Health*
http://www.nlm.nih.gov/medlineplus/ency/article/000631.htm

**See also:** Amebic dysentery; Ascariasis; Balantidiasis; *Campylobacter*; Campylobacteriosis; Cholera; Cryptosporidiosis; Developing countries and infectious disease; *Escherichia*; Fecal-oral route of transmission; Food-borne illness and disease; Gastritis; *Helicobacter*; Pigs and infectious disease; Protozoan diseases; Roundworms; *Salmonella*; *Shigella*; Travelers' diarrhea; *Vibrio*; Worm infections; Zoonotic diseases.

---

# Trichomonas

CATEGORY: Diseases and conditions
ANATOMY OR SYSTEM AFFECTED: Genitalia, genitourinary tract
ALSO KNOWN AS: Trich, trichomoniasis

### DEFINITION

Trichomonas is a common sexually transmitted disease (STD), or infection. It is a symptomatic infection of the vaginal tract in women and a usually asymptomatic infection of the urethra in men.

### CAUSES

Trichomonas is caused by infection with the single-celled protozoan parasite *Trichomonas vaginalis*, which is transmitted almost exclusively through vaginal sexual intercourse. Extremely rare cases of fomite transmission, that is, transmission through a contaminated object, have been reported.

### RISK FACTORS

Risk factors for contacting trichomonas include those things that increase the chances of contact with an infected partner. Persons with multiple sexual partners, who have unprotected sexual intercourse, and who have untreated sexual partners are at high risk.

In addition to the noted risk factors for trichomonas, associated high risks have received focused attention from researchers. Increased rates of human immunodeficiency virus (HIV) infection have been documented in women with a history of trichomonas. Biological changes associated with trichomonas may occur. Microabrasions caused by the inflammatory response associated with the organism, and possibly with itching and scratching from the discomfort caused by the infection, can make trichomonas-infected women more susceptible to seroconversion with HIV if they are exposed to infectious fluids. Pregnant women infected with *T. vaginalis* have demonstrated increased rates of complications, including premature rupture of membranes, preterm birth, and delivery of low-birth-weight neonates.

### SYMPTOMS

In women, trichomonas symptoms include a foamy grayish discharge with a foul odor; mild, moderate, or intense itching and burning that often includes pain with intercourse; and, in severe cases, erythema (redness) of the vagina and inner vulvar folds. Some women may experience pain with urination and may confuse their symptoms with that of a urinary tract infection.

Men are usually asymptomatic, but men who do have symptoms present with penile burning on urination, a reddened urethral opening, and a clear penile discharge that is often misdiagnosed as nongonococcal urethritis or chlamydia. This misdiagnosis can result in the provision of antibiotics that are effective against chlamydia but that have no treatment value for trichomonas. Men with longstanding infection may also have symptoms of prostatitis.

Symptoms may present anywhere from a few days to a month following transmission, so for persons with multiple partners, there is often no way to determine when the infection was acquired based on symptoms.

### SCREENING AND DIAGNOSIS

Trichomonas is one of the STDs for which screening tests are not widely employed. Infection in women is marked by an increased pH (acidity) of the vaginal fluid in most cases, so screening women who are undergoing vaginal speculum examinations with pH paper has been suggested.

For many years the gold standard for diagnosis has been the saline wet prep, which requires a working microscope, skill in examining wet prep specimens, and a laboratory certification for the clinical setting for provider-performed microscopy. The sensitivity (the percentage of time a positive result is identified from the testing) of vaginal wet preps for trichomonas is estimated to be between 60 and 70 percent, but the specificity is very high if only mobile trichomonads are used for identification. Specificity refers to a lack of false-positive results and is especially important for a sexually transmitted infection that can raise serious issues in a relationship. Sensitivity is increased by scanning multiple fields and by examination immediately after collection of a specimen, because the organisms may die quickly. Because of these limitations, many clinical settings have not always been able to offer wet prep testing, and laboratory diagnostic testing methodologies have become available with send-out and point-of-care testing.

Many issues remain concerning the low specificity of these DNA (deoxyribonucleic acid) probe or PCR-based tests. Commercial tests continue to enter the market. Pap screening may also produce incidental findings of trichomonal organisms, but because of a high rate of false-positive results (low specificity), this should only be treated as a screening, rather than a diagnostic finding, so confirmatory testing is required. Culture is also available in a few specialty laboratory settings, utilizing vaginal secretions in women and urine, urethral swabs, or semen in men. In laboratories that have the capability of centrifuging urine and doing a microscopic examination of the spun sediment, trichomonal organisms, or trichomonads may be identified in male urine sediment.

Diagnosis is usually made from testing symptomatic women through a wet prep of vaginal discharge. Male partners receive a presumptive diagnosis.

### TREATMENT AND THERAPY

Trichomonas is a curable sexually transmitted infection, without a high rate of relapse if partners are properly treated and if future behavioral changes can be implemented. Treatment is generally with only two approved medications: metronidazole in a single 2 gram (g) oral dose, or tinidazole in a single 2 g oral dose. Alternatively, metronidazole can be given as one 500 milligram tablet twice each day for seven days.

Persons who are treated with a one-dose regimen are given multiple tablets (often four). They need to remain abstinent for one week while the medication is eradicating the organism. They also need to abstain from alcohol for twenty-four hours before taking the medications and for twenty-four hours after completing metronidazole and for seventy-two hours after completing tinidazole, as severe symptoms can result from interaction with alcohol. If a provider has concerns about resistant infection, he or she can contact the Centers for Disease Control and Prevention. Metronidazole is safe to give during pregnancy and is preferred over tinidazole.

### PREVENTION AND OUTCOMES

Prevention of infection with *T. vaginalis* involves decreasing one's number of sexual partners, practicing mutual monogamy, and using barrier protection such as male or female condoms. Prevention is also accomplished at the community level through the contact and treatment of all potentially infected partners.

*Clair Kaplan, M.S.N., M.H.S., R.N.,*
*MT(ASCP), APRN, WHNP*

### FURTHER READING

Boston Women's Health Collective. *Our Bodies, Ourselves: A New Edition for a New Era.* 35th anniversary ed. New York: Simon & Schuster, 2005. A popular, classic book dealing with all aspects of women's sexuality, including sexually transmitted infections and safer sex.

Grimshaw-Mulcahy, Laura J. "Now I Know My STDs: Part II—Bacterial and Protozoal." *Journal for Nurse*

*Practitioners* 4 (2008): 271-281. A review article that has a comprehensive section on trichomonas.

Holmes, King K., et al., eds. *Sexually Transmitted Diseases.* 4th ed. New York: McGraw-Hill Medical, 2008. A comprehensive text covering all aspects of sexually transmitted infections and diseases.

Johnston, Victoria J., and David C. Mabey. "Global Epidemiology and Control of Trichomonas Vaginalis." *Current Opinion in Infectious Diseases* 21 (2008): 56-64. Updated information on epidemiology and treatment trends.

Szumigala, J. A., et al. "Vulvovaginitis: Trichomonas." In *Ferri's Clinical Advisor 2011: Instant Diagnosis and Treatment,* edited by Fred F. Ferri. Philadelphia: Mosby/Elsevier, 2011. Provides recommendations on clinical treatments for trichomonas infection.

Van Der Pol, Barbara, et al. "Trichomonas Vaginalis Infection and Human Immunodeficiency Virus Acquisition in African Women." *Journal of Infectious Diseases* 197 (2008): 548-555. Research article on the risks that trichomonas can pose for increased seroconversion to HIV.

## Web Sites of Interest

*Centers for Disease Control and Prevention*
http://www.cdc.gov/std/trichomonas

*National Institute of Allergy and Infectious Diseases*
http://www.niaid.nih.gov/topics/trichomoniasis

*National Women's Health Information Center*
http://www.womenshealth.gov

*Sex Information and Education Council of Canada*
http://www.sieccan.org

**See also:** Bacterial infections; Bacterial vaginosis; Chlamydia; Diagnosis of protozoan diseases; Gonorrhea; Herpes simplex infection; HIV; Horizontal disease transmission; Men and infectious disease; Pelvic inflammatory disease; Pregnancy and infectious disease; Prevention of protozoan diseases; Protozoa: Structure and growth; Protozoan diseases; Sexually transmitted diseases (STDs); Treatment of protozoan diseases; Urethritis; Vaginal yeast infection; Women and infectious disease.

# Trichophyton

CATEGORY: Pathogen
TRANSMISSION ROUTE: Direct contact

## Definition

*Trichophyton* is a genus of filamentous fungi that is a primary cause of infections of the outer layer of the skin, nail beds, and hair.

---

**Taxonomic Classification
for *Trichophyton***

**Kingdom:** Fungi
**Phylum:** Ascomycota
**Class:** Euascomycetes
**Order:** Onygenales
**Family:** Arthrodermataceae
**Genus:** *Trichophyton*
**Species:**
*T. mentagrophytes*
*T. rubrum*
*T. schoenleinii*
*T. tonsurans*
*T. verrucosum*
*T. violaceum*

---

## Natural Habitat and Features

Twenty species of *Trichophyton* have been identified. Most are distributed worldwide, although some are restricted to specific geographic regions. Among species (anthropophlic species) whose natural habitat is human beings, those most commonly associated with human infection are *rubrum, schoenleinii, tonsurans,* and *violaceum.* Among species (zoophilic species) whose natural habitat is animals, *verrucosum* (cattle and horses) and *mentagrophytes* (rodents and rabbits) are most commonly associated with human infection.

Animal-to-human transmission occurs most frequently among rural populations in less developed regions of the world. Direct human-to-human transmission occurs most frequently within families or among children in day-care or school settings. Object-to-human transmission involves wet floors in gym showers or locker rooms; shared towels; and hair, shredded skin, nails, and contaminated tools in barber shops and beauty and nail salons. Self-inoculation occurs when a person first touches an infected area of his or her own body, then touches a noninfected, vulnerable area elsewhere on the body.

Colonies of *Trichophyton* are incubated on Sabouraud's agar at between 77° and 86° Fahrenheit (25° and 30° Celsius) for from seven to fourteen days, depending on the species. Color and physical features vary depending on the species. In general, fronts are white to bright yellowish beige or red violet. The reverse may be pale yellow, brown, or reddish brown. The surface is waxy, glabrous (smooth and hairless), or cottony.

Microscopic examination of colonies of *Trichophyton* reveals septate, hyaline hyphae (partitioned and transparent tubelike filaments). Additional features vary by species. Macroconidia (large, multicelled spores) are not seen in great numbers. *Trichophyton* species are smooth, either thin- or thick-walled and are either cylindrical, shaped like a clavate (club), or shaped like a fusiform (spindle). Microconidia (small, single-celled spores) are numerous. They are solitary or arranged in clusters and are round, pyriform (pear-shaped), clavate, or irregular. Microconidia are usually the predominant type of conidia observed in *Trichophyton* species. Their presence distinguishes *Trichophyton* from *Epidermophyton*, in which microconidia are rarely observed. Arthroconidia (jointed spores) and chlamydospores (round, thick-walled spores) may also be observed, especially in older cultures.

## PATHOGENICITY AND CLINICAL SIGNIFICANCE

*Trichophyton*, along with *Epidermophyton* and *Microsporum*, is classified as a dermatophyte, a fungi that causes dermatophytosis, an infection of the outer layer of the skin (stratum corneum) and of the hair and nail beds. *Trichophyton* species are highly adapted to the nonliving outer tissue of the skin, hair shafts, and nail beds. A minor lesion, such as a paper cut or a blister, allows the fungus to penetrate the outer layer of the skin, where it grows and spreads sideways with sharp, advancing margins. Infection of the hair occurs when hyphae penetrate the hair shaft. An erythematous papule (red pimple) develops, followed by scaling and discoloration. Eventually the shaft breaks off. Infection progresses to surrounding hair in a ringlike pattern. Nail-bed infection begins with discoloration of tissue under the nail. The nail plate then hardens and discolors and may become misshapen.

## DRUG SUSCEPTIBILITY

Susceptibility methods for testing agents used to treat dermatophytosis caused by *Trichophyton* species have not been standardized. Limited testing and comparisons have shown that specific newer agents have lower minimum inhibitory concentrations (MICs) than earlier agents such as griseofulvin, amphotericin B, and fluconazole, which were once the drugs of choice. These newer agents also carry a lower risk of side effects. Fluconazole, the first azole, has been replaced by newer, broad-spectrum azoles with much lower MICs for treating dermatophytoses caused by *Trichophyton* species. These newer azoles include clotrimazole, econazole, miconazole, oxiconazole, and sulconazole, all of which are available as topical agents (creams, ointments, and solutions). Along with topical formulations of the allylamine drugs naftifine and terbinafine, these are the drugs of choice in otherwise healthy persons for treating tinea corporis (infection of the trunk, legs, and arms), tinea cruris or jock itch (infection of the groin and pubic area), tinea manuum (infection of one or both hands), and tinea pedis (athlete's foot).

For persons with spreading, persistent, or recurring skin or hair infections, oral drugs may be required in addition to or in place of topical agents. Oral terbinafine, which has an especially low MIC, is the drug of choice in these cases. Oral formulations of azoles, including itraconazole, ketoconazole, and voriconazole, may also be used. All these drugs are more effective and convenient than (and do not have the risks associated with the use of) griseofulvin. Nail bed infections (tinea unguium) caused by *Trichophyton* species are difficult to treat in all persons. These infections require long-term treatment with both a topical agent and oral griseofulvin.

*Ernest Kohlmetz, M.A.*

## FURTHER READING

Richardson, Malcolm D., and David W. Warnock. *Fungal Infection: Diagnosis and Management.* New ed. Malden, Mass.: Wiley-Blackwell, 2010.

Ryan, Kenneth J., and George Ray. *Sherris Medical Microbiology: An Introduction to Infectious Diseases.* 5th ed. New York: McGraw-Hill Medical, 2010.

White, Gary M., and Neil H. Cox. *Diseases of the Skin: A Color Atlas and Text.* 2d ed. Philadelphia: Mosby/Elsevier, 2006.

## WEB SITES OF INTEREST

*Centers for Disease Control and Prevention, Division of Foodborne, Bacterial, and Mycotic Diseases*
http://www.cdc.gov/nczved/divisions/dfbmd

*Microbiology and Immunology On-line: Mycology*
http://pathmicro.med.sc.edu/book/mycol-sta.htm

**See also:** Antifungal drugs: Mechanisms of action; Antifungal drugs: Types; Athlete's foot; Chromoblastomycosis; Dermatomycosis; Dermatophytosis; *Epidermophyton*; Fungal infections; Fungi: Classification and types; Jock itch; *Malassezia*; *Microsporum*; Mold infections; Mycoses; Onychomycosis; Prevention of fungal infections; Ringworm; Skin infections; Treatment of fungal infections.

# Tropical medicine

CATEGORY: Epidemiology
ALSO KNOWN AS: Endemic tropical disease, global medicine, neglected tropical disease

## DEFINITION

Tropical medicine is the study of diseases that occur principally in tropical regions of the world. Tropical diseases flourish predominately in hot, humid climates. The year-round hot climate and large amounts of rain in such regions afford insects and other organisms greater opportunity to transmit certain diseases to humans. Mosquitoes and flies are the most common carriers of these diseases. In areas with a cold season, these carriers hibernate each year, thus controlling and limiting infectivity.

Given that these diseases disproportionately affect poor and underdeveloped areas, poverty plays an important role in their prevalence. Therefore, tropical medicine is primarily a discipline aimed at maintaining the health of impoverished persons. The main concerns of tropical medicine are direct health care, preventive health care strategies, education, and research of diseases that disproportionately affect the world's poorest peoples.

## HISTORICAL PERSPECTIVE

Scottish physician Sir Patrick Manson is considered the founder of tropical medicine. In 1877, Manson began publishing his research findings while working in Formosa (now Taiwan) for the Chinese government. His research would lay the foundation for the study of infectious diseases and for the study of tropical medicine. Manson discovered that the filarial worm, the causative agent for elephantiasis (a tropical disease), was transmitted to humans by mosquitoes. This paved the way for further discoveries regarding insect-borne diseases, including the malaria infection cycle by English physician Sir Ronald Ross, who won the Nobel Prize in Physiology or Medicine in 1902 for his studies of malaria.

Years later, these discoveries led to the establishment of the Liverpool School of Tropical Medicine, founded in 1898. It was the first institution dedicated solely to research and education in tropical diseases. The London School of Hygiene and Tropical Medicine, now a college of the University of London, was founded the following year by Manson.

By the early twentieth century, the transmission cycles for most insect-borne diseases were known. These

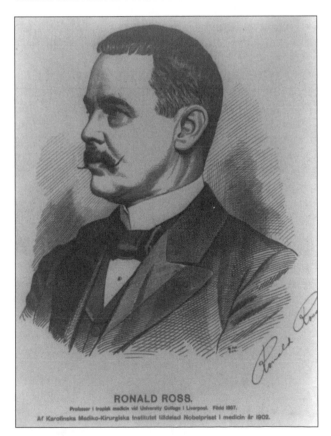

*Ronald Ross.* (LLL)

diseases would be fought with evermore sophisticated methods, using insect control, antibiotics, and advances in molecular biology.

Disease control, however, also led to a dramatic reduction in funding for research and education in tropical and preventive medicine. Concurrently, global population growth and urbanization were occurring. By the 1990's, previously controlled tropical diseases in certain populations saw a resurgence, despite warnings from experts decades earlier. While acquired immunodeficiency syndrome (AIDS), malaria, and tuberculosis received the bulk of research funding and education attention, other neglected tropical diseases flourished during the latter part of the twentieth century.

Even with advancements in combating tropical diseases worldwide, the prevalence of such diseases remains high among the poorest populations. Areas particularly affected are primarily rural, impoverished regions of Africa, Asia, and the Americas. The World Health Organization (WHO) provides funding and training for the treatment of neglected tropical diseases. These neglected tropical diseases remain the primary focus of the discipline of tropical medicine.

## MAJOR DISEASES OF TROPICAL MEDICINE

Although malnutrition, genetic blood disorders, sexually transmitted diseases, and environmental concerns are addressed by experts in tropical medicine, the treatment of infectious diseases remains the prime focus. While a few diseases once prevalent in the tropics have garnered more research and financial attention, many more tropical diseases still flourish in impoverished areas.

Tropical diseases are caused by a variety of organisms, including bacteria, viruses, and worms. These diseases cause gastrointestinal, nervous system, and cardiopulmonary disorders. The diseases of greatest concern and focus are African sleeping sickness (trypanosomiasis), the buruli ulcer (*Mycobacterium ulcerans*), Chagas' disease (American trypanosomiasis), cysticercosis, dengue fever, rabies, leishmaniasis, schistosomiasis, onchocerciasis (river blindness), lymphatic filariasis (which causes elephantiasis), cholera, Rift Valley fever, yaws, yellow fever, dracunculiasis (guinea worm disease), echinococcosis, trachoma, Ebola hemorrhagic fever, and Lassa fever.

## PREVENTION AND CONTROL

Major international health groups, including WHO, have established programs to control tropical diseases in the poorest areas of Africa, Asia, Central America, and South America. Several strategies have been implemented by these groups, including controlling the population of insects and other carriers of disease by the use of insecticides and residential sleeping nets, and by the reduction of wetland waters. Improved water sanitation is necessary to prevent the spread of disease. Affected populations need access to vaccinations and medications for the prevention and treatment of infections, and they need access to adequate health care and health education. If the spread of disease is to be halted, communities need strong human and veterinary public-health infrastructures. Poverty should be addressed through a multidisciplinary approach that includes self-sufficiency and education.

Neglected tropical diseases receive little or no attention from researchers and academic institutions, compared with the attention given to, for example, AIDS, tuberculosis, and malaria. Many of the world's largest health agencies agree that neglected tropical diseases could be controlled at a comparatively nominal cost, and WHO has called upon educational institutions and pharmaceutical companies to donate medical personnel, health services, and medications to residents of affected regions.

## IMPACT

According to WHO, more than one billion people are infected with tropical diseases worldwide. On average, two million people are killed by malaria annually and more than one-half million deaths occur yearly as a result of neglected tropical diseases. The majority of deaths are of children, particularly those who live in poverty. Physical disabilities and infant mortality are also direct results of these diseases.

To measure the epidemiological and economical impact of a disease, health experts have developed the disability-adjusted life year (DALY) measure. It is calculated by assessing the sum of the years of potential life lost because of premature mortality and the years of productive life lost because of disability. Malaria has a global DALY of 46 million life years lost annually. The neglected tropical diseases cause more than 1 billion life years lost per year. These losses result in decreased productivity, negative impacts on families, reduction of the labor force, and increased costs of health care. The medication requirements and the productivity loss from tropical disease is especially devastating for communities relying on agriculture for income and subsistence. Global health experts believe that tropical diseases are major, critical obstacles to improved economic growth in impoverished areas.

*Marie President, M.D.*

#### FURTHER READING

Cook, Gordon C., and Alimuddin I. Zumla, eds. *Manson's Tropical Diseases.* 22d ed. Philadelphia: Saunders/Elsevier, 2009. This textbook offers an extensive discussion of tropical diseases.

Hotez, Peter J. "Neglected Tropical Disease Control in the 'Post-American World.'" *PLoS Neglected Tropical Diseases* 4, no. 8 (August, 2010). Available at http://www.plosntds.org. Examines the realities of disease control as a global concern in a truly global world.

_____, et al. "Control of Neglected Tropical Diseases." *New England Journal of Medicine* 357 (2007): 1018-1027. Discusses how tropical diseases can be managed and controlled.

Jong, Elaine C., and Russell McMullen, eds. *Travel and Tropical Medicine Manual.* 4th ed. Philadelphia: Saunders/Elsevier, 2008. A useful reference manual with advice on preventing, evaluating, and managing diseases that can be acquired in tropical environments.

Kealey, Alison, and Robert Smith. "Neglected Tropical Diseases: Infection, Modeling, and Control." *Journal of Health Care for the Poor and Underserved* 21 (2010): 53-69. Focuses on the epidemiology of tropical diseases affecting the world's poor.

Lorenzo Saviol. *Working to Overcome the Global Impact of Neglected Tropical Diseases.* Geneva: World Health Organization, 2010. Addresses the wide-reaching nature of tropical diseases and the work being done to overcome them.

#### WEB SITES OF INTEREST

*American Society of Tropical Medicine and Hygiene*
http://www.astmh.org

*Global Health Council*
http://www.globalhealth.org/infectious_diseases

*Neglected Tropical Diseases Coalition*
http://www.neglectedtropicaldiseases.org

*World Health Organization*
http://www.who.int/topics/tropical_diseases

**See also:** Blood-borne illness and disease; Carriers; Developing countries and infectious disease; Disease eradication campaigns; Emerging and reemerging infectious diseases; Epidemics and pandemics: Causes and management; Epidemiology; Flies and infectious disease; Globalization and infectious disease; Insect-borne illness and disease; Mosquitoes and infectious disease; Public health; Sleeping nets; Social effects of infectious disease; Transmission routes; Vectors and vector control; World Health Organization (WHO).

---

# *Trypanosoma*

CATEGORY: Pathogen
TRANSMISSION ROUTE: Blood

#### DEFINITION

The numerous species of *Trypanosoma* cause many diseases in vertebrates, most notably Chagas' disease and trypanosomiasis in humans.

---

**Taxonomic Classification
for *Trypanosoma***

**Kingdom:** Protista
**Phylum:** Sarcomastigophora
**Class:** Zoomastigophorea
**Order:** Kinetoplastida
**Family:** Trypanosomatidae
**Genus:** *Trypanosoma*
**Species:**
 *T. brucei brucei*
 *T. brucei gambiense*
 *T. brucei rhodesiense*
 *T. evansi*

---

#### NATURAL HABITAT AND FEATURES

*Trypanosoma* is one of several genera within the order Kinetoplastida. All species are flagellate parasites that contain a special structure unique to this order called the kinetoplast, found within the kinetosome, which contains the mitochondrial DNA (deoxyribonucleic acid). Most trypanosomes are heterozenous, living one stage of their lives in the blood and tissues of a vertebrate host; in other stages they dwell within the intestines of blood-sucking (hematophagous) invertebrates.

Within the Trypanosomatidae, six life cycles occur, depending upon the genus. These life cycles are the amastigote, promastigote, choanomastigote, epimastigote, opisthomastigote, and trypanomastigote. The life-cycle designations are based upon the location of the flagellum on the body surface, the body shape, and the position of the kinetoplast/kinetosome. The life cycle that defines *Trypanosoma* is the trypanomastigote. The morphological features of this stage include a posterior position of the kinetosome; a long, whip-like flagellum running along the surface of the organism; and a set of pellicular microtubules that provide support for the parasite when the flagellum beats.

Two broad groups, or sections, of trypanosomes designated by parasitologists are the Salivaria and the Stercoraria. These designations are based upon where the parasites settle within the invertebrate vector's body. If the trypanosomes develop within the anterior portion of the invertebrate's digestive tract, they belong to the Salivaria section. These parasites will be transmitted to the vertebrate host through the invertebrate's saliva or other oral secretions. If the trypanosomes develop in the posterior portion or hind gut of the invertebrate host, they are in the Stercoraria section. Trypanosome species infect the vertebrate host through fecal material that the invertebrate vector sheds while feeding.

## PATHOGENICITY AND CLINICAL SIGNIFICANCE

Within the Salivaria section are three subspecies of trypanosomes: *T. brucei brucei*, *T. brucei gambiense*, and *T. brucei rhodesiense*. These subspecies occur in parts of Africa, specifically the area that coincides with the range of their vector, the tsetse fly (*Glossina* spp.). *T. b. brucei* is a parasite of the native antelopes and other ruminant animals of this region; the parasite causes a deadly disease called nagana in domestic livestock.

*T. b. gambiense* and *T. b. rhodesiense* are the parasites of both East and West types of trypanosomiasis (African sleeping sickness), which are transmitted by the bite of the tsetse fly. Humans are the reservoirs for *T. b. gambiense*, whereas native game animals provide the reservoirs for *T. b. rhodesiense*. In both forms of sleeping sickness, pathogenesis is similar, with the trypano-

somes entering the site of the tsetse fly's bite. A small sore develops at the spot, and within one to two weeks a widespread parasitemia develops in the bitten person. Initially, the trypanosomes live in the blood, lymph nodes, and spleen, causing intermittent fever episodes. *T. b. rhodesiense* rarely enters the central nervous system because the infected person tends to die before this can occur. *T. b. gambiense* does invade the central nervous system, causing increased somnolence, tremors, paralysis, and convulsions before coma and death ensue.

*T. cruzi*, of the Stercoraria section of trypanosomes, causes Chagas' disease. *T. cruzi* is transmitted by hemipteran insects of the family Reduviidae, which are known colloquially as kissing bugs or cone-nosed bloodsuckers. *T. cruzi* occurs throughout most of Central America and South America, and in some areas of the southern and southwestern United States. Dogs, cats, armadillos, opossums, wood rats, and a number of other domestic and wild animals serve as reservoirs for the parasite, which afflicts millions of people.

When a reduviid insect bites, it often deposits feces containing trypanosomes on the skin of the human. If the bitten person then scratches the bite or inadvertently rubs mucous membranes that contain fecal material, the trypanosomes gain entry to the body. An acute local inflammatory reaction occurs at the site, producing a red sore called a chagoma, or a swelling of the eyelid and conjunctiva (Romana's sign) if the eyelid was the infection site. The local reaction is followed in one to two weeks by a generalized parasitemia, which affects virtually every body tissue. Muscle and nerve cells are especially affected. If left untreated, Chagas' disease may cause death in three to four weeks. If the person survives, the chronic stage of the disease generally affects the heart, destroying the cardiac muscle. In some manifestations of Chagas' disease, the esophagus and colon become greatly enlarged because of the destruction of muscle and nervous tissue.

Throughout northern Africa, Asia Minor, southern Russia, India, parts of southwestern Asia, Indonesia, the Philippines, Central America, and South America, another trypanosome, *T. evansi*, causes a fatal disease generally known as surra. Horses, elephants, camels, deer, and other mammals are susceptible to infection from this disease. Horseflies (*Tabanus* spp.) are the primary vectors of *T. evansi*, although in South America, vampire bats fulfill that role.

For many years, *T. evansi* was not known to infect

humans; however, in 2005, the first case of typanoso-miasis caused by this species was diagnosed in a person in India.

## Drug Susceptibility

Trypanosomiasis in humans has proved challenging to treat because trypanosomes are continuously changing their surface antigens. Because the surface antigens of the parasites are being released into the blood of the bitten person almost constantly, large amounts of the host's immunoglobulins are being produced in an attempt to counteract the trypanosomes' attack.

In the early stage of infection by *T. b. gambiense*, treatment involves the use of the drug pentamidine or, alternatively, suramin. In later stages, if the central nervous system is involved, eflornithine, melarsoprol, or nifurtimax are used. For cases of *T. b. rhodesiense* infection, early-stage treatment is by suramin and late-stage treatment is with melarsoprol. Treatment with melarsoprol, because of its arsenical basis, may cause encephalopathy in the patient and must be used with great care.

*Lenela Glass-Godwin, M.S.*

## Further Reading

Bacchi, Cyrus J. "Chemotherapy of Human African Trypanosomiasis." *Interdisciplinary Perspectives on Infectious Diseases* (2009): 1-6. Provides an update on chemotherapeutic treatments for both forms of African sleeping sickness. Available at http://www.hindawi.com/journals/ipid/2009/195040.cta.html.

Jong, Elaine C., and Russell McMullen, eds. *Travel and Tropical Medicine Manual.* 4th ed. Philadelphia: Saunders/Elsevier, 2008. A useful reference manual with advice on preventing, evaluating, and managing diseases that can be acquired in tropical environments and countries outside the United States.

Joshi, P. P., et al. "Treatment and Follow-up of the First Case of Human Trypanosomiasis Caused by *Trypanosoma evansi* in India." *Transactions of the Royal Society of Tropical Medicine and Hygiene* 100, no. 10 (2006): 989-991. Provides details of the medical treatment of the person in India who contracted *T. evansi*.

Roberts, Larry S., and John Janovy, Jr. *Gerald D. Schmidt and Larry S. Roberts' Foundations of Parasitology.* 8th ed. Boston: McGraw-Hill, 2009. A classic work focusing on parasites of humans and domestic animals.

Seguraa, E. L., and S. Sosa-Estani. "Protozoan Diseases: Chagas' Disease." In *International Encyclopedia of Public Health*, edited by Stella Quah and Kris Heggenhougen. Boston: Academic Press/Elsevier, 2008.

## Web Sites of Interest

*American Society of Tropical Medicine and Hygiene*
http://www.astmh.org

*Centers for Disease Control and Prevention*
http://www.cdc.gov/parasites

*Emerging and Reemerging Infectious Diseases Resource Center*
http://www.medscape.com/resource/infections

**See also:** African sleeping sickness; Antiparasitic drugs: Mechanisms of action; Antiparasitic drugs: Types; Chagas' disease; Children and infectious disease; Developing countries and infectious disease; Diagnosis of protozoan diseases; Emerging and reemerging infectious diseases; Encephalitis; Flies and infectious disease; Insect-borne illness and disease; Insecticides and topical repellants; Intestinal and stomach infections; Myocarditis; Parasites: Classification and types; Prevention of protozoan diseases; Protozoa: Structure and growth; Protozoan diseases; Treatment of protozoan diseases; Tropical medicine; Trypanosomiasis; Trypanosomiasis vaccine; Vectors and vector control.

# Trypanosomiasis

**Category:** Diseases and conditions
**Anatomy or system affected:** Blood, lymphatic system, nervous system
**Also known as:** African lethargy, African sleeping sickness, Gambian sleeping sickness, trypanosomosis

## Definition

Trypanosomiasis is a tropical parasitic disease transmitted by the African tsetse fly, which infects the blood, lymphatic system, and nervous system in humans and animals.

## The Tsetse Fly

The tsetse fly acts as a carrier for trypanosomiasis, a parasite that causes sleeping sickness, which is a wasting disease. When sleeping sickness is acute, the symptoms are high temperature, anemia, fitful appetite, and swollen limbs. The infected person eventually sinks into an irritable haze, then slips into a coma and dies.

Sleeping sickness has had a long history in Africa. One subspecies of the trypanosomiasis parasite lives amicably in the bloodstream of wild animals such as antelope. However, when it gets into a cow, it makes the animal waste away and die. As a consequence, raising livestock has been difficult or impossible in much of sub-Saharan Africa. Still, the tsetse fly is cheered by conservationists because it makes so much of Africa largely uninhabitable for humans and cattle, thus preserving wildlife. However, it is estimated that disease spread by the tsetse fly threatens millions of people in Africa annually.

### CAUSES

Trypanosomiasis is caused by a bite from the tsetse fly, an insect found only in sub-Saharan Africa. This fly conveys the *Trypanosoma* parasite. Trypanosomiasis also can be transferred through the placenta during pregnancy. Additionally, laboratory workers have become infected with trypanosomiasis by accidentally pricking their skin with needles infected with *Trypanosoma*.

### RISK FACTORS

Because the vector of trypanosomiasis, the tsetse fly, is found only in rural areas of sub-Saharan Africa, those who frequent those areas, and villagers, hunters, and fishermen, are at greatest risk. Persons inhabiting rural African woodland and savannah regions, especially near bodies of water and dense vegetation, are most susceptible.

### SYMPTOMS

The symptoms of trypanosomiasis include fever, headaches, swollen lymph nodes, extreme fatigue, skin rash, itching, joint and muscle pain, weight loss, confusion, sleepiness, slurred speech, impaired coordination, and altered personality.

### SCREENING AND DIAGNOSIS

After conducting a physical examination and after questioning the patient about symptoms and medical history, a physician will draw blood and spinal fluid samples. Electron microscopy of spinal fluid is necessary to confirm a diagnosis of trypanosomiasis because trypanosomiasis frequently is asymptomatic or manifests mild symptoms in its initial stage, and because it is sometimes difficult to discern in blood.

### TREATMENT AND THERAPY

Five drugs are used to treat trypanosomiasis, depending upon the stage of the illness. Suramin and pentamidine are used to treat trypanosomiasis in its initial stage, when it is confined to the blood and lymphatic systems. If trypanosomiasis is advanced and has infected the nervous system, then melarsoprol or eflornithine, sometimes combined with nifurtimox, is administered in a hospital setting. For two years after treatment, at six-month intervals, the patient's spinal fluid is drawn and tested for trypanosomiasis because the patient may relapse or become reinfected, requiring further treatment.

### PREVENTION AND OUTCOMES

The World Health Organization has greatly reduced trypanosomiasis by treating male tsetse flies with radiation—rendering them sterile—then releasing them back into the environment, thereby lowering the number of tsetse flies. Although there is no vaccine or drug that prevents trypanosomiasis, several steps may be taken to reduce the likelihood of infection. In endemic areas, one should use netting or screens around tents or other living areas to barricade against insects. All skin, wherever possible, should be covered by medium-weight clothing to protect against insect bites. Bright and dark colors should be avoided because tsetse flies are attracted to those colors; one should instead wear light colors.

Tsetse flies bite during the daytime, but they repose in bushes during the hottest part of the day, so bushes and dense vegetation should be avoided if possible. Because tsetse flies are attracted to swirling dust created by moving vehicles on the African savannah, vehicles should be examined carefully for tsetse flies before being entered.

*Mary E. Markland, M.A.*

## FURTHER READING

Dumas, Michel, Bernard Bouteille, and Alain Buguet, eds. *Progress in Human African Trypanosomiasis, Sleeping Sickness.* New York: Springer, 1999.

Kruel, Donald. *Deadly Diseases and Epidemics: Trypanosomiasis.* New York: Chelsea House, 2007.

Maudlin, I., P. H. Holmes, and M. A. Miles, eds. *The Trypanosomiases.* Cambridge, Mass.: CABI, 2004.

World Health Organization. "African Trypanosomiasis (Sleeping Sickness)." Available at http://www.who.int/mediacentre/factsheets/fs259.

## WEB SITES OF INTEREST

*American Society of Tropical Medicine and Hygiene*
http://www.astmh.org

*Centers for Disease Control and Prevention*
http://www.cdc.gov/parasites

*Emerging and Reemerging Infectious Diseases Resource Center*
http://www.medscape.com/resource/infections

*World Health Organization*
http://www.who.int

**See also:** African sleeping sickness; Antiparasitic drugs: Mechanisms of action; Antiparasitic drugs: Types; Chagas' disease; Developing countries and infectious disease; Diagnosis of protozoan diseases; Emerging and reemerging infectious diseases; Encephalitis; Flies and infectious disease; Insect-borne illness and disease; Intestinal and stomach infections; Myocarditis; Parasitic diseases; Prevention of protozoan diseases; Protozoa: Structure and growth; Protozoan diseases; Treatment of protozoan diseases; Tropical medicine; *Trypanosoma*; Trypanosomiasis vaccine; Vectors and vector control.

---

# Trypanosomiasis vaccine

CATEGORY: Prevention

## DEFINITION

African trypanosomiasis, also known as African sleeping sickness, is a potentially fatal, vector-borne parasitic disease of sub-Saharan Africa. Protozoan parasites cause trypanosomiasis. Human disease is transmitted through the bite of a tsetse fly. Despite many years of effort, no effective vaccine has been developed to prevent trypanosomiasis in humans.

## IMMUNIZATION

Trypanosomiasis vaccine development has been thwarted by the organism's ability to evade its human host's immune system. It does this by changing its surface glycoprotein. These variable surface glycoproteins (VSGs) switch spontaneously and by immune pressure. The rapid switching of VSGs has resulted in more than one thousand unique VSG types. Because of this constantly changing surface coat, the development of any vaccine has been thought unlikely. However, more recent identification of invariant surface proteins, and DNA (deoxyribonucleic acid) vaccine technology, promise hope for a future vaccine. Vaccine prototypes are being constructed and tested against controls in animal models.

## PATHOLOGY

African trypanosomiasis occurs in thirty-six sub-Saharan countries. There are two forms of the infection. *Trypanosoma brucei gambiense*, which causes disease in western and central parts of Africa, is the most common form; it causes about 95 percent of all cases. *T. b. rhodesiense* causes infections that occur in eastern and southern Africa. The bite of the tsetse fly is often painful and results in a chancre. The bite is followed by fever, headache, muscle ache, itching, and lymphadenopathy within one to four weeks.

*T. b. gambiense* infection may occur months or years before secondary disease symptoms emerge. *T. b. rhodesiense* develops more rapidly toward secondary infection. Symptoms of secondary infection are caused by invasion of the central nervous system and include confusion, personality changes, loss of coordination, slurred speech, and seizure. Death can occur if the infection is left untreated. Disturbance of the sleep cycle results in somnolence, and in the final stages of infection, a comatose state develops, giving rise to the common name sleeping sickness.

## PATHOGENICITY

Rural populations of sub-Saharan Africa who are involved in agriculture, fishing, and herding are at greatest risk. Infected tsetse fly bites are the most common mode of transmission, but infection can also be spread from a pregnant woman to her fetus across the placenta; the infection also can be spread through blood transfusion. Domestic and wild animals may serve as a reservoir for the disease.

During the first stage of infection, called the hemolympahtic stage, symptoms are caused by hemolysis. During the second stage of disease, called the neurologic or meningoencepahlitic stage, the parasite crosses the blood-brain barrier to infect the central nervous system, eventually resulting in coma and death if not treated.

### IMPACT

Public health efforts to control trypanosomiasis have led to a drop in the number of reported cases (to below ten thousand). The latest epidemic occurred in 1970. Many cases still go unreported, so the actual number of cases is probably closer to thirty thousand.

Treatment of trypanosomiasis is complex. Once the disease crosses the blood-brain barrier, drugs become more toxic and difficult to administer. The development of an effective vaccine would help significantly in controlling this potentially fatal disease.

*Christopher Iliades, M.D.*

### FURTHER READING

Carvalho, Joanna, et al. "Developing a Vaccine for African Trypanosomiasis: Only Wishful Thinking or a Definite Possibility?" *BMC Proceedings* 2, suppl. 1 (September 23, 2008): 9.

Centers for Disease Control and Prevention. "Trypanosomiasis, African." Available at http://www.dpd.cdc.gov/dpdx/html/trypanosomiasisafrican.htm.

Jong, Elaine C., and Russell McMullen, eds. *Travel and Tropical Medicine Manual.* 4th ed. Philadelphia: Saunders/Elsevier, 2008.

Plotkin, Stanley A., Walter A. Orenstein, and Paul A. Offit. *Vaccines.* 5th ed. Philadelphia: Saunders/Elsevier, 2008.

World Health Organization. "African Trypanosomiasis (Sleeping Sickness)." Available at http://www.who.int/mediacentre/factsheets/fs259.

### WEB SITES OF INTEREST

*Centers for Disease Control and Prevention*
http://www.cdc.gov/vaccines

*Emerging and Reemerging Infectious Diseases Resource Center*
http://www.medscape.com/resource/infections

*Vaccine Research Center*
http://www.niaid.nih.gov/about/organization/vrc

*World Health Organization*
http://www.who.int/immunization

**See also:** Antiparasitic drugs: Mechanisms of action; Antiparasitic drugs: Types; Chagas' disease; Children and infectious disease; Developing countries and infectious disease; Emerging and reemerging infectious diseases; Encephalitis; Encephalitis vaccine; Flies and infectious disease; Immunity; Immunization; Intestinal and stomach infections; Myocarditis; Parasitic diseases; Tropical medicine; *Trypanosoma*; Trypanosomiasis; Vaccines: History; Vaccines: Types; Vectors and vector control; Virology.

---

# Tuberculosis (TB)

CATEGORY: Diseases and conditions
ANATOMY OR SYSTEM AFFECTED: All

### DEFINITION

Tuberculosis (TB) is a contagious infectious disease with either active or inactive forms. Although TB can affect many organ systems, it mostly affects the lungs.

### CAUSES

Tuberculosis is caused by the bacterium *Mycobacterium tuberculosis.* Persons near someone with active TB of the lungs may inhale the bacteria if the infected person coughs or sneezes. TB is easily spread in crowded conditions. It is also easily spread among people who are ill or who have weakened immune systems.

### RISK FACTORS

The factors that increase the chance of developing TB include a weakened immune system or chronic diseases (highest risk); human immunodeficiency virus infection; malnutrition; intravenous drug use;

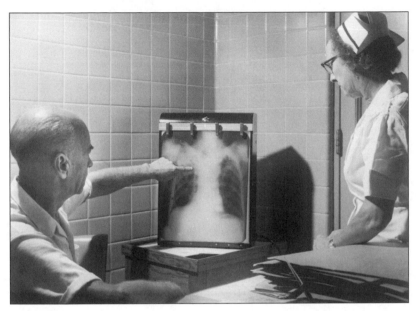

*A physician and nurse examine a chest X ray showing tuberculosis, circa 1963.* (CDC)

alcoholism; leukemia, lymphoma, and other cancers; poorly controlled diabetes mellitus; severe kidney disease; corticosteroids; some medications used for treating rheumatoid arthritis and other diseases, including etanercept, infliximab, and adalimumab; and a suppressed immune system caused by medications, such as drugs to prevent rejection of a transplanted organ.

Other risks factors include silicosis (an occupational lung disease) and living in crowded, indoor conditions (such as homeless shelters, dormitories, and military barracks). Persons at higher risk for TB are infants, young children, and the elderly.

## SYMPTOMS

Tuberculosis causes no symptoms in most persons. In others it is fatal. The bacteria lie dormant in the lungs and may remain there permanently without causing illness. During this time, the infected person cannot spread TB to others. The infection spreads only when the bacteria are active.

Other symptoms for TB are a severe cough that lasts more than two weeks, coughing up blood and sputum (mucus from deep in the lungs), pain in the chest, weakness or fatigue, unexplained weight loss, chills, fever, night sweats, and loss of appetite.

## SCREENING AND DIAGNOSIS

A skin test is used to screen for TB. A small amount of tuberculin test fluid is injected into the skin of the lower part of the arm. The test is positive if, after two to three days, a raised, firm welt appears at the injection site. The welt is 10 mm or greater in diameter (5 mm or 15 mm under some situations). A positive test means a person was exposed to TB, even if he or she never became ill. People at high risk for TB should have a skin test regularly. Also, a blood test is available to screen for TB. If a person has symptoms or signs of active TB, a doctor may order a chest X ray and also get samples of sputum to test for the presence of the bacterium.

## TREATMENT AND THERAPY

Medication can prevent TB from becoming active. It can also help cure active TB. One should take all medication as prescribed, even if the symptoms disappear. If a person does not finish the medication, he or she may develop drug-resistant TB, which is difficult to cure.

Persons who have a positive skin test but no signs of active TB may need to take medication to prevent active TB. The drug isoniazid is usually given for six months or longer. For persons with active TB, a doctor may prescribe a combination of isoniazid, rifampin, pyrazinamide, ethambutol, or streptomycin. Under special circumstances, other drugs may be prescribed.

A person with active TB must be isolated from friends, family, and coworkers until a doctor determines the person is no longer contagious. This is usually after the first several weeks of the infected person taking medication. Isolation will help prevent the spread of TB. Infected persons can resume normal activities after getting a doctor's approval and will need to continue taking the prescribed drugs until the doctor says it is okay to stop. Drugs may need to be taken for six months and, in some cases, up to two years.

## PREVENTION AND OUTCOMES

If the infected person has a positive skin test, he or she might be able to prevent active TB from developing by taking medication. A TB vaccine is available, but it is not routinely used in the United States because of the unreliable protection it provides. A person with active TB can prevent its spread by avoiding contact with people and by taking all medication as prescribed for the full course of treatment.

*Michelle Badash, M.S.;*
*reviewed by David L. Horn, M.D., FACP*

**FURTHER READING**

Centers for Disease Control and Prevention. "The Difference Between Latent TB Infection and Active TB Disease." Available at http://www.cdc.gov/tb/topic/basics.

Levitzky, Michael G. *Pulmonary Physiology.* 7th ed. New York: McGraw-Hill Medical, 2007.

Maartens, G., et al. "Tuberculosis." *The Lancet* 370 (2007): 2030.

Rom, William N., and Stuart M. Garay, eds. *Tuberculosis.* 2d ed. Philadelphia: Lippincott Williams & Wilkins, 2004.

West, John B. *Pulmonary Pathophysiology: The Essentials.* 7th ed. Philadelphia: Wolters Kluwer/Lippincott Williams & Wilkins, 2008.

**WEB SITES OF INTEREST**

*American Lung Association*
http://www.lungusa.org

*Canadian Lung Association*
http://www.lung.ca

*Centers for Disease Control and Prevention*
http://www.cdc.gov/tb

*National Institute of Allergy and Infectious Diseases*
http://www.niaid.nih.gov

**See also:** Airborne illness and disease; Bronchiolitis; Bronchitis; Coccidiosis; Contagious diseases; Croup; Diphtheria; Legionnaires' disease; Mycobacterial infections; *Mycobacterium*; Pleurisy; *Pneumocystis*; Pneumocystis pneumonia; Pneumonia; Tuberculosis (TB) vaccine; Vaccines: History; Vaccines: Types; Whooping cough.

# Tuberculosis (TB) vaccine

CATEGORY: Prevention
ALSO KNOWN AS: Bacille Calmette-Guérin vaccine, Bacillus Calmette-Guérin vaccine

**DEFINITION**

The tuberculosis (TB) vaccine is a weakened strain of live bacteria that infect cattle. The vaccine was developed by Albert Calmette and Camille Guérin to prevent TB, an infectious disease of humans and animals caused by various strains of bacteria of the genus *Mycobacterium.* The weakened strain (*M. bovis*) was obtained by repeated growth in ox bile media until a strain was produced that would not kill experimental animals and would not revert to an infectious state. The vaccine, also known as BCG (for its developers), was first used as a vaccine in 1921 after thirteen years of development.

**VACCINE ADMINISTRATION**

BCG is administered through the skin either by injection or by multiple punctures. Localized skin reactions can occur after vaccination. If drainage occurs, the wound must be covered to prevent transmission of the weakened live bacteria. Serious side effects may include bone infection and disseminated disease, especially in persons who have compromised immune systems.

**VACCINE EFFICACY**

Studies have shown that BCG protects against tuberculous meningitis and miliary (disseminated) TB in children, but that it provides inadequate prevention against pulmonary TB in adults. These variable outcomes may have been influenced by study designs, geographical location, and statistical factors. Studies also conflict on the duration of protection, ranging from ten to fifteen years to fifty to sixty years

Several factors may influence vaccine efficacy, including the immune status of vaccinated persons. For example, although persons exposed to *Mycobacterium* that is endemic to their environment have some inherent protection against *Mycobacterium* infections, their immune response to BCG is not as pronounced as in persons who have not been exposed to *Mycobacterium,* such as newborns, infants, and those who live in nonendemic areas.

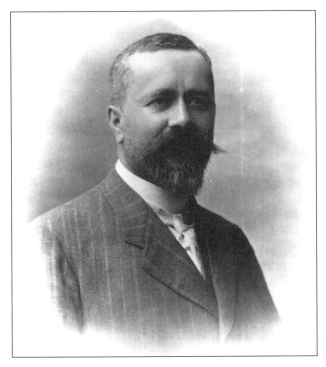

*Albert Calmette.* (LLL)

## OFFICIAL RECOMMENDATIONS

BCG is not generally recommended in the United States because of the low prevalence of TB and because of variable vaccine efficacy and interference of BCG with the tuberculin skin test (TST). Selective use of BCG is recommended in some persons, such as children, with negative TST, and who are continually exposed to either adults with untreated TB or to persons infected by strains resistant to isoniazid and rifampin. Health care workers should be considered for BCG vaccination in specific situations.

BCG vaccination should not be given to immunocompromised persons, such as those with cancer, those with viral infections such as human immunodeficiency virus (HIV), and those taking medications (such as steroids) that cause immune suppression. Pregnant women should not be vaccinated because of the presence of live bacteria in the vaccine.

## FUTURE VACCINES

A number of TB vaccines are under investigation because of the appearance of drug resistant strains, the threat of TB in immunocompromised persons, the easy spread of the disease through the air, and the increasing number of infections relative to population growth. These newer vaccines include genetically modified BCG strains, *M. tuberculosis* mutants, *M. tuberculosis* antigens introduced by viruses, and substances included in vaccine modifiers (adjuvants).

## IMPACT

The BCG vaccine is the most commonly used vaccine in the world; more than three billion people have been immunized. The vaccine confers protection, though with variable efficacy, against different manifestations of tuberculosis. A more effective vaccine against TB is needed, as it is a contagious disease that infects two billion people, approximately one-third of the world's population.

*Miriam E. Schwartz, M.D., Ph.D.,*
*and Shawkat Dhanani, M.D., M.P.H.*

## FURTHER READING

Aronson, N. E., et al. "Long-Term Efficacy of BCG Vaccine in American Indians and Alaska Natives: A Sixty-Year Follow-up Study." *Journal of the American Medical Association* 291 (2004): 2086-2091.

Dockrell, Hazel M., and Ying Zhang. "A Courageous Step Down the Road Toward a New Tuberculosis Vaccine." *American Journal of Respiratory and Critical Care Medicine* 179 (2009): 628-629.

Hoft, D. F. "Tuberculosis Vaccine Development: Goals, Immunological Design, and Evaluation." *The Lancet* 372 (2008): 164-175.

West, John B. *Pulmonary Pathophysiology: The Essentials.* 7th ed. Philadelphia: Wolters Kluwer/Lippincott Williams & Wilkins, 2008.

## WEB SITES OF INTEREST

*Centers for Disease Control and Prevention*
http://www.cdc.gov/tb

*Vaccine Research Center*
http://www.niaid.nih.gov/about/organization/vrc

*World Health Organization*
http://www.who.int/tb

**See also:** Airborne illness and disease; Bronchiolitis; Bronchitis; Coccidiosis; Contagious diseases; Croup;

Diphtheria; Legionnaires' disease; Mycobacterial infections; *Mycobacterium*; Pleurisy; *Pneumocystis*; Pneumonia; Prevention of bacterial infections; Respiratory route of transmission; Tuberculosis (TB); Vaccines: Types; Whooping cough.

# Tularemia

CATEGORY: Diseases and conditions
ANATOMY OR SYSTEM AFFECTED: All
ALSO KNOWN AS: Deer-fly fever, rabbit fever

## DEFINITION

Tularemia is a rare bacterial infection that can be deadly. Governments have studied its use as a biological weapon that releases bacteria into the air. The disease occurs naturally through exposure to infected animals or insects or to contaminated water or food.

There are different types of the disease, depending on where the exposure and symptoms occur. These types are ulceroglandular (skin), glandular (lymph nodes), oculoglandular (eye), oropharyngeal (mouth and throat), intestinal (bowels), pneumonic (lung), and typhoidal (systemwide disease).

## CAUSES

The bacterium *Francisella tularensis* causes tularemia. There are two strains of the bacterium, and one causes infection more easily than the other. The bacteria are normally found in small animals, such as mice and rabbits. The germs can survive for weeks in a cool, moist environment. A person can catch the disease if bitten by an infected animal, tick, or deer fly. Infection also can occur through contact with an infected animal's tissues or with contaminated water, food, or soil. The bacteria also can enter a person's body through the lungs, eyes, mucous membranes, or skin. The infection cannot be passed from person to person.

## RISK FACTORS

The main risk factor for tularemia is exposure to the bacteria. Exposure can occur through hunting, trapping, or butchering infected animals; working with infected animals or their tissue; working in a laboratory with the bacteria; biological terrorism; eating meat from an infected animal; and bites by an infected mosquito or tick.

## SYMPTOMS

Symptoms usually occur three to five days after exposure, but they can begin earlier or later. Symptoms vary depending on where the bacteria enter the body. Other factors include the amount of bacteria, their strength, and the ability of the infected person's immune system to fight the germs.

Pneumonic symptoms include fever, chills, fatigue, headache, body aches, sore throat, cough, and a burning sensation or pain in chest. Ulceroglandular symptoms include a raised, red bump that continues to swell. The raised area opens, drains pus, and forms an ulcer, and it may form a dark scab. Other symptoms are swollen and tender lymph nodes, a fever, and chills. Glandular symptoms include swollen, tender lymph nodes that are not sore. Oculoglandular symptoms include sensitivity to light; tearing; a puffy eyelid; swelling, redness, and sores in the eye; and swollen lymph nodes. Oropharyngeal symptoms include irritated membranes in the mouth, sore throat, ulcers in the throat or on tonsils, and swollen lymph nodes. Intestinal symptoms include fever, abdominal pain, diarrhea, and vomiting.

Typhoidal symptoms fever, chills, headache, muscle aches, poor appetite, nausea, vomiting, diarrhea, abdominal pain, and cough. Symptoms of progression from other types include swollen lymph nodes, difficulty breathing, bleeding, confusion, coma, organ failure, shock, and death.

## SCREENING AND DIAGNOSIS

A doctor will ask about symptoms, medical history, and possible source of exposure, and will perform a physical exam. Tests may include a chest X ray, examination of body fluids using special techniques and precautions, a skin test to assess immune response, a culture of body fluids to check for bacteria, and a blood test to detect antibodies to the bacteria. Other cases in the infected person's environment would alert health care workers of the possibility of a bioterrorism attack.

## TREATMENT AND THERAPY

Antibiotics typically produce a quick response to the lung disease. The drugs are injected in a muscle or given through a vein. Later in treatment, some drugs can be given by mouth. Treatment lasts ten to fourteen days. The antibiotics that might be prescribed include streptomycin, with or without chloramphenicol; gentamicin; doxycycline; and quinolone antibiotics, such as ciprofloxacin. In addition to drug therapy, the lymph nodes may require draining. All cases of tularemia are reported to public health officials.

## PREVENTION AND OUTCOMES

Antibiotics may be ordered in the event of a terrorism exposure. An affected population may be placed on "fever watch" and will receive drugs after developing a fever or flulike symptoms. A vaccine exists to help prevent tularemia, but the vaccine is only partially effective. The vaccine is not available in the United States and is not recommended for the general population. However, it is recommended for laboratory workers who are in regular, close contact with large quantities of the organism.

Measures to prevent the disease from natural causes include not handling sick or dead animals; wearing gloves, a mask, and goggles if skinning or butchering animals; completely cooking game meats; wearing protective clothing if in areas where ticks or deer flies live; using tick repellant; checking skin often for ticks; not touching a tick with one's hands; and following precautions when working in a laboratory.

*Reviewed by David L. Horn, M.D., FACP*

## FURTHER READING

Centers for Disease Control and Prevention. "Tularemia." Available at http://emergency.cdc.gov/agent/tularemia.

Farlow, Jason, et al. "*Francisella tularensis* in the United States." *Emerging Infectious Diseases* 11, no. 12 (December, 2005): 1835-1841.

Henderson, Donald A., Thomas V. Inglesby, and Tara Jeanne O'Toole. *Bioterrorism: Guidelines for Medical and Public Health Management.* Chicago: American Medical Association, 2002.

Jay, James M., Martin J. Loessner, and David A. Golden. *Modern Food Microbiology.* 7th ed. New York: Springer, 2005.

Khardori, Nancy, and Robert C. Moellering, Jr., eds. "Bioterrorism and Bioterrorism Preparedness." *Infectious Disease Clinics of North America* 20, no. 2 (June, 2006).

Mandell, Gerald L., John E. Bennett, and Raphael Dolin, eds. *Mandell, Douglas, and Bennett's Principles and Practice of Infectious Diseases.* 7th ed. New York: Churchill Livingstone/Elsevier, 2010.

Nigrovic, L. E., et al. "Tularemia." *Infectious Disease Clinics of North America* 22 (2008): 489.

Pickering, Larry K., et al., eds. *Red Book: 2009 Report of the Committee on Infectious Diseases.* 28th ed. Elk Grove Village, Ill.: American Academy of Pediatrics, 2009.

## WEB SITES OF INTEREST

*Center for Biosecurity*
http://www.upmc-biosecurity.org

*Centers for Disease Control and Prevention, Emergency Preparedness and Response*
http://emergency.cdc.gov

*National Institute of Allergy and Infectious Diseases*
http://www.niaid.nih.gov

*Todar's Online Textbook of Bacteriology*
http://www.textbookofbacteriology.net

*U.S. Department of Agriculture, Food Safety Information Center*
http://foodsafety.nal.usda.gov

**See also:** Anthrax; Arthropod-borne illness and disease; Bacterial infections; Biological weapons; Bioterrorism; Blood-borne illness and disease; Contagious diseases; Flies and infectious disease; Food-borne illness and disease; *Francisella*; Hantavirus infection; Insect-borne illness and disease; Lyme disease; Malaria; Melioidosis; Plague; Rat-bite fever; Respiratory route of transmission; Rodents and infectious disease; Soilborne illness and disease; Ticks and infectious disease; Waterborne illness and disease; Zoonotic diseases.

# Typhoid fever

CATEGORY: Diseases and conditions
ANATOMY OR SYSTEM AFFECTED: All
ALSO KNOWN AS: Enteric fever

## DEFINITION

Typhoid fever and paratyphoid fever are serious illnesses caused by *Salmonella* bacteria, either *S. typhi* or *S. paratyphi*, respectively. The illness occurs most often

## Development of Typhoid Fever

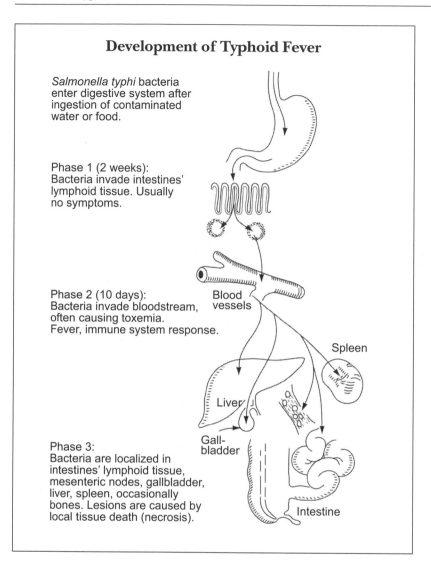

*Salmonella typhi* bacteria enter digestive system after ingestion of contaminated water or food.

Phase 1 (2 weeks): Bacteria invade intestines' lymphoid tissue. Usually no symptoms.

Phase 2 (10 days): Bacteria invade bloodstream, often causing toxemia. Fever, immune system response.

Blood vessels

Spleen

Liver

Gallbladder

Phase 3: Bacteria are localized in intestines' lymphoid tissue, mesenteric nodes, gallbladder, liver, spleen, occasionally bones. Lesions are caused by local tissue death (necrosis).

Intestine

in developing countries where sanitation is poor. Typhoid fever can be fatal, especially if not treated.

### CAUSES

Typhoid fever is caused by eating foods or drinking beverages contaminated with the *Salmonella* bacterium. Contamination can occur from food or drinks handled by someone who is sick or getting sick with typhoid fever, food or drinks handled by someone who has no symptoms but carries the bacteria, water or food contaminated by sewage, unpasteurized dairy products, and poultry products left unrefrigerated. Once bacteria enter the body, they infect the intestine. Bacteria can be carried through the bloodstream to other organs.

### RISK FACTORS

Risk factors for typhoid fever include drinking contaminated water, eating raw shellfish, eating fruits and vegetables that are raw or have been washed with contaminated water, and living in, or recent travel, to a country with poor sanitation.

### SYMPTOMS

Symptoms, which may develop within one to three weeks after exposure, include fever, often for a prolonged time; chills; severe headaches; constipation or diarrhea; abdominal pain; fatigue or lethargy; loss of appetite; rose-colored spots on the body; dizziness; muscle pain; and swelling of the neck glands, liver, or spleen.

### SCREENING AND DIAGNOSIS

A doctor will ask about symptoms and medical history and will perform a physical exam. Typhoid fever is usually diagnosed with a blood culture.

### TREATMENT AND THERAPY

Typhoid fever, which is highly contagious, is treated with antibiotics. In some cases, people may become typhoid carriers even after their illness has subsided. People who are chronic carriers can shed contagious *Salmonella* bacteria in their stool or urine. This chronic condition can be treated with antibiotics or, in unusual cases, surgery.

### PREVENTION AND OUTCOMES

There are two main ways to prevent typhoid fever: vaccination and careful food monitoring. A typhoid vaccine is recommended for persons planning to visit a country in which typhoid fever is prevalent. However, the vaccine is not always effective, and careful food monitoring is just as important. When in an area where typhoid fever is prevalent, one should always take the following precautions with food and water: Drink only bottled water or water that has been boiled for a minimum of one minute; eat foods while they are still hot and ensure that they are thoroughly cooked; avoid raw fruits and vegetables that cannot be peeled; avoid raw shellfish; and avoid unpasteurized dairy products.

*Michelle Badash, M.S.;*
*reviewed by David L. Horn, M.D., FACP*

**FURTHER READING**

Bhan, M. K., R. Bahl, and S. Bhatnagar. "Typhoid and Paratyphoid Fever." *The Lancet* 366 (August 27-September 2, 2005): 749-762.

Levine, M. M. "Typhoid Fever." In *Bacterial Infections of Humans: Epidemiology and Control,* edited by Philip S. Brachman and Elias Abrutyn. 4th ed. New York: Springer Science, 2009.

Mintz, Eric. "Typhoid and Paratyphoid Fever." In *CDC Health Information for International Travel 2010.* Available at http://wwwnc.cdc.gov/travel/yellowbook/2010/table-of-contents.aspx. (See chapter two.)

Murray, Patrick R., Ken S. Rosenthal, and Michael A. Pfaller. *Medical Microbiology.* 6th ed. Philadelphia: Mosby/Elsevier, 2009.

Tortora, Gerard J., Berdell R. Funke, and Christine L. Case. *Microbiology: An Introduction.* 10th ed. San Francisco: Benjamin Cummings, 2010.

**WEB SITES OF INTEREST**

*Centers for Disease Control and Prevention*
http://www.cdc.gov

*National Center for Emerging and Zoonotic Infectious Diseases*
http://www.cdc.gov/ncezid

*Public Health Agency of Canada*
http://www.phac-aspc.gc.ca

*World Health Organization*
http://www.who.int

**See also:** Amebic dysentery; Cholera; Contagious diseases; Developing countries and infectious disease; Food-borne illness and disease; Intestinal and stomach infections; *Salmonella; Shigella;* Shigellosis; Travelers' diarrhea; Typhoid vaccine; *Vibrio;* Waterborne illness and disease.

# Typhoid vaccine

CATEGORY: Prevention

**DEFINITION**

Typhoid vaccines prevent infection caused by *Salmonella* bacteria found in areas of poor sanitation worldwide.

**PATHOGEN AND DISEASE CHARACTERISTICS**

Typhoid fever, an acute illness of fever, rash, and malaise caused by *S. enterica,* serotype typhi (commonly known as *S. typhi*), is distinguished from typhus by its intestinal symptoms. Humans are the only source, and bacteria are spread through fecal contamination of food and water sources. An estimated 22 million cases of typhoid and approximately 200,000 deaths occur each year worldwide, but only 400 cases occur in the United States (primarily in travelers). Approximately 2 to 4 percent of people with acute fever become chronic carriers.

**VACCINE DEVELOPMENT AND DESCRIPTIONS**

Early typhoid vaccines had numerous adverse effects, poor efficacy, or low potency. An inactivated injection and an oral attenuated version are now available and are active against strains of *S. typhi,* but even these are not 100 percent effective; approximately 50 to 80 percent of recipients are protected.

Typhim VI is an inactivated cell surface polysaccharide vaccine of *S. typhi,* Ty2 strain for intramuscular administration; it contains 0.25 percent phenol preservative, is safe for ages two years and older, and should be administered a minimum of two weeks before possible typhoid exposure. Boosters are recommended every two years if necessary.

Vivotif, an oral vaccine against typhoid, contains live attenuated virus from the Ty21a strain. The four-capsule regimen should be administered a minimum of one week before possible exposure; one capsule is taken every other day. Vivotif is safe for ages six years and older and should be swallowed whole with a cool liquid, one hour before a meal. Boosters should be given every five years. Both products require refrigeration at 2° to 8° Celsius (36° to 46° Farhenheit) before use.

**VACCINATION SETTINGS AND RISK GROUPS**

Vaccination is recommended for travelers to areas

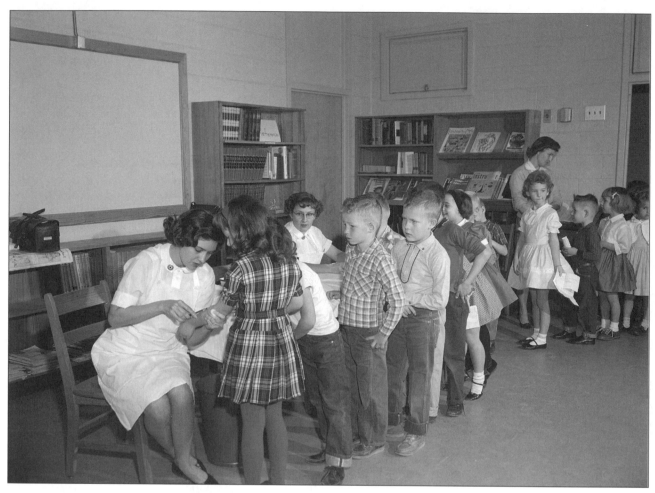

*Schoolchildren wait in line to receive a typhoid vaccine, circa 1950.* (CDC)

without proper sanitation, for persons who have contact with people who are carriers of *S. typhi*, and laboratory staff who work with pure typhoid culture. (Higher rates of fever are noted in these technicians.)

*S. typhi* is spread through unclean water sources in Africa, Asia, Central America, and South America. Disease risk is greatest for travelers to South Asia, for longer durations of travel, and for travelers visiting friends or family.

### Adverse Effects and Contraindications

Typhoid vaccines are not recommended for common use in local populations of risk areas or for treatment of chronic carriers.

Vaccine side effects are mild and typically resolve within forty-eight hours. Adverse effects of fever, headache, injection site reaction (with intramuscular administration), and gastrointestinal upset causing reduced capsule absorption (with oral vaccine) occur in less than 10 percent of cases. Immune diseases may increase the risk of any adverse events.

Vaccine contraindications are acute febrile illness and previous allergic reaction (such as hoarseness, wheezing, and anaphylaxis) to the vaccine. Live vaccine should not be given to persons with a weakened immune system (such as from human immunodeficiency virus infection), to persons with cancer or who are undergoing cancer treatments, to persons receiving immunomodulating drug treatment or corticosteroid treatment for more than two weeks, and for persons receiving certain antibiotics, such as sulfonamides, within one day of a planned vaccination.

## IMPACT

Typhoid incidence decreased dramatically with vaccine use and with improved sanitation and prevention measures. Because the vaccine is not 100 percent effective, vaccinated travelers should practice preventive measures, such as boiling raw foods, avoiding drinks with ice, and using only boiled or bottled liquids when traveling in countries without adequate sanitation.

*Nicole M. Van Hoey, Pharm.D.*

## FURTHER READING

Centers for Disease Control and Prevention. "Typhoid Fever." Available at http://www.cdc.gov/nczved/divisions/dfbmd/diseases/typhoid_fever.

"Immunization: Typhoid Vaccine." In *Mandell, Douglas, and Bennett's Principles and Practice of Infectious Diseases*, edited by Gerald L. Mandell, John E. Bennett, and Raphael Dolin. 7th ed. New York: Churchill Livingstone/Elsevier, 2010.

Levine, Myron M. "Typhoid Fever." In *Bacterial Infections of Humans: Epidemiology and Control*, edited by Philip S. Brachman and Elias Abrutyn. 4th ed. New York: Springer Science, 2009.

_____. "Typhoid Fever Vaccines." In *Vaccines*, edited by Stanley A. Plotkin, Walter A. Orenstein, and Paul A. Offit. 5th ed. Philadelphia: Saunders/Elsevier, 2008.

Mintz, Eric. "Typhoid and Paratyphoid Fever." In *CDC Health Information for International Travel 2010*. Available at http://wwwnc.cdc.gov/travel/yellowbook/2010/table-of-contents.aspx. (See chapter 2.)

## WEB SITES OF INTEREST

*Centers for Disease Control and Prevention*
http://www.cdc.gov/vaccines

*MedlinePlus. "Typhoid Vaccine"*
http://www.nlm.nih.gov/medlineplus/druginfo/meds/a607028.html

**See also:** Bacterial infections; Cholera; Developing countries and infectious disease; Food-borne illness and disease; Immunization; Intestinal and stomach infections; *Salmonella*; Salmonellosis; *Shigella*; Shigellosis; Travelers' diarrhea; Typhoid fever; Vaccines: Types; *Vibrio*; Waterborne illness and disease.

# Typhus

CATEGORY: Diseases and conditions
ANATOMY OR SYSTEM AFFECTED: Lungs, respiratory system, skin
ALSO KNOWN AS: Brill-Zinser disease, epidemic typhus, jail fever, murine typhus

## DEFINITION

Typhus is an acute fever characterized by a disseminated rash. It is caused by primitive bacteria in the genus *Rickettsia* and spread by arthropod bites. Historically, epidemic typhus has caused massive mortality during wars and famines.

## CAUSES

A minimum of two distinct diseases are classified as typhus: epidemic typhus, caused by *R. prowazekii*, and murine typhus, caused by *R. typhi*. The Rickettsiae are primitive, obligately parasitic, gram-negative bacteria that grow and reproduce entirely within the cells of their hosts. Most rickettsial diseases of humans and other mammals are spread by the bites of ectoparasitic arthropods, including lice, fleas, mites, and ticks. Lice are the principal vectors of epidemic typhus and fleas of murine typhus. Both diseases affect other species of mammals, including rodents.

## RISK FACTORS

Typhus emerges as a major health problem when people are crowded together and living in filthy, unsanitary conditions that promote the proliferation of lice, fleas, and rats, which serve as animal reservoirs. Typhus is more prevalent in temperate rather than tropical regions and among people who need heavy clothing, blankets, and enclosed spaces to keep warm but who also have no means of keeping clean.

In temperate zones, such conditions usually accompany war or famine. Typhus epidemics raged during the Irish famines of 1816-1817 and 1843-1845; the latter epidemic spread to port cities in England, Canada, and the United States when infected immigrants settled in urban slums. Typhus ravaged Eastern Europe during and immediately after World War I and killed an estimated three million people during the Russian civil war (1918-1921). It also was a major source of mortality in Nazi concentration camps during World War II. The invention of DDT (dichloro-diphenyl-trichloroethane) and its use in

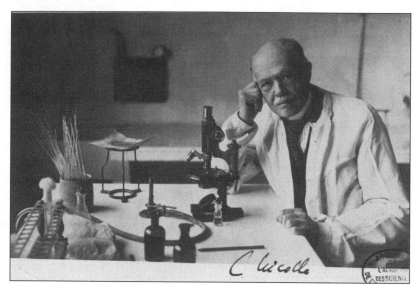

*French bacteriologist Charles Nicolle discovered, in 1909, that typhus is transmitted by lice.*

refugee camps in post-World War II Europe and Asia prevented a repeat of the epidemics that followed World War I.

A person's overall health affects the mortality rate in untreated typhus. Murine typhus has a death rate of less than 2 percent and mainly affects the elderly and others with complicating illnesses and conditions. Before the advent of antibiotics, death rates for epidemic typhus ranged from 10 percent in urban slums to 60 percent during famines.

In later years, significant numbers of human cases of epidemic typhus have occurred only in the Andes Mountains in South America and in the highlands of Burundi and Ethiopia in Africa. Cases in the United States have been traced to flying squirrels, which act as reservoirs. Murine typhus is more common and more widespread, especially in Asia, where it tends to occur in sporadic outbreaks in rural areas. It also is a concern for the homeless population in the southeastern United States.

## SYMPTOMS

The symptoms of murine typhus are a dull red rash that spreads from the abdomen, extremely high fever (105-106° Fahrenheit), abdominal pain, backache, headache, joint pain, dry and hacking cough, nausea, and vomiting. Symptoms of epidemic typhus include chills, dry and hacking cough, high fever, low blood pressure, dull red rash, sensitivity to light, severe headache, severe muscle pain, stupor, and delirium. The disease affects the permeability of small blood vessels, leading to edema in the lungs and brain.

A condition known as Brill-Zinser disease, with symptoms similar to typhus but considerably less severe, sometimes affects elderly people who have a prior history of murine or epidemic typhus. Therapies do not completely eliminate Rickettsiae from the system, so they may lie dormant for decades, resurfacing as a low-level infection when the body's immune defenses decline.

## SCREENING AND DIAGNOSIS

A positive diagnosis of either form of typhus requires a blood test to detect high levels of antibodies to the particular organism. In a clinical setting, medical personnel would be presented with an acutely ill person with a set of symptoms that strongly suggests either typhus or one of the spotted fevers. A person's recent history of exposure to rodents or a history of travel to endemic areas also aid in diagnosis.

Other diseases whose clinical manifestations might be confused with typhus include viral exanthemas, such as measles and rubella, which makes serological testing highly advisable. Epidemiologists and public health workers in some areas screen animal populations to assess the risk of human exposure and advise people on steps they can take to protect themselves.

Historical typhus epidemics can be traced through serological assay of dental pulp in skeletons. This testing has confirmed massive mortality in military operations in Europe in the early eighteenth century, which lends support to the theory that typhus is of New World origin and was imported into Europe by the conquistadores returning home.

## TREATMENT AND THERAPY

A course of the antibiotics doxycycline, tetracycline, or (less commonly) chloramphenicol usually cures typhus. The infected person may need intravenous fluids to counteract dehydration caused by fever and digestive problems. People who have recovered from typhus may have persistent neurological problems or be at risk for other infections.

## PREVENTION AND OUTCOMES

Prevention of typhus centers on the control of vectors. Washing or fumigating clothing and bedding and being vigilant in the detection and elimination of head lice are still important public health measures. Also important is controlling rodent populations in or near human dwellings. The growing resistance of vectors to common insecticides also is a matter of concern for health experts.

Vaccines have been developed for both epidemic and murine typhus. They are recommended only for people traveling to endemic areas who will be working with vulnerable populations or who will be living under less than ideal conditions in rural areas. The U.S. military does not require immunization against typhus for its members.

*Martha A. Sherwood, Ph.D.*

## FURTHER READING

Gratz, Norman. *Vector- and Rodent-Borne Diseases in Europe and North America: Distribution, Public Health Burden, and Control.* New York: Cambridge University Press, 2006. This book examines insect- and rodent-borne diseases, mechanisms to control them, and their epidemiology in Europe, the United States, and Canada.

Hechemy, Karin M., ed. *Century of Rickettsiology: Emerging, Reemerging Rickettsioses, Molecular Diagnostics, and Emerging Veterinary Rickettsioses.* Boston: Blackwell, 2006. A collection of technical papers. Information on animal reservoirs and a number of diseases related to typhus from attacks by domestic dogs and cats.

International Conference on Rickettsiae and Rickettsial Diseases 2005. *Rickettseoses, from Genome to Proteome: Pathobiology and Rickettsiae as an International Threat.* New York: Academy of Sciences Press, 2006. A collection of scientific papers, with the focus on evaluating *Rickettsiae* as a biological warfare agent. Typhus, however, is not a prime concern as a biological weapon.

Sherman, Irwin W. *The Power of Plagues.* Washington, D.C.: ASM Press, 2006. A general overview of the role of epidemic disease in history that includes a chapter on typhus.

## WEB SITES OF INTEREST

*Centers of Disease Control and Prevention*
http://www.cdc.gov/rodents

*National Center for Emerging and Zoonotic Infectious Diseases*
http://www.cdc.gov/ncezid

**See also:** Arthropod-borne illness and disease; Body lice; DDT; Emerging and reemerging infectious diseases; Epidemics and pandemics: History; Fever; Fleas and infectious disease; Head lice; Insect-borne illness and disease; Mites and chiggers and infectious disease; Parasitic diseases; Rat-bite fever; *Rickettsia*; Rodents and infectious disease; Skin infections; Ticks and infectious disease; Vectors and vector control; Zoonotic diseases.

# Typhus vaccine

CATEGORY: Prevention

## DEFINITION

The typhus vaccine is administered to prevent the spread of typhus fever, a rickettsial infection.

## DISEASE CHARACTERISTICS

Typhus and its causal bacterium, *Rickettsia*, were identified in 1909 by Charles Niccole, although the disease's symptoms of fever, red rash, and delirium were described as early as 1489. Four related types of typhus are transmitted by arthropods (such as lice, fleas, mites, and chiggers) that carry distinct strains of *Rickettsia*. A large sore and a rash spread from the bite location within four to six days and may be accompanied by swollen lymph nodes.

Symptoms of acute typhus infection are severe headache, chill, high fever, rash, and stupor. Disease spreads rapidly in crowded areas, particularly in areas of Southeast Asia and South America. Typhus is fatal if not treated. Antibiotic treatment with doxycycline, tetracycline, or chloramphenicol provides a rapid cure. Epidemic typhus, the classic disease, is caused by *R. prowazekii* and is carried by lice; the disease may cause hypotension and neurologic impairment if untreated.

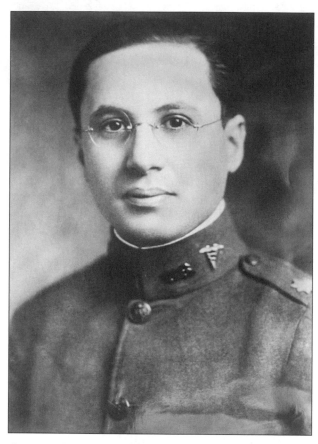

*American bacteriologist Harry Plotz developed a typhus vaccine in 1914.*

## VACCINE HISTORY AND DEVELOPMENT

Early attempts to design vaccines against rickettsial infections focused on Rocky Mountain spotted fever. In 1932, a typhus vaccine was developed by Hans Zinsser to increase the body's antibody response to dead bacteria. During World War II, vaccine need peaked in regions of fighting where the disease was endemic. By 1945, epidemics of typhus in U.S. troops were controlled by the use of the pesticide dichloro-diphenyl-trichloroethane (DDT) to kill lice in crowded, unclean living quarters, and by the use of the typhus vaccine to halt the infection's spread.

Traditionally, typhus vaccines were made with killed, inactivated, whole-cell bacteria, but the marketed typhus vaccine comprised live, attenuated *R. prowazekii* that was harvested in egg yolk sacs. Live, attenuated typhus vaccine was available in freeze-dried, single- or multi-use vials that required storage at colder than 4° Celsius (39° Fahrenheit) until reconstitution. The injection was approved for ages six months and older.

## VACCINATION RISK GROUPS AND CONTRAINDICATIONS

Typhus is transmitted easily in overcrowded populations (such as prisons). Although the vaccine is not required by any country for entry, travelers to Asia should consider typhus vaccine to prevent scrub typhus, the most common form of disease in that area. The vaccine also may be necessary in areas with endemic outbreaks, such as Africa, South America, and Asia, and in areas with diseases that are resistant to antibiotics. Typhus has not been fully eradicated worldwide, and the disease prognosis depends on the risk for complications: older adults experience up to 60 percent mortality with epidemic typhus. Contraindications for receiving a typhus vaccine include a history of egg allergy, an acute infection at time of planned vaccination, and a history of long-term corticosteroid use.

## IMPACT

The typhus vaccine was most useful during World War II, when vaccine administration prevented typhus epidemics among crowded troop populations. Vaccine use diminished greatly with the use of pesticides to kill lice and to halt epidemics. The best prevention for typhus remains repellant use and good hygienic practices (such as regular laundering) to reduce lice and tick populations. No typhus vaccines are produced or in development by U.S. manufacturers.

*Nicole M. Van Hoey, Pharm.D.*

## FURTHER READING

Chattopadhyay, S., and A. L. Richards. "Scrub Typhus Vaccines: Past History and Recent Developments." *Human Vaccines* 3 (2007): 73-80.

Plotkin, Susan L., and Stanley A. Plotkin. "A Short History of Vaccination." In *Vaccines*, edited by Stanley A. Plotkin, Walter A. Orenstein, and Paul A. Offit. 5th ed. Philadelphia: Saunders/Elsevier, 2008.

"Typhus Vaccine." *Time*, July 4, 1932. Available at http://www.time.com/time/magazine/article/0,9171,743926,00.html.

World Health Organization. "Requirements for Louse-Borne Human Typhus Vaccine." Available at http://www.who.int/biologicals/publications/trs/areas/vaccines/typhus.

## WEB SITES OF INTEREST

*Centers for Disease Control and Prevention, Division of Vector Borne Infectious Diseases*
http://www.cdc.gov//ncidod/dvbid

*National Center for Emerging and Zoonotic Infectious Diseases*
http://www.cdc.gov/ncezid

**See also** Arthropod-borne illness and disease; Body lice; DDT; Developing countries and infectious disease; Emerging and reemerging infectious diseases; Fleas and infectious disease; Head lice; Insect-borne illness and disease; Mites and chiggers and infectious disease; Parasitic diseases; *Rickettsia*; Ticks and infectious disease; Vaccines: Types; Vectors and vector control; Zoonotic diseases.

# U

---

## Urethritis

CATEGORY: Diseases and conditions
ANATOMY OR SYSTEM AFFECTED: Bladder, genitalia, genitourinary tract
ALSO KNOWN AS: Urethral infection

### DEFINITION

Urethritis is an inflammation, infection, or irritation of the urethra. The urethra is the tube that carries urine out of the body from the bladder.

### CAUSES

Urethritis is usually caused by bacteria or viruses, including organisms such as *Escherichia coli* and *Klebsiella* that cause bladder or kidney infections; organisms such as *Neisseria gonorrhoeae, Chlamydia trachomatis*, and *Trichomonas vaginalis*, which cause sexually transmitted diseases (STDs); viruses such as herpes simplex, cytomegalovirus, or human papillomavirus; and other bacteria, such as *Ureaplasma urealyticum* and *Mycoplasma genitalium*.

### RISK FACTORS

Risk factors include multiple sexual partners, a recent change in sexual partners, unprotected sex, history of other STDs, bacterial infection of other parts of the urinary tract (such as the bladder, kidney, prostate), medications that lower resistance to bacterial infection, catheter or tube placement in the bladder, acidic foods, and spermicides. Also, females are at higher risk for urethritis.

### SYMPTOMS

There may be no symptoms, especially in women. Approximately 50 percent of men infected with *C. trachomatis* have no symptoms. Symptoms that do occur include pain or burning, or both, while urinating, and blood in the urine. Another symptom is an increase in urinary frequency and urgency. Other symptoms are itching, swelling, and tenderness in the groin; pain during intercourse; discharge from the penis; blood in the semen; pain during ejaculation; and swollen or tender (or both) testicles. If left untreated, urethritis can spread and cause infection in other parts of the urinary tract, such as the bladder, ureters, or kidneys.

### SCREENING AND DIAGNOSIS

The doctor will ask about symptoms and medical history and will perform a physical exam, including a pelvic exam. Urethritis is usually diagnosed from its symptoms. Tests to confirm the diagnosis and identify the organism causing the condition may include a urethral swab for microscopic study or culture, blood and urine tests, and specific tests for gonorrhea, chlamydia, or other STDs.

### TREATMENT AND THERAPY

Urethritis is usually treated with medication. The type of medication will depend on the cause of the urethral infection. Antibiotics are used to treat urethritis caused by bacteria. Antiviral drugs are used to treat urethritis caused by a virus. If urethritis is caused by an STD, all sexual partners should be tested and treated.

### PREVENTION AND OUTCOMES

Steps to prevent urethritis include practicing safer sex by using condoms; using the barrier methods of contraception; urinating immediately after sexual intercourse; treating all sexual partners who are infected or exposed; and regularly drinking increased amounts of fluids, including cranberry juice.

*Rick Alan; reviewed by Adrienne Carmack, M.D.*

### FURTHER READING

"Diseases Characterized by Urethritis and Cervicitis." *Morbidity and Mortality Weekly Report* 55 (2006): 1-94.

Miller, K. E. "Diagnosis and Treatment of *Chlamydia trachomatis* Infection." *American Family Physician* 73 (2006): 1411-1416.

Parker, James N., and Philip M. Parker, eds. *The Official Patient's Sourcebook on Urinary Tract Infection.* San Diego, Calif.: Icon Health, 2002.

Porter, Robert S., et al., eds. *The Merck Manual Home Health Handbook*. 3d ed. Whitehouse Station, N.J.: Merck Research Laboratories, 2009.

Schrier, Robert W., ed. *Diseases of the Kidney and Urinary Tract*. 8th ed. Philadelphia: Wolters Kluwer Health/Lippincott Williams & Wilkins, 2007.

Vasavada, Sandip P., et al., eds. *Female Urology, Urogynecology, and Voiding Dysfunction*. New York: Marcel Dekker, 2005.

### Web Sites of Interest

*Centers for Disease Control and Prevention*
http://www.cdc.gov

*National Kidney and Urologic Diseases Information Clearinghouse*
http://www.niddk.nih.gov

*Our Bodies Ourselves*
http://www.obos.org

*Women's Health Matters*
http://www.womenshealthmatters.ca

**See also:** Acute cystitis; Bacterial vaginosis; Chlamydia; Cytomegalovirus infection; Epididymitis; *Escherichia coli* infection; Genital herpes; Group B streptococcal infection; Herpes simplex infection; Human papillomavirus (HPV) infections; Inflammation; Men and infectious disease; *Mycoplasma*; Neisserial infections; Pelvic inflammatory disease; Prostatitis; Sexually transmitted diseases (STDs); Trichomonas; Women and infectious disease.

# Urinary tract infections

CATEGORY: Diseases and conditions
ANATOMY OR SYSTEM AFFECTED: Bladder, genitourinary tract, kidneys, urinary system

### Definition

A urinary tract infection (UTI) is an infection of the bladder, kidneys, urethra, and uterers (which connect the bladder to the kidneys). A UTI may be limited to one area of these organs or may spread throughout the urinary tract.

### Causes

The urinary tract normally contains no microorganisms. However, sometimes bacteria or yeast from the lower gastrointestinal tract or rectal area enter the urinary tract, usually through the urethra (the tube that allows urine to pass from the bladder). A UTI is caused when these harmful organisms affect the urinary tract.

### Risk Factors

It is possible to develop a UTI with or without the following risk factors:

*Sexual activity.* Frequent sexual intercourse increases the risk of UTI. Having unprotected sex raises the risk still further.

*Medical conditions.* The following medical conditions increase the chance of UTI: urinary tract anatomical defects, vesicoureteral reflux (in which urine washes back up the ureter into the kidneys), diabetes, weakened immune system, kidney stones, enlarged prostate gland, paraplegia or quadriplegia (body paralysis), history of kidney transplant, sickle cell anemia, menopause, and nervous system disorders that make it difficult to completely empty the bladder.

*Medical devices and procedures.* For females, the following devices and procedures increase the chance of UTI: using a diaphragm for birth control; having a partner who uses condoms with spermicidal foam; having a urinary catheter inserted; and having surgery that involves the urinary tract system.

*Medications.* Taking antibiotics for other conditions can increase the risk of getting a UTI.

*Age and gender.* The rate of UTI increases with age in both men and women. The risk of infection increases even further after menopause in women and after age fifty years in men. Women have a high rate of UTI throughout their lives because the openings to the urethra and rectum in women are near one another. Also, the urethra is shorter in women than it is in men.

*Genetic factors.* Researchers are still trying to understand whether certain genetic factors might make someone more prone to UTIs. Studies seem to show that if a mother has a history of multiple UTIs, then her daughter will be more likely to have UTIs too. There also may be some factors related to blood type that increase the risk for infection.

## SYMPTOMS

Although it is possible to have a UTI without any symptoms, most people do notice symptoms, including increased frequency of urination; feeling of urgency, burning, or pain while urinating; itching in the genital area; urinating only small amounts at a time; pain over the area (the pubic area or lower abdomen) of the bladder or pain in the lower back; back and flank pain along the sides under the ribs; blood in the urine or on toilet tissue after wiping (after urination in women); cloudy looking urine, possibly signifying visible pus; unpleasant smell to urine; and new onset of incontinence (inability to hold the urine during the day or at night).

Symptoms that suggest that the infection has reached the kidneys, indicating a more serious problem, are fever and chills and severe pain in the lower back.

Children (babies in particular) may have less common symptoms of UTI, such as irritability, difficulty feeding, incontinence, loose stools, diarrhea, nausea, vomiting, and slow weight gain (failure to thrive). Older people may have more vague symptoms of infection, such as fatigue, confusion, loss of appetite, or trouble walking.

## SCREENING AND DIAGNOSIS

The purpose of screening is early diagnosis and treatment. Screening tests are usually administered to people without current symptoms, but who may be at high risk for certain diseases or conditions.

A doctor will want to discuss the infected person's medical history and current symptoms and will perform a physical examination. The patient will be asked to provide a "clean catch" urine specimen by urinating into a sterile specimen cup.

Urine tests include the following:

*Urine dip.* This test is often performed in a doctor's office. A dipstick coated with special chemicals is dipped into the patient's urine sample. Areas on the stick will change color if blood, pus, bacteria, or other materials are present.

*Microscopic urinalysis.* The urine is examined under a microscope for the presence and quantity of red blood cells, white blood cells (pus), bacteria, and other substances. Microscopic urinalysis is a more accurate way to diagnose a UTI.

*Urine culture and sensitivity test.* A urine sample is sent to a laboratory to see if bacteria will grow. Once the bacteria have been identified, an appropriate antibiotic can be prescribed.

More extensive testing of the urinary system may be necessary for men or children who develop UTIs. Additionally, the doctor may request further testing if there is a concern that the patient has a structural problem with the urinary tract system, or has other conditions, such as urinary stones, vesicoureteral reflux, enlarged prostate, tumors, or polyps. Such further tests includes kidney-ureter-bladder X ray, intravenous pyelogram, kidney ultrasound, spiral computed tomography scan, voiding cystourethrogram, nuclear cystogram, and cystoscopy.

There is no consensus as to whether healthy people should be screened for UTIs. It is common practice to regularly screen pregnant girls and women in their first trimester of pregnancy. Some doctors also screen for UTIs in persons with diabetes.

Urine dip tests and urinalysis are frequently performed as screening tests for conditions other than UTIs (such as in well-child check-ups and other routine adult physical examinations). In the process of using these tests to screen for other conditions, asymptomatic UTIs may be diagnosed. However, these infections do not always need to be treated. Treatment is sometimes required and is often not required.

## TREATMENT AND THERAPY

Urinary tract infections are primarily treated with antibiotic medications. The goals of treatment are to eliminate the bacteria causing the infection and to relieve the discomfort. Treatment involves lifestyle changes, medications, and alternative and complementary treatments. Surgery is generally not considered for treatment.

## PREVENTION AND OUTCOMES

There are a number of recommendations that may help a person prevent UTIs. Persons who have frequent UTIs may be helped by taking a small daily dose of an antibiotic or by taking cranberry tablets. Persons who tend to get an infection after sexual intercourse might be advised to take a dose of antibiotic just before or just after engaging in intercourse. Both trimethoprim-sulfamethoxazole and nitrofurantoin are used in small doses to prevent UTIs. Cranberry extract has been shown to be of similar efficacy with lower side effects.

Other ways to reduce the risk of UTI include drinking increased amounts of water (several eight-ounce glasses each day), which may help flush out the urinary system and wash out bacteria, or drinking cranberry juice too. Some studies have suggested that one to three cups per day makes the urine more acidic, which can help prevent the growth of bacteria.

It is possible that sitting in bath water (especially soapy bath water) may irritate skin tissue and make a person more susceptible to infection. Furthermore, using perfumed products, bubble bath, douches, or feminine hygiene sprays may also increase the risk of developing a UTI.

Women should carefully wipe themselves after urinating or after a bowel movement, from the labia (the front) to the rectum (the rear). This avoids contamination of the urethral or vaginal areas with bacteria from the rectum.

One should avoid holding one's urine for extended periods of time, should ensure that the bladder is emptied completely when urinating, and should urinate before and after sexual intercourse. Also, drinking an eight-ounce glass of water can help flush out bacteria that may have entered the urethra during intercourse.

Finally, one should wear cotton underwear, which is more absorbent than underwear made with artificial fibers. Cotton also wicks moisture from the skin. Artificial fibers, such as nylon and polyester, trap moisture, making an ideal growing environment for bacteria (and yeast), which can promote infections.

*Rosalyn Carson-DeWitt, M.D.*

## FURTHER READING

Alexander, Ivy L., ed. *Urinary Tract and Kidney Diseases and Disorders Sourcebook: Basic Consumer Health Information About the Urinary System.* 2d ed. Detroit: Omnigraphics, 2005. Covers diagnosis and treatment of a range of disorders, including urinary tract infections and kidney and bladder stones.

Boston Women's Health Collective. *Our Bodies, Ourselves: A New Edition for a New Era.* 35th anniversary ed. New York: Simon & Schuster, 2005. An updated discussion of topics related to women's health. A compendium of material relevant to a wide variety of issues, the book contains a well-written section dealing with urinary tract problems.

Gorbach, Sherwood L., John G. Bartlett, and Neil R. Blacklow, eds. *Infectious Diseases.* 3d ed. Philadelphia: W. B. Saunders, 2004. A textbook dealing with the general topic of infectious disease. The section covering urinary tract infections provides a thorough discussion of the subject.

Jepson, R. G., and J. C. Craig. "Cranberries for Preventing Urinary Tract Infections." *Cochrane Database of Systematic Reviews* (2008): CD001321. Available through *EBSCO DynaMed Systematic Literature Surveillance* at http://www.ebscohost.com/dynamed. A review of the medical literature on the use of cranberries in preventing UTI.

McMurdo, M. E., et al. "Cranberry or Trimethoprim for the Prevention of Recurrent Urinary Tract Infections?" *Journal of Antimicrobial Chemotherapy* 63, no. 2 (2009): 389-395. Discusses the possible use of trimethoprim for UTIs.

Parker, James N., and Philip M. Parker, eds. *The Official Patient's Sourcebook on Urinary Tract Infection.* San Diego, Calif.: Icon Health, 2002. Draws from public, academic, government, and peer-reviewed research to provide a wide-ranging handbook for persons with recurring urinary tract infections.

Schrier, Robert W., ed. *Diseases of the Kidney and Urinary Tract.* 8th ed. Philadelphia: Wolters Kluwer Health/Lippincott Williams & Wilkins, 2007. Covers a full range of the biochemical, structural, and functional correlations in the kidney and discusses urological diseases of the genitourinary tract.

## WEB SITES OF INTEREST

*American Urological Association*
http://www.auanet.org

*National Institute of Diabetes and Digestive and Kidney Diseases*
http://www2.niddk.nih.gov

**See also:** Acute cystitis; Bacterial infections; Bacterial vaginosis; *Candida*; Candidiasis; Chlamydia; *Enterococcus*; Gonorrhea; Kidney infection; Men and infectious disease; Oral transmission; Pelvic inflammatory disease; Prostatitis; Sexually transmitted diseases (STDs); Urethritis; Vaginal yeast infection; Women and infectious disease.

# U.S. Army Medical Research Institute of Infectious Diseases

CATEGORY: Epidemiology

## DEFINITION

The U.S. Army Medical Research Institute of Infectious Diseases (USAMRIID) is a branch of the Army Medical Research and Materiel Command.

## MISSION

The USAMRIID, located in Ft. Detrick, Maryland, was established in 1969 by a general order of the Office of the Surgeon General of the Army. The primary mission of the institute is to conduct medical research to develop vaccines, drugs, and specific diagnostic testing protocols to protect U.S. military personnel throughout the world from biological threats and endemic diseases. The institute serves as the main research laboratory for the Biological Defense Research Program. It is the only Department of Defense (DOD) lab that can safely study infectious disease agents that require maximum containment strategies at biosafety levels (BSL) 3 and 4.

Although the foremost mission of the institute is to support members of the Armed Forces, the institute also works closely with civilian agencies such as the Centers for Disease Control and Prevention (CDC) and the World Health Organization (WHO), particularly in epidemiological research and response but also in countering bioterrorism.

## PRIMARY RESEARCH AREAS AND ACCOMPLISHMENTS

Since its inception, the institute has developed and supplied a number of vaccines that have been crucial in controlling disease outbreaks in both military and civilian populations. For example, outbreaks of Rift Valley fever, a viral disease affecting both domestic livestock and humans, occur in areas of eastern and southern Africa, Madagascar, and parts of the Middle East. This mosquito-borne virus (prevalent during years of heavy rainfall) causes, in humans, fever, liver abnormalities, encephalitis, and ocular disease. A vaccine developed at the institute was used in treating high-risk patients in the Rift Valley fever epidemics in Egypt in 1977 and in Senegal and Mauritania in 1988.

Ribavirin, an antiviral drug, may be used to treat future outbreaks.

Tularemia, a disease caused by the bacterium *Francisella tularensis*, occurs naturally in rodent and lagomorph populations. Because *F. tularensis* can be inhaled, the use of aerosol applications of the bacterium as a biological weapon remains a threat. The institute has developed a tularemia vaccine that has been used in specific international outbreaks of the disease, but in the United States, the vaccine is available only to health care workers who routinely work with the bacterium. This vaccine, however, has been under review by the U.S. Food and Drug Administration (FDA) for perhaps more widespread use.

For two decades, the institute has conducted valuable research on Ebola viruses. Ebola hemorrhagic fever is a serious disease occurring in humans and in nonhuman primates. Initially recognized in 1976 in the Democratic Republic of the Congo (formerly Zaire), Ebola virus is one of two members of Filoviridae, a family of ribonucleic acid (RNA) viruses. The virus is responsible for a number of deaths in several African nations, including Gabon, Sudan, Ivory Coast, Uganda, Republic of the Congo, and Democratic Republic of the Congo. Institute staff members have assisted WHO and the CDC with Ebola outbreaks in Africa and have studied antiviral compounds that may be used in a vaccine.

Following the terrorist attacks of September 11, 2001, in the United States, the institute assisted several federal agencies in testing thousands of samples suspected of containing the bacterium that causes anthrax. Anthrax, an acute infectious disease caused by the bacterium *Bacillus anthracis*, can be transmitted to humans through the handling of infected mammalian carcasses or by the inhalation of spores. Because anthrax can infect humans by means of inhalation, the bacterium has been used as a biological weapon. From September, 2001, through May, 2002, institute personnel tested primarily nonmedical samples thought to be contaminated with anthrax. The lab also advised federal and state officials on area decontamination strategies. The anthrax antibiotic treatment protocol was developed at the institute's animal research facility.

In response to the global outbreak of severe acute respiratory syndrome (SARS) in 2003, the institute worked with the CDC to identify antiviral drugs that might be used to control the coronavirus that causes

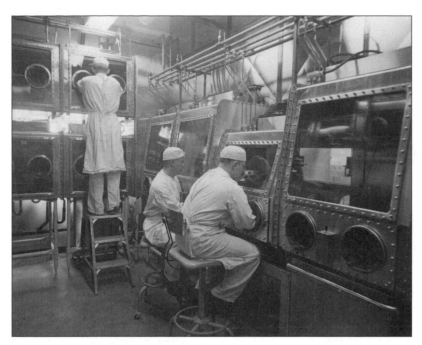

*Technicians in a laboratory at Ft. Detrick, Maryland, in the late 1960's. The U.S. Army ran a biological weapons program here from 1943 to 1969 and then formed USAMRIID to continue medical research into biological warfare. (AP/Wide World Photos)*

the disease. Around 300,000 compounds were tested by the institute's viral therapeutic branch, and of these, one has gone to clinical trials.

### Education and Future Research

The continuing and increasing threat of bioterrorism has led to the critical need for both military and civilian health care professionals to recognize and deal with a biological attack. To address this need, the institute has developed a training series, Medical Management of Biological Casualties, which covers the essential topics of managing the care of the victims of a biological attack. The training course includes classroom, laboratory, and field exercises designed to prepare health care providers with the necessary skills of personal protection and of treatment and decontamination within a biological-attack environment.

The continuing research efforts and goals of the institute include vaccine development for anthrax, plague, botulinum neurotoxins, staphylococcal enterotoxins, hantaviruses, Ebola virus, and Venezuelan equine encephalitis.

### Impact

The USAMRIID provides state-of-the-art research and development to assist health care providers both in the armed forces and in civilian realms in the United States and around the world. Many critical vaccines and treatment protocols for a number of diseases were developed at institute laboratories, and the agency's ongoing research will continue to assist in future international health care efforts.

*Lenela Glass-Godwin, M.S.*

### Further Reading

Borden Institute, Office of the Surgeon General, U.S. Army. Textbooks of Military Medicine. Washington, D.C.: Author. A comprehensive series covering virtually every aspect of military medicine. Provides an easily understood narrative for both military and civilian readers.

Centers for Disease Control and Prevention. "Update: Investigation of Bioterrorism-Related Anthrax and Interim Guidelines for Exposure Management and Antimicrobial Therapy." *Morbidity and Mortality Weekly Report* 50, no. 42 (2001): 909-919. A summary statement of anthrax cases in Florida, New York, New Jersey, Pennsylvania, and the District of Columbia following the September, 2001, terrorist attacks.

Committee on Advances in Technology and the Prevention of Their Application to Next Generation Biowarfare Threats. National Research Council. *Globalization, Biosecurity, and the Future of the Life Sciences.* Washington, D.C.: National Academies Press, 2006. This report describes the challenges in defending against bioterrorism that are posed by advances in the biological sciences.

Friedlander, A. M., and S. F. Little. "Advances in the Development of Next-Generation Anthrax Vaccines." *Vaccine* 27, suppl. 4 (November 5, 2009): D61-64. Summarizes accomplishments by the USAMRIID in improving anthrax vaccines.

Kortepeter, M. G., et al. "Managing Potential Laboratory Exposure to Ebola Virus by Using a Patient

Biocontainment Care Unit." *Emerging Infectious Diseases* 14, no. 6 (June, 2008): 881-887. Provides details of a case study of a USAMRIID scientist infected with Ebola. Outlines the federal government's biosafety level 4 laboratory precautions for other research facilities.

Murray, C. K., and L. L. Horvath. "An Approach to Prevention of Infectious Diseases During Military Deployments." *Clinical Infectious Diseases* 44, no. 3 (2007): 424-430. Examines the U.S. military's approach to deployment medicine, which emphasizes "preparation, education, personal protective measures, vaccines, chemoprophylaxis, and surveillance in an attempt to prevent infectious diseases."

## WEB SITES OF INTEREST

*Centers for Disease Control and Prevention*
http://www.cdc/gov

*Uniformed Services University of the Health Sciences*
http://www.usuhs.mil

*U.S. Army Medical Research Institute of Infectious Diseases*
http://www.usamriid.army.mil

**See also:** Anthrax vaccine; Biological weapons; Biosurveillance; Bioterrorism; Centers for Disease Control and Prevention (CDC); Developing countries and infectious disease; Disease eradication campaigns; Emerging and reemerging infectious diseases; Emerging Infections Network; Epidemics and pandemics: Causes and management; Epidemic Intelligence Service; Epidemiology; Globalization and infectious disease; Infectious disease specialists; Koch's postulates; National Institutes of Health; Outbreaks; Primates and infectious disease; Public health; Social effects of infectious disease; Tropical medicine; World Health Organization (WHO).

---

UTIs. *See* Urinary tract infections.

# V

## Vaccines: Experimental

CATEGORY: Prevention

ALSO KNOWN AS: Candidate vaccines, trial vaccines

### DEFINITION

Experimental vaccines are those vaccines that have yet to be officially approved for medical use. By definition, many experimental vaccines are never approved. Some simply do not produce an immune response, some produce a response that is too weak, and some have serious side effects that researchers consider too risky when compared with the possible benefits of the vaccine.

### HISTORY

The first experimental vaccine of the modern era was Edward Jenner's smallpox vaccine. Jenner observed that people infected with cowpox developed a mild illness but never developed smallpox, a common infection that had killed millions throughout history. In 1796, Jenner used pus from a milkmaid infected with cowpox to inoculate an eight-year-old boy. He later inoculated the boy with smallpox, and no illness ensued, proving his vaccine was successful. From such a modest beginning sprouted a medical revolution that added years to the human life span. The list of diseases against which a successful vaccine has been developed is long, but some of humanity's biggest scourges are not on this list.

Vaccines against malaria, hepatitis C, tuberculosis, and the human immunodeficiency virus (HIV) are some of the most sought after vaccines today. (A vaccine exists for tuberculosis, one that has been in use for decades, but its effectiveness is unclear and its use is controversial.) For each of these diseases, several experimental vaccines are in clinical trials and more experimental vaccines are in development. However, the specifics of each disease present practical challenges that make the development and testing of new vaccines difficult, lengthy, and expensive. For example, the malaria parasite spends little time in the blood-

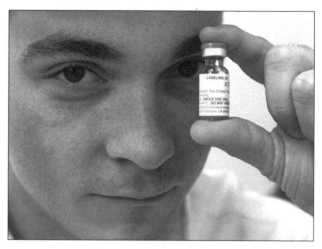

*A drug-study volunteer in 1999 holds a vial of the experimental HIV vaccine AIDSVAX. (AP/Wide World Photos)*

stream once it invades the human body; most of the parasite's development occurs in the liver. Because of this, developing a vaccine that will activate the immune system before the parasite gets into the liver, where it spends most of its time, has been an ongoing challenge.

In addition to looking for vaccines against infectious diseases, researchers are looking for vaccines against specific types of cancers, such as melanoma (a particularly deadly form of skin cancer), and for vaccines that target specific drug addictions (to cocaine and nicotine, for example). In the developing vaccine field, researchers are also trying to develop therapeutic vaccines, those vaccines given to people who are already sick, in an attempt to reduce both the severity of the illness and the risk of transmitting the illness to others.

### TESTING AND TRIALS

Jenner's method of testing his vaccine would be considered criminal today. However, not until the latter half of the twentieth century did the concept of protecting the rights of people in medical research emerge. The concept emerged slowly, but it gained momentum after World War II and even more so when evidence of serious abuse came to light.

Today, participating in clinical studies of experimental vaccines has to be voluntary. Before any volunteers are allowed to participate in a trial, the suggested trial procedure is reviewed by several regulatory and ethics committees. These reviews are designed to ensure the trial is safe and that volunteers are sufficiently informed of the possible dangers of the trial before they agree to participate. Volunteers also must meet strict health criteria to participate in vaccine trials.

## EXPERIMENTAL METHODS OF CREATING IMMUNITY

Many of the ailments for which vaccines are sought present special challenges for researchers. For example, a weakened form of HIV as a vaccine cannot be administered because of the risk that the virus will reappear at full strength. Researchers are therefore trying to create an immune response through several novel methods that do not involve using the entire organism.

One experimental method has been the insertion of some genes from a dangerous virus (such as HIV) into a weakened virus, such as a cold virus, that is known to be relatively safe in humans. When the administered weak virus forms in the body, it forms with some of the proteins of the dangerous virus. Researchers hope the immune system in such cases will learn to recognize these proteins as foreign and will then mount an attack against the dangerous virus if it infects the body. Another experimental method involves, first, identifying the proteins on the surface of a microorganism that produce an immune response and then, second, vaccinating a person with these proteins alone (instead of the whole virus) to produce an immune response.

## IMPACT

Vaccines have played a significant role in bettering human health and prolonging human life. The dreaded childhood diseases of the past, especially of the time before vaccines, no longer claim or maim thousands of young lives each year. All vaccines began as experimental vaccines. As technology advances, and as the understanding of the immune system increases, researchers are taking on bigger, more complex challenges and testing vaccines that could revolutionize medicine for generations to come.

*Adi R. Ferrara, B.S., ELS*

## FURTHER READING

Allen, Arthur. *Vaccine: The Controversial Story of Medicine's Greatest Lifesaver.* New York: W. W. Norton, 2008. Examines the history of vaccines, complete with spectacular failures and controversies, in this well-researched and well-reasoned book.

Artenstein, Andrew W., ed. *Vaccines: A Biography.* New York: Springer, 2010. A thorough history of vaccines and vaccination, with the chapters "Vaccinology in Context" and "The Future of Vaccine Discovery and Development," and chapters on specific diseases.

Offit, Paul. *Vaccinated: One Man's Quest to Defeat the World's Deadliest Diseases.* New York: HarperCollins, 2007. A look at the life of a controversial scientist who developed nine of the most important vaccines of modern times, including vaccines against measles, mumps, rubella, and hepatitis A and B.

Plotkin, Stanley A., Walter A. Orenstein, and Paul A. Offit. *Vaccines.* 5th ed. Philadelphia: Saunders/Elsevier, 2008. An excellent description of the role of vaccines in the prevention of disease. Begins with a history of immunization practices. Chapters deal with a specific disease and the role and history of vaccine production in its prevention.

Speid, Lorna. *Clinical Trials: What Patients and Volunteers Need to Know.* New York: Oxford University Press, 2010. While not specifically about vaccine trials, this book is a good reference for anyone interested in participating in important clinical trials

## WEB SITES OF INTEREST

*Centers for Disease Control and Prevention*
http://www.cdc.gov/vaccines

*College of Physicians of Philadelphia, History of Vaccines*
http://www.historyofvaccines.org

*Global Health Council*
http://www.globalhealth.org

*Vaccine Research Center*
http://www.niaid.nih.gov/about/organization/vrc

*World Health Organization*
http://www.who.int/immunization

**See also:** Centers for Disease Control and Prevention (CDC); Chickenpox vaccine; Cholera vaccine; Cowpox;

Disease eradication campaigns; DTaP vaccine; Emerging and reemerging infectious diseases; Epidemiology; Globalization and infectious disease; Hepatitis vaccines; Immunity; Influenza vaccine; Malaria vaccine; Microbiology; MMR vaccine; Polio vaccine; Public health; Smallpox vaccine; Vaccines: History; Vaccines: Types; Virology; World Health Organization (WHO).

# Vaccines: History

CATEGORY: Prevention

### DEFINITION

Vaccines are substances administered through inoculation, ingestion, or nasal inhalation to stimulate a person's immune system to fight infection.

### DEVELOPMENT HISTORY

In 1796, Edward Jenner (1749-1823) developed the first successful vaccine. Jenner, as the tale of discovery goes, had heard a milkmaid declare "I shall never have smallpox for I have had cowpox. I shall never have an ugly pockmarked face." Jenner, after hearing this, took some pus from a cowpox lesion on the hand of a milkmaid named Sarah Nelmes and used it to inoculate an eight-year-old boy. A few days later, the boy had a mild case of vaccinia, a form of cowpox contracted by humans, but he soon recovered. Six weeks later, Jenner inoculated the boy with smallpox, yet the boy was unaffected by this and subsequent exposures; he had gained immunity from smallpox through the inoculation with cowpox.

Jenner's was the first safe and successful attempt to artificially induce active immunity. To describe this particular style of inoculation, Jenner coined the term "vaccine," from the Latin word *vaccinus*, or "of cows."

About eighty years later, in 1879, Louis Pasteur (1822-1895) furthered the vaccination concept through his work in microbiology. Pasteur was employed to find a solution for chicken cholera, which could wipe out an entire flock in as few as three days. One summer, the cholera cultures used for infecting the test chickens were inadvertently stored in the heat. These cultures produced some symptoms of disease but were no longer deadly to the chickens. When subsequently inoculated with young virulent cultures, the chickens remained unaffected. Pasteur reasoned that the "stale"

cultures were actually attenuated (weakened), and with these attenuated organisms, the chickens had become immune.

In the laboratory, Pasteur learned that by prolonged growth and exposure to oxygen, the microbes could be manipulated to the ideal virulence. This experiment marked the first time a pathogenic microbe was isolated and used as a bacterial vaccine. In 1881, applying the methodology he had developed for the chicken cholera virus, Pasteur and his associates heated anthrax germs, exposed them to the oxidizing agent potassium dichromate, and inoculated a number of sheep.

The rabies vaccine was initially created by Emile Roux, a French doctor and a colleague of Pasteur who had been working with a killed vaccine produced by desiccating the spinal cords of infected rabbits. In 1885, Pasteur successfully vaccinated a shepherd boy who had been bitten fourteen times by a rabid dog. He produced his vaccine for rabies by growing the virus in rabbits and then weakening it by drying the affected nerve tissue. The vaccine had been tested only on eleven dogs before its first human trial. The delay in rabies germs reaching the brain enabled the rabies vaccine to be effective after the bite had occurred.

The first toxoid vaccine was for diphtheria. The diphtheria bacillus was discovered by Edwin Klens in 1883. In 1884, Frederick Loeffler isolated it and grew it in culture. In 1890, Emil Von Behring discovered an antitoxin and subsequently developed a vaccine with a combination of diphtheria toxin and antitoxin. However, he did not deem the vaccine safe for widespread use. In 1924, a researcher at the Pasteur Institute weakened diphtheria toxin with formaldehyde to make a "toxoid" to kill the bacteria. He was able to immunize guinea pigs with his toxoid. Mass vaccination began in New York within three years.

As vaccines continued to be developed and released (bubonic plague, 1897; cholera and typhoid, 1917; pertussis, or whooping cough, 1926; tetanus, 1927; and tuberculosis, 1927), they became more and more integral to utilitarian and public health notions of security, productivity, and protection. Licensing of vaccines began and vaccination became ever more managed by government from the municipal level to the federal level. For example, vaccination became mandatory for infants in the United Kingdom in 1853. In the United States, in 1902, the Biologies Control Act was

## Vaccines Time Line

| Year | Vaccine developed | Vaccine-related events |
| --- | --- | --- |
| 1796 | Smallpox | |
| 1879 | Cholera | |
| 1885 | Rabies | |
| 1890 | Tetanus | |
| 1896 | Typhoid fever | |
| 1897 | Bubonic plague | |
| 1921 | Diphtheria | |
| 1926 | Pertussis (whooping cough) | |
| 1927 | Tuberculosis | |
| 1932 | Yellow fever | |
| 1937 | Typhus | |
| 1945 | Influenza | |
| 1952 | Polio | |
| 1954 | Anthrax<br>Japanese encephalitis | |
| 1955 | Inactivated polio vaccine | |
| 1957 | Adenovirus-4 and 7 | |
| 1961 | Oral polio vaccine | |
| 1963 | Measles<br>Trivalent oral polio vaccine | |
| 1967 | Mumps | |
| 1970 | Rubella | |
| 1971 | Measles, Mumps, & Rubella | Routine smallpox vaccination ceases in the United States |
| 1974 | Chicken pox | |
| 1976 | | Swine flu vaccination ends in the United States |
| 1977 | Pneumonia (*Streptococcus pneumoniae*) | Last indigenous case of smallpox (Somalia) |
| 1978 | Meningitis (*Neisseria meningitidis*) | |
| 1979 | | Last case of polio caused by a wild virus in the United States |
| 1980 | | Smallpox declared eradicated from the world |
| 1981 | Hepatitis B | |
| 1985 | *Haemophilus influenzae* type B | |
| 1986 | | National Childhood Vaccine Injury Act enacted |
| 1988 | | Worldwide Polio Eradication Initiative launched |
| 1989-1991 | | Major resurgence of measles in the United States; two-dose measles vaccine recommended |

## Vaccines Time Line (continued)

| Year | Vaccine | Event |
|---|---|---|
| 1990 | *Haemophilus influenzae* type B polysaccharide conjugate (infants) | U.S. Vaccine Adverse Event Reporting System launched |
| 1991 | | Hepatitis B vaccine recommended for all infants |
| 1992 | Hepatitis A | |
| 1994 | | Polio elimination certified in the Americas<br>Vaccines for Children program launched |
| 1995 | Hepatitis A<br>Varicella | First harmonized childhood immunization schedule published |
| 1996 | Acellular pertussis (infants) | |
| 1998 | Lyme disease<br>Rotavirus | |
| 1999 | | Rotavirus vaccine withdrawn<br>FDA recommends removing mercury from all products including vaccines |
| 2000 | | Worldwide measles initiative launched<br>Measles declared no longer endemic in the United States<br>Pneumococcal conjugate vaccine recommended for all young children |
| 2001 | | United States introduces an emergency stock of smallpox vaccine |
| 2003 | Nasal (influenza) | First live attenuated influenza vaccine licensed for use in persons age five to forty-nine<br>Measles declared no longer endemic in the Americas<br>First Adult Immunization Schedule introduced |
| 2004 | | Inactivated influenza vaccine recommended for children age six to twenty-three months |
| 2005 | | Rubella declared no longer endemic to the United States |
| 2006 | Human papillomavirus | |
| 2009 | Swine flu | |

passed after the deaths of thirteen children in St. Louis, Missouri, in 1901; the children had received diphtheria antitoxin that had been accidentally contaminated with tetanus.

## GOLDEN AGE OF VACCINES

The golden age of vaccines began after World War II. Scientific knowledge had developed enough so that large-scale vaccine production was possible, and several important new vaccines were developed in a relatively short time: influenza (1945), polio (1952), measles (1963), mumps (1967), and rubella (1969). The success in preventing diseases such as polio and measles, of which parents had been terrified, was revolutionary. When the polio vaccine was licensed in 1955, its developer, Jonas Salk, was heralded as a hero. In 1967, the World Health Organization led a huge campaign against smallpox. Within ten years, smallpox had been vaccinated out of existence.

Important vaccines from the late twentieth century

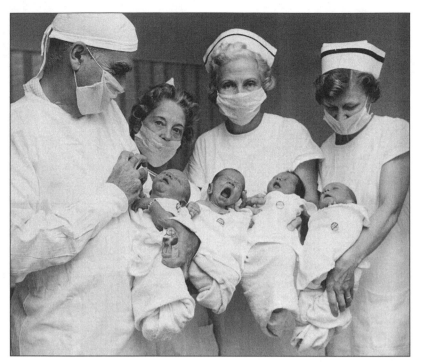

*Newborns receive the oral polio vaccine in Miami, Florida, in 1960.* (AP/Wide World Photos)

include those against meningitis (1975), chickenpox (1996), rotavirus (1998), and the first acellular vaccine (pertussis, 1997). In acellular vaccine production, only the antigenic part of the microbe (for example, the capsule, the flagella, or part of the cell wall) is used. Prompting the replacement of whole-cell pertussis vaccines by acellular variations was the potential for severe side effects after vaccination and the reported shift in the age distribution of pertussis. *Haemophilus influenzae* type B (Hib) vaccine is also acellular. Neither killed nor acellular vaccines induce the strongest immune response and may therefore require booster shots, yet they are safer for use in immunocompromised persons.

In the early twenty-first century, vaccines for adults are becoming increasingly common. For example, a shingles vaccine was licensed in 2008. Unlike childhood vaccines, adult vaccines are not mandated. The first formalized adult immunization schedule was published in 2002 and is updated annually.

## New Vaccine Development

Researchers have examined many possible approaches for vaccines against malaria. One of the most promising approaches has been a subunit vaccine. Researchers in Australia have begun testing another approach: a vaccine that combines killed parasites with an adjuvant to boost immune response.

Researchers also are trying to develop an influenza vaccine that can provide broad protection, including against future strains, so that a single shot would be enough to protect a person from the seasonal flu for ten years or longer.

The human immunodeficiency virus (HIV) is a challenging target for vaccine researchers for many reasons, not the least of which is the virus's lack of stability. The surface proteins of the virus frequently change, keeping the immune system from recognizing it and keeping researchers from pinpointing a surface protein as a successful target for a vaccine.

A number of other vaccine strategies are under experimental investigation. These include deoxyribonucleic acid (DNA) vaccination and recombinant viral vectors.

## Opposition to Vaccination

Vaccination efforts have met with some controversy since their inception. To a great extent, nation-states have responded to this opposition by articulating the right to immunize for the common good. In 1905, for example, the U.S. Supreme Court ruled that the need to protect the public health through compulsory smallpox vaccination outweighed an individual's right to privacy. This principal has been consistently reiterated and is supported by the concept of herd immunity, whereby a certain target of the population (approximately 90 percent, depending on the disease) must be immunized for protection to be conferred upon the entire group.

As a small but vocal antivaccine movement has gained ground, some rates for vaccine-preventable diseases have risen. This is of special concern because many diseases entail complications. In the case of measles, complications include pneumonia and encephalitis. The modern antivaccine movement also claims that vaccines cause autism, either from the additive thiomersal (known in the United States as thimer-osol), which has been used as a vaccine preservative since the 1930's, or from an overload of the combined mumps, measles, and rubella (MMR) vaccine.

The movement was catalyzed by a British doctor, Andrew Wakefield. In 1998, he published his study of twelve children, several of whom developed signs of autism and intestinal symptoms following MMR im-munization. He suggested that the vaccine inflamed the gut in a manner that allowed an unspecified toxic substance to cross into the bloodstream. Although he has stated that his paper does not prove an association between the MMR vaccine and autism, his paper does include parental allegations that he adopted as fact. Wakefield recommended separating the components of the injections by a minimum of one year.

The antivaccination movement gained traction be-cause parents tend to first notice symptoms of autism in their child around the time of the MMR; another factor in the movement's initial success is parental fear of mercury: Thimerosol metabolizes to ethyl mercury, which is often confused with methyl mercury, a neuro-toxin. A 2006 review of scientific studies found "no convincing evidence" that thimerosol had a causal role in the onset of autism. Also, courts have ruled that there is no connection. After a lengthy investigation by a medical fraternity, Wakefield's paper was deter-mined unethical. In February, 2010, *The Lancet* re-tracted Wakefield's 1998 article, noting that elements of his submitted manuscript had been falsified.

## Impact

Jenner's assertion "that the cow-pox protects the human constitution from the infection of smallpox" laid the foundation for modern vaccination. The principle that guided Jenner in developing vaccines is still followed; namely, develop harmless preparations that will induce immune responses and thereby pro-tect persons from pathogens.

Most vaccines today are safe, highly effective, mass produced, and administered to millions of people for long-term protection against infectious diseases. Nothing, except perhaps clean, safe water, has had a more positive effect on reducing deaths and helping populations around the world than vaccines, making vaccination one of the most important public health advances in history.

Vaccines also contribute significantly to the eco-nomic strength of nations. A study in Kenya, for ex-

ample, concluded that the Hib vaccine remains a cost-effective intervention, having saved that nation close to one million dollars in treatment costs for children born in 2004. Vaccines also enhance economic growth by protecting persons from the long-term effects of an illness on their physical, emotional, and cognitive de-velopment. For example, approximately twenty-eight thousand cases of pneumonia and meningitis, five thousand deaths, and one thousand severe neurologic complications are prevented each year in Uganda alone.

At the end of the nineteenth century, the infant mortality rate in the United States was 20 percent, and the childhood mortality rate before age five was an-other 20 percent. Infectious diseases such as measles, diphtheria, smallpox, and pertussis once topped the list of childhood killers. Many of these devastating dis-eases have been contained, especially in industrial-ized nations, because of the development and wide-spread distribution of safe, effective, and affordable vaccines.

Before the development of the diphtheria vaccine in 1923, diphtheria accounted for about 15,500 child deaths and 200,000 illnesses. However, there were only 2 reported cases of diphtheria in 2001. Likewise, in the 1950's, about 20,000 people per year in the United States were affected by polio. The number of paralytic polio cases fell to less than 100 per year after the intro-duction of the vaccine.

After a carefully orchestrated and long-fought erad-ication effort by the World Health Organization, an ef-fort that was supported by national immunization pro-grams, smallpox was eradicated from the planet in 1979. This is perhaps the greatest triumph since the development of vaccines. No naturally occurring cases of smallpox have been found since 1977, and smallpox now exists only in two laboratories: one in the United States and one in Russia. Vigorous debate exists on whether these two stores of the virus should be de-stroyed; were smallpox released into the environment, the results could be devastating. Smallpox vaccination is no longer routine, so the world's population is highly susceptible to the disease, a susceptibility rate that rises each year.

No other pathogen has been eradicated on a global scale, but diphtheria has largely been eradicated in industrialized nations. Also, in 1994, WHO declared the Western Hemisphere free of the wild-type polio virus.

Contemporary evidence of the impact of vaccination on disease incidence was clearly seen in the United Kingdom in 2000. Meningococcal group C infection had been increasing and was responsible for many deaths, particularly in adolescents. In October, 1999, the United Kingdom's health department introduced a vaccination program, and the number of new cases fell from about 145 to about 65 in one year.

Nonimmunized children still die every day from vaccine-preventable diseases. They may also be rendered physically weakened, developmentally delayed, or permanently disabled. Almost eleven million children under the age of five years die each year worldwide because they did not receive vaccinations.

*Stephanie Eckenrode, B.A.*

**FURTHER READING**

Allen, Arthur. *Vaccine: The Controversial Story of Medicine's Greatest Lifesaver.* New York: W. W. Norton, 2007. Written by a Washington journalist, this book tells the story of vaccines from the point of view of public health policy.

Artenstein, Andrew W., ed. *Vaccines: A Biography.* New York: Springer, 2010. A thorough history of vaccines and vaccination, with the chapters "Vaccinology in Context" and "The Future of Vaccine Discovery and Development," and chapters on specific diseases.

Atkinson, W., et al., eds. *Epidemiology and Prevention of Vaccine-Preventable Diseases.* 11th ed. Washington, D.C.: Public Health Foundation, 2009. A comprehensive text on vaccine-preventable diseases. This work is also available at http://www.cdc.gov/vaccines/pubs/pinkbook.

Barquet, N., and P. Domingo. "Smallpox: The Triumph over the Most Terrible of the Ministers of Death." *Annals of Internal Medicine* 127, no. 8 (1997): 635-642. A lively history of the rise and fall of smallpox, a disease that once toppled empires.

Delves, Peter J., et al. *Roitt's Essential Immunology.* 11th ed. Malden, Mass.: Blackwell, 2006. An excellent textbook on the subject of immunology. Much of the book is detailed and requires some background in biology. Nevertheless, the chapters that deal with infection and immunization are clear and contain much that will interest nonscientists.

Plotkin, Stanley A., Walter A. Orenstein, and Paul A. Offit. *Vaccines.* 5th ed. Philadelphia: Saunders/Elsevier, 2008. An excellent description of the role of vaccines in the prevention of disease. Begins with a history of immunization practices. Chapters deal with a specific disease and the role and history of vaccine production in its prevention. The text is appropriate for nonscientists.

**WEB SITES OF INTEREST**

*Centers for Disease Control and Prevention*
http://www.cdc.gov/vaccines

*College of Physicians of Philadelphia, History of Vaccines*
http://www.historyofvaccines.org

*Global Health Council*
http://www.globalhealth.org

*Vaccine Research Center*
http://www.niaid.nih.gov/about/organization/vrc

*World Health Organization*
http://www.who.int/immunization

**See also:** Centers for Disease Control and Prevention (CDC); Chickenpox vaccine; Cholera vaccine; Cowpox; Developing countries and infectious disease; Disease eradication campaigns; DTaP vaccine; Emerging and reemerging infectious diseases; Epidemics and pandemics: Causes and management; Epidemiology; Globalization and infectious disease; Hepatitis vaccines; Immunity; Immunization; Influenza vaccine; Malaria vaccine; Microbiology; MMR vaccine; Outbreaks; Polio vaccine; Public health; Smallpox vaccine; Tuberculosis (TB) vaccine; U.S. Army Medical Research Institute of Infectious Diseases; Vaccines: Experimental; Vaccines: Types; Virology; World Health Organization (WHO).

# Vaccines: Types

CATEGORY: Prevention
ALSO KNOWN AS: Immunization

**DEFINITION**

A vaccine is a suspension of immunogens (molecules that produce an immune response or stimulate production of antibodies) such as weakened or dead pathogenic (disease-causing) cells or cellular components. The act of administering a vaccine, or immunization, is called vaccination. Persons who receive a vaccine are considered immunized against a particular pathogen. Vaccines may contain a pathogen, suspending fluid, adjuvants, excipients, and preservatives.

Several types of vaccines are given to humans. These types include live attenuated, inactivated, component or subunit, toxoid, deoxyribonucleic acid (DNA), and recombinant vector vaccines. Live attenuated vaccines contain altered bacteria or viruses that do not cause disease. Inactivated or killed vaccines contain killed bacteria or inactivated viruses that do not cause disease. Component or subunit vaccines contain parts of the whole bacteria or viruses. Toxoid vaccines contain toxins (or poisons) produced by the pathogen that have been made harmless. DNA and recombinant vector vaccines are investigational. Some vaccines are combinations of pathogens for different diseases, such as the measles, mumps, and rubella (or MMR). Most vaccines are administered by injection into the muscle (intramuscular); however, some may be given into the skin (subcutaneous), by mouth, or into the nose (intranasal).

Active immunity is classified as natural (after pathogen exposure and infection) or acquired (after vaccination). Passive immunity is also classified as natural (across the placenta during pregnancy) or acquired (injection of antibodies or immunoglobulins pooled from several donors). Immunoglobulins are prepared antibodies that are given to a person who has already been infected or who is at risk of acquiring an infection, thereby providing passive immunization. In this case, the immune system does not need to produce antibodies protecting the body.

Herd immunity occurs when most of, but not all, the people in a given population are immune to a pathogen. If there is an outbreak or exposure to a pathogen, those who are immune will sometimes protect those who are not immune from getting the disease; however, those who are not immune are still more likely to get the disease and spread it to others.

## MECHANISMS OF ACTION

A vaccine is given to intentionally expose the immune system to a pathogen in a safe, controlled manner, so that the immune system can react and develop antibodies to that pathogen or antigen. Antibodies are large proteins that help fight infection and control disease. Many antibodies disappear after destroying the invading antigens, but the cells involved in antibody production remain and become memory cells. Memory cells "remember" the original antigen and then defend against it if the antigen attempts to reinfect a person. This protection is called immunity. Therefore, after sufficient antibodies have been developed, the immune system that is re-exposed to that pathogen will react within minutes to hours; the pathogen will be destroyed before a full-fledged infection and organ damage can occur. B cells are a type of lymphocyte (white blood cell) that makes antibodies. B cells use antibodies to identify, inactivate, and help destroy these pathogens.

Vaccines, which provide protection from the disease without the serious symptoms, have a high effectiveness rate (usually 95 to 99 percent). Vaccine failure, meaning that the vaccine administration did not result in antibody production, is uncommon. Several factors can lead to vaccine failure, including having a compromised immune system and the inadequate storage or administration of the vaccine. The immune response to a pathogen may decrease over time, so vaccines known as boosters are sometimes given to restore antibodies. Protective immunity lasts longer with boosters.

A suspending fluid (such as sterile water or saline) is needed to allow the vaccine to be administered. Preservatives and stabilizers, such as albumin, phenols, and glycine, keep the vaccine from being changed. Adjuvants, or enhancers, help the vaccine work. Adjuvants help promote an earlier, more potent response and a more persistent immune response to the vaccine. Antibiotics prevent the growth of bacteria during production and storage of the vaccine. Eggs are used to grow the pathogen, and egg protein is found in influenza and yellow fever vaccines. Formaldehyde is used to inactivate bacterial products for toxoid vaccines and to kill unwanted viruses and bacteria that might contaminate the vaccine during production. Monosodium glutamate and 2-phenoxy-ethanol are preservatives that help the vaccine remain unchanged during the vaccine's exposure to heat, light, acidity, or humidity. Thimerosal is a mercury-containing preservative that helps prevent contamination and growth of bacteria.

Most vaccines are given to prevent disease and are effective only if administered to the person before he or she is exposed to the pathogen or disease; most vaccines must be given by a certain age to ensure effective-

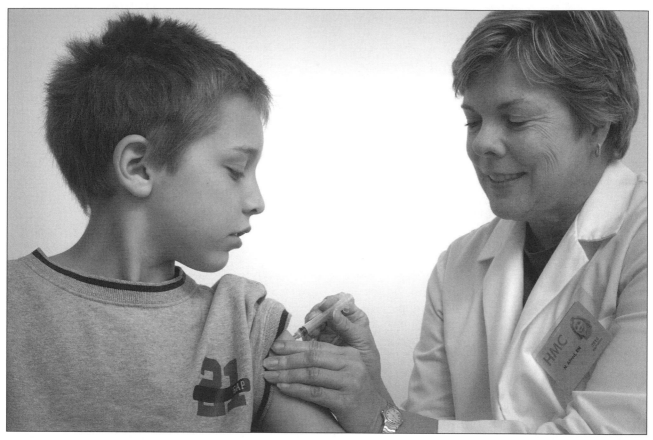

*A child receives an intramuscular vaccine.* (CDC)

ness. Also, most vaccine-preventable diseases can cause serious or life-threatening infections in infants and young children. For example, exposure and infection with polio can occur at a very young age and can cause paralysis, so the vaccine should be given to infants as soon as possible. Immunity to some pathogens can be transferred from a pregnant woman to her fetus, but this immunity wanes once the newborn is older than six months of age. Breast feeding can also help extend immunity to some diseases, but even this is limited.

Certain vaccines (such as pneumococcal or hepatitis B vaccines) are given once in a lifetime, unless a booster is needed. The seasonal influenza vaccine, however, is given annually because hundreds of influenza-like viruses exist; also, the seasonal variations or types of virus that are prevalent change every year. Vaccination schedules have been developed for children, adolescents, and adults that indicate when these persons should receive doses of required vaccinations or boosters.

## VACCINE TYPES

The selection of the type of vaccine depends on fundamental information or factors about the pathogen. These factors include how the pathogen infects cells and how the immune system responds to it. Practical considerations include the regions of the world where the vaccine would be used. Pros and cons are associated with each type of vaccine.

*Live attenuated vaccines.* Live attenuated vaccines are usually created from the naturally occurring pathogen. The pathogen's ability to cause serious infection is attenuated, or "weakened," by manipulating the virus or bacteria in a laboratory environment, but these vaccines can still induce antibody production or a protective immune response. Attenuation of the pathogen usually is done by "passing" or growing the virus or bacteria from culture to culture before it is formulated into a vaccine. Live attenuated vaccines elicit strong cellular and antibody responses and often confer lifelong immunity with only one or two doses. Not everyone can safely receive live attenuated vaccines. People with weakened immune systems cannot be given live vaccines.

These types of vaccines usually need to be refrigerated to stay potent. Proper storage then becomes critical in maintaining vaccine efficacy. Examples of live attenuated vaccines include measles, mumps, and rubella (MMR vaccine), oral polio vaccine (OPV), the nasal form of the influenza (flu) vaccine, and the varicella (chickenpox) vaccine.

*Inactivated vaccines.* Inactivated vaccines contain a killed pathogen that cannot cause the disease but can stimulate antibody production. Pathogens can be inactivated with chemicals such as formaldehyde. Inactivated vaccines are more stable and safer than live vaccines. These vaccines usually do not require refrigeration and are easily stored and transported in freeze-dried form. Most inactivated vaccines, however, produce a weaker immune response than do live vaccines. Several additional doses or booster shots, therefore, are needed to maintain immunity. Examples of inactivated vaccines include inactivated polio vaccine (IPV) and inactivated (injectable form) influenza vaccine.

*Component or subunit vaccines.* Component or subunit vaccines are made by using only parts of the pathogen. These vaccines cannot cause disease, but they can stimulate the body to produce an immune response against the disease. Component vaccines contain only the essential antigens, but not all the other molecules, of the pathogen, so the chance of an adverse reaction to the vaccine is lessened.

These vaccines can contain anywhere from one to twenty or more antigens. Identifying what antigens best stimulate the immune system can be a tricky, time-consuming process. A recombinant component vaccine has been created for the hepatitis B virus. Hepatitis B genes that code for important antigens were inserted into common baker's yeast. The yeast then produced the antigens, which were collected and purified for use in the vaccine.

A conjugate vaccine is another type of component vaccine that has been developed for bacterium that possesses an outer coating of sugar molecules called polysaccharides. The polysaccharide coating disguises the internal antigens of the bacterium so that the immune system does not recognize or respond to it. Vaccines help the immune system link the polysaccharide coating to the bacterium and, therefore, allow antibodies to produce immunity to that pathogen. Examples of component vaccines include *Haemophilus influenzae* type B (Hib) vaccine, hepatitis B (Hep B) vaccine, hepatitis A (Hep A) vaccine, and pneumococcal conjugate vaccine.

*Toxoid vaccines.* Toxoid vaccines are made by treating the toxin produced by the pathogen with heat or chemicals, such as formalin (a solution of formaldehyde and sterilized water). For pathogens that secrete toxins or harmful chemicals, a toxoid vaccine may be used when the toxoid is the main cause of illness. Toxins are inactivated and do not produce disease. Detoxified toxins are called toxoids. After vaccination with a toxoid vaccine, the immune system produces antibodies that block the toxin. Examples of toxoid vaccines include those against diphtheria and tetanus.

*DNA vaccines.* DNA vaccines, which are experimental, contain the genes that code for antigens. This requires that the genes from the pathogen be analyzed. DNA vaccines would stimulate an immune response to the free-floating antigen secreted by cells and would stimulate a response against the antigens displayed on cell surfaces. DNA vaccines would contain copies of a few of the pathogen's genes, so the vaccine would not cause disease.

DNA vaccines are relatively easy and inexpensive to design and produce. Naked DNA vaccines, which consist of DNA that is administered directly into the body, could be mixed with molecules that facilitate its uptake by the body's cells. Naked DNA vaccines for influenza and herpesviruses are being investigated.

*Recombinant vector vaccines.* Recombinant vector vaccines, also experimental, use an attenuated pathogen to introduce DNA to cells of the body. A vector in this case is a harmless virus or bacterium used as a carrier. Certain harmless or attenuated viruses are used to carry portions of the genetic material from other microbes. The carrier viruses then ferry the microbial DNA to cells and display the antigens of the pathogen on the cell's surface. The harmless organism mimics a pathogen and provokes an immune response. Recombinant vector vaccines closely mimic a natural infection, effectively stimulating the immune system. Recombinant vector vaccines for human immunodeficiency virus (HIV), rabies, and measles are under investigation.

## CONTROVERSY

State laws in the United States mandate that children in day care and students be immunized against certain diseases. Some exceptions are allowed. Still, many parents are refusing to immunize their children for fear of a link between autism, for example, and the use of vaccines containing thimerosal, a mercury-based preservative. Although scientific evidence does not support this link, thimerosal is no longer used in the production of most vaccines in the United States. To alert persons to adverse effects associated with vaccine administration, and to educate parents and others about what to expect after receiving a vaccine, an information sheet must be given to each person before he or she can be vaccinated.

## IMPACT

Disease prevention is the key to public health, and it is always better to prevent a disease than to have to treat it. Vaccination is considered one of the most important medical discoveries. Diseases can cause suffering, permanent disability, and death. Vaccines prevent disease in those who get vaccinated and protect those who come into contact with unvaccinated persons. Vaccination has controlled many infectious diseases that were once common, including polio, measles, diphtheria, pertussis (whooping cough), rubella (German measles), mumps, tetanus, and influenza.

Not all countries have the same level of vaccination requirements as the United States. Given the current global nature of travel and business, exposure to many diseases is likely. Vaccination minimizes the risk of developing a disease and its associated complications. When persons travel outside the United States, additional vaccinations may be needed. One should consult a physician within a minimum of four weeks of traveling to determine what vaccines, if any, are needed.

*Beatriz Manzor Mitrzyk, Pharm.D.*

## FURTHER READING

Centers for Disease Control and Prevention. "General Recommendations on Immunization: Recommendations of the Advisory Committee on Immunization Practices." *Morbidity and Mortality Weekly Report* 55 (December 1, 2006): 1-48. Also available at http://www.cdc.gov/mmwr/preview/mmwrhtml/rr5515a1.htm. Review article about immunizations and general recommendations for persons in the United States. Geared toward the health care provider.

_____. "Immunization Schedules." Available at http://www.cdc.gov/vaccines/recs/schedules. CDC schedules that list the age or age range when each vaccine or series of shots is recommended. For consumers and health care providers.

_____. "Understanding the Basics: General Recommendations on Immunization." Available at http://www2a.cdc.gov/nip/isd/ycts/mod1/courses/genrec/10300.asp. An educational module that describes antigens, antibodies, passive and active immunity, the different types of vaccines, and the seven general rules on immunization.

Plotkin, Stanley A., Walter A. Orenstein, and Paul A. Offit. *Vaccines.* 5th ed. Philadelphia: Saunders/Elsevier, 2008. An excellent discussion of the role of vaccines in the prevention of disease. The book begins with a history of immunization practices. Chapters deal with a specific disease and the role of vaccine production in its prevention.

## WEB SITES OF INTEREST

*Bill and Melinda Gates Children's Vaccine Program*
http://www.childrensvaccine.org

*Centers for Disease Control and Prevention*
http://www.cdc.gov/vaccines

*Immunization Action Coalition*
http://www.immunize.org

*National Institute of Allergy and Infectious Diseases*
http://www.niaid.nih.gov/topics/vaccines

*National Network for Immunization Information*
http://www.immunizationinfo.org

**See also:** Bacteriology; Immunity; Immunization; Microbiology; Parasitology; Vaccines: Experimental; Vaccines: History; Virology; Virulence; Viruses: Structure and life cycle; Viruses: Types.

# Vaginal yeast infection

CATEGORY: Diseases and conditions
ANATOMY OR SYSTEM AFFECTED: Genitalia, skin, vagina
ALSO KNOWN AS: Candida vulvovaginitis, monilial vulvovaginitis, vaginal candidiasis, vulvovaginal candidiasis, yeast infection

## DEFINITION

A vaginal yeast infection is caused by the fungus *Candida albicans*. Although yeast is common in the vagina, it can cause problems when it grows excessively. This excess growth causes the uncomfortable symptoms of a yeast infection.

## CAUSES

Yeast grows in conditions that are less acidic. Vaginal fluids are most often mildly acidic, but this fact can change. For example, acid levels can decrease during menstrual flow. Good bacteria also helps keep yeast levels in check. Conditions that decrease levels of good bacteria will also increase the chance of a yeast infection.

## RISK FACTORS

Factors that can increase the chance of a yeast infection include situations that can cause hormonal changes, such as the use of birth control pills; pregnancy; menopause; steroid use; broad-spectrum antibiotics; diabetes, especially when blood sugar is not well-controlled; a compromised immune system, such as with human immunodeficiency virus infection; perfumed feminine hygiene sprays, deodorant tampons, or bubble bath; tight jeans, synthetic underwear, or a wet swimsuit; and douching.

## SYMPTOMS

Symptoms of yeast infection include vaginal itching, ranging from mild to severe; a clumpy, vaginal discharge that may look like cottage cheese; vaginal soreness, irritation, or burning; rash or redness on the skin outside the vagina; painful urination; and painful sexual intercourse.

## SCREENING AND DIAGNOSIS

A doctor will perform a pelvic exam. Vaginal discharge, if any, will be tested. One should consult a doctor at the first onset of symptoms. Other infections have symptoms that are like those of a yeast infection. These other infections include bacterial vaginosis and trichomoniasis.

If a woman has had a yeast infection, she may be able to recognize the signs of a new infection. In this case, over-the-counter medications are safe to use.

## TREATMENT AND THERAPY

Treatment for vaginal yeast infection includes the use of medications. Various antifungal drugs are available as intravaginal creams, tablets, or suppositories. These drugs include Monistat (miconazole nitrate), Gyne-Lotrimin (clotrimazole vaginal), Fem-stat (butoconazole vaginal), Terazol (terconazole vaginal), and Mycelex (clotrimazole vaginal). The treatments come in one-day, three-day, and seven-day packs. Some of these are over-the-counter, and others (such as Terazol) may require a prescription. A doctor also can prescribe fluconazole (Diflucan), an oral medication. It is a single-dose treatment. If pregnant, one should consult a doctor before any treatment.

## PREVENTION AND OUTCOMES

To help reduce the chance of getting a yeast infection, one should take the following steps: Dry outside the vaginal area thoroughly after a shower, bath, or swim; remove a wet bathing suit or damp workout clothes as soon as possible; wear cotton underwear; avoid tight clothing; avoid douching unless instructed to do so by a health care provider (douching decreases vaginal acidity); avoid bubble baths, perfumed feminine hygiene sprays, and scented soap; and avoid frequent or prolonged use of antibiotics, if possible. Persons with diabetes should control their blood sugar levels.

*Mary Calvagna, M.S.;*
*reviewed by Ganson Purcell, Jr., M.D., FACOG, FACPE*

## FURTHER READING

Berek, Jonathan S., ed. *Berek and Novak's Gynecology.* 14th ed. Philadelphia: Lippincott Williams & Wilkins, 2007.

EBSCO Publishing. *DynaMed: Candida Vulvovaginitis.* Available through http://www.ebscohost.com/dynamed.

National Institute of Allergy and Infectious Diseases. "Vaginal Yeast Infection." Available at http://www.niaid.nih.gov/topics/vaginalyeast.

National Institutes of Health, Medline Plus. "Yeast Infections." Available at http://www.nlm.nih.gov/medlineplus/yeastinfections.html.

Richardson, Malcolm D., and Elizabeth M. Johnson. *Pocket Guide to Fungal Infection*. 2d ed. Malden, Mass.: Blackwell, 2006.

Stewart, Elizabeth Gunther, and Paula Spencer. *The V Book: A Doctor's Guide to Complete Vulvovaginal Health*. New York: Bantam Books, 2002.

## WEB SITES OF INTEREST

*American Congress of Obstetricians and Gynecologists*
http://www.acog.org

*National Women's Health Information Center*
http://www.womenshealth.gov

*Our Bodies Ourselves*
http://www.obos.org

*Women's Health Matters*
http://www.womenshealthmatters.ca

**See also:** Antifungal drugs: Types; Bacterial infections; Bacterial vaginosis; *Candida*; Candidiasis; Cervical cancer; Diagnosis of fungal infections; Endometritis; Fungal infections; Pelvic inflammatory disease; Pregnancy and infectious disease; Prevention of fungal infections; Treatment of fungal infections; Trichomonas; Urinary tract infections; Women and infectious disease.

---

Valley fever. *See* Coccidiosis.

---

# Vancomycin-resistant enterococci infection

CATEGORY: Diseases and conditions
ANATOMY OR SYSTEM AFFECTED: All
ALSO KNOWN AS: Multiply-resistant enterococci

## DEFINITION

Enterococci are bacteria that commonly live in the intestines, mouth, and female genital tract. In some cases, the bacteria can cause an infection. When this happens, the antibiotic vancomycin may be given to cure the infection.

However, some types of the bacteria are resistant to vancomycin. When the bacteria are resistant, the infection is not cured, leading to vancomycin-resistant enterococci (VRE) infection. The infection is common in hospitals and long-term care facilities, and it is dangerous to those who are critically ill.

## CAUSES

A number of species cause VRE infection, but the most common are *Enterococcus faecium* and *E. faecalis*.

## RISK FACTORS

The factors that increase the chance of developing VRE include enterococci growing (colonizing) in the body, most commonly in the intestines; contact with an infected person or contact with contaminated surfaces (such as tables and door knobs); earlier treatment with vancomycin or another antibiotic; hospitalization (such as in an intensive care unit, cancer ward, or transplant ward) or long-term institutionalization; a weakened immune system; having neutropenia or mucositis; treatment with corticosteroids, parenteral feeding, or chemotherapy; surgery (such as chest or abdominal surgery); urinary catheterization; and dialysis.

## SYMPTOMS

Symptoms depend on where the infection is found. For example, if VRE causes a urinary tract infection (most common), the patient may have a fever and chills, a frequent need to urinate, and pain in the abdomen. VRE also can cause intra-abdominal and pelvic infection (also common), surgical wound infection, bacteremia (bacterial infection of the blood), endocarditis (infection of the inner surface of the heart muscles and valves), neonatal sepsis (caused by a bacterial infection of an infant's blood), and meningitis (infection of the membranes that surround the brain and spinal cord). Each infection has its own symptoms, which the doctor will discuss with the patient.

## SCREENING AND DIAGNOSIS

A doctor will ask about symptoms and medical history and will perform a physical exam. A laboratory test is done to diagnose VRE and to rule out other conditions.

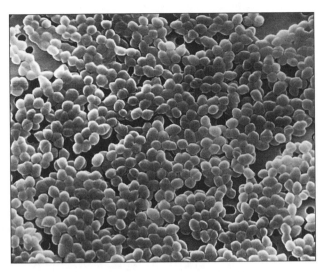

*A micrograph of Enterococcus bacteria.* (CDC)

## TREATMENT AND THERAPY

VRE can be treated with other types of antibiotics, and tests can determine which ones will work for each patient. The type that is chosen is based on the kind of infection and how severe it is. Common antibiotics used to treat VRE include linezolid (Zyvox), which is most common; quinupristin-dalfopristin (Synercid); daptomycin (Cubicin); tigecycline (Tygacil); and nitrofurantoin (Macrobid). If the infection is in the bladder, the doctor may order the placement of a catheter to drain urine from the bladder.

## PREVENTION AND OUTCOMES

The best way to reduce the chance of getting VRE is to use proper handwashing techniques. Handwashing is especially important after using a restroom, before preparing food, and after being in contact with someone who has VRE. Also, areas of the home (including bathrooms and kitchen) that may be contaminated with VRE should be cleaned and disinfected.

One should wear gloves if caring for someone with VRE. If a caregiver expects contact with the bodily fluids of the infected person, the caregiver should wear a gown over his or her clothing. Also, the ill person's room and linens should be cleaned.

If the patient is prescribed vancomycin, he or she should consult the doctor because this antibiotic increases the chance that the bacteria will colonize the patient's body and start an infection. Hospitals normally take special precautions when they know a patient is infected with VRE. In some hospitals, screening tests are done for patients at high-risk for VRE.

*Rebecca J. Stahl, M.A.;*
*reviewed by David L. Horn, M.D., FACP*

## FURTHER READING

Centers for Disease Control and Prevention. "Information for the Public About VRE." Available at http://www.cdc.gov.

_____. "Multidrug-Resistant Organisms in Non-hospital Healthcare Settings." Available at http://www.cdc.gov.

Conte, John E. *Manual of Antibiotics and Infectious Diseases: Treatment and Prevention.* 9th ed. Philadelphia: Lippincott Williams & Wilkins, 2002.

EBSCO Publishing. *DynaMed: Vancomycin-Resistant Enterococci (VRE) Infection.* Available through http://www.ebscohost.com/dynamed.

Huycke, M. M., D. F. Sahm, and M. S. Gilmore. "Multiple-Drug Resistant Enterococci: The Nature of the Problem and an Agenda for the Future." *Emerging Infectious Diseases* 4, no. 2 (April-June, 1998).

National Institute of Allergy and Infectious Diseases. "Antimicrobial (Drug) Resistance: Vancomycin-Resistant Enterococci (VRE)." Available at http://www.niaid.nih.gov/topics/antimicrobialresistance.

Walsh, Christopher. *Antibiotics: Actions, Origins, Resistance.* Washington, D.C.: ASM Press, 2003.

## WEB SITES OF INTEREST

*Centers for Disease Control and Prevention*
http://www.cdc.gov

*National Institutes of Health*
http://www.nih.gov

*Public Health Agency of Canada*
http://www.phac-aspc.gc.ca

**See also:** Antibiotic resistance; Antibiotic-associated colitis; Antibiotics: Types; Bacteria: Classification and types; Bacterial endocarditis; Bacterial infections; Drug resistance; *Enterococcus*; Hospitals and infectious disease; Iatrogenic infections; Infection; Intestinal and stomach infections; Oxazolidinone antibiotics; Transmission routes.

# Variant Creutzfeldt-Jakob disease

CATEGORY: Diseases and conditions
ANATOMY OR SYSTEM AFFECTED: Brain, muscles, musculoskeletal system, nervous system
ALSO KNOWN AS: Human mad-cow disease

## DEFINITION

Variant Creutzfeldt-Jakob disease (vCJD) is a type of prion disease. Bovine spongiform encephalopathy is a prion disease that affects cows, but there is evidence that this illness can be transmitted to humans, producing vCJD. This illness is often called human mad-cow disease.

## CAUSES

Prion diseases are a unique form of infectious diseases. The disease is not produced by a bacterial or viral infection; instead, the illness is related to progressive accumulation of prions (infectious protein particles). The central nervous system is progressively damaged as these prions accumulate.

## RISK FACTORS

Exposure to prion-containing tissue is the primary risk factor. Other risk factors include eating beef from infected cows, receiving human growth hormone (HGH) injections before the mid-1980's (changes in the preparation of HGH in the mid-1980's eliminated this risk), working with brain tissue, and receiving a corneal or dura mater (brain lining) transplantation. Five to ten percent of all cases of the nonvariant form of Creutzfeldt-Jakob are inherited.

## SYMPTOMS

The average age of persons who get this disease is twenty-nine years. Rare cases have been reported in children. Once a person is exposed, it can take up to twenty years until symptoms develop. When symptoms develop they usually follow three phases: early phase (zero to six months), in which psychiatric symptoms predominate, including depression, anxiety, withdrawal, memory problems, and difficulty pronouncing words; middle phase, in which neurologic symptoms predominate, including abnormal gait, ataxia (problems with coordination), involuntary movements (muscle jerks and stiffness), and cognitive decline (impaired speech); late phase, in which symptoms include muteness (inability to speak) and immobility. The average length of time from first symptoms to death is thirteen months (with a range of six to thirty-nine months).

## SCREENING AND DIAGNOSIS

A clinical history and physical exam are the primary diagnostic tools. If the physician suspects vCJD, additional tests may be needed. These tests include a lumbar puncture (a procedure to collect cerebrospinal fluid), a magnetic resonance imaging (MRI) scan (a scan that uses radio waves and a powerful magnet to produce detailed computer images), a computed tomography (CT) scan (a detailed X-ray picture that identifies abnormalities of fine tissue structure), an electroencephalogram (EEG; a test used to evaluate brain function or disorders), SPECT or PET scans (tests that produce images showing the amount of functional activity in the tissue; used to differentiate vCJD from other diseases), biopsy (removal of a sample of tonsil tissue to test to confirm vCJD), and blood tests and cerebrospinal fluid analysis (which may be used to distinguish this disease from other diseases, such as Alzheimer's). In many cases, final diagnosis requires autopsy and pathological studies.

## TREATMENT AND THERAPY

There is no cure for vCJD. Treatment is primarily supportive to maximize patient function and minimize patient discomfort.

## PREVENTION AND OUTCOMES

There have been more than two hundred cases of vCJD worldwide, most of which were associated with beef consumption in the United Kingdom. There is a great deal of controversy regarding safety of beef in the United States. Only a few cases of bovine spongiform encephalopathy have been detected in the United States, but no cases of vCJD have been attributed to eating beef originating in the United States. To minimize risk, it is generally recommended that people avoid eating beef products, particularly processed meat such as sausage and hotdogs, or beef items containing brain, spinal cord, or bone marrow.

*Diane Stresing;*
*reviewed by J. Thomas Megerian, M.D., Ph.D., FAAP*

## FURTHER READING

Dawidowska, K. "Where's the (Safe) Beef?" *Prevention* 56 (2004): 34.

EBSCO Publishing. *DynaMed: Churg-Strauss Syndrome.* Available through http://www.ebscohost.com/dynamed.

_____. *DynaMed: Creutzfeldt-Jakob Spongiform Encephalopathy.* Available through http://www.ebscohost.com/dynamed.

"Moo-ve Over, Beef Burgers: EN Finds Many Alternatives." *Environmental Nutrition* 27 (August, 2004): 5.

Prusiner, S. B. "Detecting Mad Cow Disease." *Scientific American* 291 (2004): 60-67.

Raloff, J. "Better Protection from Mad Cow Disease." *Science News* 165 (2004): 93.

Smith-Bathgate, B. "Creutzfeldt-Jakob Disease: Diagnosis and Nursing Care Issues." *Nursing Times* 101 (2005): 52.

Zeidler, M., et al. "The Pulvinar Sign on Magnetic Resonance Imaging in Variant Creutzfeldt-Jakob Disease." *The Lancet* 355 (2000): 1412-1419.

## WEB SITES OF INTEREST

*Creutzfeldt-Jakob Disease Foundation*
http://www.cjdfoundation.org

*National Creutzfeldt-Jakob Disease Surveillance Unit*
http://www.cjd.ed.ac.uk

*National Institute of Neurological Disorders and Strokes, Creutzfeldt-Jakob Disease Information Page*
http://www.ninds.nih.gov/disorders/cjd/cjd.htm

**See also:** Creutzfeldt-Jakob disease; Food-borne illness and disease; Iatrogenic infections; Prion diseases; Prions; Subacute sclerosing panencephalitis; Zoonotic diseases.

# Vectors and vector control

CATEGORY: Transmission

## DEFINITION

Vector-borne disease is disease caused by microorganisms, such as bacteria, viruses, or protozoa, that are transferred from one living thing (a host) to another living thing (a recipient) through a third living thing (a vector).

## TYPES AND EXAMPLES

With vector-borne disease, the host and recipient can be of the same species; a well-known example is malaria, in which the parasitic protozoan is acquired from an infected person by a mosquito during a blood meal and transferred to another human that the mosquito subsequently feeds on. The host and recipient also can be of different species. An example is western equine encephalitis, in which the host is a bird that is infected by the disease-causing species of arbovirus and the recipient is a horse or a human; as with malaria, the vector is a mosquito.

Another example of a vector-borne disease is dengue fever, in which a flavivirus is transmitted from the host to the susceptible person by a species of mosquito called *Aedes aegypti*. Another vector-borne disease, and one that is spreading in eastern North America, is Lyme disease. Caused by the bacterium *Borrelia burgdorferi*, Lyme disease is transmitted from contaminated animals, such as deer, to humans by the bite of several species of tick. Although Lyme disease is easily treated early in the infection (when its hallmark is a bulls-eye pattern at the point of the tick bite), the disease becomes difficult to treat and is debilitating if not treated promptly. Symptoms include severe fatigue, joint pain, and heart trouble that can persist for years, even if diagnosed and treated.

An ancient vector-borne disease is plague. The disease, which is caused by the bacterium *Yersinia pestis*, is described in passages of the Old Testament. Rodents harbor the bacterium. The vector that transmits the bacterium from rodents to humans is another rat or, more commonly, a flea. Both can feed on an infected rat and subsequently spread the infection to a human through a bite. Several types of plague exist, depending on the site of the infection. Infection of the lungs (pneumonic plague) is almost always fatal within one week if not treated.

A final example of a vector-borne disease is yellow fever. Also caused by a flavivirus, the disease is transferred from the host (a species of monkey) to humans through a mosquito. Yellow fever has caused huge outbreaks in tropical regions; one notable outbreak occurred during the original construction of the Panama Canal. Each year, yellow fever sickens several hundred thousand people and kills an estimated thirty thousand people.

Vector-borne diseases occur worldwide. While some diseases, such as malaria and yellow fever, are concentrated in tropical equatorial regions of the globe, the transmission of other diseases can occur in more temperate climates. An example is mosquito-borne West Nile virus disease. The West Nile virus that causes the disease also has spread to Canada, where it can be transmitted by mosquitoes during warmer months and even during the cooler days of spring by mosquitoes that have survived the cold Canadian winter.

Global warming has led to an increase in territory that is habitable for vectors such as the mosquito. The expanding geographic distribution of malaria has been documented. As global warming continues, vector-borne diseases are expected to continue to expand geographically.

### VECTOR CONTROL

Vector-borne diseases can be treated and even prevented by interrupting the vector-mediated transmission between the infected host and the susceptible person or animal. Treatment and prevention strategies for malaria focus on the mosquito vector. For example, spraying mosquito breeding grounds with insecticide can be an effective control. Indeed, mosquito control now involves the carefully controlled use of dichloro-diphenyl-trichloroethane (DDT).

Another efficient and environmentally friendly means of controlling the mosquito-borne spread of malarial protozoa is the use of mosquito netting (sleeping nets) to protect people at night. Organizations such as World Vision have patron-sponsored campaigns to supply villages in Africa with mosquito netting. Similarly, protective clothing with overlapping upper and lower layers minimizes exposed skin, which is susceptible to a bite from a vector.

A trial prevention program involved the release of laboratory-bred infertile male mosquitoes. Because malaria transmission requires female mosquitoes, it is hoped that the reduced reproductive success resulting from a greater population of infertile males will decrease the numbers of females.

Other treatment and prevention strategies include vaccine development and the use of genetic material (known as morpholino antisense oligonucleotides) to compete with viral genetic material for control of binding sites to host sites, which are critical to the formation of new virus particles.

Organizations including the World Health Organization are promoting a vector-control program known as integrated vector management, which seeks to pre-

vent disease transmission and to optimize the environment. An example of this approach is the rational design of drinking-water delivery systems to reduce the harmful presence of stagnant water (which is a breeding ground for mosquitoes), to minimize deforestation, and to optimize the protection of water quality. Implemented solutions are relevant to a particular region.

### IMPACT

That some infectious agents can be moved from one organism to another by means of another organism (a vector) is critical to disease transmission. Classic examples of this form of transmission are malaria, plague, and yellow fever, which have exacted a huge toll on human life. For example, the number of malaria infections each year is about 500 million, leading to approximately 3 million deaths. Infamously, plague led to millions of deaths worldwide in the fourteenth century. Yellow fever continues to infect hundreds of thousands of people in developing tropical countries each year, despite the existence of a vaccine capable of long-term protection.

Vector-borne diseases are difficult to treat. The vector is mobile and capable of movement over considerable distances. Additionally, as has been clear by the use of insecticides to kill mosquitoes in malaria prevention programs, one can see vector resistance to these compounds. Insects such as mosquitoes have been around for millennia, primarily because of their ready adaptation to change.

To lessen the effects of vector-borne disease, science needs to understand vector habitats, life cycles, and migratory patterns. Global climate change is another major concern in the study of vector-borne disease.

*Brian Hoyle, Ph.D.*

### FURTHER READING

Brower, Vicki. "Vector-Borne Diseases and Global Warming: Are Both on an Upward Swing?" *EMBO Reports* 2 (2001): 755-757. Examines the medical and political controversy about whether or not warmer global temperatures are increasing the incidence of vector-borne diseases.

Gratz, Norman. *Vector- and Rodent-Borne Diseases in Europe and North America: Distribution, Public Health Burden, and Control.* New York: Cambridge University Press, 2006. Details diseases that are spread by vectors. Covers the costs to public health and the control and distribution of vector-borne diseases.

Marquardt, William C., ed. *Biology of Disease Vectors*. 2d ed. New York: Academic Press/Elsevier, 2005. An excellent reference for understanding the role of vectors in the transmission of infectious diseases. Discusses prevention and control strategies and future implications.

Tolle, Michael A. "Mosquito-Borne Diseases." *Current Problems in Pediatric and Adolescent Health Care* 39 (2009): 97-140. A thorough review of the life cycles of insects as disease agents. Includes discussion of the diagnoses, treatments, and vaccines for several mosquito-borne diseases. Special focus on the impact of the diseases on pregnant women and on children.

### WEB SITES OF INTEREST

*Centers for Disease Control and Prevention, Division of Vector Borne Infectious Diseases*
http://www.cdc.gov/ncidod/dvbid

*VectorBase*
http://www.vectorbase.org

*World Health Organization, Integrated Vector Management, Directory of Resources*
http://www.who.int/heli/risks/vectors/vectordirectory

**See also:** Arthropod-borne illness and disease; Blood-borne illness and disease; Carriers; DDT; Fleas and infectious disease; Flies and infectious disease; Hosts; Insect-borne illness and disease; Insecticides and topical repellants; Mosquitoes and infectious disease; Sleeping nets; Ticks and infectious disease; Transmission routes; Zoonotic diseases.

---

Venereal diseases. *See* Sexually transmitted diseases (STDs).

---

# Vertical disease transmission

CATEGORY: Transmission
ALSO KNOWN AS: Fetomaternal transmission, maternal-fetal transmission, mother-to-child transmission, perinatal transmission

### DEFINITION

Vertical disease transmission is the passing of a disease-causing agent (pathogen) from one generation to another, as when a parent transmits a pathogen to potential offspring at conception, during the perinatal period (pregnancy), at labor and delivery, or shortly after birth. The pathogen may be transferred either in sperm, by crossing the placenta, by fetal or newborn exposure to secretions or blood, or through breast-feeding.

### DISEASE TYPES

Many of the vertically transmitted (VT) infections are first acquired by horizontal disease transmission, meaning from persons within the same generation. For instance, sexually transmitted diseases are passed between partners and then may be vertically transmitted to a fetus. Common examples of VT diseases are human immunodeficiency virus (HIV) infection, hepatitis, herpes, and syphilis. Other infections are contracted by contact with young children or animals and their feces and then vertically transmitted. These infections include cytomegalovirus, toxoplasmosis, and chickenpox. Pregnant women may be asymptomatic, but affected fetuses can have severe disease presentation after birth depending on the timing of exposure. Infections can lead to multiple medical and developmental concerns or to fetal or neonatal death.

### PERINATAL TESTING AND TREATMENT

Women (both pregnant and those planning to become pregnant) are screened on routine blood work for many of the diseases that show VT. Treatments, although specifically tailored to the individual disease, include maternal or neonatal medication (or both), changing delivery route from a vaginal delivery to a cesarean section to avoid maternal-fetal contact in the birth canal, and avoiding breast-feeding. Vaccines for certain diseases, such as hepatitis B, are administered in the newborn period to prevent disease development and VT to future generations.

### IMPACT

It is important to identify vertical disease transmission to apply appropriate preventive measures during pregnancy and labor and delivery. There is no fully effective way to avoid many perinatal infections. However, some changes in obstetrical and pediatric practice have proven effective. For example, when both maternal and neonatal treatment is administered for HIV infection, the VT rate decreases from approximately 25 to 2 percent or less. Ongoing research on animal models aims to identify the predisposing factors for disease transmission and identify possible future treatments, such as medications or vaccines.

*Janet Ober Berman, M.S., CGC*

**FURTHER READING**

American College of Obstetricians and Gynecologists. "Hepatitis B Virus in Pregnancy." Available at http://www.acog.org/publications/patient_education/bp093.cfm.

_____. "Prenatal and Perinatal Human Immunodeficiency Virus Testing: Expanded Recommendations." *Obstetrics and Gynecology* 112 (2008): 739-742.

Khare, Manjiri. "Infectious Disease in Pregnancy." *Current Obstetrics and Gynaecology* 15 (2005): 149-156.

Taverna, Paola, et al. "CMV Infection in Pregnancy: Prevention of Vertical Transmission by Means of Specific Immunoglobulin Therapy (CMV-IgG)." *Early Human Development* 85 (2009): S98-S99.

**WEB SITES OF INTEREST**

*Genetic and Rare Diseases Information Center*
http://rarediseases.info.nih.gov/gard

*National Institutes of Health*
http://www.nlm.nih.gov/medlineplus/infectionsandpregnancy

**See also:** Breast milk and infectious disease; Childbirth and infectious disease; Children and infectious disease; Horizontal disease transmission; Men and infectious disease; Pathogens; Pregnancy and infectious disease; Superbacteria; Transmission routes; Women and infectious disease.

# *Vibrio*

CATEGORY: Pathogen
TRANSMISSION ROUTE: Direct contact, ingestion

**DEFINITION**

*Vibrio*, among the most common forms of bacteria of the surface waters of the earth, is a motile aerobic rod that causes the human disease cholera, other forms of gastroenteritis, and some extraintestinal infections.

---

**Taxonomic Classification for *Vibrio***

**Kingdom:** Bacteria
**Phylum:** Proteobacteria
**Order:** Vibrionales
**Family:** Vibrionaceae
**Genus:** *Vibrio*
**Species:**
*V. cholerae*
*V. parahaemolyticus*
*V. vulnificus*
*V. mimicus*
*V. hollisae*
*V. fluvialis*
*V. alginolyticus*
*V. damsela*

---

**NATURAL HABITAT AND FEATURES**

Vibrios are gram-negative bacteria with a curved rod shape. They are aerobic and motile, with a polar flagellum. Vibrios are common in salt water and fresh water around the world. The bacteria can be carried by numerous animals that live in the sea and may be ingested through human consumption of crabs, clams, and oysters. *V. cholerae* is the most medically important species, as it causes the disease cholera, which is endemic to India and Southeast Asia.

Vibrios produce smooth, rounded colonies that are opaque when exposed to light. They grow well at 98.6° Fahrenheit (37° Celsius) on thiosulfate-citrate-bile-sucrose agar and on many other media. When cultured over time, the curved rods may become straight and resemble gram-negative intestinal bacteria. *Cholerae* grows rapidly on blood agar with a pH (acidity) level near 9. Typical colonies are identifiable in about eighteen hours.

Vibrios are differentiated from other intestinal gram-negative bacteria by being oxidase positive. A positive oxidase test is important in preliminary identification of *cholerae* and other vibrios. They grow well in high pH but are rapidly killed by acid. For this reason, any condition or medication that decreases stomach acidity may predispose a person to infection.

Antigenic structures of vibrios include a single

heat-labile flagellar H antigen. *Cholerae* has O lipo-polysaccharides that define serologic specificity. (A minimum of 139 O-antigen groups exist.) Antibodies to O antigens may protect some animals from infection. Enterotoxins produced by *cholerae* can cause prolonged hypersecretion of water and electrolytes in humans, causing profuse diarrhea. Cholera enterotoxin may stimulate the production of neutralizing antibodies. Although an attack of cholera may be followed by immunity, the duration and degree is unpredictable.

## PATHOGENICITY AND CLINICAL SIGNIFICANCE

*Cholerae* is pathogenic only in humans. It is not an invasive infection. It remains in the intestinal tract attached to the microvilli of intestinal epithelial cells, where it releases toxins but does not enter the bloodstream. Up to 60 percent of infections may be asymptomatic. The development of symptoms depends on the size of the inoculum. When symptoms do occur, they follow an incubation period of one to four days. Typically, symptoms develop suddenly and may include cramping, abdominal pain, nausea, vomiting, and profuse diarrhea. The term "rice water diarrhea" is used to describe the stools, which contain copious mucus, epithelial cells, and large numbers of vibrios. Diarrhea and vomiting lead to rapid depletion of fluid and electrolytes.

Untreated cholera may result in profound dehydration, anuria, circulatory collapse, and death. Mortality rates as high as 50 percent may be seen during an epidemic. Diagnosis of epidemic or endemic cholera is not difficult, but sporadic or isolated cases may be confused with other causes of gastroenteritis.

Other vibrios causing human disease include *para-haemolyticus*, which causes gastroenteritis following ingestion of *Vibrio*-infected seafood. Incubation is twelve to twenty-four hours, which is followed by nausea, vomiting, fever, and diarrhea that may be bloody. The symptoms usually subside without treatment in one to four days. *Parahaemolyticus* does not produce a toxin. It is present worldwide and may infect humans who eat raw seafood.

*Vulnificus* is a free-living organism found in ocean estuaries worldwide. In the United States, *vulnificus* is found predominantly along the Gulf Coast. People swimming in these waters with an open wound may become infected, and the infection may cause sepsis. *Vulnificus* may be found in oysters during warm months and may cause gastroenteritis if eaten raw. Although wound infections may be mild, *vulnificus* may have a mortality rate as high as 50 percent if sepsis develops. Other vibrios that may cause diarrhea include *mimicus*, *hollisae*, and *fluvialis*. Other vibrios that cause wound infections include *damsela* and *alginolyticus*.

## DRUG SUSCEPTIBILITY

Vibrio gastroenteritis is usually self-limited, and most people will recover as long as adequate hydration and nutrition are available. Most vibrios are sensitive to antibiotics, but antibiotic therapy may not shorten the course of intestinal illness. Antibiotics are more important in vibrio wound infection or in bacteremia. In these cases, intensive medical therapy, including intravenous antibiotics, management of septic shock, and aggressive surgical debridement, may be needed.

Antibiotics that are effective against cholera include tetracycline and ciprofloxacin. In wound infections and bacteremia caused by noncholera *Vibrio* species, the combination of doxycycline, ceftazidime, and a broad-spectrum type penicillin, such as ticarcillin, is the treatment of choice. Many *Vibrio* species have developed resistance to commonly used antibiotics. Vibrios have been found to be susceptible to several novel antibiotics, such as tigecycline, daptomycin, and linezolid.

*Christopher Iliades, M.D.*

## FURTHER READING

Brooks, George F. and Carroll, Karen C. *Jawetz, Melnick, and Adelberg's Medical Microbiology.* 25th ed. New York: McGraw-Hill, 2010. Chapter 17 of this textbook gives an excellent introduction to the vibrios including their morphology, identification, antigenic structure, and growth characteristics.

Fauci, Anthony, et al., eds. *Harrison's Principles of Internal Medicine.* 17th ed. New York: McGraw-Hill, 2008. Chapter 149 covers cholera and other vibrio infections. Includes a good discussion of vibrio infections other than cholera gastroenteritis.

Ho, Hoi. "Vibrio Infections." Available at http://emedicine.medscape.com/article/232038-overview. Examines vibrio infection, including aggressive treatment of noncholera wound infection and bacteremia.

Vaseeharan, B., et al. "In Vitro Susceptibility of Antibiotics Against *Vibrio* spp. and *Aeromonas* spp. Isolated from *Penaeus monodon* Hatcheries and Ponds." *Journal of Antimicrobial Agents* 26 (2005): 285-291. Provides a good background on antibiotic susceptibilities of *Vibrio* species and the emergence of resistant strains.

### WEB SITES OF INTEREST

*Centers for Disease Control and Prevention, Division of Foodborne, Bacterial, and Mycotic Diseases*
http://www.cdc.gov/nczved/divisions/dfbmd

*Todar's Online Textbook of Bacteriology*
http://www.textbookofbacteriology.net

**See also:** Bacteria: Classification and types; Cholera; Cholera vaccine; Developing countries and infectious disease; Food-borne illness and disease; Intestinal and stomach infections; Parasites: Classification and types; Pathogens; Sepsis; Tropical medicine; Waterborne illness and disease; Wound infections.

# Vincent's angina

CATEGORY: Diseases and conditions
ANATOMY OR SYSTEM AFFECTED: Gums, jaw, mouth, pharynx, throat, tissue, tonsils
ALSO KNOWN AS: Acute necrotizing ulcerative gingivitis, trench mouth, Vincent's disease, Vincent's stomatitis

### DEFINITION

Vincent's angina, named for French physician Jean Hyacinthe Vincent, is a severe bacterial infection of the gums, mouth, pharynx, and tonsils, resulting in swelling, bleeding, pain, and ulceration of the gums, mouth, and jaw.

### CAUSES

Vincent's angina is caused by the build up of *Fusobacterium* and spirochetes in the mouth, primarily because of poor oral hygiene. The normal balance of bacteria in the mouth becomes seriously compromised, resulting in a pronounced infection that ravages the gums, throat, and tonsils. Poor overall health, improper diet, smoking, lack of dental care, stress, and a weakened immune system all contribute to cre-

ating an extreme imbalance in the otherwise healthy level of oral bacteria.

### RISK FACTORS

Those who live in extreme poverty are at greatest risk for Vincent's angina because they often lack the means to practice adequate oral hygiene, are malnourished, and receive little or no dental care. Smoking also greatly increases the likelihood of Vincent's angina. People under increased emotional stress are more susceptible to developing the disease, and persons with weakened immune systems, especially those with diabetes or acquired immunodeficiency syndrome, are at much greater risk of developing Vincent's angina.

### SYMPTOMS

Vincent's angina symptoms include red, swollen, or bleeding gums accompanied by severe pain, bad breath, fever, difficulty swallowing and chewing, oral ulcers, and swollen lymph glands in the throat and neck.

### SCREENING AND DIAGNOSIS

After a visual exam, a throat swab culture is taken and examined for increased levels of *Fusobacterium* and spirochetes in the mouth. Also, dental and facial X rays are ordered to determine how much tissue of the gums, bone, or teeth has already been destroyed by the infection.

### TREATMENT AND THERAPY

Treatment begins by prescribing good oral hygiene and providing demonstrations of proper oral care. If fever, severe gum pain, and bleeding are present, antibiotics, particularly penicillin, are administered. Lidocaine applied directly to the gums will help reduce pain and swelling. Hydrogen peroxide is used to rinse the mouth and gums regularly, clearing away damaged tissue. Additional salt-water rinses of the mouth several times per day help to soothe the gums and decrease pain. All hot, spicy foods should be avoided while undergoing treatment, so that the symptoms of Vincent's angina will not be exacerbated. After the gums have become less painful and less tender, a dentist or dental assistant should clean the teeth, scraping away plaque to assist further healing.

### PREVENTION AND OUTCOMES

Good oral hygiene, involving brushing and flossing the teeth a minimum of twice per day, is the best prevention for Vincent's angina. Regular professional cleaning of the teeth by a dentist or dental assistant is also a deterrent. Stopping smoking, eating a more nutritious diet, exercising, and reducing emotional stress are also effective in helping prevent Vincent's angina.

*Mary E. Markland, M.A.*

### FURTHER READING

Chow, Anthony W. "Infections of the Oral Cavity, Head, and Neck." In *Mandell, Douglas, and Bennett's Principles and Practice of Infectious Diseases*, edited by Gerald L. Mandell, John F. Bennett, and Raphael Dolin. 7th ed. New York: Churchill Livingstone/ Elsevier, 2010.

Galgut, Peter N., Sherie A. Dowsett, and Michael J. Kowolik. *Periodontics: Current Concepts and Treatment Strategies*. London: Martin Dunitz, 2001.

Langlais, Robert P., and Craig S. Miller. *Color Atlas of Common Oral Diseases*. 4th ed. Philadelphia: Lippincott Williams & Wilkins, 2009.

### WEB SITES OF INTEREST

*American Academy of Periodontology*
http://www.perio.org

*American Dental Association*
http://www.ada.org

*Canadian Dental Association*
http://www.cda-adc.ca

**See also:** Abscesses; Acute necrotizing ulcerative gingivitis; Gangrene; Gingivitis; Mouth infections; Tooth abscess.

---

# Viral gastroenteritis

CATEGORY: Diseases and conditions
ANATOMY OR SYSTEM AFFECTED: Abdomen, digestive system, gastrointestinal system, intestines, stomach
ALSO KNOWN AS: Stomach bug, stomach flu

### DEFINITION

Viral gastroenteritis is an infection of the intestines caused by a virus.

### CAUSES

Viral gastroenteritis is caused by one of several viruses that assault the intestines. The viruses are usually spread through contact with someone who is infected or with something the infected person touched. Viral gastroenteritis also can spread through food or water that is contaminated.

### RISK FACTORS

Risk factors for viral gastroenteritis include one's age (children and the elderly) and location, especially child-care centers and nursing homes, and in other group settings (such as on cruise ships, in college dormitories, and at campgrounds).

### SYMPTOMS

The symptoms of viral gastroenteritis usually begin one to two days after exposure to the virus. The illness usually lasts one to two days, but it can last up to ten days. Symptoms may include watery diarrhea, nausea, vomiting, abdominal cramps, fever, muscle aches, and headache. Vomiting and diarrhea can lead to dehydration, especially in children.

### SCREENING AND DIAGNOSIS

A doctor will ask about symptoms and medical history and will perform a physical exam. Blood tests and a stool culture may be ordered by the doctor. The stool culture will check for bacteria in a stool sample, which would indicate a different type of illness and one that is not caused by a virus.

### TREATMENT AND THERAPY

There is no specific medical treatment for viral gastroenteritis. (Antibiotics are not helpful for infections caused by any virus.) However, there are a number of things one can do to be more comfortable and avoid dehydration.

One should ingest fluids to replace those lost during the illness by having small sips of water, by sucking on ice chips, or by drinking clear soda or decaffeinated sports drinks (such as Gatorade). Children should be given an oral rehydration solution (such as Pedialyte) instead of water.

One should gradually begin to eat bland foods, such as toast, crackers, bananas, rice, chicken, and potatoes, and should avoid dairy products, caffeine, fatty foods, and spicy foods until feeling better. Breastfeeding infants who are sick should continue with breast-feeding; if the sick infant is bottle-fed, he or she should receive oral rehydration solution or formula.

One should rest while sick and should contact a doctor if unable to keep fluids down for twenty-four hours or if having symptoms such as vomiting blood, bloody diarrhea, or a fever higher than 101° Fahrenheit. Other symptoms requiring medical attention are vomiting for more than two days and having signs of dehydration (such as dizziness or light-headedness, excessive thirst or dry mouth, or dark urine or little or no urine).

For children, one should contact a doctor if the child is under six months of age, has a fever of 102° F or higher, seems tired or irritable, has bloody diarrhea, has stomach pain, or has signs of dehydration (such as unusual drowsiness or dry lips and mouth, no tears when crying, dark urine or not urinating much for example, no wet diaper in three hours or feeling thirsty but vomiting after drinking fluids).

## PREVENTION AND OUTCOMES

There are several steps one can take to prevent viral gastroenteritis. If possible, one should avoid contact with people who have the condition; wash hands thoroughly with warm water and soap (and help children wash their hands thoroughly); use bleach to disinfect contaminated surfaces in the home, including toilets and sink faucets; and avoid sharing personal items such as toothbrushes, towels, and drinking glasses.

Also, one should take special care when traveling to countries that are more likely to have contaminated food and water. Experts recommend that travelers drink only bottled water, avoid ice cubes, and avoid eating raw foods, including vegetables.

*Diane W. Shannon, M.D., M.P.H.;*
*reviewed by Daus Mahnke, M.D.*

## FURTHER READING

Blaser, Martin, eds. *Infections of the Gastrointestinal Tract.* 2d ed. Philadelphia: Lippincott Williams & Wilkins, 2002.

Blum, Richard H., and W. LeRoy Heinrichs. *Nausea and Vomiting: Overview, Challenges, Practical Treatments, and New Perspectives.* Philadelphia: Whurr, 2000.

Centers for Disease Control and Prevention. "Viral Gastroenteritis." Available at http://www.cdc.gov/ncidod/dvrd/revb/gastro/faq.htm.

"Infectious Diarrheal Diseases and Bacterial Food Poisoning." In *Harrison's Principles of Internal Medicine,* edited by Joan Butterton. 17th ed. New York: McGraw-Hill, 2008.

Kapadia, Cyrus R., James M. Crawford, and Caroline Taylor. *An Atlas of Gastroenterology: A Guide to Diagnosis and Differential Diagnosis.* Boca Raton, Fla.: Parthenon, 2003.

Kirschner, Barbara S., and Dennis D. Black. "The Gastrointestinal Tract." In *Nelson Essentials of Pediatrics,* edited by Karen J. Marcdante et al. 6th ed. Philadelphia: Saunders/Elsevier, 2011.

## WEB SITES OF INTEREST

*American Academy of Family Physicians*
http://familydoctor.org

*Centers for Disease Control and Prevention*
http://www.cdc.gov

**See also:** Airborne illness and disease; Amebic dysentery; Antibiotic-associated colitis; Ascariasis; Diverticulitis; Enteritis; Food-borne illness and disease; Gastritis; Giardiasis; Hookworms; Intestinal and stomach infections; Norovirus infection; Peptic ulcer; Peritonitis; Travelers' diarrhea; Tropical medicine; Waterborne illness and disease.

# Viral hepatitis

CATEGORY: Diseases and conditions
ANATOMY OR SYSTEM AFFECTED: Gastrointestinal system, liver

## DEFINITION

Viral hepatitis is an infection of the liver caused by a virus. Viral hepatitis leads to liver inflammation and can also lead to liver cancer. There are five types of viral hepatitis infection: A, B, C, D, and E.

## CAUSES

Progressive and chronic viral hepatitis is caused by toxins and by heavy drinking of alcohol.

## RISK FACTORS

It is possible to develop viral hepatitis with or without the common risk factors listed here. However, the more risk factors, the greater the likelihood that a person will develop viral hepatitis. The risk factors for hepatitis vary, depending on the type of hepatitis.

Persons at a greater risk include infants born to women with hepatitis B or C and children in day-care centers. Also at greater risk are child-care workers (especially if one changes diapers or toilet-trains toddlers), first aid and emergency workers, funeral home staff, health care workers, dentists and dental assistants, firefighters, and police personnel.

The following behaviors are risk factors for developing hepatitis: close contact with someone who has the disease; using household items that were used by an infected person and were not properly cleaned; anal sex; sexual contact with multiple partners; sexual contact with someone who has hepatitis or a sexually transmitted disease (STD); injecting drugs, especially with shared needles; using intranasal cocaine; and getting a tattoo or body piercing (because the needles may not be properly sterilized). For hepatitis A or E, risk factors include traveling to (or spending long periods of time in) a country where hepatitis A or E are common or where there is poor sanitation.

Health conditions and procedures that increase the risk of hepatitis include hemophilia or other disorders of blood clotting, kidney disease requiring hemodialysis, receiving a blood transfusion, receiving multiple transfusions of blood or blood products, receiving a solid-organ transplant, persistent elevation of certain liver function tests (found in people with undiagnosed liver problems), and having an STD.

## SCREENING AND DIAGNOSIS

The purpose of screening is early diagnosis and treatment. Screening tests are usually administered to people without current symptoms but who may be at high risk for certain diseases or conditions.

The Centers for Disease Control and Prevention recommends screening for hepatitis in pregnant women at their first prenatal visit and in people at high risk for the disease. Screening for hepatitis is a method of finding out if a person has hepatitis before he or she begins to have symptoms. Screening involves assessing the person's medical history and behaviors that may increase or decrease the risk of hepatitis and undergoing tests to identify early signs of hepatitis, including blood tests for hepatitis antigens and antibodies.

## TREATMENT AND THERAPY

Treatment for hepatitis involves behavioral changes, medications, and alternative and complementary therapies. There are no surgical procedures to treat viral hepatitis.

## PREVENTION AND OUTCOMES

Hepatitis is a contagious disease that is preventable. Basic preventive principles include avoiding contact with other people's blood or bodily fluids and practicing good sanitation. In addition, vaccines are available to prevent some types of hepatitis. They are given to people at high risk of contracting the disease.

Infected blood and bodily fluids can spread hepatitis. To avoid contact, one should avoid sharing drug needles, avoid sex with partners who have hepatitis or other STDs, practice safer sex (such as using latex condoms) or abstain from sex, limit one's number of sexual partners, avoid sharing personal hygiene products (such as toothbrushes and razors), and avoid handling items that may be contaminated with hepatitis-infected blood. Also, one should donate his or her own blood before elective surgery so it can be used if a blood transfusion is necessary.

Health care professionals should always follow routine barrier precautions and safely handle needles and other sharp instruments and dispose of them properly. One should wear gloves when touching or cleaning up bodily fluids on personal items, such as bandages, tampons, sanitary pads, diapers, and linens and towels. One should cover open cuts or wounds and use only sterile needles for drug injections, blood draws, ear piercing, and tattooing.

Women who are pregnant should have a blood test for hepatitis B. Infants born to women with hepatitis B should be treated within twelve hours of birth.

When traveling to countries where the risk of hepatitis is higher, one should follow proper precautions, such as drinking bottled water only, avoiding ice cubes, and avoiding certain foods, such as shellfish, unpasteurized milk products, and fresh fruits and vegetables. Good sanitation too can prevent the transmission of some forms of hepatitis.

Vaccines are available for hepatitis A and B. Hepatitis A vaccine is recommended for all children age twelve months and older. The following people also should be vaccinated: persons traveling to areas where hepatitis A is prevalent, persons who engage in anal sex, drug users, people with chronic liver disease or blood-clotting disorders (such as hemophilia), children who live in areas where hepatitis A is prevalent, and people who will have close contact with an adopted child from a medium- or high-risk area. Hepatitis B vaccine is recommended for all children and for adults who are at risk.

An immunoglobulin injection, if recommended, is available for hepatitis A and B. Immunoglobulin contains antibodies that help provide protection. This shot is usually given before exposure to the virus or as soon as possible after exposure to the virus.

*Debra Wood, R.N.;*
*reviewed by David L. Horn, M.D., FACP*

## FURTHER READING

Boyer, Thomas D., Teresa L. Wright, and Michael P. Manns, eds. *Zakim and Boyer's Hepatology: A Textbook of Liver Disease.* 5th ed. Philadelphia: Saunders/Elsevier, 2006. A thorough compendium on most aspects of liver disease. The section on hepatitis contains a complete clinical description of the disease and of the biology of the hepatitis viruses.

Feldman, Mark, Lawrence S. Friedman, and Lawrence J. Brandt, eds. *Sleisenger and Fordtran's Gastrointestinal and Liver Disease: Pathophysiology, Diagnosis, Management.* New ed. 2 vols. Philadelphia: Saunders/Elsevier, 2010. A clinical text that covers basic liver anatomy, disorders and diseases of the liver (including hepatitis), and related topics.

Humes, H. David, et al., eds. *Kelley's Textbook of Internal Medicine.* 4th ed. Philadelphia: Lippincott Williams & Wilkins, 2000. A medical textbook that contains an extensive section on liver diseases, including a concise description of viral hepatitis. The discussion of hepatitis viruses is thorough and clear.

Plotkin, Stanley A., and Walter A. Orenstein, eds. *Vaccines.* 5th ed. Philadelphia: Saunders/Elsevier, 2008. An excellent description of the role of vaccines in the prevention of disease. The book begins with a history of immunization practices. Chapters deal with specific diseases and the role and history of vaccine production in its prevention.

Specter, Steven, ed. *Viral Hepatitis: Diagnosis, Therapy, and Prevention.* Totowa, N.J.: Humana Press, 1999. This clearly written and readable review of viral hepatitis provides useful information for family physicians and general readers. Each chapter is divided into sections for quick access to desired information.

## WEB SITES OF INTEREST

*American Liver Foundation*
http://www.liverfoundation.org

*Centers for Disease Control and Prevention*
http://www.cdc.gov/hepatitis

*Hepatitis Foundation International*
http://www.hepfi.org

*National Institute of Diabetes and Digestive and Kidney Diseases*
http://www.niddk.nih.gov

*World Health Organization*
http://www.who.int/csr/disease/hepatitis/whocdscsrncs20011

**See also:** AIDS; Blood-borne illness and disease; Childbirth and infectious disease; Contagious diseases; Hepatitis A; Hepatitis B; Hepatitis C; Hepatitis D; Hepatitis E; Hepatitis vaccines; HIV; Iatrogenic infections; Immunodeficiency; Liver cancer; Saliva and infectious disease; Sexually transmitted diseases (STDs); Viral infections.

# Viral infections

CATEGORY: Diseases and conditions
ANATOMY OR SYSTEM AFFECTED: All

## DEFINITION

Viral infections are illnesses that arise from the presence of pathogens known as viruses in the cells of living organisms, including plants, birds, humans, and nonhuman animals. Unlike bacteria, viruses are not living things but are tiny protein-covered bits of genetic matter, composed of either deoxyribonucleic acid (DNA) or ribonucleic acid (RNA). Because they do not absorb or metabolize nutrients to sustain themselves, as do bacteria, they need living cells in which to carry out their only function, reproduction. Because they cannot reproduce on surfaces or in the air, they do not survive more than twenty-four to forty-eight hours.

Infection in humans occurs when viruses release their DNA or RNA into a human cell, replacing that of the organism they have invaded. Viruses do this repeatedly, not to kill cells but to reproduce in them and to do so rapidly. Viruses continue this process until they have taken over their unwitting host or a specific organ system in the body, often interrupting normal organ function. Different parts of the body may be affected by viruses, and persons can be affected in different ways, depending on the nature of the virus and on the person's overall health.

Familiar viral infections are the childhood diseases measles (rubella) and chickenpox (herpes zoster), genital and oral herpes (herpes simplex, or HSV), upper respiratory infections such as the common cold (rhinoviruses and coronaviruses), sinusitis and bronchial infections (influenza, H1N1, respiratory syncytial virus, rhinovirus, and coronavirus), stomach or intestinal infections, and certain sexually transmitted diseases (STDs), such as human papilloma virus (HPV) and genital herpes. Shingles is another herpes zoster virus that affects the nerves and skin.

Viruses, such as West Nile, also can affect the nervous system; other viruses cause diseases such as rabies and encephalitis. The human immunodeficiency virus (HIV) is a particularly aggressive virus. It affects people around the world and has killed millions since the early 1980's, when the virus was discovered. The hepatitis viruses include hepatitis A, B, C, D, and E, of which hepatitis C results in the most prevalent blood-borne illness globally. Some viruses remain in human cells, resulting in lifelong episodes of infection and alternating with long periods of inactivity.

## CAUSES

Many different types of viruses cause viral infections. The Universal Virus Database, an international compilation of viruses that is updated often by the International Committee on Taxonomy of Viruses to include newly discovered viruses, lists hundreds of virus families and their members, sometimes dozens in one family. Specific viruses cause specific types of illness because they characteristically infect a specific type of cell. Cold viruses, for example, infect cells in the respiratory tract and certain enteroviruses affect the intestinal tract. Viruses spread from person to person through direct human contact (skin, sexual, or blood transfusion) or through being inhaled or ingested in airborne droplets expelled during a sneeze or cough. Insects and parasites, such as mosquitoes and ticks, also carry and transmit certain viruses.

## Types of Viral Infection

| Family | | Conditions |
|---|---|---|
| Adenoviruses |  | Respiratory and eye infections |
| Arenaviruses |  | Lassa fever |
| Coronaviruses |  | Common cold |
| Herpesviruses |  | Cold sores, genital herpes, chickenpox, herpes zoster (shingles), glandular fever, congenital abnormalities (cytomegalovirus) |
| Orthomyxoviruses |  | Influenza |
| Papovaviruses |  | Warts |
| Paramyxoviruses |  | Mumps, measles, rubella |
| Picornaviruses |  | Poliomyelitis, viral hepatitis types A and B, respiratory infections, myocarditis |
| Poxviruses |  | Cowpox, smallpox (eradicated), molluscum contagiosum |
| Retroviruses |  | AIDS, degenerative brain diseases, possibly various kinds of cancer |
| Rhabdoviruses |  | Rabies |
| Togaviruses |  | Yellow fever, dengue, encephalitis |

## RISK FACTORS

Any person can be infected with a virus, but risk is increased in persons with a weakened immune system (those who are immunodeficient or immunocompromised), including infants, young children, and the elderly; those with a chronic disease, such as AIDS; and persons taking immunosuppressive drugs to treat cancer or to deter organ rejection following organ transplantation.

## SYMPTOMS

Symptoms vary widely depending on which virus has caused infection and what part of the body it has affected. Respiratory infections in the nose, throat, sinuses, and lungs may produce symptoms such as a sore throat, runny nose, painful sinuses, cough, and production of phlegm that can block the upper airways. Viruses affecting the skin may produce warts or a rash or skin eruptions and inflammation.

## SCREENING AND DIAGNOSIS

Screening for certain viruses is applied especially to blood donors to rule out hepatitis, STDs, and HIV, and in sexually active persons who wish to know their own status regarding sexually transmitted viruses such as HIV, herpes, and HPV to protect their sexual partners. Diagnosis relies generally on laboratory tests and cultures of infected material and specific antibody tests (polymerase chain reaction, or PCR), which may identify corresponding proteins (antigens) on the causative viruses, indicating the virus responsible. With the outbreak of a viral epidemic, such as influenza, the prevailing symptoms among other cases may help identify the virus in new cases.

## TREATMENT AND THERAPY

Viruses are difficult to approach with medications because they have built-in protection from the walls of the cells within which they are encased. Because they live inside human cells, they also do not respond to most antibiotics, which are designed to kill living bacteria that reproduce outside cells. Often used instead are antiviral drugs, which do not destroy the virus directly but interfere with the ability of viruses to reproduce. These drugs are exceptionally potent and may exhibit toxic effects against human cells, resulting in nausea, headache, diarrhea, rashes, and (rarely) seizures or kidney problems, Other antiviral drugs work by reinforcing the body's own immune response to the virus (interferons and immunoglobulin), which also deter the viruses from reproducing.

## PREVENTION AND OUTCOMES

The body's own defense system includes physical barriers such as the skin that preclude easy access for viruses. Cells already occupied by viruses manufacture substances called interferons, which can increase the resistance of unoccupied cells to virus infection. Immune defenses include the release of infection-fighting white blood cells (lymphocytes, monocytes, and specialized killer T cells), which can defeat the virus attack and protect against subsequent exposure to the same virus. Immunity can also be established by receiving vaccines (such as influenza, HPV, chickenpox, rabies, and hepatitis); however, vaccines have not yet been developed for all viruses.

*L. Lee Culvert, B.S., CLS*

## FURTHER READING

Kane, Melissa, and Tatyana Gotovkina. "Common Threads in Persistent Viral Infections." *Journal of Virology* 84 (2010): 4116-4123. Examines how some viruses establish a permanent host relationship and recurrent infection by avoiding immune system actions.

Knipe, David M., and Peter M. Howley, eds. *Fields' Virology*. 5th ed. Philadelphia: Wolters Kluwer Health/Lippincott Williams & Wilkins, 2007. Covers later discoveries concerning the replication, molecular biology, pathogenesis, and medical aspects of viruses.

National Library of Medicine. "Viral Infections." Available at http://www.nlm.nih.gov/medlineplus/viralinfections.html.

Schaffer, Kirsten, Alberto M. LaRosa, and Estella Whimbey. "Respiratory Viruses." In *Cohen and Powderly Infectious Diseases*, edited by Jonathan Cohen, Steven M. Opal, and William G. Powderly. 3d ed. Philadelphia: Mosby/Elsevier, 2010. Describes viruses responsible for respiratory conditions, including prevalence and manifestation of respiratory virus infection.

Sompayrac, Lauren M. *How Pathogenic Viruses Work*. Sudbury, Mass.: Jones and Bartlett, 2002. An engaging exploration of the basics of virology. The author examines twelve of the most common viral infections to demonstrate how viruses devise various solutions to stay alive.

"Systemic Viral Infection." In *Textbook of Family Medicine*, edited by Robert E. Rakel. 7th ed. Philadelphia: Saunders/Elsevier, 2007. Discusses the characteristics of viruses that cause systemic infection in the body rather than affecting only one organ system.

Wagner, Edward K., and Martinez J. Hewlett. *Basic Virology*. 3d ed. Malden, Mass.: Blackwell Science, 2008. An undergraduate text covering issues of virology and viral disease, properties of viruses and virus-cell interaction, working with viruses, and replication patterns of specific viruses.

## WEB SITES OF INTEREST

*Centers for Disease Control and Prevention*
http://www.cdc.gov

*International Committee on Taxonomy of Viruses*
http://www.ictvonline.org

*Universal Virus Database*
http://www.ictvdb.org

**See also:** Antiviral drugs: Mechanisms of action; Antiviral drugs: Types; Carriers; Diagnosis of viral infections; Hosts; Immune response to viral infections; Infection; Insect-borne illness and disease; Pathogenicity; Pathogens; Prevention of viral infections; Transmission routes; Treatment of viral infections; Virology; Virulence; Viruses: Structure and life cycle; Viruses: Types.

# Viral meningitis

CATEGORY: Diseases and conditions
ANATOMY OR SYSTEM AFFECTED: Brain, central nervous system, spinal cord, tissue

## DEFINITION

The brain and spinal cord are encased by layers of tissue called the meninges. Certain viruses can cause an infection in these layers. This infection is called viral meningitis. Some types of viral meningitis can be less serious than bacterial meningitis.

## CAUSES

A number of viruses can cause viral meningitis, including enteroviruses, herpesviruses, mumps, varicella virus (chickenpox), measles, rubella viruses, and West Nile virus. Most of these viruses can also cause encephalitis, an inflammation of the brain tissue. It is a much more serious condition.

Viruses that cause meningitis can be spread in numerous ways. Enteroviruses are spread through direct contact with respiratory secretions of an infected person, and through feces. Other viruses (mumps, herpes, chickenpox) are spread through close personal contact or through the air. Some viruses (such as West Nile) that cause encephalitis are spread by insects.

## RISK FACTORS

Risk factors for viral meningitis include conditions that weaken the immune system, such as human immunodeficiency virus infection (which itself can lead to meningitis and encephalitis); immunosuppressive treatments; crowded, unsanitary conditions; and the months of summer and early fall.

## SYMPTOMS

Classic symptoms of viral meningitis include high fever, headache, stiff, sore neck, nausea, vomiting, sensitivity to bright lights, and sleepiness. In newborns and infants, symptoms include inactivity, high fever (especially unexplained high fever), irritability, vomiting, feeding poorly or refusing to eat, tautness or bulging of soft spots between skull bones, and difficulty awakening.

## SCREENING AND DIAGNOSIS

A doctor will ask about symptoms and medical history and will perform a physical exam. The doctor will focus on the nervous system. To help rule out other causes of the inflammation, such as a tumor, the doctor may order a magnetic resonance imaging (MRI) scan (a scan that uses radio waves and a powerful magnet to produce detailed computer images) or a computed tomography (CT) scan (a detailed X-ray picture that identifies abnormalities of fine tissue structure).

To rule out bacterial meningitis, the doctor may order a lumbar puncture (spinal tap), which removes fluid from the lower spinal column to be tested for bacteria (bacterial cultures), or the doctor may order other cultures, such as blood, urine, mucus, and pus from skin infections.

## TREATMENT AND THERAPY

Treatment includes rest and fluids, nonsteroidal anti-inflammatory drugs, and aspirin. Aspirin, however, is not recommended for children with a current or recent viral infection. Antibiotics may be given for two to three days while waiting for bacterial cultures to be reported as negative. If encephalitis is present, the doctor may prescribe IV antiviral drugs and other medications.

## PREVENTION AND OUTCOMES

To help prevent infection, one should wash his or her hands often if in close contact with an infected person, after changing the diaper of an infected infant, or if working in a child-care setting; and should regularly wash objects and surfaces touched by children using a diluted bleach solution. Persons who have not had measles, mumps, rubella, or chickenpox should consider being vaccinated.

Some forms of viral meningitis are spread by mosquito bites. One should follow public health recommendations for reducing mosquitoes near one's home and should take steps to avoid being bitten by mosquitoes.

If thinking about pregnancy, one should ensure protection (such as a chickenpox vaccine) from common diseases. Also, one should avoid all contact with rodents during pregnancy because lymphocytic choriomeningitis virus can be acquired from pet hamsters, mice, or other rodents. Pregnant women who have a pet rodent should consider finding another home for the rodent for the duration of the pregnancy.

*Rick Alan; reviewed by David L. Horn, M.D., FACP*

## FURTHER READING

Ferreiros, C. *Emerging Strategies in the Fight Against Meningitis.* New York: Garland Science, 2002.

Logan, Sarah A. E., and Eithne MacMahon. "Viral Meningitis." *British Medical Journal* 336 (January 5, 2008): 36-40.

National Institute of Neurological Disorders and Stroke. "Meningitis and Encephalitis Fact Sheet." Available at http://www.ninds.nih.gov.

Shmaefsky, Brian. *Meningitis.* Rev. ed. Philadelphia: Chelsea House, 2010.

Strauss, James, and Ellen Strauss. *Viruses and Human Disease.* 2d ed. Boston: Academic Press/Elsevier, 2008.

Wagner, Edward K., and Martinez J. Hewlett. *Basic Virology.* 3d ed. Malden, Mass.: Blackwell Science, 2008.

## WEB SITES OF INTEREST

*Centers for Disease Control and Prevention*
http://www.cdc.gov

*Meningitis Research Foundation*
http://www.meningitis.org

*National Center for Emerging and Zoonotic Infectious Diseases*
http://www.cdc.gov/ncezid

**See also:** Airborne illness and disease; Bacterial meningitis; Chickenpox; Echovirus infections; Encephalitis; Enterovirus infections; Fecal-oral route of transmission; Herpesviridae; Herpesvirus infections; Immunodeficiency; Inflammation; Insect-borne illness and disease; Measles; Mosquito-borne viral encephalitis; Mosquitoes and infectious disease; Mumps; Poliomyelitis; Pregnancy and infectious disease; Respiratory route of transmission; Rodents and infectious disease; Rubella; Vectors and vector control; Viral infections; West Nile virus.

# Viral pharyngitis

CATEGORY: Diseases and conditions
ANATOMY OR SYSTEM AFFECTED: Pharynx, throat, upper respiratory tract
ALSO KNOWN AS: Sore throat, viral sore throat

## DEFINITION

Viral pharyngitis is a sore, inflamed throat caused by infection with a virus.

## CAUSES

The viruses most likely to cause a sore throat are adenovirus, rhinovirus, parainfluenza virus, coxsackie virus, herpes simplex virus, Epstein-Barr virus, cytomegalovirus, and the human immunodeficiency virus (HIV).

## RISK FACTORS

Risk factors for viral pharyngitis include cigarette smoking or exposure to secondhand smoke; living or working in close quarters (such as day care, school, or military); diabetes; lowered immunity caused by excess fatigue, poor eating habits, and poor hygiene; and recent illness. Also, children are at greatest risk.

## SYMPTOMS

Symptoms of viral pharyngitis include a sore, red, swollen throat; trouble swallowing; decreased appetite; fatigue; and swollen, tender lymph nodes in the neck and behind the ears.

## SCREENING AND DIAGNOSIS

A doctor will ask about symptoms and medical history and will perform a physical exam. Most viral sore throats are diagnosed based on the symptoms and examination of the throat. Often, the throat will be swabbed to rule out a strep infection, which would require treatment with antibiotics. A viral sore throat is a diagnosis of exclusion; that is, it is made when a sore throat is present and strep is unlikely. Even in the absence of strep, some types of sore throats need further tests or treatment.

## Treatment and Therapy

There are no treatments to cure a viral sore throat. Most cases of viral pharyngitis heal on their own within about one week. A sore throat, however, may be the initial symptom of an HIV infection.

Treatments to relieve symptoms until the infection heals include over-the-counter pain medication, such as acetaminophen or ibuprofen. Aspirin, however, is not recommended for children or teens with a current or recent viral infection because of the risk of Reye's syndrome. One should consult a doctor about medicines that are safe for children.

Other treatments are gargling with warm salt-water and using throat lozenges every couple of hours; drinking increased amounts of fluids (including hot drinks and soups); and running a cool-mist humidifier, which can help keep nasal passages moist and reduce congestion, two factors that can worsen a sore throat.

## Prevention and Outcomes

To reduce the chance of getting a viral sore throat, one should practice good hygiene, including careful handwashing; should avoid sharing food or beverages; and should avoid areas where people are smoking. One should seek medical care if the sore throat worsens; if the sore throat is associated with new or serious symptoms, especially difficult breathing, weakness, or chills; or if the sore throat does not get better within the time frame predicted by a doctor.

*Rosalyn Carson-DeWitt, M.D.;*
*reviewed by Elie Edmond Rebeiz, M.D., FACS*

## Further Reading

Ferrari, Mario. *PDxMD Ear, Nose, and Throat Disorders.* Philadelphia: PDxMD, 2003.

Kimball, Chad T. *Colds, Flu, and Other Common Ailments Sourcebook.* Detroit: Omnigraphics, 2001.

Pechère, Jean Claude, and Edward L. Kaplan, eds. *Streptococcal Pharyngitis: Optimal Management.* New York: S. Karger, 2004.

Vincent, Miriam T. "Sore Throat-Strep Throat? When to Worry." *Pediatrics for Parents* 21, no. 8 (August 1, 2004): 11-12.

## Web Sites of Interest

*American Academy of Family Physicians*
http://familydoctor.org

*American Academy of Otolaryngology—Head and Neck Surgery*
http://www.entnet.org

*Centers for Disease Control and Prevention*
http://www.cdc.gov

*College of Family Physicians of Canada*
http://www.cfpc.ca

*Public Health Agency of Canada*
http://www.phac-aspc.gc.ca

**See also:** Adenovirus infections; Children and infectious disease; Common cold; Coxsackie virus infections; Cytomegalovirus infection; Epstein-Barr virus infection; Genital herpes; Herpes simplex infection; Herpesvirus infections; HIV; Inflammation; Influenza; Laryngitis; Mononucleosis; Nasopharyngeal infections; Orthomyxoviridae; Parotitis; Parvovirus infections; Pharyngitis and tonsillopharyngitis; Respiratory syncytial virus infections; Rhinovirus infections; Strep throat; Streptococcal infections; Thrush; Viral infections; Viral upper respiratory infections.

# Viral upper respiratory infections

**Category:** Diseases and conditions
**Anatomy or system affected:** Ears, lungs, muscles, nose, throat, upper respiratory tract
**Also known as:** Cold, common cold, influenza, the flu

## Definition

Viral upper respiratory infection comprises the common cold and influenza. A common cold is a viral infection that irritates the upper respiratory tract (nose and throat). Colds are commonly mistaken for influenza, a more severe viral disease that affects the respiratory system and includes a high fever and extreme fatigue, among other symptoms.

## CAUSES

The common cold is caused by any of about two hundred viruses, including rhinovirus, coronavirus, adenovirus, coxsackie virus, paramyxovirus, parainfluenza virus, and respiratory syncytial virus. There are two significant types of influenza viruses: A and B (influenza virus type C causes minor infections).

The vast majority of the population in any given area may get colds or influenza during the course of a year. The average rate for adults in the United States is three or four infections per person per year. Children get even more.

## RISK FACTORS

Risk factors for getting a cold include being near someone who has a cold; touching one's nose, mouth, or eyes with contaminated fingers; having allergies (which lengthens the duration of the cold); smoking or being near cigarette smoke (because of decreased resistance); and stress (because of decreased resistance). Another risk factor for the common cold (and influenza) is living in crowded conditions.

For the seasonal flu, people younger than age five years or older than age sixty-five years are most at risk for contracting the flu, as are health care workers. Several groups of people are at high risk for complications from the flu. According to the Centers for Disease Control and Prevention (CDC), high-risk groups include pregnant women, people with certain chronic medical conditions (such as heart disease or diabetes), people whose immune system is weakened or suppressed (such as persons with human immunodeficiency virus infection), young children, and people older than age fifty years.

## SYMPTOMS

Common cold symptoms, which usually resolve on their own within one to two weeks, include a sore or scratchy throat; stuffy nose (hard to breathe through nose); runny nose; sneezing; itchy, stuffed sensation in the ears; watery eyes; slight cough; headache; aches and pains; low energy and malaise; and low-grade fever.

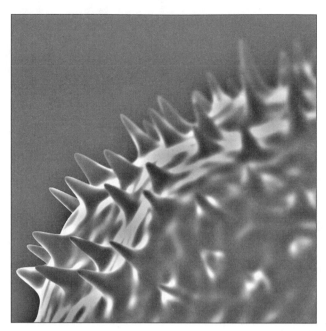

*An illustration of the surface of an influenza virion, or virus particle. Influenza is one type of viral upper respiratory tract infection.*

The classic symptoms of the flu, which can take up to four days (in adults) from the time of infection to appear, are high fever and chills, sore throat, dry cough, runny nose, watery eyes, severe muscle aches, severe fatigue and malaise, decreased appetite, and headache. The headache can be severe enough to cause sensitivity to light. Muscle aches are most common in the legs, though they can appear anywhere in the body.

Nausea, vomiting, and diarrhea can occur in people with the flu and are especially common in children. Most flu symptoms disappear in five to six days, though full recovery takes longer; the fatigue may last several weeks.

Most people are familiar with cold and flu symptoms; however, one should be aware of a few specifics. Having a runny nose in which the discharge is yellow or green and combined with a fever, sore face or teeth, and persistent symptoms may signal the onset of a sinus infection. Blood in the mucus or phlegm and a headache are even more likely to be the result of a sinus infection.

A dry cough is much less problematic than a wet cough. Colored sputum, be it yellow, green, or bloody, could be a sign of bronchitis or pneumonia; in such cases, one should contact a doctor, especially if the infected person is a smoker.

If the glands near the throat are swollen or if the throat is bright red or covered with yellow or white discharge, the infected person may have strep throat. Strep throat should be treated with penicillin (to prevent rheumatic fever).

### SCREENING AND DIAGNOSIS

The purpose of screening is early diagnosis and treatment. Screening tests are usually administered to people without current symptoms, but who may be at high risk for certain diseases or conditions. There are no screening tests for colds and influenza. Diagnosis and treatment begin with the onset of symptoms.

Based on symptoms and a physical examination, a doctor can diagnose a cold or influenza. In some situations, tests, such as a throat culture or blood count, may be ordered to characterize the severity of the condition and identify other related problems.

Identification of the specific virus causing the symptoms is not usually necessary because it usually does not make a difference in treatment. However, if influenza A virus is suspected, on the basis of the time of year and community public health reports, persons who are at high risk for infection may be treated specifically for that virus.

Diagnosis may include the following: taking one's temperature every six to eight hours to help define the severity of the illness; a urinalysis to check for conditions (such as diabetes) that may make an acute case of cold or influenza worse (this is not usually done for colds or flu unless there is another reason to suspect urinary infection); a blood count to assess general health and the ability to fight the illness (also not done routinely in colds or flu); a throat culture if there are signs or symptoms of sore throat (to rule out strep throat); and a chest X ray if the doctor suspects that the infection has spread to the lungs (which could indicate pneumonia).

### TREATMENT AND THERAPY

The treatment and management of colds and influenza mainly involves alleviating symptoms, though the symptoms ordinarily resolve on their own. Persons with a chronic health condition, particularly diabetes and chronic heart and lung diseases, could see their condition worsen during a cold or flu. Occasion-ally, viral upper respiratory infections develop into complications such as ear or sinus infections or pneumonia.

Treatment includes pain relievers for body aches and headaches and medicine to reduce fever. Many over-the-counter, multisymptom flu treatments are available. They treat the worst cold symptoms and can bring relief, though they will not cure the flu. Treatments for the common cold include pain relievers (for aches and pains and fever) such as acetaminophen (Tylenol), ibuprofen (Motrin), and aspirin. Another treatment for the cold is the use of nasal sprays, which can shrink nasal passages and decrease mucous production. Nasal sprays should be used for two to three days only.

Medications against the flu virus are called antiviral medications. Two classes of antivirals are available against the flu virus: Neuraminidase inhibitors are effective against influenza A and B. They interfere with the release of the virus from infected cells. Two drugs are available in this class: oseltamivir (Tamiflu) and zanamivir (Relenza). Amantadines are effective only against (some) influenza A viruses, and viral resistance to this class of antivirals is high. Two drugs are available in this class: amantadine (Symmetrel) and rimantadine (Flumadine).

### PREVENTION AND OUTCOMES

The most important way to keep from getting or spreading a cold is by washing one's hands, and to do so well and often. Other ways to keep from getting a cold include keeping hands away from one's nose, mouth, and eyes, and avoiding people who have a cold.

Vaccination is the best protection against the flu. Because the flu viruses that circulate in the population change every year, it is important to get the flu vaccine each year. Vaccination is especially important in people who are at high risk for serious complications from influenza. It is also important that people who care for or live with a person in any of the risk groups be vaccinated to prevent giving the disease to the person at high risk. Health care workers should receive the vaccine every year.

The primary way of spreading both colds and influenza is person-to-person contact. Handwashing is the most neglected, yet most effective, method of disease containment. Using alcohol-based hand gels when washing is not possible is another effective method.

Persons at high risk of catching a cold or influenza or are at risk for developing complications from these infections should avoid crowded areas and contacting people who are obviously sick during the influenza season.

Each year, the World Health Organization tries to determine what strains of the influenza virus will be most dangerous in the upcoming influenza season. Vaccines are developed for these seasonal strains.

The seasonal flu vaccine has been associated with fewer hospitalizations and deaths from influenza or pneumonia among the elderly living in community settings (such as nursing homes or residential care). There are two types of seasonal flu vaccines. One is the flu shot, which is approved for use in people older than six months of age. The shot is made from an inactivated, killed virus. It is given by injection, usually into the arm. Another type of seasonal flu vaccine is the nasal spray flu vaccine, which is approved for healthy people between the ages of two and forty-nine years (and who are not pregnant). It is made from live, weakened flu viruses.

A possible side effect of the vaccines is a mild flu-like reaction, including fever, aches, and fatigue. Up to 5 percent of people experience these symptoms after getting the seasonal influenza vaccine.

*Ricker Polsdorfer, M.D.;*
*reviewed by David L. Horn, M.D., FACP*

**FURTHER READING**

Beigel, John, and Mike Bray. "Current and Future Antiviral Therapy of Severe Seasonal and Avian Influenza." *Antiviral Research* 78 (2008): 91-102. Article discusses the use of antiviral medications against influenza viruses.

Belshe, R. B., et al. "Live Attenuated Versus Inactivated Influenza Vaccine in Infants and Young Children." *New England Journal of Medicine* 356, no. 7 (2007): 685-696. Discusses the differences between influenza vaccine types.

Cowling, B. J., et al. "Facemasks and Hand Hygiene to Prevent Influenza Transmission in Households." *Annals of Internal Medicine* 151, no. 7 (2009): 437-446. Discussion of handwashing and the use of masks to prevent the spread of the flu.

Eccles, Ronald, and Olaf Weber, eds. *Common Cold.* Boston: Birkhäuser, 2009. A general text examining all aspects of the common cold.

National Institute of Allergy and Infectious Diseases. "Common Cold." Available at http://www.niaid.nih.gov/topics/commoncold. Good introduction to the common cold.

Pappas, D. E., et al. "Symptom Profile of Common Colds in School-Aged Children." *Pediatric Infectious Disease Journal* 27 (2008): 8-11. Details common symptoms of the cold in children who are in school environments.

Schaffer, Kirsten, Alberto M. LaRosa, and Estella Whimbey. "Respiratory Viruses." In *Cohen and Powderly Infectious Diseases*, edited by Jonathan Cohen, Steven M. Opal, and William G. Powderly. 3d ed. Philadelphia: Mosby/Elsevier, 2010. Describes viruses responsible for respiratory conditions, including prevalence and manifestation of respiratory virus infection.

Strauss, James, and Ellen Strauss. *Viruses and Human Disease.* Burlington, Mass.: Elsevier, 2008. Detailed discussion of animal viruses with emphasis on those associated with human disease. Includes accounts of the history of human viruses.

*2011 PDR for Nonprescription Drugs, Dietary Supplements, and Herbs.* Toronto, Ont.: Thomson Health Care, 2010. The basic drug reference book for health care professionals, this PDR guide to nonprescription drugs is updated yearly with information about commonly used OTCs, organized alphabetically by manufacturer's name.

**WEB SITES OF INTEREST**

*American Lung Association*
http://www.lungusa.org

*Centers for Disease Control and Prevention*
http://www.cdc.gov

*Clean Hands Coalition*
http://www.cleanhandscoalition.org

*Flu.gov*
http://www.flu.gov

*National Foundation for Infectious Diseases*
http://www.nfid.org

*World Health Organization*
http://www.who.int/topics/influenza

**See also:** Adenovirus infections; Airborne illness and disease; Allergic bronchopulmonary aspergillosis; Atypical pneumonia; Bronchiolitis; Bronchitis; Children and infectious disease; Common cold; Contagious diseases; Coronavirus infections; Coxsackie virus infections; Epiglottitis; Home remedies; Influenza; Influenza vaccine; Laryngitis; Paramyxoviridae; Parvovirus infections; Pharyngitis and tonsillopharyngitis; Pneumonia; Respiratory syncytial virus infections; Rhinovirus infections; Seasonal influenza; Sinusitis; Strep throat; Viral infections; Viral pharyngitis; Whooping cough.

# Virology

CATEGORY: Epidemiology

## DEFINITION

Virology is the study of viruses and their role in disease. The science includes human, animal, insect, plant, fungal, and bacterial virology. Researchers may work in clinical, ecological, biological, or biochemical fields.

## HISTORY

The first studies of viruses and their role in causing disease began thousands of years ago in China, when an early form of vaccination against smallpox was developed. This early process involved applying tiny amounts of secretions from a person who had smallpox to those who had not yet been infected to keep them from becoming infected. Viruses received closer study in 1892, when Russian bacteriologist Dmitri Ivanovsky noticed in an experiment that the agent that carried tobacco mosaic disease could pass through filters that kept out bacteria. Though the question still existed as to what exactly this agent was, it was soon discovered by Dutch microbiologist Martinus Beijerinck that the agent grew in the host and, therefore, was not a toxin. However, the agent had other characteristics not found in bacteria. Louis Pasteur then experimented with immunizations using viruses, and others continued these studies throughout the nineteenth century and into the twentieth century.

The modern study of virology began early in the twentieth century with the discovery of bacterio-phages, viruses that infect bacteria. Plant viruses and bacteriophages are fairly easy to grow in a laboratory environment, so it became easier to experiment with and observe these viruses. Animal viruses normally require a living host, which impeded study in virology until 1931, when it was demonstrated that the influenza virus could be grown in fertilized chicken eggs. This method is still used to develop flu vaccines.

Already in 1903, discussions had begun about how viruses caused cancer by transduction (by transferring genetic material from one bacterium to another using a bacteriophage). Peyton Rous described this type of oncovirus in chickens in 1911, and it was later determined to be a retrovirus, a type that includes the human immunodeficiency virus.

By 1937, the yellow fever virus was being grown in chicken eggs, and vaccines were being developed with many different viruses. With the introduction of the electron microscope in the 1940's came the ability to see viruses.

Viruses have been the cause of many of the epidemics and pandemics that have occurred worldwide. These epidemics include the yellow fever epidemics

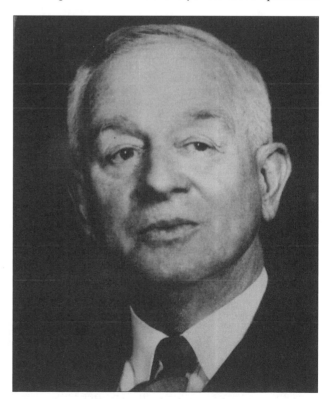

*Peyton Rous.* (The Nobel Foundation)

of 1793 and 1878 and the Spanish flu pandemic of 1918. Late twentieth and twenty-first century viruses have caused epidemics and pandemics of human immunodeficiency virus (HIV) infection, severe acute respiratory syndrome (SARS), and H1N1 influenza.

## VIROLOGISTS

As undergraduates, virologists generally studied biology or chemistry, with a focus on biochemistry and cell biology. (The biology of viruses is closely tied to cell biology.) Other common areas of study are epidemiology, behavioral and social sciences, and the humanities because of the impact of viruses on human health. Virologists have extensive science backgrounds and also may take courses in physics, mathematics, molecular biology, immunology, and structural biology.

Most virologists continue their education to earn a medical degree (M.D.). They attend medical school for four years, complete a residency of three years, and train in postdoctoral research for three to five years. Others earn a doctoral degree (Ph.D.) by attending graduate school for four to six years and then training in postdoctoral research for three to five years. Graduates may then pursue research in a variety of areas, including human health, infectious diseases, and epidemiology. Virologists who intend to teach often substitute formal teacher-training for postdoctoral research.

## IMPACT

Each year, public health officials, including virologists, attempt to determine, for example, what types of influenza viruses are likely to cause the most infections during the yearly flu season. Virologists help to craft a vaccine to keep these viruses from spreading.

Virology also is studying how a bundle of proteins called interferon, which are produced during a viral infection of a cell, triggers an immune response. These proteins somehow inhibit the replication of the virus in the cell. Virology also is looking at how viruses may cause some types of cancers and at how viruses cause the body's immune response to occasionally malfunction and develop autoimmune disorders.

Viruses have an interesting role in genetics too because of their ability to carry extra genetic material into host cells. This ability has been studied by virologists through transferring material specifying a particular enzyme into the nucleus of host cells that lack the ability to synthesize that enzyme. This method has particular interest for those studying hereditary enzyme-deficiency diseases, such as diabetes, because these gene transfers may help to cure such diseases.

*Marianne M. Madsen, M.S.*

## FURTHER READING

Carter, John, and Venetia Saunders. *Virology: Principles and Applications.* Hoboken, N.J.: John Wiley & Sons, 2007. Basic virology textbook with an "at-a-glance" feature for each chapter, a list of abbreviations, and a glossary.

Dimmock, N. J., A. J. Easton, and K. N. Leppard. *Introduction to Modern Virology.* 6th ed. Hoboken, N.J.: Wiley-Blackwell, 2007. Includes the definition of viruses and discusses laboratory techniques and the evolution of viruses. Chapters focus on specific groups of viruses.

Norkin, Leonard. *Virology: Molecular Biology and Pathogenesis.* Washington, D.C.: ASM Press, 2010. A detailed account of virus structure and replication and the basis for disease pathology.

Shors, Teri. *Understanding Viruses.* Sudbury, Mass.: Jones and Bartlett, 2008. Includes historical perspectives on viruses and treatment and prevention information.

## WEB SITES OF INTEREST

*American Society for Virology*
http://www.asv.org

*Pan American Society for Clinical Virology*
http://www.virology.org

*U.K. Clinical Virology Network*
http://www.clinical-virology.org

*Virology.net*
http://www.virology.net

**See also:** Biochemical tests; Diagnosis of viral infections; Disease eradication campaigns; Emerging and reemerging infectious diseases; Epidemics and pandemics: Causes and management; Epidemiology; Immune response to viral infections; Microbiology; Outbreaks; Pathogenicity; Prevention of viral infections; Public health; Serology; Transmission routes; Tuberculosis (TB) vaccine; Viral infections; Virulence; Viruses: Structure and life cycle; Viruses: Types.

# Virulence

CATEGORY: Epidemiology
ALSO KNOWN AS: Infectiousness, pathogenicity

## DEFINITION

The term "virulence" means the disease-producing (pathogenic) capabilities and mechanisms of a microorganism and also the inherent potential of an infection to cause harm.

## DISEASE-CAUSING AGENTS

The human body is populated by a multitude of bacteria, viruses, fungi, and parasites. Most pathogens, except viruses, are harmless, and some are even beneficial. These microorganisms live, feed, and grow in or on the body, the host. Microorganisms that take from the host or change it in some way, that contribute nothing to the host's survival, and that harm the host by causing infection, are known collectively as pathogens or parasites. These abilities, mechanisms, and potentials define a pathogen's virulence.

Infection virulence is characterized by its effect on the host and is measured by degrees. For example, an infection that causes death is considered more virulent than an infection that causes disability. Mortality rate is another way to measure the virulence of an infection.

The properties and mechanisms of virulence in many pathogens are well known to medical biologists. By understanding the capacity of virulence in microorganisms, medical biologists can estimate the likelihood of a particular microorganism causing infection, the rate at which an infection will likely spread through a population, the capacity of a pathogen to invade and damage the host, the severity and impact of an infection on individual hosts and entire populations, and the mortality rate of an infection. However, a complete understanding of virulence in many pathogens remains elusive because of the evolution of pathogens, both outside and inside the human body, and because of the many factors involved in virulence.

## VIRULENCE FACTORS

Virulence factors refer to the properties and mechanisms that enable a microorganism to enter a host and cause harm. Virulence factors operate at the molecular and genetic levels. A single pathogen may have one or many virulence factors, and there are huge variations in virulence among pathogens. Some bacteria species, for example, engender different diseases by combining different virulence factors. Some of the more common, and easy-to-understand, virulence factors are discussed here.

*Adherence.* To cause infection, pathogens must first adhere to certain cells on the surface of tissue in the host. If they do not adhere, they will be flushed away by mucus and other fluids that naturally rid the body of foreign invaders. Bacteria, in particular, have evolved mechanisms that allow them to attach themselves to host cells. Dental plaque, for example, is caused by bacteria with the power to stick fast to the teeth and gums.

*Colonization.* Bacteria and viruses are most harmful when they work cooperatively, or colonize, as all bacteria or all viruses, in huge numbers called colonies. These colonies provide benefit among members, but they harm the host.

*Adaptation.* Some pathogens produce specific enzymes (proteins that speed up chemical changes) in response to their environment that enable them to flourish and produce infection. Some enzymes cut into cells, allowing the pathogen to enter. Some dissolve the glue between cells, allowing the pathogen to spread. Others protect the pathogen from the body's natural defenses. For example, the fungus *Cryptococcus gatti* (which causes a deadly but rare lung disease) develops a thick outer coating after it enters the lungs. Also, some bacteria can produce enzymes to counter the effects of antibiotics; this ability of bacteria is known as antibiotic resistance.

*Toxicity.* Some pathogens manufacture toxins (poisons) inside the body that immobilize, damage, or destroy vital components or functions of the host, allowing the pathogen to thrive. The agents that cause cholera, botulism, anthrax, and tetanus are examples of this type of pathogen. Toxins produced by bacteria outside the body cause many of the diseases commonly known as food poisoning, including *Salmonella* infection and *Escherichia coli* infection.

Virulence factors in pathogens and the virulence of infections are parts of the equation only. The final part involves factors within the host.

## HOST FACTORS

Virulence involves a complex interaction of the pathogen, infection, and host. Various factors inherent in or acquired by the host influence the effects of a pathogen or infection. Host factors include age, gender, genetic makeup, nutritional status, immune system status, and acquired immunity.

The status of the immune system is particularly important. Persons (hosts) with weakened immune systems, such as those with cancer or human immunodeficiency virus (HIV) infection; the morbidly obese; and drug addicts, are susceptible to microorganisms not normally harmful to healthy people. People with weakened immune systems also contract more infectious diseases, experience more severe symptoms, have more chronic infections, and heal more slowly from injuries and wounds than do healthy people.

Acquired immunity is powerful protection against infection. Humans acquire immunity, or resistance, to some pathogens and infections through previous exposure to them. That exposure can come from contracting an infectious disease or through acquired immunological resistance (vaccination). After acquiring immunity, the immune system becomes stimulated when encountering certain pathogens, and it can reduce the virulence of an infection to such low levels that no symptoms appear.

## IMPACT

Virulence from both pathogens and infections has affected the course of civilizations. The great plague epidemics in Europe in the Middle Ages and the smallpox epidemics that decimated Native American peoples are two examples of the power of virulence.

On the positive side, the systematic study of virulence has contributed to advances in the biological sciences and to a better understanding of pathogens and infections. Researchers have unraveled the genomes of many pathogens, and based on an understanding of the makeup and evolution of pathogen virulence, medical biologists are finding ways to manage virulence by selecting for mild strains of infection, thus forcing the more virulent strains into extinction. Also, specific antigens (substances that stimulate the immune response) are being created for active immunity against some of the most dangerous pathogens.

*Wendell Anderson, B.A.*

## FURTHER READING

Dieckmann, Ulf, et al., eds. *Adaptive Dynamics of Infectious Diseases: In Pursuit of Virulence Management.*

New York: Cambridge University Press, 2005. An introductory text for infectious disease researchers.

Ewald, Paul W. "The Evolution of Virulence and Emerging Diseases." *Journal of Urban Health* 75 (1998) 480-491. Provides insights into the evolution of virulence.

Madigan, Michael T., and John M. Martinko. *Brock Biology of Microorganisms.* 12th ed. Upper Saddle River, N.J.: Pearson/Prentice Hall, 2010. This text outlines many common bacteria and describes their natural history, pathogenicity, and other characteristics.

Myers, Judith H., and Lorne E. Rothman. "Virulence and Transmission of Infectious Diseases in Humans and Insects: Evolutionary and Demographic Patterns." *Trends in Ecology and Evolution* 10 (1995): 194-198. A discussion of the evolution of diseases.

Perlman, R. L. "Life Histories of Pathogen Populations." *International Journal of Infectious Diseases* 13 (2009): 121-124. Argues that the virulence of pathogens should be rethought as a feature of pathogen populations, or groups, rather than as a feature of individual microorganisms within these populations.

Wilson, Michael, Brian Henderson, and Rod McNab. *Bacterial Disease Mechanisms: An Introduction to Cellular Microbiology.* New York: Cambridge University Press, 2002. Based on research advances in microbiology, molecular biology, and cell biology, this work describe the interactions between bacteria and human cells both in health and during infection.

## WEB SITES OF INTEREST

*Microbiology and Immunology On-line*
http://pathmicro.med.sc.edu/book/welcome.htm

*National Institute of Allergy and Infectious Diseases*
http://www.niaid.nih.gov

*Todar's Online Textbook of Bacteriology*
http://www.textbookofbacteriology.net/pathogenesis

**See also:** Antibiotics: Types; Antibodies; Bacteria: Classification and types; Bacteriology; Carriers; Contagious diseases; Drug resistance; Fungi: Classification and types; Hosts; Immunity; Immunodeficiency; Incubation period; Koch's postulates; Parasites: Classification and types; Pathogenicity; Pathogens; Virology; Viruses: Structure and life cycle; Viruses: Types.

# Viruses: Structure and life cycle

CATEGORY: Pathogen

### DEFINITION

A virus is a parasitic pathogenic microorganism consisting of a protein coat called a capsid that surrounds genetic material, which can be either deoxyribonucleic acid (DNA) or ribonucleic acid (RNA). Each virus type carries out a life cycle tailored to that particular organism, but in general, the process begins with the entrance of the virus's genetic material into the host cell, the replication of the viral genome, and the viral genome's packaging within newly produced capsid proteins.

### STRUCTURAL CHARACTERISTICS

The individual virus particle, known as a virion, consists of genetic material, either DNA or RNA, surrounded by a protein coat called a capsid. Some viruses also include an external lipid envelope generally obtained by budding through a cell membrane during the assembly process. Both the morphology (physical shape) or appearance of the virus and the presence of a viral envelope are genetically determined. The morphology of virus particles encompasses many sizes, ranging from 20 nanometers (nm) in diameter for the smallest viruses, such as those that are the etiological agents for the common cold (rhinoviruses) or certain forms of hepatitis (hepatitis A virus), to the largest and most complex viruses in the 500 nm range (smallpox virus). The poxviruses are large enough to be observed with conventional light microscopes. By comparison, the average-size bacterium is approximately 1 to 2 micrometers (µm) in diamcter, or roughly two to four timcs largcr than the largest viruses, and a blood cell is approximately 20 µm in diameter.

Viruses are limited in the quantity of genetic material they carry. Consequently, the most efficient means to encode the proteins that will be used for the capsid is to utilize repeating protein units known as protomers, which can self-assemble into the subunits, or capsomeres, of the capsid. The result of utilizing re-

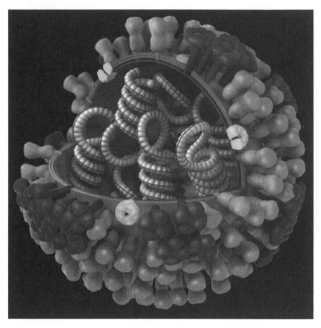

*An illustration of the structure of an influenza virion, or virus particle.* (CDC)

peating units is that the morphological symmetry will be one of two forms: icosahedral (cuboidal) or helical. The only exception is found among the large poxviruses that exhibit a more complex symmetry, reflecting their ability to encode more than two hundred proteins.

Helical capsids resemble long hollow tubes in which the genome is in the center and capsomeres are arranged in a helical fashion around the core. All known helical viruses contain RNA as the genetic material. Examples of helical viruses include some bacterial viruses, the tobacco mosaic virus (TMV), influenza virus, and measles virus. The helical capsid for some viruses, including measles and influenza, is enclosed within a viral envelope.

Icosahedral-shaped viruses have twenty faces, each an equilateral triangle, and twelve corners or vertices. These viruses exhibit what is known as 5:3:2 symmetry, representing the symmetry exhibited by respective axes of the virus. Capsomeres on the faces consist of six protomers (hexons), while capsomeres that make up the vertices consist of five protomers (pentons). The precise numbers of protomers and the diameter of the virus particle are functions of the size of the genome. Icosahedral viruses include the papilloma (wart) viruses, poliovirus, rhinoviruses (common cold), and herpesviruses. The herpesviruses also contain an external envelope. The largest viruses, including the poxviruses, exhibit a more complex structure that is neither helical nor icosahedral. The poxviruses also contain complex internal structures.

The viral capsid in many viruses is enclosed within a lipid membrane called the envelope. With the exception of the poxviruses, the envelope is derived entirely from host cell membranes. Viruses such as the herpesviruses, which replicate in the nucleus of the cell, acquire an envelope by budding through the inner nuclear membrane. Viruses such as influenza and measles obtain their envelope by budding through cytoplasmic membranes. Viral envelopes usually have protein projections, viral encoded spikes or peplomers, on their surface that determine the host range for the virus. For example, influenza viruses have two sets of spikes embedded within their envelopes: the hemagglutinin (H) antigen protein, which attaches the virus to the target cell, and a neuraminidase (N) protein, which is used for release from the cell.

## VIRAL GENOMES

The structures of viral genetic molecules encompass numerous categories. Viral genomes may be either single-stranded DNA (parvoviruses, which are associated with fifth disease in humans), double-stranded DNA (adenoviruses and herpesviruses), single-stranded RNA (poliovirus, influenza, measles, rabies, and human immunodeficiency virus), or double-stranded RNA (rotaviruses). The genome in some RNA viruses may consist of a single segment (poliovirus, measles, and rabies) or may consist of multiple individual segments (influenza and rotaviruses). The genome in human immunodeficiency virus (HIV) is diploid, consisting of two identical copies of the RNA. The Baltimore classification scheme used to categorize or classify viruses is based upon the type of genome and its replication strategy.

## VIRAL INFECTION

Viral infection begins with the adsorption of the particle to the host cell, with the variety of targets referred to as the host range. Attachment is dependent upon the interaction between viral surface molecules and specific receptors on the target cell. Cells that lack such receptors cannot be infected by that virus.

For example, HIV infects a class of lymphocytes called T cells that express the CD4 receptor protein. The rhinoviruses attach to a molecule on the surface of respiratory mucosal tissues called the intercellular adhesion molecule-1 (ICAM-1). Influenza H antigen attaches to a class of carbohydrates on the surface of respiratory cells. Most viruses are species-specific, infecting members only within the same species. Influenza virus is an exception. Because many organisms, including humans and birds, express the same carbohydrates on respiratory tissues, influenza has a wide host range that crosses species lines.

The ability of a virus to infect specific tissues is dependent on the expression of receptors by the host cell, leading to the question of why evolution does not select for cells that no longer express those receptor molecules. The answer lies in why cells express such receptors in the first place. The molecule is required for normal functions of the cell, particularly in its interactions with other cells. For example, the CD4 HIV receptor on T lymphocytes is critical for lymphocyte interactions with other classes of white blood cells. ICAM-1 molecules likewise facilitate cell-cell interactions and serve as a signal mediator in immune functions.

Attachment is followed by penetration of the viral capsid into the cell. If the virus has an envelope, fusion of the viral and cell membranes, analogous to two oil droplets fusing, allows the capsid to penetrate into the cell cytoplasm. Alternatively, if the virus lacks an envelope (and sometimes with viruses that do contain an envelope), the particle enters though a process called endocytosis, in which the cell membrane flows around or "envelops" the attached viral particle. Once inside the cell, the capsid is disassembled, releasing the genome. DNA viruses such as the herpesviruses generally travel to the nucleus for replication, while RNA viruses such as poliovirus and rhinoviruses replicate in the cytoplasm.

## VIRAL MULTIPLICATION

Once the viral capsid has been disassembled, the expression and replication of the viral genome begin. The process used by DNA viruses differs from that in the replication of RNA viruses; cells already contain the basic machinery for the replication and expression of DNA, while no cellular enzymes are present for the replication of RNA.

The proteins necessary for duplication (DNA polymerases, DNA ligases, and other auxiliary molecules) and transcription (RNA polymerase) of viral DNA are already present in the nucleus of the cell. The processes of viral DNA replication and expression differ little from those that normally take place in the cell, and for smaller viruses cellular proteins are sufficient. Some larger viruses, such as the herpesviruses and poxviruses, have the genetic capacity to encode some of their own replication enzymes. For example, both herpesviruses and poxviruses synthesize their own specific DNA polymerases and are not dependent on the cellular enzymes.

Transcription and translation of genetic material immediately following infection results in the production of proteins utilized in the duplication of viral DNA. These are referred to as early genes, reflecting the timing of their expression. Genes expressed after DNA duplication are referred to as late genes and primarily encode structural or capsid proteins.

Because the cell lacks any machinery for duplication of RNA, RNA viruses must encode their own enzymes for duplication of their genetic material. The Baltimore classification scheme for RNA viruses roughly classifies these viruses on the nature or polarity of the RNA genome. Messenger RNA (mRNA), the RNA that is directly translated by cell ribosomes into protein, is defined as having a positive (+) polarity; RNA that is complementary to mRNA is defined as a minus (-) polarity. The + and - symbols here refer only to the orientation of the molecule and do not reflect a positive or negative charge. Positive-stranded viruses have a genome that is identical to mRNA, while minus- or negative-stranded viruses possess a genome that is complementary to their mRNA.

Positive-stranded RNA viruses include the rhinoviruses, poliovirus, hepatitis A virus, and some of the mosquito-borne encephalitis viruses. Following entry into the cell and removal of the capsid, the RNA immediately attaches cell ribosomes and begins the process of translation of viral proteins. Among the enzymes being synthesized is a viral-specific RNA transcriptase used to replicate the viral genome.

The category of negative-stranded RNA viruses includes the influenza viruses; measles, mumps, and rubella viruses; and rabies virus. Because the RNA is complementary to mRNA, it cannot be directly translated following cell penetration. Negative-stranded viruses incorporate the viral transcriptase directly into the progeny capsids during assembly. Following infec-

tion, the viral mRNA is then transcribed by the RNA transcriptase, which the virus carries. The transcriptase also functions in copying the positive mRNA into the progeny (or negative) strands for the next generation of viral particles.

HIV, the etiological agent of acquired immunodeficiency syndrome (AIDS), is in an unusual class of viruses called the retroviruses. Other viruses in this class include the RNA tumor viruses, the agents associated with tumors and leukemia primarily in nonhuman animals. The genome in the retrovirus is a diploid plus-stranded RNA. However, the genome does not function directly as the mRNA following infection. The particle carries within its capsid an enzyme referred to as a reverse transcriptase, the function of which is to copy the RNA genome into a double-stranded DNA. The viral DNA integrates within the host cell chromosome from which the viral mRNA is transcribed, producing capsid proteins and copies of the reverse transcriptase enzyme for progeny virions.

## ASSEMBLY AND RELEASE

Viral assembly is largely nonenzymatic and results from charge interactions among the structural proteins that make up the capsomeres. Animal viruses begin the assembly process in the region of the cell in which replication of the genome has taken place: RNA viruses in the cytoplasm and DNA viruses in the nucleus of the cell. Expression of the genes for structural proteins occurs primarily after the genome has been replicated. Capsid assembly begins as individual capsomeres commence forming scaffolds around the progeny genomes. The complexity of the process depends upon the coding capacity of the virus; larger and more complex viruses utilize a greater variety of assembly proteins, while smaller viruses may utilize only two or three protein molecules. The assembly of protein capsids is generally associated with a final cleavage step, in which capsid precursor proteins are cut to produce the final protein products.

Assembly and release of enveloped particles require an additional step: budding through a cell membrane. Some viruses, such as measles and influenza, encode a matrix or membrane protein (M) and those proteins that make up the spikes. The matrix and spikes are then inserted into the cell membrane. Assembly of the capsid is completed in association with the M protein, followed by a reverse endocytosis (exocytosis) as the virus buds through the membrane and acquires the envelope. Budding and release of influenza virus requires activity of the viral neuraminidase (N protein) that separates the envelope proteins on progeny viruses that would otherwise remain attached to carbohydrate residues on the cell surface. Some anti-influenza drugs act by inhibiting this enzyme activity. Maturation of the HIV capsid also requires a final proteolytic step using a viral encoded protease. Certain anti-HIV drugs target this reaction.

The effect of viral infection on the cell itself depends upon two factors: the extent of damage to the cell and whether cell processes are shut down. Productive infection by DNA viruses usually results in cell death. Viral products inhibit both transcription and translation of cell proteins, and release of progeny virions coincides with cell lysis. Alternatively, herpesvirus infections may result in a latent infection in which the virus does not carry out a complete cycle and is retained in a nonreplicative form within the cell. The cell remains functional while the virus is carried by the human host throughout his or her life. Enveloped viruses are released from the cell by budding through the cell membrane, a process that may damage or kill the host cell. The complete replication cycle for RNA viruses generally takes place in twelve to twenty-four hours, whereas DNA viruses require a slightly longer time, ranging from twenty-four to forty-eight hours.

## IMPACT

Viruses are a class of strict intracellular parasites. Unlike bacteria, viruses are largely devoid of metabolic and enzymatic reactions and are therefore dependent on enzymes and other molecules provided by the host cell. For decades following the discovery of viruses, experts believed the inert nature and dependence of viruses on host functions precluded development of antibiotics specifically targeting these organisms. However, in 1967, Joseph Kates and Brian McAuslan reported the presence of a viral polymerase in the capsid of poxviruses. In subsequent years, numerous viral encoded enzymes were discovered in infected cells, including the reverse transcriptase, an enzyme that copies viral genomic RNA into complementary DNA in cells infected with HIV and with RNA tumor viruses. The presence of enzymes and other molecules unique to viruses and required for their replication meant that antiviral compounds targeting viruses specifically could be developed.

Because many viruses utilize their own encoded polymerases for replication of their genomes, the first generation of antiviral antibiotics targeted these molecules. DNA analogs such as acyclovir and ganciclovir, molecules resembling normal nucleotides but that block genome replication, proved effective in treating herpesvirus infections. Amantadine was shown to block influenza virus infection and has proven effective in treating that illness. Two of the drugs targeting influenza, zanamivir and Tamiflu, act at the level of virus release, inhibiting the cleavage reaction involving the viral neuraminidase.

Several generations of drugs have been effective in controlling HIV replication. These include DNA analogs such as zidovudine (or azidothymidine, AZT) and protease inhibitors that block assembly of the virus. Although viruses do utilize host macromolecules for replication, the production of molecules unique to the virus has provided an opportunity for the application of antiviral drugs.

*Richard Adler, Ph.D.*

## FURTHER READING

Levine, Arnold. *Viruses.* New York: Scientific American Library/W. H. Freeman, 1992. Although an older source, this helpful book provides numerous photographs and a useful summary of virus structures and replication strategies.

Norkin, Leonard. *Virology: Molecular Biology and Pathogenesis.* Washington, D.C.: ASM Press, 2010. Using the framework of the Baltimore classification scheme, the author provides a detailed account of virus structure and replication and of the basis for disease pathology.

Strauss, James, and Ellen Strauss. *Viruses and Human Disease.* 2d ed. Boston: Academic Press/Elsevier, 2008. Detailed discussion of animal viruses with emphasis on those associated with human disease. Includes accounts of the history of human viruses.

Tidona, Christian, and Gholamreza Darai, eds. *The Springer Index of Viruses.* New York: Springer, 2002. An index for most major viruses that includes representative photographs and structure and replication strategy and history.

Wagner, Edward K., and Martinez J. Hewlett. *Basic Virology.* 3d ed. Malden, Mass.: Blackwell Science, 2008. An undergraduate text covering issues of virology and viral disease, properties of viruses and virus-cell interaction, working with viruses, and replication patterns of specific viruses.

Willey, Joanne, Linda Sherwood, and Christopher Woolverton. *Prescott's Microbiology.* 8th ed. New York: McGraw-Hill, 2011. Chapters in this general microbiology text cover structural and replication strategies of viruses. Includes numerous photographs and a glossary.

**WEB SITES OF INTEREST**

*Big Picture Book of Viruses*
http://www.virology.net/big_virology

*Centers for Disease Control and Prevention*
http://www.cdc.gov

*Universal Virus Database*
http://www.ictvdb.org

*Viral Zone*
http://www.expasy.org/viralzone
·,

**See also:** Antiviral drugs: Mechanisms of action; Antiviral drugs: Types; Immune response to viral infections; Microbiology; Parasites: Classification and types; Pathogens; Vaccines: Types; Viral infections; Virology; Viruses: Types.

---

# Viruses: Types

CATEGORY: Pathogen

### DEFINITION

Viruses are intracellular, parasitic, pathogenic organisms that consist of either deoxyribonucleic acid (DNA) or ribonucleic acid (RNA), either of which can be single-stranded or double-stranded depending on the virus type. Both types are surrounded by a protein coat called the capsid; the combination of genome and capsid is referred to as the nucleocapsid. Some viruses also have an outer envelope with embedded spikes acquired by budding through a cellular membrane.

### CLASSIFICATION

The morphology (physical shape) of the virus particle represents one broad category of viral classification. Most viruses are limited in the quantity of ge-

---

## Cross-Species Viruses

Viruses are smaller and less complex than cells, and they generally contain only a protein coat surrounding either deoxyribonucleic acid (DNA) or ribonucleic acid (RNA) as the genetic material. Some viruses may also have a covering membrane derived from the plasma membrane of the host cell from which they budded out during replication.

DNA viruses include adenoviruses (respiratory infections), herpesviruses (cold sores, genital herpes, pox infections, mononucleosis), papillomaviruses (certain warts), and hepatitis B virus. Viruses with genetic information in RNA include hepatitis A and C, myxoviruses (measles, mumps, influenzas), picornaviruses (polio, respiratory infections), rabies virus, and retroviruses (acquired immunodeficiency syndrome, or AIDS, and some types of leukemia).

Viruses that infect animals without causing disease may jump species to infect humans or mutate to produce major disease epidemics, such as influenzas from recombinant bird or pig viruses or infections with Ebola virus or the human immunodeficiency virus (HIV). In some cases, the animal source or reservoir is known, while often it is unknown. Many emerging diseases in human populations have originated in animals native to rainforest jungles or other habitats that humans have encroached upon, encountering previously unknown viruses.

---

netic material they encode. Consequently, the most efficient means to encode the proteins that will be used for the capsid is to utilize repeating protein units known as protomers, which can self-assemble into the subunits, or capsomeres, of the capsid. The result of utilizing repeating units is that the morphological symmetry will be one of two forms: icosahedral (cuboidal) and helical. The only exception is found among the large poxviruses that can encode more than two hundred proteins, allowing for a significantly greater complexity of structure.

Helical capsids resemble long hollow tubes in which the genome is in the center. Capsomeres are arranged in a helical fashion around the core. All known helical viruses contain RNA as the genetic material. The helical nucleocapsid for some viruses, such as rabies, measles, and influenza, is enclosed within a viral envelope. Icosahedral viruses have twenty faces, each an equilateral triangle, and twelve corners or vertices. Icosahedral viruses include the papilloma (wart) viruses, poliovirus, rhinovirus (which causes the common cold), and herpesvirus. The herpesviruses also contain an external envelope.

The host range of the virus, the species the virus can infect, is determined by proteins on the surface of the virus (the capsid on nonenveloped viruses or the spikes on enveloped particles) and viral receptors on the surface of the host cell. As a rule, viruses are species-specific: Human rhinoviruses, measles, and herpesviruses infect humans only. In some cases different species share common types of receptors, which explains why certain viruses, such as influenza and rabies, may cross species lines. Likewise, viruses may exhibit specific cell tropisms within the species, infecting only those tissues that express certain receptors. Influenza is a respiratory virus and does not infect other tissues; the popular term "stomach flu" is a misnomer because it involves neither the influenza virus nor the stomach.

## Viral Genomes

The disadvantage of classifying viruses on the basis of morphology is the failure of this method to take into account evolutionary relationships. Viruses, which are closely related genetically, may produce radically different pathologies; respiratory viruses like the rhinoviruses are genetically related to poliovirus and hepatitis A virus, even though the methods of transmission and the sites of infection differ.

In the early 1970's, David Baltimore, then a virologist at the Massachusetts Institute of Technology, proposed a method of classification in which virus families were grouped according to the structure and replication strategy of the genome. Viruses within the same class generally shared a genetic relationship, even though their pathologies differed. Baltimore proposed six classes: double-stranded or single-stranded DNA, classes I and II respectively; double-stranded RNA (class III); single-stranded RNA of positive (+) polarity (class IV); single-stranded RNA of negative (-) polarity (class V); and RNA viruses, which replicate through a DNA intermediate (class VI). Class VII was later added, representing double-stranded DNA viruses that use an RNA intermediate. The positive and negative polarities refer not to any charge, but to the orientation of the genome with respect to messenger RNA (mRNA). mRNA is defined as being a positive strand. Genomes that are positive-stranded are iden-

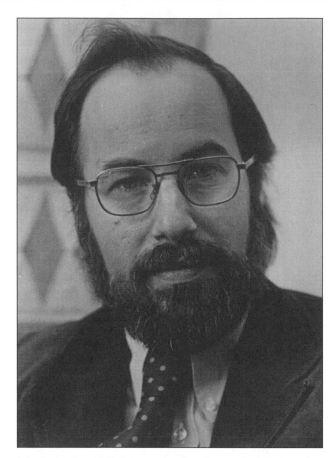

*Virologist David Baltimore developed a method of classification that grouped virus families.* (The Nobel Foundation)

tical to the mRNA, while negative-stranded genomes are complementary to mRNA.

Within each class, viruses are grouped in subcategories of families in which the suffix *viridae* denotes a family. For example, all herpesviruses are within the family Herpesviridae. The viral genus is denoted by the suffix *virus*, as in "rhinovirus" or "herpesvirus." The Baltimore classes are as follows:

*Class I: Double-stranded DNA viruses.* These include both nonenveloped viruses (Polyomaviridae, Papillomaviridae, and Adenoviridae) and two enveloped families (Herpesviridae and Poxviridae). The polyomaviruses that make up the family are highly species-specific, and most are not associated with human infections. The ability of several members of this family to cause neoplastic changes, or cancers, in cultured cells has led to extensive research into mechanisms of cell regulation. There is no evidence, however, that these viruses pose a threat to humans. One member of the family in particular, simian virus 40 (SV40), generated concern because it was a contaminant in early poliovirus vaccines grown in rhesus monkey cells; no evidence has been found to suggest the virus poses a threat to humans. However, two variants of the SV40 virus, JC virus and BK virus, are associated with rare neurological disease in immunocompromised persons.

The Papillomaviridae are well known as the etiological agents of human warts. More than one hundred serotypes of the human papilloma virus (HPV) are known, the vast majority causing only benign growths called condylomas (warts). Because genital HPV is so common, genital warts represent one of the most common types of sexually transmitted diseases. About one dozen HPV serotypes, however, are capable of malignant transformation of cervical cells, resulting in cervical cancer, the second leading cause of cancer deaths in women. Gardisil, the cervical cancer vaccine, is a quadrivalent vaccine directed against the four most common HPV serotypes associated with cervical cancer.

The Adenoviridae, or adenoviruses, are associated with respiratory infections in humans. More than one hundred serotypes are known, about one-half of which are associated with human infections. In the majority of cases, infections appear in children as either a mild infection or an illness associated with sore throats or fever, or both.

The Herpesviridae family includes eight known types of human herpesviruses (HHV). While the illnesses associated with these viruses vary, all exhibit latency in which following recovery, the infected person harbors the virus in a nonreplicative state for the remainder of his or her life. The virus may periodically become reactivated in some people, resulting in illness that may be mild to severe. The best known of these viruses include HHV-1,2, often called herpes simplex types 1 and 2, which are associated with cold sores. HHV-3, or varicella zoster virus, is the agent of chickenpox. Reactivation of the virus from a latent state results in the localized rash known as shingles. HHV-4, the Epstein-Barr virus (EBV), is associated with infectious mononucleosis. EBV has generated significant research, as it is also a potential cancer virus, the etiological agent of Burkitt's lymphoma and nasopharyngeal carcinoma, and possibly the etiological agent of Hodgkin's disease.

The largest group morphologically of double-stranded DNA viruses are the poxviruses. It is estimated that variola (smallpox) virus killed an estimated 400,000 persons annually in Europe before the development of an effective vaccine by English physician Edward Jenner. Smallpox is the only viral disease eradicated from human civilization, the result of an effective vaccination campaign in the 1970's.

*Class II: Single-stranded DNA viruses.* The Parvoviridae (*parvo* means "small") contain linear single-stranded DNA genomes. The only parvovirus known to be associated with human disease is B19, the etiological agent for erythema infectiosum, or fifth disease, a common rash in children.

*Class III: Double-stranded RNA viruses.* The only family of double-stranded RNA animal viruses are the Reoviridae ("reo" stands for "respiratory enteric orphan"). The name originally reflected its isolation from both the gastrointestinal and respiratory tracts and the mistaken belief that it was of no clinical significance. The evolution of the original classification of reovirus as an enteric virus to its own family reflected the increasing role of molecular biology in the study of viruses during the 1960's. The virus was later discovered to contain a distinctive genome, both double-stranded and existing in the form of ten to twelve segments. Reoviruses are nonenveloped viruses, with a double-layered icosahedral capsid.

Most members of the family cause no significant clinical disease. The most important pathogen is rotavirus, arguably one of the most important causes of gastrointestinal disease in young children. Estimates are that nearly 100 percent of children worldwide are infected early in childhood, with some one-half million deaths, caused primarily by the combination of severe diarrhea and poor health care throughout much of the world.

*Class IV: Single-stranded, positive-stranded RNA viruses.* Four major families are placed in this class, two icosahedral nonenveloped families (Picornaviridae, or picornaviruses, and Caliciviridae) and two families on enveloped icosahedral viruses (Togaviridae and Coronaviridae).

The term "picornavirus" refers to a "small" (*pico*) RNA virus. These viruses include the first animal virus discovered (foot-and-mouth-disease virus) and polioviruses, hepatitis A virus, and rhinoviruses, which is associated with the common cold. The development of the first Salk vaccine and, subsequently, of the

Sabin oral vaccine for the prevention of poliomyelitis have ranked among the most important in the control of infectious disease. From its peak annual incidence of greater than fifty thousand cases of polio in the United States in the early 1950's, the disease was largely eradicated worldwide by the twenty-first century. The rhinoviruses, which include more than 120 serotypes, are the etiological agents for most colds. The existence of many serotypes is the primary reason that people average two to three colds each year until well into the adult years.

The term "hepatitis" refers to a clinical condition and is associated with infection by several different, and unrelated, types of viruses. Hepatitis A virus, like poliovirus and several other types of picornaviruses, is transmitted through a fecal-oral route and begins as a gastrointestinal infection.

The caliciviruses (calyx- or cup-shaped structures on the viral surface) include the norovirus (Norwalk virus), which is among the most common causes of gastroenteritis in adults. The Norwalk virus is frequently the cause of intestinal illnesses on cruise ships, in schools, and in nursing homes.

The togaviruses, named for the toga or coat appearance of the envelope, include primarily arthropod-borne viruses such as those associated with viral encephalitis, yellow fever, West Nile virus, and hepatitis C virus. Yellow fever was the first viral disease demonstrated to be transmitted by mosquitoes. The building of the Panama Canal during the first decade of the twentieth century was made possible in large part by the Walter Reed Commission's program for control of mosquitoes in Cuba and Panama. Not all togaviruses are arthropod-borne. Rubella virus, associated with German measles, is a respiratory transmitted virus classified within the togaviruses because of its molecular similarity.

Coronaviruses contain a single RNA genome that is the largest known among the RNA viruses. Human infections are relatively common, probably second only to those caused by rhinoviruses, and they often result in symptoms resembling those of the common cold. The SARS (severe acute respiratory syndrome) epidemic that appeared in early 2003 represented an unusually virulent strain of the virus.

*Class V: Single-stranded, negative-stranded RNA viruses.* The negative-stranded RNA viruses include four major enveloped families: Orthomyxoviridae (influenza viruses), Paramyxoviridae (measles, mumps), Filoviridae (Ebola virus), and Rhabdoviridae (rabies). Only the myxoviruses have segmented genomes.

The myxoviruses (myxa or mucus) include all the influenza viruses. The type of influenza (A, B, and C) refers to the proteins of the nucleocapsid: Type A is the most common cause of epidemics. The viral envelope includes two types of spikes: the hemagglutinin (H) protein, which is used to attach the target cell, and the neuraminidase (N), which is used for release from the cell. The particular strain of the virus is indicated by one of the sixteen types of H protein and nine types of N protein. For example, the 2009 swine influenza was the H1N1 type. Because the genome of influenza viruses is segmented, coinfection of cells by different strains of the virus may result in reassortment of segments, creating an entirely new strain, as happened with the swine influenza virus.

Measles virus is similar to those viruses that cause illnesses in animals: distemper and rinderpest viruses. Genetic analysis has suggested all three viruses originated from a common ancestor, and humans became infected from cross-species infection and adaptation as animals were domesticated.

The filoviruses include the Marburg virus, discovered in Marburg, Germany, in 1967 when workers were infected from handling monkey tissue, and the Ebola virus, discovered following an outbreak near the Ebola River in northern Congo. Both viruses cause life-threatening hemorrhagic fevers.

*Class VI: RNA viruses with DNA intermediate.* The Retroviridae or retroviruses contain a positive-stranded RNA but replicate through a DNA intermediate. Following infection, the RNA is copied by a viral reverse transcriptase into a double-stranded DNA, which is then integrated into the host genome. Expression of the viral genes and production of progeny virus utilizes only the integrated "provirus."

Three subclasses of retroviruses are known: RNA tumor viruses, originally discovered by Peyton Rous early in the twentieth century; lentiviruses (slow viruses, reflecting the slow progression of disease) such as human immunodeficiency virus (HIV); and "foamy" viruses, which are not associated with known human disease.

The RNA tumor viruses were critical in the discovery of the role played by oncogenes in creating cancer cells, but with few exceptions, they are not associated with human cancers. Those viruses that are, such as human T-cell lymphotropic viruses (HTLV-1,2), do not actually kill the cell but disrupt regulation. HIV, the agent of acquired immunodeficiency syndrome, ultimately kills the infected cell. Because the target cell, the T lymphocyte, is critical to the regulation of the immune response, the result is a complete breakdown of the immune system. HIV likely originated from similar viruses in chimpanzees that jumped species and became adapted to humans.

*Class VII: DNA retroviruses.* The newest members of the Baltimore classification system, the Hepadnaviridae (hepatitis DNA viruses), contain a double-stranded DNA genome that replicates using an RNA intermediate. The RNA is generated using a cellular RNA polymerase that copies the viral genome. In turn, the RNA is copied by a viral reverse transcriptase into progeny DNA.

The most important member of the group is hepatitis B virus, the primary cause of severe viral liver disease and of hepatocellular carcinoma, or liver cancer. An estimated 500 million persons worldwide are believed to carry the virus, which causes nearly two million deaths annually.

## IMPACT

The ability to sequence the genomes of an increasing number of viruses has led to an understanding of the phylogenetic relationships among these organisms, despite the seemingly unrelated array of diseases with which they are associated. Viruses within the same family have been shown to share common ancestry. Among the questions that can be addressed is that of the origin of human viruses, many of which began as zoonotic diseases in other animals. As human civilization began to encroach into new animal habitats and began the domestication of animals such as dogs and ruminants (cattle and sheep), viruses adapted to new hosts. The process continues, as virus infections associated with newly discovered agents such as Ebola virus, hantavirus, and even HIV have moved from nonhuman hosts, such as rodents, and from nonhuman primates into the human population.

*Richard Adler, Ph.D.*

## FURTHER READING

Norkin, Leonard. *Virology: Molecular Biology and Pathogenesis.* Washington, D.C.: ASM Press, 2010. Using the framework of the Baltimore classification scheme, the author provides a detailed account of virus structure and replication and of the basis for disease pathology.

Strauss, James, and Ellen Strauss. *Viruses and Human Disease.* 2d ed. Boston: Academic Press/Elsevier, 2008. Detailed discussion of animal viruses with emphasis on those associated with human disease. Includes accounts of the history of human viruses.

Wagner, Edward K., and Martinez J. Hewlett. *Basic Virology.* 3d ed. Malden, Mass.: Blackwell Science, 2008. An undergraduate text covering issues of virology and viral disease, properties of viruses and virus-cell interaction, working with viruses, and replication patterns of specific viruses.

Willey, Joanne, Linda Sherwood, and Christopher Woolverton. *Prescott's Microbiology.* 8th ed. New York: McGraw-Hill, 2011. Chapters in this general microbiology text cover structural and replication strategies of viruses. Includes numerous photographs and a glossary.

## WEB SITES OF INTEREST

*Big Picture Book of Viruses*
http://www.virology.net/big_virology

*Centers for Disease Control and Prevention*
http://www.cdc.gov

*Universal Virus Database*
http://www.ictvdb.org

*Viral Zone*
http://www.expasy.org/viralzone

**See also:** Antiviral drugs: Mechanisms of action; Antiviral drugs: Types; Immune response to viral infections; Microbiology; Parasites: Classification and types; Pathogens; Vaccines: Types; Viral infections; Virology; Viruses: Structure and life cycle.

# W

Walking pneumonia. *See* Atypical pneumonia; Mycoplasma pneumonia; Pneumonia.

## Warts

CATEGORY: DISEASES and conditions
ANATOMY OR SYSTEM AFFECTED: Genitalia, skin

### DEFINITION

Warts are usually painless, harmless growths on the skin caused by a virus that can be disfiguring, embarrassing, and occasionally itchy and uncomfortable. Different types of warts include common warts, which usually appear on hands but can appear anywhere; flat warts, which usually appear on the face and forehead and are common in children and teenagers but rarely seen in adults; genital warts, which are usually found on the genitals, in the pubic area, and in the area between the thighs, but can also appear inside the vagina and anal canal; plantar warts, found on the soles of the feet; and subungual and periungual warts, which appear under and around the fingernails or toenails.

### CAUSES

The typical wart is a raised round or oval growth on the skin with a rough surface caused by a virus. This virus includes dozens of types of the human papilloma virus (HPV).

### RISK FACTORS

Most warts are harmless and are more of a nuisance than a threat, but genital warts are the main cause of cervical cancer. Although not a danger, warts around and under nails are much more difficult to cure than warts elsewhere.

### SYMPTOMS

Warts are named by their clinical appearance and location; different forms are linked to different HPV types. Common warts (verrucae vulgaris) are caused by HPV 1, 2, 4, 27, and 29. They are usually asymptomatic but sometimes cause mild pain, especially when they are located on a weight-bearing surface. Flat warts, caused by HPV 3, 10, 28, and 49, are smooth, flat-topped, yellow-brown papules, most often located on the face and along scratch marks. Genital warts manifest as discrete flat to broad-based smooth to velvety papules on the perineal, perirectal, labial, and penile areas. Infection with high-risk HPV types (most notably 16 and 18) is the main cause of cervical cancer.

### SCREENING AND DIAGNOSIS

Diagnosis of warts is based on clinical appearance; biopsy is rarely needed. A primary sign of warts is the absence of skin lines crossing their surface and the presence of pinpoint black dots (thrombosed capillaries) or bleeding when warts are shaved. Differential diagnosis includes corns (clavi), lichen planus, seborrheic keratosis, skin tags, and squamous cell carcinomas. DNA (deoxyribonucleic acid) typing is available in some medical centers but is generally not needed.

Some warts will disappear without treatment, although they can sometimes remain for a couple of years. Treated or not, warts that go away often reappear. Genital warts are contagious, while common, flat, and plantar warts are much less likely to spread from person to person. All warts can spread from one part of the body to another. Treatment is often sought because people generally consider warts unsightly and because the appearance of warts is often stigmatized.

### TREATMENT AND THERAPY

Standard treatment for warts includes freezing (cryotherapy, or liquid nitrogen therapy), treatment with cantharidin (a substance extracted from the blister beetle), and minor surgery that may involve cutting away the wart tissue or destroying it by using an electric needle in a process called electrodessication and curettage.

Other possible treatments include self-care approaches such as salicylic acid and patches available at drugstores. Another approach is the use of duct tape to cover warts for six days, followed by their soaking in warm water and rubbing them with an emery board or pumice stone. Other therapies include injection with bleomycin or the use of retinoids.

### PREVENTION AND OUTCOMES

Avoiding the following behaviors will help to reduce the risk of getting or spreading warts: brushing, clipping, combing, or shaving areas that have warts; using on healthy nails the same file or nail clipper used on warts; biting fingernails near warts; and picking at warts. One should also keep hands as dry as possible, wash hands carefully after touching warts, and use footwear in public showers or locker rooms.

*Margaret Ring Gillock, M.S.*

### FURTHER READING

American Academy of Dermatology. "Warts." Available at http://www.aad.org/public/publications/pamphlets/common_warts.html.

Androphy, E. J., et al. "Warts." In *Fitzpatrick's Dermatology in General Medicine*, edited by K. Wolff et al. 7th ed. New York: McGraw-Hill Medical, 2008.

Berger, T. G. "Dermatologic Disorders." In *Current Medical Diagnosis and Treatment 2011*, edited by Stephen J. McPhee and Maxine A. Papadakis. New York: McGraw-Hill, 2011.

Dehghani, F., et al. "Healing Effect of Garlic Extract on Warts and Corns." *International Journal of Dermatology* 44 (2005): 612.

Egawa, K., et al. "Topical Vitamin D3 Derivatives for Recalcitrant Warts in Three Immunocompromised Patients." *British Journal of Dermatology* 150 (2004): 367.

### WEB SITES OF INTEREST

*American Academy of Dermatology*
http://www.aad.org

*Centers for Disease Control and Prevention*
htto://www.cdc.gov

**See also:** Cancer and infectious disease; Genital warts; Human papillomavirus (HPV) infections; Human papillomavirus (HPV) vaccine; Molluscum contagiosum; Plantar warts; Skin infections; Social effects of infectious disease; Viral infections.

# Water treatment

CATEGORY: Prevention
ALSO KNOWN AS: Water purification

### DEFINITION

Water treatment is the process of removing contaminants from water to make it safe for drinking, cooking, bathing, and swimming. Without water treatment, waterborne pathogens such as *Cryptosporidium* species, *Escherichia coli*, hepatitis A virus, and *Giardia intestinalis* (also known as *G. lamblia*) can proliferate and cause illness and death, often from the dehydration that follows diarrhea.

Clean water is expected to be clear, colorless, odorless, and tasteless. This requires that water be free of particulates (minute substances). Treating water involves the killing of microbes such as bacteria, viruses, and parasites, and the binding and removal of minerals such as iron, calcium, magnesium, manganese, and sulphur.

To clean water, a series of specific processes must be performed: physical separation of solids by settling and filtration; chemical reactions of coagulation and disinfection; and biological methods such as aeration, bacterial digestion of sludge, and filtration through natural materials. The choice of processes depends on the nature and volume of the water to be purified. An analytical survey must be performed initially.

Two original sources of water exist: surface water and ground water. Surface water comprises rivers, lakes, streams, and ponds. Ground water is accessible by digging wells. Ground water generally requires less water treatment than surface water, which contains more debris and pollutants.

### TREATMENT PROCESSES

*Coagulation.* When water is first received at a water-treatment plant, large pieces of solid material, such as sewage, are removed by a coarse screen and then discarded. Smaller solid particles are then induced to bind together so that they will form into larger particles through coagulation. Ions with multiple charges (polyelectrolytes) change the pH (acidity) of the water and trigger chemical reactions that cause aggregation. Alum is frequently added to attract dirt particles, which may contain herbicides and pesticides. Lime and soda ash cause calcium and magnesium to precipitate, thus softening the water.

## Facts: Water Quality, Health, and Disease

- Almost one billion people lack access to an improved supply of drinking water.

- Two million annual deaths from diarrheal diseases are attributable to unsafe water, poor sanitation, and poor hygiene.

- More than fifty countries still report cases of cholera to the World Health Organization.

- An estimated 260 million persons are infected with schistosomiasis worldwide.

- The increasing use of wastewater in agriculture is associated with serious public health risks.

*Source:* World Health Organization

*Sedimentation.* The material resulting from coagulation, called floc, has sufficient weight that it sinks to the bottom of settling tanks. This separation of solids by sedimentation is time-consuming. Algae eventually rise to the surface, where they may be skimmed. The clearer water on the surface is then slowly siphoned for filtration. Aerobic and anaerobic bacteria may be added to the withheld solids (sludge) to digest organic waste matter and to neutralize pollutants. Carbon dioxide, ammonia, and methane gases are generated. The digested sludge may then be used as a fertilizer supplement in farming.

*Filtration.* Remaining particles in the water may be removed by filters made of artificial membranes, nets, or natural materials. Water may be filtered by passing it through beds of sand, gravel, or pulverized coal. Activated charcoal may be added to the water first to remove color, odor, taste, and radioactivity. In another method of removing calcium and magnesium, water may be passed through ion exchange columns, in which sodium ions compete with these cations for binding to porous material.

Aeration is used to remove dissolved elements such as iron, sulphur, and manganese. Air is forced into the water to remove carbon dioxide, hydrogen sulfide, and other gases. In diffused aeration, air is bubbled through the water. In spray aeration, water is sprayed through the air.

The process of removing salt from the water, called desalination, is often used to make ocean water drinkable in places where fresh water is scarce. The salt is removed by microfiltration and by reverse osmosis.

*Disinfection.* Disinfection is the general method of killing pathogens (bacteria, viruses, and parasites). The most common method of water disinfection is chlorination with sodium hypochlorite bleach. Used less frequently are ultraviolet light and ozone aeration. (To disinfect water in one's home in an emergency, one should boil the water to kill microbes.)

### STORAGE

Treated water must then be stored and delivered under clean conditions to prevent recontamination. The water is stored in closed tanks or reservoirs; from there, it is piped to homes, businesses, and other facilities. Minimal chlorine may be added at this stage to maintain cleanliness. Fluoride also may be added to the treated water as a method to prevent tooth decay.

### IMPACT

The U.S. Safe Drinking Water Act of 1974 established national drinking-water standards, which includes maximum acceptable contaminant levels. The act was amended in 1986 and 1996 to protect natural water sources. The original act was intended to address drinking water as it flowed in homes, businesses, and public drinking fountains. The amendments address water safety as it flows from the original water source to the faucet.

Most water-treatment plants are not prepared to remove pharmaceuticals, including natural and synthetic hormones, that are flushed down the sink or toilet. Those treatment plants that use chemical oxidative processes to remove estrogen and other medications generate disinfection by-products in the water supply that pose potential risks to human health. Communities are organizing collections of unused and unwanted over-the-counter and prescription medications for disposal by authorized incineration.

*Bethany Thivierge, M.P.H.*

### FURTHER READING

Amjad, Zahid, ed. *Science and Technology of Industrial Water Treatment.* Boca Raton, Fla.: CRC Press, 2010. This text by the International Water Association features discussion of the "fundamental and practical aspects of industrial water treatment."

Binnie, Chris, and Martin Kimber. *Basic Water Treat-*

*ment.* 4th ed. Cambridge, England: Royal Society of Chemistry, 2009. A comprehensive textbook on water quality standards and practices in the United States and in Europe.

Brettar, Ingrid, and Manfred G. Hofle. "Molecular Assessment of Bacterial Pathogens: A Contribution to Drinking Water Safety." *Current Opinion in Biotechnology* 19 (2008): 274-280. A summary of detection methods for bacterial pathogens in drinking water.

Centers for Disease Control and Prevention. "Safe Water System: A Low-Cost Technology for Safe Drinking Water." Available at http://www.cdc.gov/safewater/publications_pages/fact_sheets/WW4.pdf.

Edzwald, James K., ed. *Water Quality and Treatment: A Handbook on Drinking Water.* 6th ed. New York: McGraw-Hill, 2011. This text by the American Water Works Association discusses "state-of-the-art technologies, water quality from source to tap, conventional and advanced methods and processes in water treatment, and drinking water standards and regulations."

Morris, Robert D. *Blue Death: True Tales of Disease, Disaster, and the Water We Drink.* New York: HarperCollins, 2007. An epidemiologist who specializes in waterborne diseases discusses the history of water purification and the drinking water industry without avoiding controversy.

Symons, James M. *Plain Talk About Drinking Water.* 5th ed. Denver, Colo.: American Water Works Association, 2010. Provides consumers with clear information about drinking water in a question-and-answer format written in easily understood language.

## Web Sites of Interest

*American Water Works Association*
http://www.awwa.org

*International Water Association*
http://www.iwahq.org

*U.S. Environmental Protection Agency*
http://water.epa.gov/drink

*Water Supply and Sanitation Collaborative Council*
http://www.wsscc.org

**See also:** Bacteria: Classification and types; Bacteria: Structure and growth; Chemical germicides; Disinfectants and sanitizers; Fungi: Classification and types; Fungi: Structure and growth; Hygiene; Microbiology; Parasites: Classification and types; Pathogens; Public health; Viruses: Types; Waterborne illness and disease.

---

# Waterborne illness and disease

Category: Transmission

### Definition

Waterborne illnesses and diseases are transmitted primarily through the ingestion of water that is contaminated (infested) by microorganisms or toxins. Contact with infested water that allows pathogens to enter through broken skin is another method of disease transmission.

There are four primary types of waterborne illness: waterborne disease, which is contracted by ingesting contaminated drinking water; water-washed disease, which is spread through an improper or inadequate sewage system; water-based disease, which is transmitted by an organism that lives in the water, such as a worm or fish; and water-related vector-borne disease, which is transmitted by vectors (such as mosquitoes) that breed in water.

### Global Reach

Waterborne illness is a major global health problem, as nearly 900 million people worldwide do not have access to potable (drinkable) water and 2.5 billion people live without basic sanitation. Diarrheal diseases contracted as a result of inadequate sanitation are the leading cause of illness and death globally. Approximately 2 million people worldwide, most of whom are children less than five years of age, die each year from waterborne diarrheal illnesses.

Waterborne illnesses are common in developing areas in the world, where poverty, political conflict, and other factors prevent the construction of infrastructures that provide adequate sanitation and sewage treatment facilities. Sporadic outbreaks of waterborne diseases still occur, however, in countries with well-established water-purification and sewage systems.

Water may be contaminated either at the source or at post-purification as it travels through the drinking water supply system (DWSS). Although waterborne illnesses are commonly associated with drinking water

## Water-Related Diseases by Type of Pathogen

| BACTERIAL | PARASITIC | VIRAL |
|---|---|---|
| Campylobacteriosis | Acanthamoeba infections | Adenovirus infections |
| Cholera | Ascariasis | Coxsackievirus infections |
| *Escherichia coli* infection | Elephantiasis | Dengue fever |
| Legionnaires' disease | Giardiasis | Eastern equine encephalitis |
| Legionellosis | Hookworm | Hepatitis A |
| Leptospirosis | Lice, Crab | Hepatitis E |
| Mycobacterial infections | Lice, Body | Molluscum contagiosum |
| *Pseudomonas* infections | Lice, Head | Norovirus infection |
| Salmonellosis | Malaria | Rift Valley fever |
| Shigellosis | Onchocerciasis | Rotavirus infection |
| Staphylococcal infections | Pinworms | Viral gastroenteritis |
| Trachoma | Scabies | West Nile virus |
| Typhoid fever | Toxoplasmosis | Yellow fever |

*Source:* Centers for Disease Control and Prevention

and sanitation, other points of human contact with water also can cause infection and disease. Humans can become infected through water-based recreation, bathing, food production, and irrigation.

### UNSAFE DRINKING WATER

Although considered a basic human right by the United Nations, one in six people worldwide do not have access to potable water. Most of the diseases transmitted through drinking water are spread through fecal-oral transmission and are therefore directly linked to poor sanitation. The major microorganisms causing waterborne diseases through contaminated drinking water are bacteria, viruses, and protozoa. More than 1,415 species of pathogenic microorganisms have been identified as causing waterborne disease; however, in countries with adequate sanitation systems and clean drinking water, most of these diseases are not of special concern for public health officials.

The major bacterial contaminants of drinking water that cause illness in humans are *Escherichia coli*, *Enterococcus faecalis*, *Salmonella* species (spp.), *Shigella* spp., *Aeromonas* spp., *Vibrio cholerae*, *Yersinia enterocolitica*, *Campylobacter* spp., *Legionella pneumophila*, *Leptospira* spp., and various mycobacteria. Most of these organisms cause gastroenteritis and diarrhea, although several *Salmonella* strains and *Leptospira* spp. cause infectious

fevers; *L. pneumophila* and mycobacteria cause respiratory infections. All of these organisms are excreted in human feces, with the exception of *L. pneumophila*, *Leptospira* spp., and mycobacteria.

Major viral human pathogens in drinking water include enterovirus (polio, coxsackie, and echo), rotavirus, adenovirus, hepatitis A and E, and norovirus. All of these pathogens have the potential to cause fatal diseases, with rotavirus being one of the most dangerous gastrointestinal viruses for children. All are transmitted by human feces except the norovirus, which is carried through water and can be deposited on and retrieved from inanimate objects (fomites). The enteroviruses cause meningitis, polio, and encephalitis. Adenoviruses and rotaviruses cause gastroenteritis, while the hepatitis viruses cause infectious hepatitis (hepatitis A) and liver damage. Viruses are difficult to detect in drinking water because they are not identifiable by traditional cell-culture techniques.

The pathogenic protozoa of concern for drinking water are *Cryptosporidium parvum*, *Cyclospora cayetanensis*, *Entamoeba histolytica*, *Giardia intestinalis* (also known as *G. lamblia*), and *Toxoplasma gondii*. All of these pathogens cause diarrhea or dysentery in humans, except *T. gondii*. Most pathogenic protozoa are transmitted through human or animal feces into water in the cystic phase of the life cycle, making them highly resistant to chlorination. Furthermore, bac-

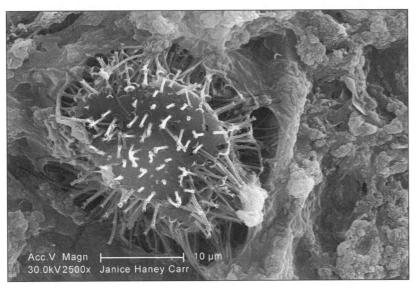

*A micrograph of a water specimen extracted from a flood-control stream. The sample includes bacteria and protozoa, which can cause serious water-borne illness and disease in humans.* (CDC)

teria may live within protozoa, protecting the bacteria from chlorination.

In the United States and other developed countries, most water contamination occurs after the purification process. That is, contamination occurs in the water system, at the distribution point (tap or fountain), during the transfer and processing of water to be bottled, or during storage. In 2005-2006, a reported 612 cases of waterborne illness in the United States were caused by water for drinking, resulting in four deaths. More than one-half of the waterborne illnesses were caused by organisms introduced after disinfection, and the majority of these cases were caused by *Legionella*.

Bacterial infections were contracted by a reported 135 people. Most of the illnesses were caused by *Legionella* spp., 32 were caused by *Campylobacter* spp., and the remainder were caused by other pathogens. All four deaths were caused by *Legionella*, which regrows in warm-water systems, and all occurred in hospitals or long-term care facilities. Viral pathogens were the causative agents of 212 cases of illness, 196 from norovirus and 16 from hepatitis A. These outbreaks were associated with untreated well or spring water at private residences. *G. intestinalis* and *Cryptosporidium* spp. were associated with 41 and 10 cases of illness, respectively.

## WATER-BASED DISEASES

Water-based diseases are transmitted by an organism that lives in the water, such as a worm or a fish, and are contracted by contacting or ingesting the water. The most recognized examples of water-based diseases are schistosomiasis and ascariasis. Both of these infections are common in developing countries and are caused by trematodes and helminths, respectively. Humans usually contract these diseases when bathing or playing in contaminated water, where larvae or eggs enter the body through broken skin. As the parasites reproduce, they cause severe abdominal and intestinal symptoms that can be fatal.

Waterborne illnesses can also be transmitted through bodies of water used for recreational activities, such as lakes, reservoirs, pools, and water parks. Recreational lakes and reservoirs can contain fecal contaminants from humans and animals, especially *E. coli*, *Shigella* spp., *Salmonella* spp., enterococci, norovirus, *Cryptosporidium* spp., and *G. intestinalis*. Contaminants enter the water from improperly treated or leaking wastewater from residential areas and farms, from already-infected swimmers, and from wildlife. In 2005 and 2006 in the United States, there were 245 cases (6 percent of total cases) of waterborne diseases contracted at untreated water facilities. The primary bacteria involved were *Leptospira* spp. and *Shigella sonnei*. *Cryptosporidium* spp. accounted for most of the protozoan infections, and norovirus was the causative agent of all of the viral infections. Because of the types of activities involved, these illnesses result in not only intestinal infections but also skin, eye, ear, nose, throat, and respiratory infections.

Waterborne illnesses at treated water parks accounted for 94 percent of all cases reported in 2005 and 2006 in the United States. The overwhelming majority of these cases (87 percent) was caused by protozoa, as protozoa are difficult to kill with chlorination; 98 percent of all protozoan infections were cryptosporidiosis. Only 6 percent of cases was caused by bacterial pathogens and 2 percent by viral pathogens. The bacterial pathogens were transmitted either in swimming pools, in which a number of toddlers wearing diapers were present, or in warm-water spas for adults. *Cryptosporidium* spp. transmission occurred in several splash parks and water parks across the United States that did not have ozone or ultraviolet light disinfection units (which can kill cysts) as a backup to chlorination. In these and other outbreaks, the cryptosporidiosis could be attributed to already-infected visitors to the park contaminating the water supply. Cryptosporidiosis is highly infectious and can be transmitted with the ingestion of as few as ten cysts.

## WATER-RELATED VECTOR-BORNE DISEASES

Water-related vector-borne diseases are transmitted by insect vectors that breed in stagnant pools of water. These diseases include malaria and West Nile virus infection, both of which are transmitted by mosquitoes that lay eggs in stagnant water.

## PREVENTION

Chlorination (chlorine, chloramines, chlorine dioxide) is used to disinfect drinking water. This method is usually sufficient, provided the source water is reasonably clear. Along with chlorination is filtration, which removes particulate matter, and microfiltration, which removes protozoa in the cyst phase. Many water-treatment facilities use a combination of purification methods to ensure that all types of microorganisms have been eliminated.

According to the World Health Organization (WHO), ozone is the most effective disinfection method because it can eliminate *Cryptosporidium* species. WHO recommends a combination of ozone and chlorine for maximum purity of drinking water. In developing countries, thermal or ultraviolet disinfection is a potential option because of its relatively low cost and because of the lack of chemical additives. In poor areas where power is unavailable at the household level for boiling water or for ultraviolet disinfection, WHO proposes that disinfection can be performed using solar heating. Other less common methods of water purification include precipitation of impurities with coagulation agents, adsorption of impurities onto organic materials, ion-exchange treatment, and treatment with acids or bases.

A main source of contamination of drinking water after purification is sewage influx from industrial and residential areas; cities pose the greatest risks. Other sources of post-purification contamination include flood waters, which introduce sewage overflow; micro-

organisms resistant to disinfectant procedures; increased virulence of pathogens; and emerging new pathogens. Drinking water can also be recontaminated through biofilms. As water flows through the DWSS, solid materials settle onto pipes, providing a surface onto which microorganisms can adhere and grow; this adherence leads to the formation of biofilms. Biofilms comprise a small ecosystem of various types of interacting microorganisms. Because of their complexity, biofilms present a challenge to keeping water clean in the DWSS.

Pathogens that were previously nonthreatening to human health also present concern for public health officials. Changes in the climate or environment may alter the microbial composition of the source water, requiring a change in the purification process. Previously controlled pathogens may develop resistance to disinfection procedures or may become more virulent, meaning that a smaller number of organisms are required to cause disease. Emerging pathogens (such as Epsilonproteobacteria and *Helicobacter pylori*) that have not been considered a threat to the drinking water supply are now being monitored. All of these circumstances require changes to the purification and monitoring protocols.

In the United States, public drinking water quality is regulated by the Environmental Protection Agency (EPA). Limitations have been established for more than ninety microbiological and other contaminants. For the disease-causing microorganisms *Cryptosporidium* spp., *G. intestinalis*, *L. pneumophila*, and viruses, the requirement is 99.9 percent removal/inactivation. Other nonpathogenic bacteria commonly found in source water are also tested to evaluate the maintenance of the water system (no requirement). Tests for coliforms including *E. coli* are performed as indicators of the presence of other pathogens (limit 5 percent).

Recreational water facilities in the United States are variously regulated. For treated water facilities, including water parks and swimming pools, state and local agencies are responsible for the development and oversight of any health codes. Untreated recreational areas are regulated by EPA guidelines. For fresh-water recreational areas, the EPA limits are 33 colony-forming units (CFU) per 100 milliliters (mL) for enterococci and 126 CFU per 100 mL for *E. coli*. For ocean beaches, the guideline is 33 CFU per 100 mL for enterococci, with each locality having final authority over closure of swimming areas.

## IMPACT

The impact of waterborne diseases worldwide is staggering, as they currently account for 4 percent of the global disease burden. Approximately two million people worldwide die each year from waterborne diarrheal illnesses, 75 percent of whom are children. Cholera is still present in more than fifty countries, causing 3 to 5 million cases and 100,000 deaths annually. From 2004 to 2008, the number of cholera cases increased 24 percent, indicating an increase in the number of people living in crowded, unsanitary conditions.

Schistosomiasis infects 207 million people worldwide, causing about 200,000 deaths per year, mainly in sub-Saharan Africa. Ascariasis infects up to 10 percent of people in developing countries, leading to approximately 60,000 deaths per year. Both diseases target children who frequently play in infested waters.

Water quality has been the focus of the health improvement programs of several global health organizations. In the forefront is the United Nations, which addresses water quality in the seventh of its 2015 Millennium Development Goals. One component of this goal is to cut by one-half by 2015 "the proportion of the [world's] population [that lives] without sustainable access to safe drinking water and basic sanitation." The U.N. is on track to meet this goal, having provided 86 percent of the world's population access to safe drinking water. However, the goal to provide basic sanitation will likely not be met.

Demands for clean water are exceeding the supply of potential fresh-water sources, as the world's population continues to increase. The increased diversion of water supplies for agriculture has resulted in less water for human consumption and in higher contamination of drinking water with farm wastewater. Experts also predict that climate change will adversely affect drinking water sources globally.

*Deborah A. Appello, M.S.*

## FURTHER READING

Ashbolt, Nicholas J. "Microbial Contamination of Drinking Water and Disease Outcomes in Developing Regions." *Toxicology* 198 (2004): 229-238. Summary of the most common pathogens causing waterborne diseases and of the extent of these diseases in developing nations.

Brettar, Ingrid, and Manfred G. Hofle. "Molecular Assessment of Bacterial Pathogens: A Contribution to Drinking Water Safety." *Current Opinion in Biotechnology* 19 (2008): 274-280. A summary of detection methods for bacterial pathogens in drinking water.

Bridge, Jonathan W., et al. "Engaging with the Water Sector for Public Health Benefits: Waterborne Pathogens and Diseases in Developed Countries." *Bulletin of the World Health Organization* 88 (2010): 873-875. A brief overview of waterborne illnesses as a public health issue and of recent outbreaks in developed countries.

Percival, Steven L., et al. *Microbiology of Waterborne Diseases.* San Diego, Calif.: Academic Press/Elsevier, 2004. Major pathogenic waterborne microorganisms are described in terms of physiology, reproduction, clinical features and treatment of infection, and survival in the environment.

Snelling, William J., et al. "Bacterial-Protozoa Interactions and Update on the Role These Phenomena Play Towards Human Illness." *Microbes and Infections* 8 (2006): 578-587. Discusses the bacterial-protozoan interactions in water systems that hinder the detection and eradication of pathogenic organisms in drinking water.

Soller, Jeffrey A., et al. "Estimated Human Health Risks from Exposure to Recreational Waters Impacted by Human and Non-human Sources of Faecal Contamination." *Water Research* 44 (2010): 4674-4691. This study compared the risks associated with human, gull, chicken, pig, and cattle fecal contamination of recreational swimming areas.

Woodall, C. J. "Waterborne Diseases: What Are the Primary Killers?" *Desalination* 248 (2009): 616-621. A brief review of frequently reported causative agents of waterborne diseases.

## WEB SITES OF INTEREST

*Charity: Water*
http://www.charitywater.org

*Neglected Tropical Diseases Coalition*
http://www.neglectedtropicaldiseases.org

*UN-Water*
http://www.unwater.org/discover.html

*U.S. Environmental Protection Agency*
http://water.epa.gov

*Water Supply and Sanitation Collaborative Council*
http://www.wsscc.org

*World Health Organization*
http://www.who.int/water_sanitation_health/diseases

**See also:** Bacteria: Classification and types; Bacteria: Structure and growth; Children and infectious disease; Cholera; Decontamination; Developing countries and infectious disease; Disinfectants and sanitizers; Epidemiology; Fecal-oral route of transmission; Globalization and infectious disease; Hygiene; Intestinal and stomach infections; Malaria; Mosquitoes and infectious disease; Parasites: Classification and types; Parasitic diseases; Pathogens; Public health; Tropical medicine; Viruses: Types; Water treatment; Worm infections.

# West Nile virus

CATEGORY: Diseases and conditions
ANATOMY OR SYSTEM AFFECTED: All

## DEFINITION

West Nile virus, typically transmitted by mosquitoes, first appeared in the United States in 1999. It has been found most often in Africa, Asia, the Middle East, and Europe. Most infections with this virus cause no illness. However, about 20 percent of people infected with the virus suffer flulike symptoms, including fever, nausea, vomiting, headache, and fatigue.

About 1 in every 150 people infected with the virus develops neurologic symptoms, including encephalitis (inflammation of the brain), meningitis (inflammation of the membrane covering the brain and spinal cord), and poliomyelitis (paralysis combined with fever and meningitis).

## CAUSES

West Nile infection is caused by a virus. Most cases occur after a bite from an infected mosquito. The mosquito picks up the disease from biting an infected bird. It then passes the virus on when it bites a person, horse, dog, or some other animal. An increase in dead birds may signal an increased risk for the transmission of this virus.

West Nile virus may also be passed through blood transfusions or organ transplants. Infected donors may not have any symptoms. Tests to screen blood for this virus may be used. In one reported case, West Nile virus was passed through breast milk. Experts are studying this possible route. Breast-feeding women who feel ill or suspect that they have West Nile infection should contact a doctor.

## RISK FACTORS

Being bitten by an infected mosquito poses the greatest threat. However, a small risk is associated with receiving a blood transfusion or receiving an organ transplant. Risk factors for a more severe case of the disease include being more than fifty years of age and having a condition that weakens the immune system, such as diabetes or human immunodeficiency virus infection.

## SYMPTOMS

Most people who become infected with West Nile virus have no symptoms. About 20 percent develop a mild condition called West Nile fever, which lasts about three to six days. One in 150 people develop a serious neurologic disease. It may last weeks. Some effects, such as fatigue, memory loss, difficulty walking, or muscle weakness, may be permanent. About 12 percent of hospitalized patients do not survive. The majority of West Nile cases develop in late summer and early fall.

One should seek immediate medical care if the following symptoms are present: fever, malaise, lack of appetite, nausea, vomiting, headache, body aches, eye pain, muscle pain, swollen lymph nodes, and rash. Symptoms of serious neurologic disease include high fever, stiff neck, a change in mental status, confusion or disorientation, stupor, severe muscle weakness, and paralysis.

## SCREENING AND DIAGNOSIS

A doctor will ask about symptoms and medical history and will perform a physical exam. He or she may inquire if the patient has had any recent mosquito bites. The doctor also will ask about outdoor activities, the use of insect repellent, and travel to areas where West Nile is present.

Some symptoms of this disease may be caused by other conditions. A doctor may order the following to determine the cause of the symptoms: blood tests (for antibodies to the virus and to check for abnormalities associated with West Nile infection), a lumbar puncture (spinal tap; removal of a small amount of fluid from the spinal column to check for signs of infection), a magnetic resonance imaging (MRI) scan (a scan that uses radio waves and a powerful magnet to produce detailed computer images, in this case of the brain), an electroencephalogram (EEG; a test that records the brain's activity by measuring electrical currents through the brain), and electromyography and nerve conduction studies (in which an electrical current is measured in a muscle or passed through a nerve to determine the condition of that nerve and to determine the reason for muscle weakness).

## TREATMENT AND THERAPY

No definitive treatment exists for West Nile infection. The treatment given is supportive. Patients with severe cases may need a machine to help with breathing. Care includes intravenous fluids and the prevention of other infections. Two drugs (alpha-interferon and Ribavirin) have been studied as possible medicines to shorten the length of symptoms or to decrease the disease's severity.

## PREVENTION AND OUTCOMES

The best preventive measure is to avoid mosquito bites. Tips to do so include avoiding the outdoors at dawn or dusk; wearing long pants and long-sleeved shirts when outdoors; using an insect repellent with the chemical DEET (NN-diethyl metatoluamide); repairing window and door screens to prevent mosquitoes from entering one's home; removing standing water, such as birdbaths, to prevent mosquito breeding; and cleaning clogged rain gutters to remove pooled water.

Other prevention tips include donating one's own blood before elective surgery, but not donating blood if feeling ill or if one has a fever, and not touching dead birds unless wearing disposable gloves. One should notify the local public health department if a dead bird is found.

*Reviewed by David L. Horn, M.D., FACP*

## FURTHER READING

Despommier, Dickson D. *West Nile Story*. New York: Apple Tree, 2001.

*Emerging Infectious Diseases Journal* 7, no. 4 (August, 2001).

Giesecke, Johan. *Modern Infectious Disease Epidemiology*. 2d ed. New York: Oxford University Press, 2002.

Lashley, Felissa R. "West Nile Virus." In *Emerging Infectious Diseases: Trends and Issues*, edited by Felissa R. Lashley and Jerry D. Durham. 2d ed. New York: Springer, 2007.

Oldstone, Michael B. A. *Viruses, Plagues, and History: Past, Present, and Future*. New York: Oxford University Press, 2010.

Petersen, L. R., and A. A. Marfin. "West Nile Virus: A Primer for the Clinician." *Annals of Internal Medicine* 137 (2002): 173-179.

Petersen, L. R., J. T. Roehrig, and J. M. Hughes. "West Nile Virus Encephalitis." *New England Journal of Medicine* 347 (2002): 1225-1226.

Sfakianos, Jeffrey N. *West Nile Virus*. Rev. ed. Philadelphia: Chelsea House, 2005.

White, Dennis J., and Dale L. Morse, eds. *West Nile Virus: Detection, Surveillance, and Control*. New York: New York Academy of Sciences, 2003.

## WEB SITES OF INTEREST

*American Society of Tropical Medicine and Hygiene*
http://www.astmh.org

*Centers for Disease Control and Prevention*
http://www.cdc.gov

*National Institute of Allergy and Infectious Diseases*
http://www.niaid.nih.gov

*Public Health Agency of Canada*
http://www.phac-aspc.gc.ca

*U.S. Food and Drug Administration*
http://www.fda.gov

**See also:** Birds and infectious disease; Blood-borne illness and disease; Dengue fever; Emerging and reemerging infectious diseases; Encephalitis; Iatrogenic infections; Inflammation; Insect-borne illness and disease; Mosquito-borne viral encephalitis; Mosquitoes and infectious disease; Poliomyelitis; Sleeping nets; Viral infections; Viral meningitis; Yellow fever.

# Whipple's disease

CATEGORY: Diseases and conditions
ANATOMY OR SYSTEM AFFECTED: All

## DEFINITION

Whipple's disease is a rare, chronic, systemic infection caused by a gram-positive actinomycete, *Tropheryma whipplei.*

## CAUSES

The bacterium *T. whipplei* is found ubiquitously in the general environment. However, its source and transmission is not well established.

## RISK FACTORS

Whipple's disease may occur in all age groups but mainly affects middle-aged Caucasian men. (The male-to-female ratio is estimated at 8:1 to 9:1.) Several hundred clinical cases have been reported, mostly from North America and Western Europe. Persons with Whipple's disease have characteristic immunological defects associated with reduced Th1 and Th2 response (which are promoted by T lymphocytes).

## SYMPTOMS

The prodromal stage of the disease is characterized by nonspecific symptoms that last an average of six years. The progressive stage manifests by a broad spectrum of symptoms. The main clinical features include weight loss, arthralgia, diarrhea, abdominal pain, and, in some cases, fever, anemia, skin pigmentation, and lymphadenopathy. Cardiac involvement (such as chest pain, endocarditis, pericarditis, valve insufficiency, and heart failure) has been reported in 20 to 40 percent of cases. Pulmonary involvement (with a chronic cough, pleural effusion, pulmonary infiltration, or granulomatous mediastinal adenopathy) has been reported in 30 to 40 percent of cases. Neurological symptoms (such as memory impairment, confusion, depression, sleep disturbances, nystagmus, ataxia, seizures, and symptoms of cerebral compression) are found in up to 40 percent of affected persons. Ocular movement disturbances (such as progressive supranuclear ophthalmoplegia with oculomasticatory myorhythmia or oculofacioskeletal myorhythmia) are pathognomonic. Uveitis, retinitis, vitritis, keratitis, optic neuritis, and papilloedema may be present.

Hearing loss and blurred vision has occasionally been reported. Rarely, hepatosplenomegaly and hepatitis may occur. If left untreated, the disease may be fatal, usually within one year.

## SCREENING AND DIAGNOSIS

Diagnosis is based on medical history, physical examination, and laboratory evaluations. The initial diagnostic procedure requires an upper endoscopy with a small bowel mucosal biopsy, which shows periodic acid-Schiff-positive inclusions in the macrophages of lamina propria, representing the causative bacteria. *T. whipplei* can also be detected through specific polymerase chain reaction, immunohistochemistry, and electron microscopy. Whipple's disease should be distinguished from malabsorptive and rare disorders such as celiac disease, Crohn's disease, lymphoma, acquired immunodeficiency syndrome enteropathy, parasitic disorders, amyloidosis, hypogammaglobulinemia, and abetaproteinemia.

## TREATMENT AND THERAPY

The management of Whipple's disease is focused on reducing morbidity, preventing complications, and eradicating the infection. Treatment usually starts with intravenous antibiotics, such as ceftriaxone at 2 grams daily for two weeks, that achieve high levels in the central nervous system. Penicillin, other cephalosporins, carbapenems, or chloramphenicol may be used in cases of allergy or insufficient response to ceftriaxone. The induction therapy is followed by continuous treatment for one to two years with oral cotrimoxazole, twice daily. Doxycycline in combination with hydroxychloroquine, or cefixime alone, may be considered as possible alternatives to long-term cotrimoxazole.

In a majority of treated persons, diarrhea and fever resolve within one week, while other symptoms resolve within a few weeks. The disease relapses in up to 40 percent of treated cases. Patients with severe neurological manifestations may respond poorly to treatment. In these cases, additional treatment with corticosteroids or interferon gamma may be suggested.

## PREVENTION AND OUTCOMES

Humans are the only known host. The reservoir of *T. whipplei*, the transmission mechanisms, and the significance of asymptomatic carriers remain to be established. Fecal-oral transmission has been suggested, and there has been no evidence of person-to-person transmission or of epidemic outbreaks.

*Katia Marazova, M.D., Ph.D.*

## FURTHER READING

Fenollar, Florence, Xavier Puéchal, and Didier Raoult. "Whipple's Disease." *New England Journal of Medicine* 356 (2007): 55-66.

Marth, Thomas, and Thomas Schneider. "Whipple Disease." *Current Opinion in Gastroenterology* 24 (2008): 141-148.

Roberts, Ingram M. "Whipple Disease." Available at http://emedicine.medscape.com/article/183350-overview.

Schneider, Thomas, et al. "Whipple's Disease: New Aspects of Pathogenesis and Treatment." *Lancet Infectious Diseases* 8 (2008): 179-190.

## WEB SITES OF INTEREST

*Actinomycetales Group Database*
http://www.broadinstitute.org/annotation/genome/streptomyces_group

*Centers for Disease Control and Prevention, Division of Foodborne, Bacterial, and Mycotic Diseases*
http://www.cdc.gov/nczved/divisions/dfbmd

*Genetic and Rare Diseases Information Center*
http://rarediseases.info.nih.gov/gard

*Todar's Online Textbook of Bacteriology*
http://www.textbookofbacteriology.net

**See also:** Bacteria: Classification and types; Bacteria: Structure and growth; Bacterial infections; Immunodeficiency; T lymphocytes.

---

# Whipworm infection

CATEGORY: Diseases and conditions
ANATOMY OR SYSTEM AFFECTED: Gastrointestinal system, intestines, stomach
ALSO KNOWN AS: Trichuriasis

## DEFINITION

Whipworm, or trichuriasis, is an infection caused by the roundworm *Trichuris trichiura*, a common soil inhabitant primarily of tropical regions. Whipworms can infect mammals other than humans, particularly dogs and pigs, but these infections are caused by a different species of whipworm.

## CAUSES

Whipworms are commonly found in the soil of tropical regions of the world and may also be found in warm locations in temperate regions. They tend to be tolerant of extremes in temperature and moisture and are typically associated with areas of poor sanitation. If a person ingests food or soil or has hand to mouth contact after touching something that has been contaminated with whipworm eggs, he or she is likely to become infected. Once ingested, the whipworm eggs will hatch in the small intestine, travel to the large intestine, and attach themselves to the intestinal lining. As part of the worm's life cycle, large quantities of whipworm eggs are shed in the feces of infected persons. If the infected feces are not properly disposed of, the resulting contamination of the environment will likely lead to infection in other persons.

## RISK FACTORS

People living in tropical areas with poor sanitation are at the greatest risk of infection with whipworms. Children are the most susceptible to whipworm infections because of their greater likelihood of contact with contaminated soil.

## SYMPTOMS

Mild infections may be asymptomatic. If a heavy infection is present, particularly in children, symptoms may include abdominal pain, diarrhea, loss of appetite, weight loss, and anemia. Severe infections may lead to rectal prolapse. Chronic whipworm infection in children (frequently in conjunction with other intestinal worms) can lead to developmental delays, both physically and mentally.

## SCREENING AND DIAGNOSIS

Diagnosis of whipworm infection is done by microscopic analysis of stool samples for eggs.

## TREATMENT AND THERAPY

If whipworm infection is diagnosed, it is typically treated with mebendazole or albendazole, either as a single dose or over the course of three days. Neither drug should be used to treat pregnant women.

## PREVENTION AND OUTCOMES

Whipworm infection is best prevented by using good personal hygiene and properly disposing of human waste. Thoroughly washing one's hands before eating and washing produce (vegetables and fruits) can help to prevent exposure to whipworm eggs. One should teach children the importance of keeping their hands away from their mouths and to properly wash their hands to minimize the chance of infection.

*Susan Gifford, M.S.*

## FURTHER READING

Bethony, Jeffrey, et al. "Soil-Transmitted Helminth Infections: Ascariasis, Trichuriasis, and Hookworm." *The Lancet* 367 (May 6, 2006): 1521-1532.

Garcia, Lynne Shore. *Diagnostic Medical Parasitology.* 5th ed. Washington, D.C.: ASM Press, 2007.

Geissler, P. W., et al. "Geophagy as a Risk Factor for Geohelminth Infections: A Longitudinal Study of Kenyan Primary Schoolchildren." *Transactions of the Royal Society of Tropical Medicine and Hygiene* 92, no. 1 (January/February, 1998): 7-11.

Hotez, Peter J., et al. "Emerging and Reemerging Helminthiases and the Public Health of China." *Emerging Infectious Diseases* 3, no. 3 (1997): 303-310.

_____. "Helminth Infections: Soil-Transmitted Helminth Infections and Schistosomiasis." In *Disease Control Priorities in Developing Countries.* 2d ed. New York: Oxford University Press, 2006.

Roberts, Larry S., and John Janovy, Jr. *Gerald D. Schmidt and Larry S. Roberts' Foundations of Parasitology.* 8th ed. Boston: McGraw-Hill, 2009.

## WEB SITES OF INTEREST

*Clean Hands Coalition*
http://www.cleanhandscoalition.org

*Disease Control Priorities Project*
http://www.dcp2.org/pubs/dcp/24/section/3296

*Emerging and Reemerging Infectious Diseases Resource Center*
http://www.medscape.com/resource/infections

*Global Network for Neglected Tropical Diseases*
http://globalnetwork.org/about-ntds/factsheets/trichuriasis

**See also:** Antiparasitic drugs: Types; Developing countries and infectious disease; Fecal-oral route of transmission; Flukes; Food-borne illness and disease; Hookworms; Intestinal and stomach infections; Parasites: Classification and types; Pinworms; Ringworm; Roundworms; Soilborne illness and disease; Tapeworms; Tropical medicine; Waterborne illness and disease; Worm infections.

# Whooping cough

CATEGORY: Diseases and conditions
ANATOMY OR SYSTEM AFFECTED: Lungs, respiratory system
ALSO KNOWN AS: Pertussis

## DEFINITION

Whooping cough is a bacterial infection of the respiratory tract. The bacteria invade the lining of the respiratory tract and airways, causing inflammation and increasing the secretion of mucus. It is contagious, and in some cases can be serious.

## CAUSES

Whooping cough is caused by the bacterium *Bordetella pertussis*. It is spread by inhaling droplets from the sneeze or cough of a person with whooping cough or by direct contact with the respiratory secretions of a person infected with whooping cough.

## RISK FACTORS

Risk factors for whooping cough include not being immunized; living or working with someone infected with whooping cough; living in close quarters (such as a dormitory or nursing home); living in crowded, unsanitary conditions; and pregnancy. Also at risk are children in late infancy and young children.

## SYMPTOMS

Symptoms usually begin one to two weeks (at most, three weeks) after exposure to the bacterium. Initial symptoms last about seven to fourteen days and include runny nose and congestion; sneezing; watery, red eyes; mild fever; and dry cough, which marks the onset of the second stage. In the second stage, the cough becomes progressively worse over days to weeks (usually lasting two to six weeks). Prolonged coughing spells come on suddenly and frequently end with a forceful inhale or whoop. The whoop is not often heard in infants, who might gasp for breath or might gag.

In severe cases, coughing may cause a person to have trouble breathing or to turn blue from lack of oxygen. Vomiting because of coughing is also common.

Complications may include seizures; periods of apnea, or no breathing (more common in infants); pneumonia; collapsed lungs, rarely; abdominal and inguinal hernias; and bleeding, swelling, or inflammation of the brain, possibly causing neurologic damage. Death is rare and occurs more commonly in infants. The mortality rate is 1 to 2 percent before the age of one year.

The final stage is marked by slowly decreasing duration and severity of coughing spells. The average duration of illness is about six weeks, with a range of three weeks to three months. Fits of coughing may recur for months. In the majority of cases, patients fully recover.

## SCREENING AND DIAGNOSIS

A doctor will ask about symptoms and medical history and will perform a physical exam. He or she may order blood tests, swabs of the nose and throat for culture, or a chest X ray.

Whooping cough can be difficult to diagnose, especially in older children and in adults, because, initially, symptoms are like those of the common cold. Later symptoms can be like those of bronchitis (especially in adults).

## TREATMENT AND THERAPY

Antibiotics, usually erythromycin or azithromycin, are most effective when started in the early stages. Also, to help reduce vomiting and lessen the chances of dehydration, the patient should eat small, frequent meals and should drink increased amounts of water, fruit juice, and clear soup.

Hospitalization may be necessary for those who develop pneumonia. Patients are usually isolated to prevent spreading the disease to other people.

## PREVENTION AND OUTCOMES

The best means of prevention is immunization. DTaP (for younger children) and Tdap (for adolescents and adults) are vaccines that protect against diphtheria, tetanus, and pertussis (whooping cough). The vaccine is given as a series of shots, which is usu-

ally started when an infant is two months of age. Children seven years of age and older and adults who have not been vaccinated should also receive the series.

People in close contact with someone infected with whooping cough may be advised to take preventive antibiotics, even if they have been vaccinated. This is especially important in households with members at high risk for severe disease, such as children under one year of age.

*Rick Alan; reviewed by Kari Kassir, M.D.*

## FURTHER READING

Centers for Disease Control and Prevention. "Recommended Immunization Schedules for Persons Aged 0-18 Years—United States, 2008." *Morbidity and Mortality Weekly Report* 57 (2008): Q1-Q4. Available at http://www.cdc.gov/mmwr/preview/mmwrhtml/mm5701a8.htm.

Chung, Kian Fan, John G. Widdicombe, and Homer A. Boushey, eds. *Cough: Causes, Mechanisms, and Therapy*. Malden, Mass.: Blackwell, 2008.

EBSCO Publishing. *DynaMed: Pertussis*. Available through http://www.ebscohost.com/dynamed.

Gregory, D. S. "Pertussis: A Disease Affecting All Ages." *American Family Physician* 74, no. 3 (2006): 420-426.

Hewlett, E. L. "Whooping Cough and Other *Bordetella* Infections." In *Andreoli and Carpenter's Cecil Essentials of Medicine*, edited by Thomas E. Andreoli et al. 8th ed. Philadelphia: Saunders/Elsevier, 2010.

Kimball, Chad T. *Childhood Diseases and Disorders Sourcebook: Basic Consumer Health Information About Medical Problems Often Encountered in Pre-adolescent Children*. Detroit: Omnigraphics, 2003.

Long, S. S. "Pertussis." In *Nelson Textbook of Pediatrics*, edited by Richard E. Behrman, Robert M. Kliegman, and Hal B. Jenson. 18th ed. Philadelphia: Saunders/Elsevier, 2007.

Versteegh, F. G. A., et al. "Pertussis: A Concise Historical Review Including Diagnosis, Incidence, Clinical Manifestations, and the Role of Treatment and Vaccination in Management." *Reviews in Medical Microbiology* 16, no. 3 (2005): 79-89.

## WEB SITES OF INTEREST

*American Academy of Pediatrics*
http://www.healthychildren.org

*Centers for Disease Control and Prevention*
http://www.cdc.gov

*WhoopingCough.net*
http://www.whoopingcough.net

**See also:** Airborne illness and disease; Allergic bronchopulmonary aspergillosis; *Aspergillus*; Atypical pneumonia; Bacterial infections; *Bordetella*; Bronchiolitis; Bronchitis; Children and infectious disease; Common cold; Contagious diseases; Diphtheria; DTaP vaccine; Immunization; Inflammation; Influenza; Pneumonia; Respiratory route of transmission; Tetanus; Vaccines: Types.

---

# Women and infectious disease

CATEGORY: Epidemiology

## DEFINITION

The most common infectious diseases that affect women are pelvic infections, maternal infections, and perinatal infections. Infectious diseases are caused by exposure to viruses, bacteria, fungi, or parasites. The initial inflammation or infection caused by exposure to a pathogen can persist until a person's health condition becomes chronic and manifests in a disease state that needs strong and specific treatments.

Women are especially susceptible to infections for a number of reasons, including social. A common role for women in most societies around the world is that of caregiver to the sick and needy, including those who have infectious diseases. Women also lack social power in most societies, including societies in poorer, developing countries with inadequate and unhygienic living conditions and where sexually transmitted diseases (STDs) are more widespread.

## INFECTIOUS DISEASE TYPES

STDs pose a great risk to women in parts of Asia, Africa, and Eastern Europe, where rape and prostitution and arranged marriages between older men and girls and young women are common. Children spread infections directly to their mothers and other women in traditional roles as teachers, nurses, and caregivers. These factors make women at high risk for STDs and diseases that spread among the general population. Several diseases also can be carried by pregnant women and transmitted to her fetus during pregnancy and to her child at birth.

Pelvic infections in women lead to the following diseases:

*Vaginitis.* Vaginitis is usually diagnosed initially by the presence of inflammation, itching, or discharge in the area of the vagina or cervix. There are several types of vaginitis caused by infections, including yeast infections, cervicitis, lichen simplex chronicus, bacterial vaginosis, trichomoniasis, chlamydia, gonorrhea, and genital herpes. Organisms can be transmitted from person to person, leading to gynecological and other diseases because of the proximity of the vagina to the gastrointestinal tract. Once any type of viral, bacterial, or fungal pathogen enters the female gastrointestinal tract, pelvic infection is possible, including pelvic blastomycosis, schistosomiasis, actinomycosis, shigellosis, amebiasis, and listeriosis.

*Listeriosis.* Almost two-thirds of the cases of listeriosis occur when a woman is pregnant and, therefore, has decreased immunity to the *Listeria monocytogenes* bacterium. Men can carry this bacterium without symptoms and can transmit it to women during sexual intercourse. The bacteria can lead to infection, especially when the female's immune system is compromised during, for example, pregnancy. Symptoms include fever, abdominal pain, and other flulike symptoms. Listeriosis transmitted to a fetus through the placenta can develop into granulomatosis infantiseptica, which results in death for the infant. Treatment of listeriosis includes a minimum of two weeks of penicillin, ampicillin, tetracycline, erythromycin, or other antibiotic.

*Schistosomiasis.* Schistosomiasis is a type of infection caused by the presence in the blood of flatworms of the class Trematoda. This type of infection continues to increase worldwide, with more than 200 million persons infected at any given time. The most common initial symptom is a skin rash, often called swimmer's itch, which is visible within twenty-four hours of entering the human body. About one month after infection, symptoms will include fever, sweating, chills, headache, and cough. Treatment with the drugs niridazole or stibocaptate is recommended. If not treated, cervical ulcers, cervical cancer, infertility, and death may result. A fetus may become infected by the pregnant woman. Typical diagnosis includes analysis of the urine or a rectal biopsy.

*Amebiasis and shigellosis.* Amebiasis and shigellosis can be caused by members of the Enterobacteriaceae family, which are gram-negative organisms in contaminated water. These organisms can cause dysentery, diarrhea, abdominal pain, fever, and chills. Limiting exposure to unhealthy water is the best way to prevent the development of these infections. The most effective treatments are the tetracycline or ampicillin antibiotics. If, however, the bacteria strain proves to be resistant to these antibiotics, then trimethoprim and sulfamethoxazole can be effective.

*Intrauterine-device-related infections.* The gram-positive bacterium *Actinomyces israelii* is often associated with the usage of intrauterine devices (IUDs), which are used as contraception. *A. israelii* can establish a colony within the pelvis of a female, leading to gynecological infections such as actinomycosis. Initial symptoms include fever and severe abdominal pain. Diagnosis is accomplished by either examination of the IUD after it has been removed from the female, or by a Pap test. If treated with antibiotics such as penicillin, erythromycin, tetracycline, or chloramphenicol within one week of infection, the prognosis is good. Otherwise, the required treatments can involve blood transfusion. Death may result if the infection is severe.

*Blastomycosis and coccidioidomycosis.* Blastomycosis and coccidioidomycosis are fungal infections that gain entry to the female body either through inhalation or through a skin abrasion. These infections are especially dangerous to pregnant women because they can quickly spread to many organs throughout the body. Symptoms of the two infections are similar and include coughing, chest pain, and wartlike skin lesions that continue to spread. Blastomycosis is caused by the *Blastomyces (Ajellomyces) dermatitidis* fungus, which can be found in the Ohio, Mississippi, and St. Lawrence River systems. If not treated, blastomycosis will be fatal.

Coccidioidomycosis, however, is not fatal, is usually self-limiting, and is without a progressive nature. The fungus *Coccidiodes immitis* causes this infection. This fungus is found in the soil of the southwestern United States and in some areas of South America and Central America.

Both infections can be diagnosed by testing body fluids or antigen-based skin tests and can be treated with the medication amphotericin B. Because blastomycosis can be fatal if not treated, the drug 1-hydroxystilbamidine can also be used if necessary.

*Pelvic inflammatory disease.* Pelvic inflammatory disease (PID) is caused by the *Chlamydia trachomatis* bac-

terium and transmitted through sexual intercourse. Colonies of these bacteria can gain strength and grow in size when a pregnant woman has a cesarean section, leading to severe PID. Antibiotics that include tetracycline, doxycycline, and erythromycin are effective treatments after definitive diagnosis. Diagnosis has become much more efficient since the development of the tissue culture technique in 1965. The *C. trachomatis* bacterium also can cause several other diseases, including urethritis, salpingitis, neonatal pneumonia, and endemic trachoma. Also, pregnant women are susceptible to stillbirth and abortion because of these bacteria.

*Cytomagalic inclusion disease.* Cytomagalic inclusion disease (CID) occurs in the fetus of a pregnant woman who is infected by a cytomegalovirus. The results can be pneumonia, hepatitis, seizure disorders, deafness, retardation, and anemia. The woman may have very few symptoms other than fever or malaise. Therefore, diagnosis of a pregnant woman is made after seeing the results of blood tests, urinalysis, or immunofluorescent tests on the blood of an infant's umbilical cord.

*Chancroid. Hemophilus ducreyi* is a bacterium that causes the sexually transmitted disease chancroid. The first symptoms include fever and malaise, followed by pain in the lymph nodes. Tissue cultures and Gram staining are definitive methods of diagnosis. Although this type of bacteria is resistant to penicillin, other antibiotics, such as tetracycline, erythromycin, and streptomycin, are effective. Washing with soaps and disinfectants does not help to prevent infection, but condom usage does.

*Group B* Streptococcus *infection.* Group B *Streptococcus* (GBS) infections are those infections caused by the *Streptococcus agalactiae* bacterium. Infection by this bacterium can lead to a variety of diseases, including skin infections, peritonitis, arthritis, meningitis, urinary tract infection, gangrene, and pneumonia. Colonies of these bacteria can cause death in pregnant women following a cesarean section. Infected women pass the bacterium during childbirth in approximately 33 percent of cases, and more than 50 percent of infected newborns die within the first five days of birth. To detect the presence of GBS, a doctor will order urine, blood, or cerebral-spinal fluid tests, followed by a bacterial culture. Ampicillin and penicillin G are effective antibiotics, but the tetracycline antibiotics are not effective.

*Maternal infections.* Maternal infections include puerperal and intraamniotic infections, both of which cause more than 13 percent of the deaths in the United States each year, making them the fourth leading cause of death among pregnant women. Several terms are used to describe intra-amniotic infection, including "amnionitis," "clinical choricamnionitis," and "amniotic fluid infection." Regardless of the name used, the primary risk factors for acquiring these types of infections are a complicated pregnancy involving prelabor rupture of membranes, excessive internal fetal monitoring, prolonged labor lasting more than twelve hours, and abortions. These complications make a pregnant woman more susceptible to group B *Streptococcus* growth and colonization. Additional risk factors include the presence of bacterial vaginosis and the occurrence of preterm births. Bacterial vaginosis, which is present in a minimum of 20 percent of all pregnant women, can be caused by exposure to *Mycoplasma hominis* and *Gardnerella vaginalis* during sexual intercourse.

Prolonged labor and sexual intercourse are just two of the risk factors that contribute to the incidence of infectious diseases in women because the vagina itself has a huge supply of organisms that have the potential to become virulent. There are millions of these microbial organisms within the vagina of the average woman. Thus, the rupture of any number of membranes of the placenta, uterus, or vagina, and also cesarean delivery and multiple cervical examinations, can lead to these severe infections. The most prevalent of these infections that become severe after childbirth is endometritis. As with most of these infections, the best treatment is the use of antibiotics.

*Perinatal infections.* Perinatal infections can occur in pregnant women with few symptoms, and they can be transmitted to the fetus, often resulting in severe illness or in death for the fetus. The most common of these infectious diseases are toxoplasmosis; "other" diseases, specifically syphilis, hepatitis, and zoster; rubella; cytomegalovirus; and herpes simplex. They are usually referred to by the acronym TORCH.

The protozoan parasite *Toxoplasma gondii*, which is transmitted by rodents and cats, is the cause of toxoplasmosis. Almost 80 percent of infected humans show only nonspecific, mononucleosis symptoms. Thus, the relatively high incidence of infection that ranges from one of every five to one of every two persons is generally overlooked. However, approximately one-half of infected pregnant women will transmit this disease to their fetuses, with an 85 percent mortality rate; those fetuses who do survive will endure permanent visual and neurological disabilities after birth. If diagnosed early, treatment with the drugs sulfadiazine and pyrimethamine is effective. Diagnostic methods include immunofluorescent antibody tests, enzyme-linked immunoabsorbent assay (ELISA) tests, and the polymerase chain reaction (PCR) method.

Although the rubella vaccine has been a factor in lowering the incidence rate of rubella in the general population, pregnant women who acquire rubella during the first trimester of pregnancy will have a spontaneous abortion in more than one-half of cases. If the fetus does survive until birth, a minimum of 33 percent of these babies will die. Also, in more than 70 percent of cases, the infant will develop deafness, cataracts, heart disease, pneumonitis, and additional severe disorders. The most effective diagnostic tool is hemagglutination inhibition (HI) titer, which is an antibody test.

Of the TORCH infections, cytomegalovirus (CMV) is the most common. The mode of transmission is contact with infected saliva, urine, or blood. Generally, adults have very few symptoms, and the symptoms that do occur are fever, headache, and malaise, which certainly are not diagnostic because they could easily indicate many other conditions. Therefore, although definitive diagnosis is usually made using ELISA, antibody tests, or virus isolation methods, many children are born with this infection. Typical health problems include mental retardation, visual and hearing losses, and seizures; the death rate is 20 to 30 percent. The only drug in usage is ganciclovir, but it is not a completely effective treatment.

## OTHER INFECTIOUS DISEASES

Human immunodeficiency virus (HIV) infection is the primary cause of death for adults, including women, age twenty-five to forty-four years. In 2007, 33.2 million people were infected with HIV, up from 29 million in 2001. Many rapid, easy-to-use tests, such as OraQuick and Reveal, are available, along with ELISA and Western blot analysis of antibodies to HIV. Several drugs are used for treatment, with zidovudine (ZDV or AZT) most useful for treating pregnant women to avoid transmission of the virus to her fetus.

Gram-negative bacteria cause an increase in the growth of cytokines and prostaglandin E2 because of the products of an endotoxin called lipopolysaccharide. Eventually, the gums and bones that support a person's teeth become damaged, leading to periodontal disease. Extended periodontal disease causes diabetes and cardiovascular and pulmonary diseases in both women and men. Pregnant women are even more severely affected because preterm birth or spontaneous abortions may occur. As a result, further bacterial growth can lead to additional infections.

Tuberculosis (TB) has generally been decreasing in developed countries since the early twentieth century, but approximately one-half of the populations of developing countries, and India, are infected. The bacterium *Mycobacterium tuberculosis* is the cause of TB. The lungs are the primary area infected; the second most common TB infection involves the female genital tract. Specifically, the Fallopian tubes are infected 90 to 100 percent of the time. From the Fallopian tubes, the infection generally spreads to the uterus and ovaries, causing infertility in 85 percent of the cases of genital tract TB. Symptoms of genital tract TB include menstrual disorders with excessive bleeding and lower abdominal pain. Several antituberculous drugs are used for treatment.

## IMPACT

According to a 2003 report by the World Health Organization, infectious disease is the leading cause of death for women worldwide. More than fifteen million women die each year from infectious diseases.

The most common infectious diseases that affect women are HIV infection, which leads to acquired immunodeficiency syndrome (AIDS), and malaria. The mortality rate for women is higher in economically undeveloped nations because of the combination of poor hygiene, lack of available medical care and treatments, and restrictive cultural norms. In sub-Saharan Africa, for example, women are 30 percent more likely than men to be infected with HIV. Worldwide, more than 50 percent of persons infected with HIV are women. Women are also disproportionally affected when their partners become infected by HIV. In Uganda, more than 25 percent of the women who lost their spouses to HIV/AIDS also lost their property. Children of women who die from infectious diseases also suffer economically, psychologically, and socially.

*Jeanne L. Kuhler, Ph.D.*

## FURTHER READING

Faro, Sebastian, and David Soper, eds. *Infectious Diseases in Women.* Philadelphia: Saunders, 2001. This book is an excellent source of clinical information on gynecological infections.

Hollier, Lisa D., and George D. Wendel, Jr. *Infectious Diseases in Women.* Philadelphia: Saunders/Elsevier, 2008. Discusses the latest research into infectious diseases common to women. Also provides useful clinical information.

Martin, Richard J., Avroy A. Fanaroff, and Michele C. Walsh, eds. *Fanaroff and Martin's Neonatal-Perinatal Medicine: Diseases of the Fetus and Infant.* 2 vols. 8th ed. Philadelphia: Mosby/Elsevier, 2006. This classic reference work includes discussions of the practice of neonatal-perinatal medicine.

Murthy, Padmini, and Clyde Lanford Smith. *Women's Global Health and Human Rights.* Sudbury, Mass.: Jones and Bartlett, 2010. A comprehensive work that examines the state of women's health around the world. Includes the chapter "Infectious Diseases and Women's Human Rights."

## WEB SITES OF INTEREST

*Centers for Disease Control and Prevention*
http://www.cdc.gov

*Infectious Diseases Society for Obstetrics and Gynecology*
http://www.idsog.org

*National Women's Health Information Center*
http://www.womenshealth.gov

*Our Bodies Ourselves*
http://www.obos.org

*Women's Health Matters*
http://www.womenshealthmatters.ca

**See also:** Blastomycosis; Childbirth and infectious disease; Coccidiosis; Developing countries and infectious disease; Endometritis; HIV; Listeriosis; Pelvic inflammatory disease; Pregnancy and infectious disease; Puerperal infection; Schistosomiasis; Sexually transmitted diseases (STDs); Shigellosis; Streptococcal infections; Vaginal yeast infection.

# World Health Organization (WHO)

CATEGORY: Epidemiology

## DEFINITION

The World Health Organization (WHO) is a unit of the United Nations that is devoted to global health issues. WHO coordinates and provides leadership and directions on health matters through health research programs, guidelines, and standards. The organization also provides technical support to governments to help them address global health problems and to improve the well-being of their respective populations.

The organization is governed by a constitution that has eighty-one articles or principles. The objective of WHO (described in chapter I, article 1) is "the attainment by all peoples of the highest possible level of health."

The WHO constitution came into force on April 7, 1948. Soon thereafter, the first World Health Assembly (WHA), the highest WHO decision-making body, called for the creation of a World Health Day to mark the founding of the organization. Since 1950, World Health Day has been celebrated on April 7 annually around the world. A theme, which highlights a priority area of concern, is chosen each year to focus on key public health issues that affect the international community.

## MEMBERSHIP

Any country that is a member of the United Nations may become a member of WHO by accepting the WHO constitution. Other countries may be admitted as members following the approval of their application by a simple majority vote of the WHA. Associate membership may be granted to territories not responsible for the conduct of their international relations when applications are made on their behalf by a member or other authority that is responsible for their international relations. There are 193 member states within WHO, and they are grouped according to regional location and offices.

## STRUCTURE

WHA's main function is to determine WHO policies. The assembly meets yearly in May at its headquarters in Geneva, Switzerland, with delegates from member states. The WHA appoints a director-general, who supervises the financial policies of WHO and reviews and approves the proposed program budget for a given year.

The executive board, whose members are elected to three-year terms, comprises members who have technical qualifications in health fields. The main function of the executive board is to facilitate the work of the WHA by approving their decisions and policies.

The secretariat of WHO is staffed by about eight thousand health and other experts and support staff on fixed-term appointments. The staff works at the headquarters in Geneva, in the six regional offices, and in member countries. WHO is headed by a director-general, who is appointed by WHA on the nomination of the executive board. Since the inception of WHO in 1948, eight directors-general have served. Brock Chisholm, from Canada, was the first director-general and served from 1948 through 1953. Director-general Margaret Chan, from the People's Republic of China, was appointed in November of 2006. The organization is financed by dues contributed by member states, by voluntary donations from private nongovernment organizations and foundations, and by partnership with research and pharmaceutical companies.

## REGIONAL OFFICES

There are six WHO regional offices, each of which is headed by a regional director. The regional director manages a staff of health and other experts at the regional headquarters and in specialized centers within a given region.

The director is elected to a five-year term by a regional committee that consists of all heads of health departments in the governments of the member states within the given region. The tenure of the regional director is renewable once. The committee also implements the health policy guidelines that are outlined by WHA. The committee also monitors all WHO activities and operations within its respective region.

WHO regional offices represent Africa, the Americas, Southeast Asia, Europe, the eastern Mediterranean, and the western Pacific. The Regional Office for Africa (AFRO) is headquartered in Brazzaville, the Republic of Congo, and has forty-six members, which includes most of the nations of Africa.

The Regional Office for the Americas (AMRO) is headquartered in Washington, D.C. The region has thirty-five member nations and was established before the founding of WHO as the Pan American Health Organization, the oldest international public health organization in the Western Hemisphere. The Regional Office for South East Asia (SEARO) is headquartered in New Delhi. This region consists of eleven member nations in Southeast Asia and includes North Korea. The Regional Office for Europe (EURO) is headquartered in Copenhagen. The region consists of fifty-three member nations in the European Union. The Regional Office for the Eastern Mediterranean (EMRO) is headquartered in Cairo. The region consists of twenty-one member nations, including the African nations of Egypt, Sudan, Tunisia, Libya, and Morocco, and the countries of the Middle East (except Israel).

The Regional Office for the Western Pacific (WPRO) is headquartered in Manila. The region consists of twenty-seven member nations, including the countries in Oceania and South Korea and Asian countries that are not served by SEARO or EMRO.

### Liaison and Country Offices

In addition to the six WHO regional offices, the organization has country offices and liaison and specialist offices at critical international institutions. The country offices are usually located in a country's capital and may also involve the establishment of satellite offices. Country offices are headed by WHO representatives, who most often are trained physicians but are not citizens of the host country. These physicians typically hold diplomatic rank and are accorded diplomatic privileges and immunities similar to those of a nation's ambassador or high commissioner.

WHO country offices serve as the primary advisers on health and pharmaceutical policies to the host government. The international liaison offices have functions similar to country offices, but on a smaller scale; they are usually located in countries with an adequate health system but who nonetheless request the presence and cooperation of WHO.

There are nine liaison and specialists' offices in Africa, Japan, Europe, and North America, headed by liaison officers, who are citizens of the host country and who do not hold diplomatic rank. These offices are the International Agency for Research on Cancer and the Office for National Epidemic Preparedness and Response, both in Lyon, France; the Centre for Health Development in Kobe, Japan; the Liaison Of-

fice and the Office at the World Bank and the International Monetary Fund, both in Washington, D.C.; the Mediterranean Centre for Vulnerability Reduction in Les Berges du Lac, Tunisia; the Office at the African Union and the Economic Commission for Africa in Addis Ababa, Ethiopia; the Office at the European Union in Brussels; the Office at the United Nations, New York; and WHO collaborating centers.

### Collaborating Centers

WHO collaborating centers are institutions such as those conducting research that are designated by the WHO director-general to carry out activities in support of WHO programs at the country, regional, and global levels. The centers also participate in the strengthening of country resources according to WHO policy and its strategy of technical cooperation.

There are more than eight hundred WHO collaborating centers in more than eighty member states that are actively working in areas such as food safety and nutrition, nursing and midwifery, traditional medicine, injury and violence prevention, occupational health, health promotion, communicable diseases, nutrition, mental health, chronic diseases, and health technologies.

The second WHA, in 1949, adopted a policy that prevents WHO from establishing its own international research institutions but allows it to coordinate and make use of the activities of existing institutions to advance health research. A department or laboratory within an institution or a group of facilities for reference, research, or training that belongs to a different institution may be designated as a WHO collaborating center.

Designation as a collaborating center is made with the agreement of the head of the establishment to which the institution is attached or with the agreement of the director of the institution, if it is independent, and after consultation with the national government. An institution is designated initially for a term of four years; the designation may be renewed for the same or a shorter period. A WHO collaborating center may be jointly designated by WHO and by other competent and specialized international bodies. Networks, working groups, partnerships, and programs, or nongovernmental organizations and similar bodies with a membership structure, including professional associations or foundations are not eligible for designation as WHO collaborating centers.

Other center activities include collecting and disseminating information; standardizing terminology and nomenclature of technology, substances, methods, and procedures; participating in collaborative training and research training; and the coordination of activities carried out by affiliates' institutions.

The collaborating centers help to facilitate the fulfillment of WHO-mandated activities through using resources in the respective countries and regions. The exchange of information and research findings, for example, is enhanced by regular meetings and by a database that is accessible through the Internet. This database serves as the official source of information on the centers.

### ANNUAL EVENTS

World Health Day is an annual WHO event. A theme is selected each year that focuses on a particular health issue or program. The theme for the 2010 World Health Day was urbanization and health, and its slogan was 1000 Cities-1000 Lives. Events were organized globally with a call on cities to open streets for health-related activities. In 2009, the theme was Save Lives—Make Hospitals Safe in Emergencies, which focused on the safety of health care facilities and on the readiness of health workers who handle emergencies.

WHO also observes a series of annual events that focus on specific health issues or themes. Events for 2010 included World Cancer Day on February 4, World Water Day on March 22, World TB Day on March 24, World Health Day on April 7, World No Tobacco Day on May 31, and World Blood Donor Day on June 14.

### REPORTS AND PUBLICATIONS

Beginning in 1995, WHO began publishing its *World Health Report*, considered by many to be the organization's leading publication. Each report focuses on a specific subject and combines expert assessment of global health and informative statistics about member countries. The report provides countries, donor agencies, international organizations, and others with the information and data to help make adequate policy and funding decisions. It is also a good source for researchers and journalists and for general readers with an interest in international health issues.

*The World Health Report 2010: Health Systems Financing: The Path to Universal Coverage* promotes the importance of good health to human welfare and to sustained economic and social development. The report maps out what countries can do to modify their financing systems to be able to move quickly toward the goal of universal health coverage while sustaining the progress that has been achieved.

The report also builds on new research and on lessons learned. It provides an agenda for countries at all stages of development and proposes ways that the international community can better support efforts in low income countries to achieve universal coverage and improve the health of their respective populations.

The first *World Health Report*, in 1995, with the theme of "Bridging the Gaps," focused on how poverty wields a destructive and often deadly influence at every stage of human life. The report describes WHO's efforts in helping to bridge the widening gaps between the rich and poor and between those with and without access to adequate health care.

### INTERNATIONAL HEALTH REGULATIONS

WHO's International Health Regulations (IHR) 2005 is an international legal instrument that is binding on 194 countries across the globe, including WHO member states. The IHR came into force in June of 2007.

The aim of the IHR is to help the international community prevent and respond to acute public health risks that have the potential to cross borders and threaten people worldwide. The IHR was developed in response to the exponential increase in international travel and trade and to the emergence and reemergence of disease threats and other health risks on a global scale.

The IHR calls for member countries to build up their capacity to prevent, protect against, and control disease outbreaks, and it defines the rights and obligations of countries to report to WHO certain disease outbreaks and public health events. The IHR also establishes a number of procedures that WHO must follow in helping to maintain global public health.

*Oladayo Oyelola, Ph.D., SC(ASCP)*

### FURTHER READING

Leach, Melissa, Ian Scoones, and Andrew Stirling. "Governing Epidemics In an Age of Complexity: Narratives, Politics, and Pathways to Sustainability." *Global Environmental Change* 20 (2010): 369-377.

Lee, Kelley. *The World Health Organization* (WHO). New York: Routledge, 2009. Part of the Global Institutions series, this brief but comprehensive book examines the organization from its founding through the first decade of the twenty-first century.

St. Georgiev, Vassil. *Impact on Global Health.* Vol. 2 in *National Institute of Allergy and Infectious Diseases, NIH*, edited by Vassil St. Georgiev, K. A. Western, and J. J. McGowan. Totowa, N.J.: Humana Press, 2009.

World Health Organization. "Constitution of the World Health Organization." Available at http://apps. who.int/gb/bd/pdf/bd47/en/constitution-en.pdf. The WHO constitution, formatted for easy printing.

———. *The World Health Report 2010: Health Systems Financing: The Path to Universal Coverage.* Geneva: Author, 2010.

## WEB SITES OF INTEREST

*Centers for Disease Control and Prevention*
http://www.cdc.gov

*Global Health Council*
http://www.globalhealth.org

*Health Protection Agency*
http://www.hpa.org.uk

*World Health Organization*
http://www.who.int

**See also:** Biosurveillance; Centers for Disease Control and Prevention (CDC); Developing countries and infectious disease; Disease eradication campaigns; Emerging and reemerging infectious diseases; Emerging Infections Network; Epidemic Intelligence Service; Epidemics and pandemics: Causes and management; Epidemics and pandemics: History; Epidemiology; Globalization and infectious disease; National Institute of Allergy and Infectious Diseases; National Institutes of Health; Outbreaks; Public health; Tropical medicine; U.S. Army Medical Research Institute of Infectious Diseases.

---

# Worm infections

CATEGORY: Diseases and conditions
ANATOMY OR SYSTEM AFFECTED: All

## DEFINITION

Parasitic worms are pathogenic organisms that attach to the internal structures of their hosts, including humans. Worm infections can range from mild discomfort to severe illness and death. Worms usually enter the body in the form of eggs or cysts; they then mature within the tissues they infect, including the intestines, liver, muscles, lungs, and brain, and in the bloodstream.

Worm infections are rare in the United States and Europe but are common in developing nations in Asia, Africa, Central America, and South America. Parasitic worms are classified by their shape as either roundworms (nematodes and nemathelminths) or flatworms (flukes and platyhelminths).

## CAUSES

A worm has three life stages: egg, larva, and adult. Some worms form cysts within a host's body that can develop into larvae when circumstances are favorable. Eggs or larvae of parasitic worms can enter the body (or host) through the mouth or through skin surfaces. Some are transmitted through an insect bite. This intermediate insect host is known as a vector. Examples of worm infections include tapeworm, hookworm, liver fluke, trichinosis, filariasis, and pinworm.

*Tapeworm.* Tapeworm infections occur from eating the raw or undercooked meat of animals infected with the larvae of these flatworms. Tapeworm infections mainly occur in Southeast Asia, Africa, the Middle East, Mexico, South America, Russia, and areas of the former Yugoslavia. In the United States, some forms may be acquired by swallowing the infected fleas of infected dogs or cats.

*Taenia saginata* infects beef and *T. solium* infects pigs. The larvae attach to the intestinal wall and mature into adult tapeworms, which can grow to be more than twelve feet long and live many years. Segments of the worm, which contain eggs, are released and then pass from the body in feces. Animals eat the feces, the grass, or other contaminated foods, thus perpetuating the cycle.

*Hookworm.* Hookworms are roundworms existing as two types: *Ancylostoma duodenale* and *Necator americanus. A. duodenale* is found in North Africa, the Middle East, and India; in the past, the worm was present in southern Europe. *N. americanus* is present in the Americas, Southeast Asia, China, Indonesia, and sub-Saharan Africa.

## Endoparasitic Infections and Causal Worms

| Common name | Scientific name | Affected body part | Prevalence |
|---|---|---|---|
| Anisakis | *Anisakis* sp. | intestines; also cause allergic reactions | worldwide (highest where raw fish is consumed) |
| Elephantiasis | *Wuchereria bancrofti* | lymphatic system | tropical and subtropical regions |
| Guinea worm | *Dracunculus medinensis* | muscles, subcutaneous tissue | Sudan |
| Hookworm | *Ancylostoma duodenale* *Necator americanus* | blood, lungs, small intestine | tropical regions |
| Loa loa filariasis | *Loa loa* | connective tissue, eyes, lungs | West African rainforest |
| Lung fluke | *Paragonimus* sp. | lungs | East Asia |
| Mansonelliasis | *Mansonella streptocerca* | subcutaneous tissues | West Africa |
| Onchocerciasis | *Opisthorchis viverrini* | eye tissue, skin | Africa, Central America, South America, Yemen |
| Parasitic gallbladder infection | *Clonorchis sinensis* *C. viverrini* | gallbladder | worldwide (endemic to China, Japan, and Southeast Asia) |
| Parasitic kidney infection | *Dioctophyme renale* | kidneys | worldwide |
| Parasitic pneumonia | *Strongyloides stercoralis* | intestines, lungs, skin | tropical and subtropical regions |
| Pinworm | *Enterobius vermicularis* *E. gregorii* | anus, intestines | worldwide |
| Schistosomiasis | *Schistosoma japonicum* *S. mekongi* *S. mansoni* *S. haematobium* | bladder, intestines, kidneys, liver, lungs, spleen, ureters | worldwide |
| Tapeworm | *Diphyllobothrium latum* *Echinococcus granulosus* *E. multilocularis* *E. vogeli* *E. oligarthrus* *Taenia saginata* *T. solium* | blood, intestines, kidneys, liver, lungs, spleen | worldwide |
| Toxocariasis | *Toxocara cani* *T. cati* | brain, eyes, liver | worldwide |
| Trichinosis | *Trichinella* sp. | muscles, small intestines | worldwide |
| Whipworm | *Trichuris trichiura* *T. vulpis* | anus, large intestine | worldwide |

Hookworm larvae live in moist soil. The larvae are able to penetrate the soles of the feet or other skin areas that contact soil. The larvae then enter small veins and the lymphatic system, work their way to the lungs, and enter the alveoli (sacs) in the lung. They are then coughed up into the infected person's mouth and passed down into the intestines, where they mature into adults. The adult worms release eggs, which pass out of the person's body in the feces. If the feces are deposited in the soil, the cycle repeats.

*Liver fluke.* Liver flukes (*Fasciola hepatica*) are flatworms that infect the liver of humans and other mammals. They are present in temperate areas where sheep are raised because these flukes use sheep and humans as a host. Most human infections occur in Southeast Asia, northern Africa, South America, and Cuba. Occasional infections occur in the United Kingdom, southern Europe, and Australia. The flukes require an intermediate host such as *Galba truncatula*, an aquatic snail, to complete its life cycle. Larvae enter the snail and develop into what is known as metacercariae; these organisms leave the snail and attach to plants such as water chestnuts and watercress. When eaten, further development of the parasite occurs; these organisms then burrow through the intestinal wall and into the liver; they then enter the bile ducts and mature into the adult form. The adults lay eggs, which pass through the bile duct into the intestines; they are then excreted, completing the life cycle.

*Trichinosis.* Trichinosis is caused by the roundworm *Trichinella spiralis*. Infections were once common in the United States; however, they are now quite rare. Infections are more common in developing nations and in eastern Europe. Pigs become infected with trichinosis when they eat infected rodents or meat from other pigs. Humans become infected when they eat infected pork. The infection is passed in the form of cysts within skeletal muscles. When infected muscle is eaten, the cysts develop into adults and mate in the small intestine. Their eggs develop into larvae, which pierce the small intestine and enter the bloodstream and migrate to other structures such as the heart or eye, or to the lymphatic system. The skeletal musculature is the only place where they can survive and form cysts.

*Filariasis.* Lymphatic filariasis, also known as elephantiasis, is caused by the roundworms *Brugia malayi*, *B. timori*, and *Wuchereria bancrofti*. About one-third of infected persons live in Africa, about one-third in India, and the rest in other parts of Asia, the Americas, and the Pacific Islands. The disease is transmitted from human to human by some species of mosquitoes. Mosquito species that can transmit the disease are *Culex quinquefasciatus* and some *Anopheles* species; *Brugia* roundworms are primarily transmitted by *Mansonia* mosquitoes. Another type of filariasis is a tropical skin and eye disease, *Loa loa* filariasis, which is also known as African eye worm. It is contracted through the bite of a deer fly or mango fly.

In filarial infections, the parasites enter the bloodstream as microfilariae and develop into adults. The adults mate and produce more microfilariae. If a person is bitten by a host insect, the microfilariae infect that insect and, thus, complete the life cycle. The microfilariae travel from the bloodstream into the lymphatic system, which is a network of vessels that maintain a delicate fluid balance between body tissue and the bloodstream. They lodge in the lymphatic system, where they mature into adult worms. These worms live for four to six years and produce millions of immature microfilariae that circulate in the blood. The adult worms block the normal flow of lymphatic fluid, damaging the lymphatic system. Adult *Loa loa* worms often travel to the conjunctiva (just below the surface of the eyeball); the worms transit the eyeball in about fifteen minutes, causing much pain; however, the transit does not usually affect vision.

*Pinworm.* The pinworm (*Enterobius* species) is a roundworm that is a common intestinal parasite worldwide. It is most common in children. Persons are infected by eating food contaminated with the eggs. The eggs hatch in the duodenum (the first portion of the small intestine). The eggs develop into larvae and migrate toward the colon (the large intestine). The larvae become adults in the ileum (the lower part of the small intestine) and mate. After mating, the males die and pass from the body in the stool. The pregnant females attach themselves to the ileum and the first portion of the large intestine, where they feed on the intestinal contents. The female body becomes filled with eleven thousand to sixteen thousand eggs. The females then migrate to the infected person's anus, where they release the eggs and die.

## RISK FACTORS

The major risk factor for many parasitic worm infections is living in an area where the worms are endemic (always present). Infections are more common in slums and poor communities. Poor personal hygiene and poor sanitation increase the risk of infection. Contact with fecal material increases the risk of infection with intestinal worms. In developing nations, humans defecate on the soil or use fecal material (night soil) as fertilizer. Going barefoot in contaminated areas can result in a hookworm infection. Eating raw or incompletely cooked pork increases the risk of trichinosis. Pinworms are more common among people in close contact (such as in a classroom or in crowded living conditions). Immigrants from areas where parasitic infections are endemic can expose the persons of the new country or region to these infections.

### Symptoms

The symptoms of worm infection vary, depending on the type of worm involved.

*Tapeworms.* Often, tapeworm infections do not have any specific symptoms. Weight loss and anemia can occur. Sometimes, a person will notice tapeworm segments in the stool. Rarely, tapeworms can cause intestinal obstruction, which produces nausea, vomiting, and severe abdominal pain. On occasion, cysts can form in the brain and the meninges (the tissues surrounding the brain). If this occurs, the patient may experience neurologic symptoms such as headaches, seizures, and confusion. On rare occasions, cysts can form in the eyes, which can cause blindness, or in the spinal cord, which can result in muscle weakness or paralysis.

*Hookworms.* General symptoms, such as itching on the soles of the feet, can occur soon after infection. Cough and pneumonitis (lung inflammation) can occur when the worms break into the alveolae in the lungs. When the larvae enter the small intestine, diarrhea and gastrointestinal discomfort can occur. Heavy infestations result in iron deficiency anemia from intestinal blood loss and malnutrition. Long-term blood loss can result in facial edema (swelling). Children with chronic hookworm infections can suffer from growth retardation and intellectual impairment.

*Liver flukes.* Infected persons suffer from abdominal pain, nausea, vomiting headaches, and anemia. Some develop jaundice (yellowing of the skin), hives, and muscle pains. Over time, blockage of the bile ducts can occur.

*Trichinosis.* Within a week after becoming infected, persons experience gastrointestinal symptoms such as nausea, heartburn, and diarrhea. After the larvae mi-

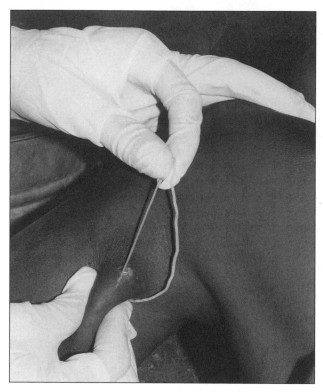

*A guinea worm* Dracunculus medinensis *is removed from the leg of a person with dracunculiasis.* (CDC)

grate from the intestines to the muscles, symptoms include fatigue, muscle pain, fever, and edema (swelling). A characteristic sign of a trichinosis infection is periorbital edema (swelling around the eyes). Splinter hemorrhages in the nails may occur. These appear as narrow, red to reddish-brown lines of blood beneath the nails. Occasionally, the worms invade the central nervous system (the brain and the spinal cord), where they can produce serious neurological conditions such as ataxia (a lack of muscle coordination), respiratory paralysis, and death.

*Filariasis.* In lymphatic filariasis, the adult worms block the normal flow of lymphatic fluid, damaging the lymphatic system. This blockage produces tremendous enlargement of the arms, legs, or genitals, which may swell up to several times the normal size. The worms also lodge in the kidneys, causing damage. *Loa loa* filariasis can also produce swelling of the extremities. Transit of the worm across the eyeball is a unique sign of this disease. Lymphedema (swelling of the limbs) can occur if the worms block lymphatic channels in the arms and legs. Intermittent swelling, known as Calabar swellings, of the arms can occur because of an allergic reaction. Calabar swellings may be accompanied by urticaria (rash) and pruritus (itching).

*Pinworms.* Itching around the anus is a common symptom. The skin around the anus may also be inflamed. Vaginal itching can occur in young girls if the worms enter the vagina rather than the anus.

### SCREENING AND DIAGNOSIS

Many worm infections produce an allergic response. Often, these infections will cause an increase in the eosinophils in the bloodstream, causing a condition known as eosinophilia. A complete blood count (CBC), including a differential count, reveals the number of eosinophils present in the bloodstream. Eosinophils are a type of white blood cell, which increases with an allergic response. A blood test, which can be done in most medical laboratories, may reveal specific antibodies to the type of worm present. A more complex but highly accurate test can be done in a genetics laboratory that can conduct deoxyribonucleic acid (DNA) sequencing for parasite-specific DNA in a blood sample.

In cases of suspected tapeworm infection, a stool sample will reveal tapeworm eggs or body segments containing eggs. For hookworms, except for early infections, a stool sample will contain hookworm eggs. For liver flukes, a stool sample is often positive for eggs. Adult worms can sometimes be present in a sputum sample or in vomit.

Trichinosis can be diagnosed after learning the infected person has eaten contaminated meat. If a sample of the meat is available, microscopic examination will reveal cysts. The characteristic signs of periorbital edema and splinter hemorrhages in the nails aid the diagnosis. As in many other worm infections, eosinophilia is present.

For cases of filariasis, examination of a blood sample may reveal the presence of microfilariae. Their presence in the bloodstream is periodic; thus, the sample must be drawn when the microfilaria are likely to be present. Visualization of a worm transiting the eyeball is diagnostic for *Loa loa* filariasis. A simple card test detects antigens to lymphatic filariasis; however, antibody tests are not particularly helpful with *Loa loa* filariasis because cross-reactivity between *Loa loa* and other worm infections often occurs.

For pinworm infections, the worms are seen in the anus, particularly at night when they lay their eggs.

Placing a piece of tape against the anus will collect eggs for microscopic examination.

### TREATMENT AND THERAPY

A number of anthelmintic (antiworm) medications are available to treat worm infestations. Inasmuch as many worm infections can produce anemia, iron supplements are helpful.

Tapeworms can be treated with a single-dose oral medication. Niclosamide is the drug of choice; however, praziquantel and albendazole are also effective.

While still in the skin, hookworm infections can be treated by cryotherapy (localized freezing). During migration to the intestines and while in the intestines, albendazole (Albenza) or mebendazole are effective. Triclabendazole is the drug of choice to treat liver flukes. Resistant strains, however, have been reported in Ireland and Australia.

If given early, albendazole or mebendazole can eradicate the intestinal worms and larvae in trichinosis. These medications are less effective after cysts form; however, they are beneficial if the larvae enter the central nervous system, heart, or lungs. Analgesics (pain relievers) are given for muscular pain. Over time, the cysts often calcify; this destroys the larvae, and the muscle pain and fatigue resolve. Corticosteroids are given to reduce allergic reactions and inflammation when dead or dying larvae release chemicals within the muscles.

The drug of choice for filariasis (both lymphatic and *Loa loa*) is diethylcarbamazine (DEC); ivermectin is also effective. Doxycycline is under investigation as a supplementary agent to use with DEC. DEC is most effective against the microfilariae; it is less effective against the adult worms. Sometimes, after receiving a course of medication, the surviving worms are surgically excised. For pinworms, a single dose of either albendazole or mebendazole is effective. These medications are available by prescription and over the counter.

### PREVENTION AND OUTCOMES

Tapeworm infections can be prevented by avoiding raw meat and by cooking meat to a core temperature greater than 140° Fahrenheit for five minutes. Freezing meat to −4° F for twenty-four hours will also kill the eggs. Self-reinfection can be prevented by good hygiene and thorough handwashing after using the toilet.

Hookworm infections can be avoided by not walking barefoot in any area suspected of having infected soil, by defecating only into a toilet connected to a sewage system, and by avoiding the use of human feces for fertilization.

Liver fluke infections can be prevented by the avoidance of eating raw vegetables from any region inhabited by aquatic snails, such as *G. truncatula*. Filariasis infections can be prevented by avoiding the fly bites that spread *Loa loa*. Spraying homes with the pesticide dieldrin is an effective method of destroying the insect vectors.

Pinworm infections can be prevented by thorough handwashing before meals and after using the toilet, cleaning toilet seats daily, washing bed linens twice a week, keeping fingernails short and clean, and by not scratching infected areas around the anus.

*Robin Wulffson, M.D., FACOG*

### FURTHER READING

Bogitsh, Burton J., Clint E. Carter, and Thomas N. Oeltmann. *Human Parasitology.* 3d ed. Boston: Academic Press/Elsevier, 2005. An upper-level textbook that provides succinct coverage of medical parasitology in an easy-to-read format.

Gittleman, Ann Louise. *Guess What Came to Dinner? Parasites and Your Health.* Rev. ed. New York: Putnam, 2001. A thorough study of the parasite world, particularly its relation to human health and nutrition. Covers parasitic illnesses and their diagnosis, treatments, and prevention.

Leventhal, Ruth, and Russell F. Cheadle. *Medical Parasitology: A Self-Instructional Text.* 5th ed. Philadelphia: F. A. Davis, 2002. A systematic introduction to the biology and epidemiology of human parasitic diseases. Includes graphics, color plates, and study exercises.

Matthews, Bernard E. *An Introduction to Parasitology.* New York: Cambridge University Press, 1998. An introductory undergraduate textbook that provides a concise, clear overview of parasite biology for students and nonspecialists.

Muller, Ralph. *Worms and Human Disease.* 2d ed. New York: CABI, 2002. An advanced-student textbook that covers all human worm infections with emphasis on diagnosis, treatment, clinical manifestations, pathogenesis (disease development), epidemiology, and control.

Nagami, Pamela. *The Woman with a Worm in Her Head,* *and Other True Stories of Infectious Disease.* New York: St. Martin's Griffin, 2002. A physician's description of cases of worm infestation, "flesh-eating" strep, and acquired immunodeficiency syndrome (AIDS). The cases illustrate hidden dangers and the challenges facing physicians who treat these diseases.

Roberts, Larry S., and John Janovy, Jr. *Gerald D. Schmidt and Larry S. Roberts' Foundations of Parasitology.* 8th ed. Boston: McGraw-Hill, 2009. A graduate-level textbook covering all aspects of parasitology. The text is highly technical and intended for the informed reader. The book is well illustrated.

### WEB SITES OF INTEREST

*National Center for Emerging and Zoonotic Infectious Diseases*
http://www.cdc.gov/ncezid

*Neglected Tropical Diseases Coalition*
http://www.neglectedtropicaldiseases.org

*U.S. Department of Agriculture, Food Safety Information Center*
http://foodsafety.nal.usda.gov

*World Health Organization*
http://www.who.int/zoonoses

**See also:** Antiparasitic drugs: Types; Developing countries and infectious disease; Flukes; Hookworms; Intestinal and stomach infections; Parasites: Classification and types; Pigs and infectious disease; Pinworms; Ringworm; Roundworms; Skin infections; Soilborne illness and disease; Tapeworms; Tropical medicine; Waterborne illness and disease; Whipworm infection.

# Wound infections

CATEGORY: Diseases and conditions
ANATOMY OR SYSTEM AFFECTED: Skin, tissue
ALSO KNOWN AS: Surgical wound infection

### DEFINITION

Wound infections involve injury marked by the division of tissue or the rupture of membranes. These injuries develop infections caused by bacteria, viruses, or fungi. For surgical cases, wound infections are specific to the surgical site.

## INTRODUCTION

Wounds caused by trauma or obtained during surgical procedures (invasive and noninvasive surgery) can become breeding grounds for infections. The majority of wound infections are caused by bacteria such as staphylococci and streptococci. Many surgical infections are caused by *Staphylococcus aureus* or *S. epidermis*. Symptoms of wound infection include pain, swelling, and redness, and drainage from the wound area. An accompanying fever means the infection has spread through the body.

Specific types of wounds are more likely to be susceptible to tetanus (*Clostridium tetani*) infection, including puncture wounds, burns, and frostbite. Tetanus results from bacteria spores present in soil. These spores invade the wound, resulting in neurologic conditions, particularly spasms, and fever. Gas gangrene is a tissue-destroying infection caused by *Clostridium* species and can result in septic shock.

Types of wound infection of special concern are methicillin-resistant *S. aureus* (MRSA) infection and vancomycin-resistant *Enterococcus* (VRE) infection, which are prevalent in hospitals and are resistant to treatment with antibiotics. Hospitalized persons are especially susceptible because they may already have a compromised immune system and are sometimes exposed to germs from other sick patients. MRSA and VRE are common in community spaces, especially day-care centers, dormitories, and athletic facilities. Skin infections can occur in a rash or wound. Wounds exposed to fresh water or sea water are often susceptible to waterborne organisms such as *Aeromonas, Pseudomonas*, and *Vibrio vulnificus*.

## RISK FACTORS

Some studies have demonstrated that certain characteristics render persons more susceptible to wound infections, compared with persons who do not have these factors. Obesity and diabetes have high wound infection rates. Specific surgical-infection risk factors include diabetes, obesity, the receipt of a blood transfusion during surgery, older age, hypertension, hyperlipidemia, length of surgery, and smoking.

## PREVENTION

Tetanus infection is completely preventable with vaccine, which is effective for ten to twelve years. MRSA, VRE, and other infections occurring commonly in clinics and hospitals can be reduced by practicing universal precautions, which are instrumental in preventing infection when treating the wounded. Universal precautions involve treating biologic fluids as though they were infected with the human immunodeficiency virus or another pathogen, treating each patient cautiously to avoid exposing oneself and others, thorough handwashing, sterilizing instruments, wearing protective gear, and properly disposing of medical waste.

Instrument sterilization, however, can be less effective than one might think. At any step of the sterilization process, it is possible to reintroduce bacteria. Some hospitals are opting to use new, unused instruments for each surgery. Debate continues about whether wearing face masks during surgery protects patients; however, it does protect medical staff from blood spatter to the face. Prophylactic antibiotics before, during, and after surgery are often helpful in reducing infection rate, such as for knee or hip replacement.

## TREATMENT

Depending on the type of infection, a lack of treatment may result in blood poisoning, gangrene (tissue death), or death. According to the World Health Organization, one should never close up an infected wound. A protocol of washing, debridement (removing any dirt and dead tissue), and saline irrigation should be followed and the wound should be left open but covered with dressing; the dressing should be changed a minimum of once per day. If the wound is not open but it does have pus under the surface, it is critical to drain the subcutaneous pus. Intravenous antibiotics should be used to treat bacterial infection, preferably tailored to the type of infection (if testing is available at the site) to reduce unnecessary overexposure to antibiotics.

## IMPACT

Infected wounds affect millions worldwide and can result in debilitation or death. Appropriate preventive measures and effective treatments are essential in reducing the widespread effects of wound infection.

*Dawn M. Bielawski, Ph.D.*

FURTHER READING

Al-Buhairan, B., D. Hind, and A. Hutchinson. "Antibiotic Prophylaxis for Wound Infections in Total Joint Arthroplasty." *Journal of Bone and Joint Surgery* 90-B (2007): 915-919. A review of the evidence from twenty-six studies, reporting on the effectiveness of prophylactic antibiotics in reducing infections in persons having total knee or total hip replacement.

Downie, Fiona, et al. "Barrier Dressings in Surgical Site Infection Prevention Strategies." *British Journal of Nursing* 19 (2010): S42-S46. This clinical article provides a multifaceted model for preventing surgical infections. Focuses largely on vapor-permeable dressings postsurgery.

Matros, Evan, et al. "Reduction in Incidence of Deep Sternal Wound Infections: Random or Real?" *Journal of Thoracic and Cardiovascular Surgery* 139 (2010): 680-685. Analyzes trends in the risk factors associated with deep sternal wound infections.

Olsen, Margaret A., et al. "Risk Factors for Surgical Site Infection Following Orthopaedic Spinal Operations." *Journal of Bone and Joint Surgery* 90 (2008): 62-69. Discusses a retrospective, case-control study of risk factors associated with spinal surgery.

Perry, Christine, ed. *Infection Prevention and Control.* Malden, Mass.: Blackwell, 2007. An evidence-based guide that describes in detail areas such as urinary catheter care, pediatric care, and wound prevention and management.

WEB SITES OF INTEREST

*Association for Professionals in Infection Control and Epidemiology*
http://www.knowledgeisinfectious.org

*Centers for Disease Control and Prevention*
http://www.cdc.gov/mrsa

*Clean Hands Coalition*
http://www.cleanhandscoalition.org

**See also:** Antibiotic resistance; Antibiotics: Types; Bacterial infections; Bloodstream infections; Disinfectants and sanitizers; Epidemiology; Fever; Fever of unknown origin; Fungal infections; Gangrene; Hospitals and infectious disease; Hygiene; Iatrogenic infections; Methicillin-resistant staph infection; Necrotizing fasciitis; Opportunistic infections; Primary infection; Prosthetic joint infections; Public health; Secondary infection; Septic shock; Superbacteria; Tetanus; Transmission routes; Vancomycin-resistant enterococci infection; Viral infections.

# Y

## Yaws

CATEGORY: Diseases and conditions

ANATOMY OR SYSTEM AFFECTED: Bones, joints, musculoskeletal system, skin

ALSO KNOWN AS: Bouba, frambresia tropica, parangi, pian, polypapilloma tropicum, thymiosis, treponematosis

### DEFINITION

Yaws is a chronic infection of the skin, bones, and joints caused by exposure to the bacterium *Treponema pallidum pertenue*. The bacterium is spread through direct physical contact.

### CAUSES

Yaws is spread by physical contact with another person who is infected with *T. pallidum pertenue*, principally through exposure to the open sores associated with the disease. Unlike the closely related disease syphilis, yaws is not spread through sexual contact. The bacterium responsible for yaws infections thrives in tropical, humid climates, especially in areas where extreme poverty, overpopulation, unsanitary living conditions, poor physical hygiene, and inadequate medical care are prevalent.

### RISK FACTORS

Indigenous peoples who live in extreme poverty in tropical climates, with unsanitary living conditions, poor physical hygiene, and overcrowded populations are at greatest risk for contracting yaws. Children, particularly age two to fifteen years, are most vulnerable to infection by yaws, but all persons are susceptible. Although massive campaigns by the World Health Organization between 1950 and 1970 largely eradicated yaws worldwide, many pockets of yaws-infected populations still exist, especially among isolated peoples in Indonesia, Africa, Latin America, and the Caribbean. Persons who visit areas where yaws is endemic also risk infection and should ensure that all precautions are taken to reduce exposure.

### SYMPTOMS

Five to eight weeks after initial exposure to the *T. pallidum pertenue* organism, initial lesions, called mother yaws, form at the site of infection, usually on the legs. The lesions, purple and shaped like raspberries, become large, ulcerative, and itchy, but they heal after about six months. Shortly thereafter, a new manifestation of yaws erupts all over the body that includes very painful lesions on the palms of the hands and soles of the feet, lasting for approximately five years. The final phase of yaws manifests five to ten years later in skin, joint, and bone destruction and disfigurement.

### SCREENING AND DIAGNOSIS

After a physical examination, blood and lesion samples are collected and tested using dark-field microscopy. Blood tests such as rapid plasma reagin will appear positive for all four subspecies of the microbe *T. pallidum*, so close examination of lesion samples is required to identify the spirochete *T. pallidum pertenue* organism responsible for yaws.

### TREATMENT AND THERAPY

In the early stages of yaws, treatment with long-acting penicillin is effective. Persons who are allergic to penicillin are prescribed erythromycin, chloramphenicol, and tetracycline to successfully eliminate the disease. Late-stage destruction of bones and joints by yaws is largely irreversible, however.

### PREVENTION AND OUTCOMES

Avoiding skin-to-skin contact with sores from those infected with yaws and receiving immediate treatment with penicillin if infected are the best ways to prevent the spread of the disease. Sanitary personal hygiene and living conditions also help prevent yaws.

*Mary E. Markland, M.A.*

### FURTHER READING

Aufderheide, Arthur, and Conrado Rodriguez-Martin. *The Cambridge Encyclopedia of Human Paleopathology.* New York: Cambridge University Press, 1998.

Feigin, Ralph D., et al., eds. *Textbook of Pediatric Infectious Diseases.* 6th ed. Philadelphia: Saunders/Elsevier, 2009.

Mann, Robert, and David Hunt. *Photographic Regional Atlas of Bone Disease: A Guide to Pathologic and Normal Variation in the Human Skeleton.* Springfield, Ill.: Charles C Thomas, 2005.

Nassar, Naiel N., and Justin David Radolf. "Nonvenereal Treponematoses: Yaws, Pinta, and Endemic Syphilis." In *Kelley's Textbook of Internal Medicine,* edited by H. David Humes et al. 4th ed. Philadelphia: Lippincott Williams & Wilkins, 2000.

Roberts, Charlotte, and Keith Manchester. *The Archaeology of Bone Disease.* Ithaca, N.Y.: Cornell University Press, 2007.

**WEB SITES OF INTEREST**

*American Society of Tropical Medicine and Hygiene*
http://www.astmh.org

*Neglected Tropical Diseases Coalition*
http://www.neglectedtropicaldiseases.org

*Virtual Museum of Bacteria*
http://www.bacteriamuseum.org

*World Health Organization*
http://www.searo.who.int/en/section10.htm

**See also:** Bacterial infections; Children and infectious disease; Developing countries and infectious disease; Pinta; Skin infections; Syphilis; *Treponema*; Tropical medicine.

# Yellow fever

CATEGORY: Diseases and conditions
ANATOMY OR SYSTEM AFFECTED: All

## DEFINITION

Yellow fever is a disease carried by female mosquitoes of two species (*Aedes* and *Haemogogus*). Mosquitoes pass yellow fever to humans through a small amount of saliva when they bite. The species of mosquito that carry yellow fever are native to sub-Saharan Africa and South America.

Yellow fever can cause flulike symptoms, yellowing of both the skin and the whites of the eyes, and death. Yellow fever is a rare disease in travelers because many people get the vaccine, but it is endemic to impoverished areas because most people cannot afford to get vaccinated or because the vaccines are not available.

## CAUSES

The yellow fever virus is the cause of yellow fever. The yellow fever virus is transmitted to humans when an infected mosquito bites a person. Yellow fever is not communicable, or contagious, meaning it cannot be passed directly from one person to another.

## RISK FACTORS

The following factors increase the chance of getting yellow fever: living, working, or traveling in jungle or urban areas with yellow fever, including sub-Saharan Africa (thirty-three countries in Africa have consistent cases of yellow fever); and South America (Bolivia, Brazil, Colombia, Ecuador, and Peru provide greatest risk). Another risk factor is failing to take precautions, including receiving the yellow fever vaccine, reducing contact with mosquitoes (by using sleeping nets, long-sleeved clothing, and screens), and using insect repellents.

## SYMPTOMS

Yellow fever has two phases: acute and toxic. All persons infected with yellow fever will experience the acute phase. Fifteen percent of people with yellow fever will progress into the toxic phase.

One should not assume that the following symptoms are caused by yellow fever. Many of them also occur with other, less serious illnesses, such as influenza. However, persons who experience any of these symptoms should seek medical attention.

During the acute phase, the symptoms are fever, headache, muscle pain, backache, chills, loss of appetite, and nausea or vomiting (or both). During the toxic phase, the symptoms are high fever; abdominal pain; bleeding from the gums, nose, eyes, or stomach; black vomit (vomit that appears black because of blood content); low blood pressure; liver failure, which may lead to jaundice, or yellowing of the skin and whites of the eyes; kidney failure; confusion; seizure; coma; and death. Approximately 50 percent of toxic-phase patients die.

Yellow fever symptoms appear three to six days after a person is bitten by an infected mosquito. Typi-

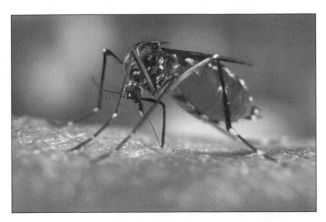

*The* Aedes aegypti *mosquito is a yellow fever vector.* (CDC)

cally, acute phase symptoms will persist for three to four days and then disappear. If an infected person is going to progress into the toxic phase, toxic-phase symptoms will begin within twenty-four hours of the end of the acute phase. When a person recovers from yellow fever, he or she is considered to have lifetime immunity from the disease.

### SCREENING AND DIAGNOSIS

A doctor will ask about symptoms, medical history, and travel history, and will then perform a physical exam. Blood tests may be ordered to screen for signs of yellow fever in the blood.

### TREATMENT AND THERAPY

Medications or treatments specifically for yellow fever are not available. However, there are treatments that can be given at a hospital to ease some symptoms of yellow fever. One should keep the body hydrated with fluids containing electrolytes and salts. These fluids may be given orally or may be injected through a vein to prevent dehydration. Cool water or fever-reducing medications (such as acetaminophen, or Tylenol) may be given to reduce fever.

In toxic-phase cases, dialysis may be needed to help the kidneys filter waste. Also, a transfusion may be needed to replace blood cells and clotting agents lost through bleeding.

Fighting yellow fever may cause a person's immune system to become temporarily weak. A weakened immune system cannot guard against bacterial infections as it normally would, so infections occur more easily. Antibiotics may be given to fight bacterial infec-tions associated with yellow-fever illness. Antibiotics cannot be given to treat yellow fever because yellow fever is caused by a virus, and viruses do not respond to antibiotics.

### PREVENTION AND OUTCOMES

Vaccination is the best way to prevent yellow fever. However, like any vaccine, it is not for everyone. People with compromised immune systems, the elderly, and women who may be pregnant should not receive the vaccine. If a person lives, works, or travels in areas where yellow fever is common, he or she should ask a doctor if vaccination is recommended.

Persons who cannot receive the vaccine or who would like to reduce their risk of being bitten by a mos-quito should take the following precautions: Stay in air-conditioned or well-screened areas, wear long-sleeved clothing and long pants, use sleeping nets, and remove or destroy mosquito-breeding areas. Mosqui-toes lay their eggs in standing pools of water, such as the insides of old tires, flower pots, and small puddles. Another preventive measure is to use insect repellents that contain NN-diethyl metatoluamide (DEET) and permethrin on clothes, exposed skin, and bed nets for extra protection.

*Jen Rymaruk; reviewed by David L. Horn, M.D., FACP*

### FURTHER READING

Delaporte, François. *The History of Yellow Fever: An Essay on the Birth of Tropical Medicine.* Translated by Arthur Goldhammer. Cambridge, Mass.: MIT Press, 1991.

Jong, Elaine C., and Russell McMullen, eds. *Travel and Tropical Medicine Manual.* 4th ed. Philadelphia: Saunders/Elsevier, 2008.

Mandell, Gerald L., John E. Bennett, and Raphael Dolin, eds. *Mandell, Douglas, and Bennett's Principles and Practice of Infectious Diseases.* 7th ed. New York: Churchill Livingstone/Elsevier, 2010.

Marquardt, William C., ed. *Biology of Disease Vectors.* 2d ed. New York: Academic Press/Elsevier, 2005.

World Health Organization. "Yellow Fever." Available at http://www.who.int/mediacentre/factsheets/fs100.

### WEB SITES OF INTEREST

*American Society of Tropical Medicine and Hygiene*
http://www.astmh.org

*Centers for Disease Control and Prevention*
http://www.cdc.gov

*World Health Organization*
http://www.who.int

**See also:** Blood-borne illness and disease; Dengue fever; Developing countries and infectious disease; Eastern equine encephalitis; Encephalitis; Fever; Insect-borne illness and disease; Insecticides and topical repellants; Japanese encephalitis; Malaria; Mosquito-borne viral encephalitis; Mosquitoes and infectious disease; Sleeping nets; Tropical medicine; Vaccines: Types; Vectors and vector control; Viral infections; West Nile virus; Yellow fever vaccine.

# Yellow fever vaccine

CATEGORY: Prevention

## DEFINITION

The yellow fever vaccine was developed to fight yellow fever, which is an acute infectious disease transmitted by mosquitoes and caused by a flavivirus. Yellow fever remains endemic to parts of South America and in Africa. The reported risk of contracting yellow fever, when in an endemic area, is approximately 1 in 267; of those infected, up to 40 percent will die. No antiviral treatment is effective against the yellow fever virus, so a vaccine was developed to prevent people from contracting the disease. The vaccine is prepared from the 17D strain of the disease, which is live but attenuated (weaker). More than four hundred million doses of yellow fever vaccine have been administered worldwide.

## HISTORY

As was first thought, yellow fever was conclusively identified as a virus rather than as a bacteria in 1928. Max Theiler, a South African-born virologist working at New York's Rockefeller Foundation, developed the yellow fever vaccine in 1937. He initially passed the virus through laboratory mice and found that the weakened form of the virus provided immunity to Rhesus monkeys. During his work with the virus, Theiler contracted yellow fever but survived and consequently developed immunity. Theiler was awarded

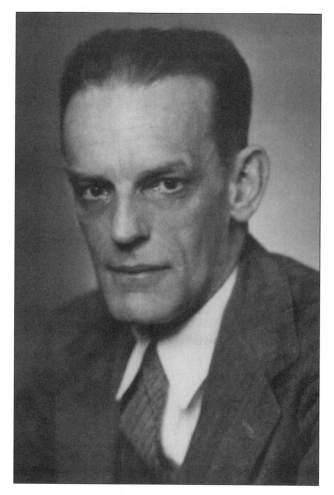

*Max Theiler.* (The Nobel Foundation)

the Nobel Prize in Physiology or Medicine in 1951 for developing the yellow fever vaccine.

## ADMINISTRATION

Persons traveling to or planning to live in areas where yellow fever is endemic should receive the vaccine. People routinely exposed to yellow fever virus, such as researchers and laboratory staff, are also encouraged to receive the vaccine. The vaccine, however, is not recommended for newborns younger than four months of age or for women during their first trimester of pregnancy. The yellow fever vaccine is administered in a single injection by a health care professional. Effective protection from the virus begins after ten days and protection lasts a minimum of ten years.

## DOCUMENTATION

To legally enter some countries, people must carry internationally recognized proof of receiving the yellow fever vaccine. This proof is established with a stamped document, the International Certificate of Vaccination Against Yellow Fever.

## SIDE EFFECTS

The yellow fever vaccine is safe. As with any drug or vaccine, strict regulations are enforced during its development and manufacturing. Common physical reactions to the vaccine include soreness and tenderness or redness at the site of the injection. Also, a slight headache, low-grade fever, or aching muscles can occur five to ten days after receiving the vaccine.

*April Ingram, B.S.*

## FURTHER READING

Bloom, Barry R., and Paul-Henri Lambert, eds. *The Vaccine Book*. San Diego, Calif.: Academic Press, 2002.

Centers for Disease Control and Prevention. "Yellow Fever Vaccine." Available at http://www.cdc.gov/ncidod/dvbid/yellowfever/vaccine.

Frierson, J. Gordon. "The Yellow Fever Vaccine: A History." *Yale Journal of Biology and Medicine* 83, no. 2 (June, 2010): 77-85.

Jong, Elaine C., and Russell McMullen, eds. *Travel and Tropical Medicine Manual*. 4th ed. Philadelphia: Saunders/Elsevier, 2008.

Norrby, Erling. "Yellow Fever and Max Theiler: The Only Nobel Prize for a Virus Vaccine." *Journal of Experimental Medicine* 204, no. 12 (November 26, 2007): 2779-2784.

World Health Organization. "Yellow Fever." Available at http://www.who.int/mediacentre/factsheets/fs100.

## WEB SITES OF INTEREST

*American Society of Tropical Medicine and Hygiene*
http://www.astmh.org

*Centers for Disease Control and Prevention, Division of Vector Borne Infectious Diseases*
http://www.cdc.gov/ncidod/dvbid

*World Health Organization: Vaccines, Immunization, and Biologicals*
http://www.who.int/vaccines/en/yellowfever.shtml

**See also:** Blood-borne illness and disease; Dengue fever; Developing countries and infectious disease; Encephalitis; Hemorrhagic fever viral infections; Insect-borne illness and disease; Insecticides and topical repellants; Malaria; Mosquito-borne viral encephalitis; Mosquitoes and infectious disease; Tropical medicine; Vaccines: Types; Vectors and vector control; Viral infections; West Nile virus; Yellow fever.

# *Yersinia*

CATEGORY: Pathogen
TRANSMISSION ROUTE: Ingestion, inhalation, skin

## DEFINITION

Three species of *Yersinia* affect humans, two causing intestinal infections and one causing the plague, an acute, contagious disease.

---

### Taxonomic Classification for *Yersinia*

**Kingdom:** Bacteria
**Phylum:** Proteobacteria
**Order:** Enterobacteriales
**Family:** Enterobacteriacae
**Genus:** *Yersinia*
**Species:**
*Y. aldovae*
*Y. aleksiciae*
*Y. bercovieri*
*Y. enterocolitica*
*Y. frederiksenii*
*Y. intermedia*
*Y. kristensenii*
*Y. mollaretii*
*Y. pestis*
*Y. pseudotuberculosis*
*Y. rohdei*
*Y. ruckeri*

---

## NATURAL HABITAT AND FEATURES

*Yersinia* bacteria are rod shaped (at times approaching a spherical shape) and are usually 0.5 micrometers (μm) in diameter and 1 to 3 μm in length. *Yersinia* are gram-negative. They are motile below 86° Fahrenheit (30° Celsius) with the exception of some

*Y. ruckeri* strains and *Y. pestis*, which is never motile. The optimal temperature for these bacteria is 82° to 86° F (28° to 30° C), although *Y. enterocolitica* is often found in cold climates.

*Yersinia* occur in a variety of habitats, including soil, water, and foods such as dairy products, and are present in birds, animals (especially rodents), and humans. Most species are occasional human pathogens. *Y. ruckerii* causes red mouth in fish; three species (*pestis, pseudotuberculosis,* and *enterocolitica*) cause infections in humans and other mammals.

Draft sequencing of the various *Yersinia* species indicates that genes have been horizontally transferred and that virulence determinants have been gained and lost over time. There is a high degree of genetic redundancy among the *Yersinia* species. Later scientific developments have led to the ability to distinguish among the various species with a high degree of accuracy. A close evolutionary relationship exists among the *enterocolitica* clade (descendant) strains. Four species (*bercorieri, mollaretii, aldovae,* and *ruckeri*) evolved from *Y. enterocolitica. Y. pestis* evolved from *Y. pseudotuberculosis* as early as twenty thousand years ago with significant branching; this resulted in a clear split around 6,500 years ago.

## PATHOGENICITY AND CLINICAL SIGNIFICANCE

Three species of *Yersinia* pose health threats to humans. The three species can be distinguished from each other by laboratory tests and by their symptoms. Most notable is *Y. pestis,* the causative agent of the plague. There have been three plague pandemics, dating from the plague of Justinian in the sixth century. The second, often referred to as the Black Death, first appeared in southern Europe in 1347 and then spread over much of the continent during the next four years. It is estimated that this pandemic killed between 30 and 60 percent of the population of Europe. Plague remained endemic to European society, with periodic epidemics until the early eighteenth century. The third pandemic began in western China in the 1860's, spread to Hong Kong by 1894, and to India, Java, Egypt, and San Francisco by 1900, killing more than one hundred million persons worldwide. Plague remains endemic to some parts of the world, such as Mongolia and the Four Corners region of the United States. The first plague pandemic probably originated in Africa; the later ones came from Asia. Alexander Yersin identified *Y. pestis* as the agent of plague during the third plague pandemic. Although most scholars credit *Y. pestis* as the causative agent of the first and second plague pandemics, the diagnosis is disputed by some.

Three varieties of plague exist: bubonic, septicemic, and pneumonic. Bubonic is the most common form and is transmitted by infected fleas, which bite humans after having bitten infected rats or other animals. Left untreated, bubonic plague has a mortality rate between 40 and 70 percent.

Septicemic plague arises as a secondary infection from a primary bubonic infection and is generally fatal. Pneumonic plague often occurs as a secondary infection but may also be a primary infection that is spread from human to human through nasal discharge. Untreated, it is fatal.

The incubation period for bubonic usually ranges from two to six days and is followed by the sudden onset of chills, fever, and headache, followed by body ache and possibly diarrhea. Painful swollen lymph glands, often in the groin, are a telltale sign of bubonic plague. Septicemic plague arises from a bubonic infection producing nausea and diarrhea. Buboes are uncommon in septicemic plague. The patient soon becomes moribund, has multiorgan failure, and dies. Pneumonic plague is often secondary to bubonic or septicemic plague, but is also spread human to human. It exhibits sudden-onset fever with chest pain and purulent sputum; death often follows. Often, also, no buboes are present.

*Y. entercolitica* is the most common form of *Yersinia* pathogen. It produces acute bacterial gastroenteritis that especially affects the young. A food-borne pathogen, it colonizes the small intestine and may exhibit symptoms similar to other intestinal ailments.

*Y. pseudotuberculosis* is also a food-borne pathogen, although it is less common than *Y. enterocolitica.* It often mimics appendicitis and generally does not cause diarrhea. Together, *Y. entercolitica* and *Y. pseudotuberculosis* cause about seventeen thousand cases of yersiniosis every year.

## DRUG SUSCEPTIBILITY

Infections from *Y. enterocolitica* and *Y. pseudotuberculosis* are often managed without antimicrobials. Antibiotic regimes, however, may be prescribed for some persons. Ampicillin is prescribed at times for *Y. pseudotuberculosis,* and ciprofloxacin is prescribed for *Y. entercolitica.*

Early antibiotic treatment is essential for the treatment of plague, as untreated cases often have a high mortality risk. Outside the United States, streptomycin is often prescribed. Gentamicin is comparable or superior to streptomycin and is often used in the treatment of plague. Doxycycline is used for persons who cannot take aminoglycosides. It is also recommended for mass casualties, such as those from an act of bioterrorism. Drug-resistant cases have been reported, however, in Madagascar.

Vaccines have been developed for use against the plague, although no country requires them. Killed whole-cell plague vaccines may cause severe side effects, require a six-month course of vaccination, and are ineffective against pneumonic plague. Largely because of the threat of the use of plague as a biological weapon by terrorists, scientists are working to develop second and third generation vaccines that avoid the problems of the first generation vaccines.

*John M. Theilmann, Ph.D.*

## FURTHER READING

Betts, Robert F., Stanley W. Chapman, and Robert L. Penn, eds. *Reese and Betts' A Practical Approach to Infectious Disease.* 5th ed. Philadelphia: Lippincott Williams & Wilkins, 2003. A standard handbook for infectious disease.

Carniel, Elisabeth. "Evolution of Pathogenic *Yersinia*: Some Lights in the Dark." In *The Genus "Yersinia,"* edited by Mikael Skurnick and José Antonio Bengoechea. New York: Kluwer Academic, 2003. A good summary of the latest knowledge of the bacteria by a leading researcher.

Inglesby, Thomas V., et al. "Plague as a Biological Weapon: Medical and Public Health Management." *Journal of the American Medical Association* 283 (2000): 2281-2290. A good article on the use of plague as a weapon of terror; from a respected medical journal.

Mandell, Gerald L., John E. Bennett, and Raphael Dolin, eds. *Mandell, Douglas, and Bennett's Principles and Practice of Infectious Diseases.* 7th ed. New York: Churchill Livingstone/Elsevier, 2010. A standard reference textbook of infectious diseases with a chapter on plague. Includes maps and illustrations.

Orent, Wendy. *Plague.* New York: Free Press, 2004. A useful historical treatment of plague with detailed attention to the biology of the disease.

## WEB SITES OF INTEREST

*American College of Gastroenterology*
http://www.acg.gi.org

*Center for Biosecurity*
http://www.upmc-biosecurity.org

*Centers for Disease Control and Prevention*
http://www.bt.cdc.gov/agent/plague

*PathoSystems Resource Integration Center*
http://www.patricbrc.org

**See also:** Airborne illness and disease; Arthropodborne illness and disease; Bacterial infections; Biological weapons; Bioterrorism; Bubonic plague; Contagious diseases; Endemic infections; *Enterobacter*; Fleas and infectious disease; Food-borne illness and disease; Intestinal and stomach infections; Lassa fever; Plague; Rat-bite fever; Respiratory route of transmission; Rodents and infectious disease; Vectors and vector control; *Yersinia pseudotuberculosis*; Yersiniosis; Zoonotic diseases.

# *Yersinia pseudotuberculosis*

CATEGORY: Diseases and conditions

## DEFINITION

One of the three main *Yersinia* bacterium species, *Y. pseudotuberculosis* causes an animal-transmitted or food-borne gastroenteritis whose symptoms mimic appendicitis.

Microscopically, *Y. pseudotuberculosis* shows as an ovoid-shaped cell (coccobacillus) that stains gram-negative (red) during a Gram's stain. If cultured from infected persons, it tends to grow slowly and form small, translucent, gray colonies. The cells have multiple flagella that allow them to move rapidly at low temperatures, but at higher temperatures that approximate that of the human body (95 degrees Fahrenheit, or 35 degrees Celsius), the species is nonmotile.

## CAUSES

Upon introduction to the gastrointestinal tract, the organism invades the wall of the lower small intestine and usually colonizes the lymphatic system associated with the intestines (causing mesenteric lymphadenitis).

## RISK FACTORS

*Y. pseudotuberculosis* normally lives in warm-blooded animals. Mammals such as dogs, cats, cattle, horses, rabbits, deer, and rodents, and birds (such as turkeys, geese, ducks, cockatoos, and canaries) can act as reservoirs of this organism. Contact with animals that carry *Y. pseudotuberculosis* can cause zoonotic infections (diseases that are transmitted from animals to humans). Likewise, the consumption of food prepared from animals that harbor the bacterium can cause food-borne infections. Drinking water from wells, streams, or other water sources, including those contaminated with bacterium-containing soil, also can lead to *Y. pseudotuberculosis* infections.

## SYMPTOMS

The symptoms of *Y. pseudotuberculosis* infection are a triad of abdominal pain in the lower right quadrant, a fever, and sometimes a skin rash, but diarrhea is rather uncommon. Symptoms usually appear five to ten days after infection and can last one to three weeks in healthy persons in the absence of treatment.

In persons with poorly functioning immune systems or with liver disorders that cause excessive blood-iron concentrations, the organism can colonize the blood, leading to sepsis. In such cases, mortality rates exceed 75 percent.

## SCREENING AND DIAGNOSIS

Because of the location of the abdominal pain, *Y. pseudotuberculosis* gastroenteritis is commonly confused with appendicitis.

## TREATMENT AND THERAPY

Most *Y. pseudotuberculosis* infections do not require antibiotic treatment, but drug therapy is essential for children or adults with preexisting conditions that makes sepsis likely.

Aminoglycoside antibiotics such as streptomycin sulfate, tobramycin, and gentamicin, can treat *Y. pseudotuberculosis* infections, but the toxicity of these drugs to the kidneys and ears limits their long-term usefulness. Bacterial cell-wall inhibitors such as the beta-lactam antibiotic pipericillin or the third-generation cephalosporin cefotaxime show consistent activity against *Y. pseudotuberculosis*. The bacterial protein-syn-thesis inhibitor chloramphenicol is effective against *Y. pseudotuberculosis* but should be used only as a last resort because it can damage bone marrow and cause aplastic anemia.

Combinations of antibiotics are also efficacious against *Y. pseudotuberculosis* infections. For example, a combination of cefotaxime and the quinolone antibiotic levofloxacin has effectively treated persons with bacteremia caused by *Y. pseudotuberculosis*.

## PREVENTION AND OUTCOMES

Prevention involves proper hygiene and food preparation and the avoidance of other sources of infection.

*Michael A. Buratovich, Ph.D.*

## FURTHER READING

Carniel, Elisabeth. "Evolution of Pathogenic *Yersinia*: Some Lights in the Dark". In *The Genus Yersinia*, edited by Mikael Skurnick and José Antonio Bengoechea. New York: Kluwer Academic, 2003.

Jay, James M., Martin J. Loessner, and David A. Golden. *Modern Food Microbiology*. 7th ed. New York: Springer, 2005.

Krauss, Hartmut, et al. *Zoonoses: Infectious Diseases Transmissible from Animals to Humans*. 3d ed. Washington, D.C.: ASM Press, 2003.

Robins-Browne, Roy M., and Elizabeth L. Hartland. "*Yersinia* Species." In *International Handbook of Food-borne Pathogens*, edited by Marianne D. Miliotis and Jeffrey W. Bier. New York: Marcel Dekker, 2003.

Ryan, Kenneth J., and C. George Ray, eds. *Sherris Medical Microbiology: An Introduction to Infectious Diseases*. 5th ed. New York: McGraw-Hill, 2010.

## WEB SITES OF INTEREST

*American College of Gastroenterology*
http://www.acg.gi.org

*Centers for Disease Control and Prevention*
http://www.cdc.gov

*National Center for Emerging and Zoonotic Infectious Diseases*
http://www.cdc.gov/ncezid

**See also:** Appendicitis; Bacteria: Classification and types; Bacterial infections; Bubonic plague; *Enterobacter*; Food-borne illness and disease; Intestinal and stomach infections; Pathogens; Plague; Respiratory route of transmission; Rodents and infectious disease; Sepsis; Waterborne illness and disease; *Yersinia*; Yersiniosis; Zoonotic diseases.

# Yersiniosis

CATEGORY: Diseases and conditions
ANATOMY OR SYSTEM AFFECTED: Gastrointestinal system, intestines, stomach

## DEFINITION

Yersiniosis is a food-borne infection of the intestines caused by ingesting the bacterium *Yersinia enterocolitica*, which is often in infected pork products and in infected unpasteurized (raw) milk.

## CAUSES

Yersiniosis is principally caused by eating raw or undercooked meat, especially pork, in the form of chitterlings. However, yersiniosis may be spread by processing pork chitterlings before cooking, by not washing hands afterward, and by then disseminating the bacteria through direct physical contact with others. Furthermore, cross-contamination of food may occur by preparing infected pork on the same cutting board as other food prepared in the kitchen. Drinking unpasteurized milk or untreated water that has been infected with the bacterium *Y. enterocolitica* also causes yersiniosis. Touching infected animals or their feces spreads yersiniosis. Rarely, yersiniosis may be transmitted through blood transfusion.

## RISK FACTORS

Anyone may contract yersiniosis by ingesting raw or undercooked meat, particularly pork, but children are at greatest risk for infection by yersiniosis through the drinking of infected unpasteurized milk. Because drinking infected untreated water may also cause yersiniosis, those living in poverty and in developing countries are highly susceptible to the disease caused by unsanitary water conditions. Having a weakened immune system greatly increases potential bacterial infection by yersiniosis. Touching infected animals can also spread yersiniosis, so farmers, veterinarians, and stockyard workers are also vulnerable to infection.

## SYMPTOMS

Symptoms of yersiniosis include abdominal and joint pain, cramps, fever, nausea, diarrhea, and bloody stool. Yersiniosis is sometimes mistaken for appendicitis because both diseases cause severe pain on the right side of the abdomen.

## SCREENING AND DIAGNOSIS

After a physical examination, a stool sample is collected and tested for the presence of *Y. enterocolitica*. However, the bacterium may also be detected by examining the person's throat culture, urine, blood, joint fluid, or bile, confirming an infection of yersiniosis.

## TREATMENT AND THERAPY

Most cases of yersiniosis resolve themselves in one to three weeks; however, severe cases of yersiniosis can reemerge approximately four weeks after infection as severe arthritic joint pain, especially in the wrists, knees, and ankles, with an accompanying skin rash. Antibiotics, particularly doxycycline, are prescribed by a physician for seven to fourteen days to eliminate the disease.

## PREVENTION AND OUTCOMES

Drinking only pasteurized milk and treated water is the primary way to prevent yersiniosis infection. All meat that is ingested, particularly pork chitterlings, should be refrigerated properly and then cooked thoroughly. Anyone involved in the preparation of chitterlings should wear rubber gloves if possible, wash hands often, use a separate cutting board and utensils for the preparation of the pork, and avoid touching one's eyes, nose, or mouth during food preparation. Those who work with animals, such as farmers, veterinarians, and stockyard workers, should wear gloves to avoid being infected by animals, and children should wash hands thoroughly after touching animals at petting zoos or other locations.

*Mary E. Markland, M.A.*

## FURTHER READING

Hunter, Beatrice. *Infectious Connections: How Short-Term Foodborne Infections Can Lead to Long-Term Health Problems.* Laguna Beach, Calif.: Basic Health, 2009.

Juneja, Vijay, and John Sofos. *Pathogens and Toxins in Foods: Challenges and Interventions.* Washington, D.C.: ASM Press, 2010.

Parker, James. *The Official Patient's Sourcebook on Yersiniosis.* San Diego, Calif.: Icon Health, 2002.

**WEB SITES OF INTEREST**

*Center for Science in the Public Interest: Food Safety*
http://cspinet.org/foodsafety

*U.S. Department of Agriculture, Food Safety and Inspection Service*
http://www.fsis.usda.gov

**See also:** Bacterial infections; Developing countries and infectious disease; Fecal-oral route of transmission; Food-borne illness and disease; Intestinal and stomach infections; *Salmonella*; Waterborne illness and disease; *Yersinia*.

# Z

---

## Zoonotic diseases

CATEGORY: Epidemiology

### DEFINITION

Domestic and wild animals, and their ecosystems, contribute to human health and well-being. Animals provide protein-rich nutrients, transportation, fuel, recreation, and companionship. With the many benefits people derive from animals (including arthropods) comes health risks at this human, animal, and ecosystem interface. This interface can be described as a continuum of direct or indirect human exposure to animals, their products, and their ecosystems.

Zoonotic diseases, also known as zoonoses, are diseases caused by infectious agents (viruses, bacteria, and parasites such as worms and protozoa) transmitted or shared by animals and humans. These diseases are caused by a diverse group of pathogenic microorganisms that ordinarily live among animals. Some zoonotic diseases are transmitted directly from animals to humans, some result from contamination of the environment by animals, and others require a vector, such as a tick or mosquito.

### VIRAL INFECTIONS

Arthropod-borne viruses include any of a large group of ribonucleic acid (RNA) viruses that are transmitted primarily by arthropods. There are more than four hundred species of arboviruses. Zoonotic diseases caused by viruses include the following:

*Encephalitis.* Encephalitis is inflammation of the brain caused by infection. All arboviral encephalitides are zoonotic. They are maintained in complex life cycles involving a nonhuman primary vertebrate host and a primary arthropod vector. Many arboviruses that cause encephalitis have a variety of vertebrate hosts, and some are transmitted by more than one vector.

Four main flavivirus agents of encephalitis exist in the United States: eastern equine encephalitis, western equine encephalitis, St. Louis encephalitis, and La Crosse encephalitis, all of which are transmitted by mosquitoes. Most human infections are asymptomatic or may result in nonspecific flulike symptoms. In some infected persons, infection may progress to full-blown encephalitis, with permanent neurologic damage or even death. Because the arboviral encephalitides are viral diseases, antibiotics are not effective for treatment; no effective antiviral drugs have been developed. There are no commercially available human vaccines for these diseases, so treatment is supportive.

*West Nile virus.* West Nile virus (WNV) is a flavivirus commonly found in Africa, West Asia, the Middle East, and the United States. The virus can infect humans, birds, mosquitoes, horses, and other mammals. WNV was first diagnosed in the United States in 1999.

Most human infections are asymptomatic or may result in a nonspecific flulike syndrome. Approximately 80 percent of people who are infected with WNV will not show any symptoms. Up to 20 percent of infected people develop swollen lymph glands or a skin rash on the chest, stomach, and back. About 1 in 150 infected persons will develop severe illness, with symptoms that can include high fever, headache, neck stiffness, stupor, disorientation, coma, tremors, convulsions, and muscle weakness.

There is no specific treatment for WNV infection. In milder cases, symptoms resolve on their own. In more severe cases, infected persons should seek supportive treatment in a hospital.

*Hantavirus pulmonary syndrome.* Hantavirus pulmonary syndrome (HPS) is contracted from rodents and has been identified throughout the United States. Rodent infestation in and around the home remains the primary risk factor for hantavirus exposure. In the United States, deer mice, cotton rats, rice rats, and white-footed mice carry hantaviruses that cause HPS.

Although rare, HPS is potentially deadly. Humans can contract the disease when they come into contact with infected rodents or their urine and droppings or when they breathe in the hantavirus from the air. HPS cannot be transmitted from one person to another.

Early symptoms include fatigue, fever, muscle aches, headaches, dizziness, chills, and abdominal problems.

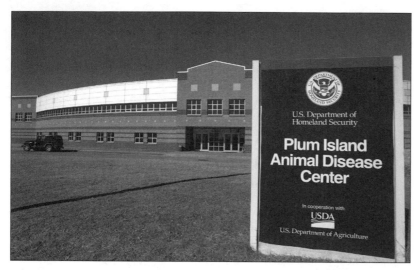

*The Plum Island Animal Disease Center in New York is a facility of the U.S. Department of Homeland Security and the U.S. Department of Agriculture. (AP/Wide World Photos)*

Four to ten days later, additional symptoms appear. These symptoms include coughing and shortness of breath, as the lungs fill with fluid. There is no specific treatment or vaccine for hantavirus infection. Supportive care is the basis for therapy.

*Lymphocytic choriomeningitis.* Lymphocytic choriomeningitis (LCM) is a rodent-borne viral disease that appears as aseptic meningitis (inflammation of the membrane that surrounds the brain and spinal cord), encephalitis, or meningoencephalitis (inflammation of the brain and meninges). LCM is caused by the lymphocytic choriomeningitis virus (LCMV). The common house mouse, *Mus musculus*, is the primary host. The virus is found in the saliva, urine, and feces of infected mice, and people become infected when exposed to these substances. Other types of rodents, such as hamsters, can become infected with LCMV in pet stores.

Initial LCM symptoms include fever, malaise, lack of appetite, muscle aches, headache, nausea, and vomiting. In the second phase of the infection, persons have symptoms of meningitis (fever, headache, and stiff neck) or characteristics of encephalitis (drowsiness, confusion, and sensory disturbances), or have symptoms such as motor abnormalities (for example, paralysis). LCM is usually not fatal. Aseptic meningitis, encephalitis, or meningoencephalitis require hospitalization. Anti-inflammatory drugs, such as corticoste-

roids, may be helpful in treating the disease.

*Monkeypox.* Monkeypox is a rare viral disease that usually occurs in central and western Africa. It is caused by the monkeypox virus, which was first found in 1958 in laboratory monkeys. In June, 2003, several people in the United States contracted monkeypox after having contact with pet prairie dogs that were sick with monkeypox. The disease was traced to a shipment of Gambian rats that were imported to the United States and later kept near prairie dogs at an Illinois animal vendor.

People can get monkeypox if they are bitten by an infected animal or if they touch the animal's blood or body fluids. The disease also can spread from person to person. After infection, symptoms include fever, headache, muscle aches, backache, and swollen lymph nodes. A few days later, symptoms include a skin rash that develops into raised bumps filled with fluid; these bumps will eventually fall off the skin. The illness usually lasts two to four weeks. There is no specific treatment for monkeypox.

*Rabies.* Rabies is a viral disease of mammals transmitted through the bite of a rabid animal. Transmission is through the virus-containing saliva of an infected host. The majority of rabies cases occur in wild animals such as raccoons, skunks, bats, and foxes.

The rabies virus infects the central nervous system of humans, ultimately involving the brain and leading to death. Early symptoms include fever, headache, and general weakness. As the disease progresses, more specific symptoms appear, including insomnia, anxiety, confusion, partial paralysis, hallucinations, hypersalivation (increased saliva), difficulty swallowing, and hydrophobia (fear of water). Once clinical signs of rabies appear, the disease is nearly always fatal, and treatment is mainly supportive.

Several tests are required for the diagnosis of rabies. Thorough wound cleansing has been shown to markedly reduce the likelihood of contracting rabies. A tetanus shot should be given if the infected person has not received one within the previous ten years. A doctor will determine if antibiotics should be used.

Persons not previously vaccinated should receive a postexposure vaccination against rabies that includes administration of both passive antibody and vaccine.

## Bacterial Infections

Zoonotic diseases caused by bacterial infections include the following:

*Anthrax.* Anthrax is an acute infectious disease caused by the bacterium *Bacillus anthracis.* It most commonly occurs in wild and domestic mammals such as cattle, sheep, and goats, but it also can occur in humans who are exposed to infected animals or to tissue from infected animals. *B. anthracis* spores can survive in the soil for many years. Humans can become infected by handling products from infected animals or by inhaling anthrax spores in contaminated animal products. Anthrax can also be contracted by eating undercooked meat from infected animals.

Anthrax infections can be of three types: cutaneous (skin), inhalation, and gastrointestinal. Most cutaneous infections occur when the bacterium enters a cut or abrasion on the skin. About 20 percent of untreated cases of cutaneous anthrax result in death, but death is rare with antimicrobial therapy. The first symptoms of inhalation infection resemble a common cold, but after several days, the symptoms may progress to severe breathing problems. Inhalation anthrax is usually fatal. The gastrointestinal form of anthrax follows the eating of contaminated meat and is followed by an acute inflammation of the intestinal tract. Intestinal anthrax results in death in 25 to 60 percent of cases of infection. Antibiotics are used to treat all three types of anthrax. Early identification and treatment are critical.

*Lyme disease.* Lyme disease is caused by the bacterium *Borrelia burgdorferi* and is transmitted to humans by the bite of infected blacklegged ticks. The Lyme disease bacterium lives in deer, mice, squirrels, and other small animals, and ticks become infected by feeding on these animals. In the northeastern and north-central United States, Lyme disease is transmitted by the deer tick *Ixodes scapularis.* In the Pacific Northwest, the disease is spread by the Western black-legged tick (*I. pacificus*).

In approximately 70 to 80 percent of infected persons, the first sign of infection is usually a circular rash that appears three to thirty days after the tick bite. This "bull's eye" rash gradually expands in several days, reaching up to twelve inches in diameter. Other early symptoms include fever, chills, headache, fatigue, swollen lymph nodes, and joint and muscle aches. If Lyme disease is left untreated, it can spread to other parts of the body. Symptoms of late-stage Lyme disease include painful, swollen joints; severe headaches and neck stiffness from meningitis; and nervous system problems, such as impaired concentration and memory loss.

Several laboratory tests for Lyme disease are available to measure antibodies to the infection. These tests may return false-negative results in persons with early disease, but they are reliable for diagnosing later stages of disease. Most cases of Lyme disease can be treated and cured with antibiotics.

*Plague.* Plague is an infectious disease of animals and humans caused by the bacterium *Yersinia pestis.* It is transmitted from animal to animal and from animal to human by the bites of infected fleas. Humans usually contract plague from being bitten by a rodent flea that is carrying the plague bacterium or by handling an infected animal. Plague is also transmitted by inhaling infected droplets expelled by the coughing of an infected person or animal, especially domestic cats, which may become infected by eating infected wild rodents. Fleas become infected by feeding on rodents, such as chipmunks, prairie dogs, ground squirrels, mice, and other mammals that are infected with the bacterium. Fleas transmit the plague bacterium to humans and other mammals during the feeding process.

The characteristic sign of plague is a very painful, swollen lymph node called a bubo. This sign, accompanied with fever, extreme exhaustion, headache, and a history of possible exposure to rodent fleas, should lead to suspicion of plague. The disease progresses rapidly; the bacteria can then invade the bloodstream and produce severe illness called plague septicemia and lung infection. Once a human is infected, a progressive and potentially fatal illness generally results unless specific antibiotic therapy is given. The plague vaccine is no longer commercially available in the United States.

*Rocky Mountain spotted fever.* Rocky Mountain spotted fever (RMSF) is the most severe tickborne illness in the United States. It is caused by infection with the bacterial organism *Rickettsia rickettsii*, which is transmitted by the bite of an infected tick. The American dog tick (*Dermacentor variabilis*) and Rocky Mountain wood tick (*D. andersoni*) are the primary arthropod vectors in the United States.

The early symptoms of RMSF are often nonspecific. Initial symptoms may include severe headache, lack of appetite, muscle pain, nausea, and fever. Later signs and symptoms include diarrhea, joint pain, abdominal pain, and rash. RMSF can be a severe illness, and the majority of infected persons are hospitalized. Diagnosis is based on a combination of clinical signs and symptoms and laboratory tests. It is best treated using a tetracycline antibiotic, usually doxycycline.

*Salmonellosis.* Salmonellosis is an infection with the bacterium *Salmonella*, which lives in the intestinal tracts of humans, animals, and birds. *Salmonella* is usually transmitted to humans through foods contaminated with animal feces. Contaminated foods are usually of animal origin and include beef, poultry, milk, and eggs, but any food, including vegetables, may become contaminated. *Salmonella* is killed by thorough cooking. *Salmonella* may also be found in the feces of some pets. Reptiles, such as turtles, lizards, and snakes, and chicks and young birds, are particularly likely to carry *Salmonella* in their feces. People should always wash their hands immediately after handling one of these animals, even if it appears healthy. Most persons infected with *Salmonella* develop diarrhea, fever, and abdominal cramps twelve to seventy-two hours after infection. The illness usually lasts four to seven days, and most persons recover without treatment.

## PARASITIC INFECTIONS

Zoonotic diseases caused by parasitic infections include the following:

*Cryptosporidiosis.* Cryptosporidiosis is a disease caused by parasites of the genus *Cryptosporidium.* Both the disease and the parasite are known as crypto. Many species of crypto infect humans and a wide range of animals. The parasite is protected by an outer shell that allows it to survive outside the body for long periods of time. Crypto is one of the most frequent causes of waterborne disease among humans in the United States and throughout the world. Crypto lives in the intestines of infected humans or animals. An infected person or animal passes the parasites in the stool. Crypto is found in soil, food, water, or surfaces that have been contaminated with the feces from infected humans or animals. Some people with crypto have no symptoms, but the most common symptom is watery diarrhea. Other symptoms include stomach cramps, dehydration, diarrhea, nausea, fever, or weight loss.

Diagnosis is made by examination of stool samples. Most people who have healthy immune systems will recover without treatment.

*Cysticercosis.* Cysticercosis is an infection caused by the pork tapeworm *Taenia solium.* Infection occurs when the tapeworm larvae enter the body and form cysticerci (cysts). When cysticerci are found in the brain, the condition is called neurocysticercosis. The tapeworm that causes cysticercosis is most often found in rural, developing countries where pigs are allowed to roam freely and eat human feces.

When pigs swallow pork tapeworm eggs, the eggs are passed through the bowel movement. The eggs are subsequently spread by people who ingest contaminated food or water. Once inside the stomach, the tapeworm egg hatches, penetrates the intestine, travels through the bloodstream, and may develop into larvae in the muscles, brain, or eyes. Although rare, larvae may float in the eye and cause swelling or detachment of the retina. Symptoms of neurocysticercosis can include seizures, headaches, confusion, lack of attention, or difficulty with balance. Death can occur suddenly with heavy infections.

Diagnosis is usually made by magnetic resonance imaging or computed tomography brain scans. Infections are generally treated with antiparasitic drugs in combination with anti-inflammatory drugs.

*Trichinellosis.* Trichinellosis, also called trichinosis, is caused by eating the raw or undercooked meat of animals infected with the larvae of a species of worm called *Trichinella.* Infection occurs commonly in domestic pigs. When an animal eats meat that contains *Trichinella* cysts (larvae), their stomach acid dissolves the hard covering of the cyst and releases the worms. The worms migrate into the small intestine and mature in one to two days. After mating, adult females lay eggs that develop into immature worms and travel through the arteries to muscles. Inside the muscles, the worms curl into a ball and become enclosed in a capsule. Infection in humans occurs when these capsules are consumed in undercooked meat.

The first symptoms of trichinellosis include nausea, diarrhea, vomiting, fatigue, fever, and abdominal discomfort. These first symptoms are later followed by headaches, fevers, chills, cough, eye swelling, aching joints, muscle pains, itchy skin, or diarrhea. In severe cases, death can occur. For mild to moderate infections, most symptoms subside within a few months, although fatigue, weakness, and diarrhea may last for months afterward. Several effective prescription drugs are available to treat trichinellosis.

## IMPACT

Zoonotic diseases have the potential to spread efficiently across international boundaries, thereby affecting not only human health and well-being but also international travel and trade. More than 60 percent of the newly identified infectious agents that have affected people since the mid-twentieth century have been caused by pathogens originating from animals or animal products. Of these zoonotic infections, 70 percent originated from wildlife.

*Gerald W. Keister, M.A.*

## FURTHER READING

Hugh-Jones, Martin E., William T. Hubbert, and Harry V. Hagstad. *Zoonoses: Recognition, Control, and Prevention.* Ames: Iowa State University Press, 2000. Preceding synopses of parasitic, fungal, and viral agents are sections on the principles and history of zoonoses recognition, newer disease agents, and advances in control and prevention.

Krauss, Hartmut, et al. *Zoonoses: Infectious Diseases Transmissible from Animals to Humans.* 3d ed. Washington, D.C.: ASM Press, 2003. Discusses the myriad infections introduced by human-animal contact.

Mandell, Gerald L., John E. Bennett, and Raphael Dolin, eds. *Mandell, Douglas, and Bennett's Principles and Practice of Infectious Diseases.* 7th ed. New York: Churchill Livingstone/Elsevier, 2010. This thorough two-volume textbook provides comprehensive coverage of infectious diseases, including zoonotic diseases.

Romich, Janet A. *Understanding Zoonotic Diseases.* Clifton Park, N.Y.: Thomson Delmar, 2008. A good introduction to zoonotic diseases in humans.

Schlossberg, D., ed. *Clinical Infectious Disease.* New York: Cambridge University Press, 2008. A detailed presentation of infectious diseases, their causes, epidemiology, symptoms, and treatments.

## WEB SITES OF INTEREST

*Centers for Disease Control and Prevention, Division of Vector Borne Infectious Diseases*
http://www.cdc.gov/ncidod/dvbid

*National Center for Emerging and Zoonotic Infectious Diseases*
http://www.cdc.gov/ncezid

*National Institute of Allergy and Infectious Diseases*
http://www.niaid.nih.gov/topics/vector

**See also:** Arthropod-borne illness and disease; Bacterial infections; Bats and infectious disease; Birds and infectious disease; Carriers; Cats and infectious disease; Dogs and infectious disease; Fecal-oral route of transmission; Fleas and infectious disease; Flies and infectious disease; Food-borne illness and disease; Hosts; Insect-borne illness and disease; Mites and chiggers and infectious disease; Mosquitoes and infectious disease; Parasitic diseases; Parasitology; Pigs and infectious disease; Primates and infectious disease; Protozoan diseases; Reptiles and infectious disease; Rodents and infectious disease; Ticks and infectious disease; Transmission routes; Vectors and vector control; Viral infections; Worm infections.

Zoster virus infection. *See* Herpes zoster virus infection.

# Zygomycosis

CATEGORY: Diseases and conditions
ANATOMY OR SYSTEM AFFECTED: Eyes, lungs, respiratory system, vision
ALSO KNOWN AS: Mucormycosis

## DEFINITION

Zygomycosis is a rapidly spreading fungal infection caused by Zygomycetes, a class of ubiquitous fungi found on fruits and breads and in soil and decaying vegetation. This rare, potentially fatal, infection primarily affects the sinuses, brain, and lungs in persons with immune disorders.

## CAUSES

Two orders of Zygomycetes cause human disease: Mucorales and Entomophthorales. Most infections are linked to the *Rhizopus* species within the Mucorales order. Infection occurs through inhalation of mold spores, through ingestion, or through local skin trauma. These opportunistic fungi grow rapidly, targeting arteries to impede blood flow, causing blood clots (thrombosis), and premature tissue death (necrosis). Rhinocerebral zygomycosis is the most common form of infection affecting the nose, eyes, sinuses, and brain. Infection of the lungs, causing pulmonary zygomycosis, is also common. Cutaneous, gastrointestinal, and widespread (disseminated) zygomycosis occur but with less frequency.

### RISK FACTORS

Exposure to these fungi occurs regularly, but many healthy persons have a natural immunity. Immunocompromised persons are more susceptible to this type of invasive infection. Conditions most commonly associated with a risk for zygomycosis include uncontrolled diabetes, malnutrition, bodily burns, steroid or intravenous drug use, metabolic acidosis, organ or stem-cell transplantation, leukemia or lymphoma, deferoxamine (iron chelator) treatment, and acquired immunodeficiency syndrome.

### SYMPTOMS

Rhinocerebral zygomycosis is indicated by fever, face pain, sinus congestion, headaches, eye swelling, visual disturbances, and nasal discharge. Infections affecting the brain are associated with seizures, paralysis, and coma. Symptoms of pulmonary zygomycosis include fever, chest pain, cough, and difficulty breathing. Gastrointestinal zygomycosis is indicated by abdominal pain and swelling, stomach upset, vomiting, diarrhea, and bloody stools, and it typically results in stomach and colon necrosis. Symptoms of cutaneous zygomycosis include a painful hardening of the skin with a blackened center. Disseminated zygomycosis usually begins in the lungs and spreads to the nervous system and includes fever, headaches, visual problems, and changes in brain function.

### SCREENING AND DIAGNOSIS

Zygomycosis is a very serious and aggressive fungal infection. Immunocompromised persons should seek immediate medical care if disease symptoms appear. Primary care physicians should consult with an infectious disease or ear-nose-throat specialist for diagnosis and treatment. Diagnostic tests may include computed tomography or magnetic resonance imaging scans. Conclusive diagnosis of zygomycosis requires the isolation, analysis, and identification of the fungus in culture.

### TREATMENT AND THERAPY

Persons with zygomycosis should be treated promptly to avoid blindness, thrombosis, nerve injuries, extensive surgery, disfigurement, and death. Intravenous amphotericin B is the antifungal therapy of choice, along with surgery to remove dead and infected tissue. Even with intensive treatment, zygomycosis has a high mortality rate, which varies with infection type and with the condition of the infected person's immune system.

### PREVENTION AND OUTCOMES

The fungi that cause zygomycosis are everywhere in the environment. The best preventive measures involve better management of underlying illnesses associated with the disease, improvement of culture-based detection of the disease, and close monitoring of at-risk persons for the earliest possible diagnosis.

*Rose Ciulla-Bohling, Ph.D.*

### FURTHER READING

Ahmad, Iqbal, et al. *Combating Fungal Infections: Problems and Remedy*. New York: Springer, 2010.

Ribes, Julie A., Carolyn L. Vanover-Sams, and Doris J. Baker. "Zygomycetes in Human Disease." *Clinical Microbiology Reviews* 13 (2000): 236-301.

St. Georgiev, Vassil. *Opportunistic Infections: Treatment and Prophylaxis*. Totowa, N.J.: Humana Press, 2003.

Vazquez, Jose A. "Zygomycosis." Available at http://emedicine.medscape.com/article/232465/overview.

### WEB SITES OF INTEREST

*Centers for Disease Control and Prevention, Division of Foodborne, Bacterial, and Mycotic Diseases*
http://www.cdc.gov/nczved/divisions/dfbmd

*Mycology Online*
http://www.mycology.adelaide.edu.au

**See also:** Allergic bronchopulmonary aspergillosis; Aspergillosis; *Aspergillus*; Coccidiosis; Cryptococcosis; Diagnosis of fungal infections; Fungal infections; Histoplasmosis; Mucormycosis; Opportunistic infections; Paracoccidioidomycosis; Respiratory route of transmission; *Rhizopus*; Soilborne illness and disease.

# APPENDIXES

## REFERENCE TOOLS

# Glossary

**abacterial:** free of bacteria.

**abnormal:** opposed to normal.

**abscess:** a collection of pus that causes swelling and inflammation.

**acanthamoeba keratitis:** an eye infection caused by microscopic amebas; normally associated with contact-lens wear; severe infections may lead to blindness.

**acetaminophen:** an over-the-counter pain reliever and fever reducer.

**acquired immunodeficiency syndrome (AIDS):** the final stage of human immunodeficiency virus (HIV) infection in which the body is unable to fight disease; treated with antiretroviral drugs; no cure available.

**active disease:** a previously dormant disease that again attacks an infected person.

**acute:** brief disease exposure of high intensity.

*aden-, adeno-, adren-, adreno-:* gland.

**adjunctive therapy:** treatment used to assist primary treatment.

**adjuvant:** a substance used with antigens to enhance immune response.

**adolescent:** a male or female between the age of ten and nineteen years.

**afebrile:** without fever.

**affinity:** attraction.

**agnogenic:** undetermined origin.

**AIDS:** See acquired immunodeficiency syndrome.

*-alge-, -algesi, -algia:* pain, painful condition.

**alanine aminotransferase (ALT):** an enzyme; normally present in large quantities during hepatitis infection.

**alkaline phosphatase (ALP):** a protein found in all body tissues; structure varies by tissue type.

**alkaline phosphatase (ALP) isoenzyme test:** a test that measures the amount of ALP in the blood; used to diagnose liver, bone, biliary, and parathyroid disease.

**allogeneic cell:** cell genetically different from other cells of the same culture.

**antibiotic:** any substance produced naturally by a microorganism that inhibits the growth of other microorganisms; important in the treatment of bacterial infections.

**antibiotic resistance:** See drug resistance.

**antibody:** a protein produced by the body's immune system when it detects antigens.

**antigen:** any molecule that is capable of being recognized by an antibody or of provoking an immune response; a harmful substance that stimulates antibody production.

**antiretroviral therapy:** group of drugs used to treat retroviral infections, such as human immunodeficiency virus (HIV); work by slowing the growth of the virus.

**antiseptic:** any chemical substance used to eliminate pathogens.

**antitoxin:** a vaccine containing antibodies against a specific toxin.

**apogee:** the most advanced stage of a disease.

**apoptosis:** cell "suicide" occurring after a cell is too old to function properly, as a response to irreparable genetic damage, or as a function of genetic programming; apoptosis prevents cells from developing into a cancerous state and is a natural event during many parts of organismal development.

**arbovirus:** an arthropod-borne virus spread by blood-sucking insects, normally mosquitoes.

**arthralgia:** generalized joint pain.

**asepsis:** the absence of living pathogenic organisms.

**asymptomatic:** without evident symptoms of disease.

**autoimmune disorder:** chronic disease that arises from a breakdown of the immune system's ability to distinguish between the body's own cells and foreign substances; leads to a person's immune system attacking that person's own organs and tissues.

**autoimmune response:** an immune response of an organism against its own cells.

**avidity:** binding strength of an antibody to an antigen.

**azithromycin:** antibiotic used in the treatment of chlamydia infection.

**B cells:** a class of white blood cells (lymphocytes) derived from bone marrow and responsible for antibody-directed immunity.

**bacteremia:** the presence of bacteria in the blood.

**bacteria:** See bacterium.

**bacterial vaginosis:** condition that originates as a result of a disturbance in the levels of bacteria present in the vagina; may be accompanied by discharge, odor, pain, itching, and burning; treated with antibiotics.

**bacteroid:** resembling bacteria.

**bacteriophage:** a virus that infects bacterial cells.

**bacterium:** plural bacteria; a unicellular (single-cell)

microorganism that can be commensal, parasitic, or pathogenic. See commensal, parasite, pathogen.

**benign:** not malignant, noncancerous.

**biological weapon:** a delivery system or weaponization of such pathological organisms as bacteria and viruses to cause disease and death in people, animals, or plants.

**bioterrorism:** use of organisms as instruments or weapons of terror; for example, the deliberate introduction of smallpox, anthrax, or other diseases in civilian populations.

*-blast-, -blasto, -blastic:* bud, germ

**blockade:** blocking of cell receptors.

**blood count:** average number of red or white blood cells found in a cubic millimeter of blood.

**blood smear:** a test performed to determine the number and shape of blood cells.

**boil:** a localized infection of the skin.

**bone marrow cell (B cell):** lymphocyte; cells that mature in the bone marrow and develop into plasma cells after antigen stimulation; essential during immunologic response.

*bronch-, bronchi-:* bronchus (large airway that leads from the trachea, or windpipe, to a lung).

**bubo:** swelling of the lymph nodes, usually around the groin area.

**capsid:** the protective protein coating of a virus particle.

**case detection rate:** number of new cases of a disease reported to the World Health Organization (WHO) during a specific year, divided by the total number of estimated new cases for that same year.

*-cele:* bulge.

*-centesis:* surgical puncture to remove fluid.

*cephal-, cephalo-:* head.

**cercaria:** parasite larva from a trematode worm that swims freely in open bodies of water and causes the disease schistosomiasis.

**chancre:** a small, painless, open sore found on the genitals, mouth, skin, or rectum.

**chancroid:** a sexually transmitted disease caused by the bacterium Haemophilus ducreyi; symptoms include small bumps in the genitals that become ulcers, and enlarged lymph nodes; normally treated with antibiotics, but symptoms may improve on their own.

**chickenpox:** a disease caused by the varicella zoster virus (VZV); highly infectious and usually associated with children; transmission occurs by direct

contact with an infected person; in most cases, medications are not used; antihistamines may be given for itching.

**chlamydia:** a sexually transmitted disease; mostly asymptomatic; affects the urinary tract and reproductive system; treated with antibiotics.

*chrom-, chromato-:* color.

**chronic:** describes the length of a disease state that continues for long periods of time, most often for more than three months.

**chronic fatigue syndrome (CFS):** a disorder characterized by extreme fatigue and tiredness not relieved by rest or sleep; limits a person's ability to perform ordinary, daily activities; its cause is not known; no treatment is available.

**commensal bacteria:** helpful, nonpathogenic bacteria.

**complete blood count (CBC) test:** a common screening blood test that checks for diseases, infections, and the presence of blood components.

**computed tomography (CT) scan:** an X-ray procedure that produces cross-sectional and three dimensional images of body organs and structures.

**congenital transmission:** disease transmission from a woman to her fetus or newborn either in the womb or at birth, respectively.

**cotrimoxazole:** an antibiotic; a sulfa drug made from the combination of trimethoprim and sulfamethoxazole; used in treating AIDS in children.

*crani-, cranio-:* brain.

*cutane-:* skin.

*cyst-, cysti-, cysto-:* bladder, sac

*cyt-, -cyte, -cytic, cyto-:* cell.

**dead-end host:** the final host for an infection that is no longer contagious.

**dehydration:** excessive reduction of water content in the body.

**dendritic cell:** a cell that belongs to the immune system; triggers antigen production.

**deoxyribonucleic acid:** See DNA.

**diphtheria:** an infectious disease that primarily affects the pharynx, nose, and other tissues of the upper respiratory system by inflaming the mucous membrane; a vaccine is available.

**diphtheria, cutaneous:** accounts for 33 percent of diphtheria cases; found among people with poor hygiene; affects the skin and creates an ulcer that is slow to heal and numb to the touch; treated with antibiotics.

*diplo-:* double.

**disability-adjusted life year:** the measurement of healthy years lost because of disability or illness and to premature mortality.

**discrimination:** in the context of infectious diseases, discrimination is the deliberate neglect or exclusion of a person infected with a disease.

**disease control:** the regulation of disease measured by a return to normal or a reduction of infection and illness.

**DNA:** the carrier of genetic information found in all cells; DNA consists of nitrogenous bases, sugar, and phosphate.

**dormant:** inactive.

**doxycycline:** antibiotic used to treat chlamydia.

**droplet infection:** an infection resulting from contact with infected respiratory droplets (such as from a cough or sneeze).

**drug resistance:** a phenomenon in which pathogens no longer respond to drug therapies that once controlled them.

*-dynia:* pain, swelling.

*dys-:* difficult, abnormal.

**dysuria:** pain or difficulty urinating.

**E. coli O157:H7:** a bacterium found in contaminated food and water; causes severe diarrhea, abdominal cramps, and dehydration, and can lead to kidney failure.

*ect-, ecto-, exo-:* outer, outside.

*-ectasis:* expansion, dilation.

*-ectomy:* cut out, removal.

**ectoparasites:** parasites that live on the surface of the host organism.

**elimination of disease:** the complete reduction of the number of disease cases and new infections.

**ELISA test:** enzyme-linked immunoabsorbent assay; a blood test that diagnoses, among other infections, human immunodeficiency virus (HIV) infection; false-positive results have been observed with the presence of syphilis, lupus, and Lyme disease.

**emerging disease:** a disease whose incidence in humans or other target organisms has increased.

*-emia:* blood condition.

**encephalitis:** inflammation of the brain resulting from a viral infection.

*end-, endo-, ent-, enter-, entero-:* inner, within.

**endemic:** prevalent and recurring in a particular geographic region; for example, an organism that is specific to a particular region is characterized as endemic to that region.

**endemic diseases:** diseases native (indigenous) to or found in a particular area of the world.

**endoparasites:** parasites that live inside a host organism.

**endophthalmitis:** inflammation of the intraocular tissues.

**endoscope:** an instrument used to inspect the interior of hollow organs during an endoscopy; consists of a long flexible tube with an attached camera.

**endoscopy:** a medical examination of the upper digestive system with the use of an endoscope.

**enteric viruses:** a group of viruses that affect the gastrointestinal tract.

**enzyme immmonoassay (EIA):** a biochemical test used to detect and quantify antigens, specifically the ones associated with cancer and autoimmune disorders.

**epidemic:** the outbreak of a disease at significantly higher numbers than normal; may be concentrated in a particular geographic region or among a certain population.

**epidemiology:** the study of populations to determine the distribution and risk frequency of a disease.

**Epstein-Barr virus (EBV):** a virus that can cause, among other infections, mononucleosis in adolescents and young adults.

**eradication:** the complete elimination of a disease.

*erythr-, erythro-:* red.

**Escherichia coli:** bacterium, commonly referred to as E. coli, that is normally found in the intestines of humans and healthy cattle; most strains are harmless, with the exception of O157:H7.

*-esis:* state, condition.

**etiology:** the study of the cause and origin of a disease or disorders.

*eu-:* good, well.

**eukaryote:** a cell with a nuclear membrane surrounding its genetic material (a characteristic of a true nucleus) and a variety of subcellular, membrane-bound organelles; eukaryotic organisms include all known organisms except bacteria, which are prokaryotic. See prokaryote.

**expectorate:** to spit.

**fecal:** excrement, feces.

**fecal occult blood test:** test that checks hidden blood in the stool.

*fibr-, fibro-:* fiber.

**first-line drug:** a drug of choice against a disease.

**flu:** See influenza.

**flu, H1N1:** also known as swine flu; a newer and severe form of the influenza virus that has claimed many lives around the world; antiviral medications have been reported to reduce the effects of the virus, and vaccination is the recommended prophylactic treatment.

**flu shot:** a vaccine that contains three different inactivated strings of the influenza virus; protects against the strings of virus present in the vaccine.

**flu vaccine, nasal-spray:** a vaccine against the influenza virus that contains a live, weakened form of the virus; administered through the nose.

**food-borne disease:** a disease transmitted by the ingestion of contaminated food.

**fungi:** single-celled or multicelled microorganisms that include yeasts and molds.

**furuncle:** a boil involving a hair follicle and surrounding skin.

**gastroenteritis:** also known as stomach flu; the irritation and or inflammation of the stomach and intestines; may be caused by bacteria, viruses, or parasites in spoiled food or contaminated water; if the infection is bacterial, it is treated with antibiotics.

**genital warts:** also called venereal warts or condylomata acuminata; flat, flesh-colored, popular growths that can be found in the genitalia, anus, and mouth of men and women; transmitted sexually by the human papillomavirus (HPV).

**genomic array footprinting (GAF):** a technique used to identify genes needed by a bacterium during different stages of infection.

**German measles:** See rubella.

**GI:** gastrointestinal.

**giardia:** infection of the small intestine caused by the protozoan Giardia; characterized by abdominal pain and severe diarrhea; can be contracted by drinking water that is contaminated with raw sewage.

*gluco-, glycol-:* glucose, sugar.

**gonorrhea:** a sexually transmitted disease caused by the bacterium Neisseria gonorrheae; affects both men and women.

*-gram, -graph, -graphy:* a recording, written.

**gram-positive:** bacteria with thick peptidoglycan cell walls that when tested by Gram staining, retain the crystal violet stain color.

**gumma:** a condition that appears in the late stages of syphilis; a mass of dead fiber and tissue, normally found in the liver.

**hand hygiene:** ensuring that one's hands are clean.

**helper T cells:** a class of white blood cells (lymphocytes) derived from bone marrow that prompts the production of antibodies by B cells in the presence of an antigen.

*hem-, hema-, hemat-, hemato-, hemo-:* blood.

**hemodialysis or haemodialysis:** treatment for kidney failure; removal of extra fluids and waste from the blood.

**hepatitis:** inflammation of the liver caused by viruses, drugs, or alcohol; can express itself in many forms (A, B, C, D, E, or G).

**hepatitis A:** caused by the hepatitis A virus, which is spread through contact with fecal-infected food or water; blood-borne infection is rare.

**hepatitis B:** caused by the hepatitis B virus, which is transmitted through blood and body fluids, needle sticks, body piercing, or tattooing with unsterilized instruments; symptoms include fatigue, jaundice, nausea, vomiting, dark urine, and light stools; treatments include antiviral drugs and hepatitis B immunoglobulin.

**hepatitis C:** caused by the hepatitis C virus; transmission occurs primarily from contact with infected blood through needle sticks but may also occur from sexual contact; also congenital; most infections lead to cirrhosis; interferon and antiviral drugs are used for treatment.

**hepatitis D:** caused by the hepatitis D virus; this form of hepatitis can occur only in the presence of hepatitis B; transmission of hepatitis D occurs the same way as hepatitis B; pegylated interferon is used for treatment.

**hepatitis E:** caused by the hepatitis E virus; this form of hepatitis is similar to hepatitis A; transmission occurs through fecal or water contamination and is commonly found in developing countries; international travelers are at the highest risk of infection; treatment is not necessary because it resolves itself.

**hepatitis G:** the newest form of the hepatitis virus; transmission is believed to occur through contact with infected blood, particularly during intravenous drug use and in persons with hemophilia or in persons who require hemodialysis; treatment is not available.

*hepat-, hepatico-, hepato-:* liver.

**herpes genitalis:** an infection caused by the herpes

simplex viruses (type 2 is the most common); spread by sexual contact; symptoms include painful blisters and open sores in the genital area; sores disappear within a few weeks of infection; additional outbreaks are common yet less severe; antiviral medications are given to shorten the outbreaks.

**herpes simplex type 1:** also known as human herpes virus 1 (HHV-1); causes cold sores, fever blisters, and, on rare occasions, herpes genitalis.

**herpes simplex type 2:** also known as human herpes virus 2 (HHV-2); causes genital herpes.

**herpes zoster:** also known as shingles; a viral infection of the nerves that causes a painful blistering rash on a patch of skin anywhere on the body; caused by the varicella zoster virus; usually disappears on its own.

*hist-, histio-, histo-:* tissue.

**HIV:** See human immunodeficiency virus (HIV).

**hormone:** a chemical produced in the body to regulate cells and organ function.

**HPV:** See human papillomavirus (HPV).

**human immunodeficiency virus (HIV):** a virus most commonly transmitted by sexual contact or needle-sharing with an infected person; reduces the body's ability to fight infections. See acquired immunodeficiency syndrome (AIDS).

**human papillomavirus (HPV):** common viruses, mostly harmless; the active forms of the virus are sexually transmitted and are divided into low-risk types, which cause warts, and high-risk types, which may lead to cancer.

**hygiene:** practices, such as handwashing, that promote or preserve health.

*hyper-:* above, beyond, excessive.

**hypersalivation:** also called ptyalism and sialorrhea; the increase of saliva production.

*hypo-:* under, deficient.

*-ia:* condition.

*-iasis:* condition, formation of.

**idiopathic:** of unknown cause.

**IgG:** immunoglobulin, class G; the most common and abundant immunoglobulin (antibody); reacts against bacteria and viruses. See antibody.

**immune response:** the reaction of the immune system to foreign substances, such as viruses and harmful bacteria.

**immunity:** the body's ability to resist a particular disease by preventing a pathogen from developing, or by counteracting its effects.

**immunization:** also known as vaccination; the process by which a person becomes immune to a disease; normally accomplished through vaccination.

**immunocompromised:** See immunodeficient.

**immunodeficient:** also known as immunocompromised; having a weakened immune system.

**immunoglobulin:** See antibody, IgG.

**immunopathology:** a branch of science concerned with immune responses to disease.

**immunosuppression:** deliberate suppression of the immune system by drugs or radiation.

**impetigo:** a common skin infection caused by Streptococcus (strep) or Staphylococcus (staph) bacteria; mild infections are treated with prescription antibacterial creams, and more severe cases require antibiotics.

**incidence:** frequency in which a disease appears in a particular area or period of time.

**incidence rate:** the number of persons infected with a disease within a specific time, divided by the number of persons at risk.

**incubation:** time between infection and disease onset.

**infection:** the development and growth of a parasitic organism inside the body; leads to disease.

**influenza:** also known as the flu; a highly infectious viral respiratory tract infection; virus type A causes most flu outbreaks; viruses B and C are milder and less common.

**inoculation:** the introduction of a vaccine to the body for immunity.

**interferon:** naturally occurring glycoprotein that helps enhance the immune system by stopping viral replication and modulating cellular function.

**intracellular:** inside the cell.

**intraocular:** within the eye.

*iso-:* equal, like.

*-ites, -itis:* inflammation.

*-ium:* structure, tissue.

**killer T cells:** lymphatic cells that attack harmful microbes and the cells they affect. See lymphocytes.

*kin-, kine-, kinesi-, kinesio-, kino-:* movement.

**latent infection:** an infection in which symptoms are not yet visible or active.

**lethargy:** abnormal drowsiness.

*leuk-, leuko-:* white.

**live attenuated influenza vaccine:** a vaccine with a live yet weakened influenza virus.

**Lyme disease:** a multistage disease caused by the bacterium Borrelia burgdorferi; transmitted by a tick bite; symptoms include a characteristic bull's-eye type rash at the location of the bite; early symptoms resemble the flu; normally treated with antibiotics.

**lymphocytes:** sensitized cells of the immune system that recognize and destroy harmful agents via antibody and cell-mediated responses that include B lymphocytes (B cells) from the bone marrow and T lymphocytes (T cells) from the thymus.

**lymphocytosis:** high lymphocyte count in the blood or an increase in the white blood cell count; may be a result of infection.

*-lysis, -lytic, lyso-, lys-:* break down, destruction, dissolving.

**macrophage:** a microbe-ingesting tissue cell that destroys antigens. See phagocyte.

**magnetic resonance imaging (MRI) scan:** radiologic instrument that uses magnetism and radio waves to produce highly detailed, computer-generated images.

*mal-:* bad, abnormal.

**malaise:** general feeling of being ill.

**malaria:** a disease caused by sporozoites transmitted person-to-person by the bite of an infected Anopheles mosquito; sporozoites develop into merozoites in the liver of the infected person and attack red blood cells; antimalaria drugs are available for treatment, and the drug used depends on the area of the world the patient is treated; if left untreated, the disease can be fatal.

**mastitis:** infection of the breast tissue caused by the Staphylococcus aureus bacterium; normally occurs when women are breast-feeding; the breast becomes swollen, red, and tender; antibiotics are used for treatment.

**measles:** also known as rubeola; a very contagious viral disease characterized by a distinct rash, bloodshot eyes, and fever; spread through airborne droplets; no specific treatment is available.

*-megaly:* enlargement.

*melan-, melano-:* black.

*mening-, meningo-:* meninges (membranes that surround brain and spinal cord).

**meningitis:** swelling and inflammation of the membranes that cover the brain and spinal cord; caused by a bacterium or a virus; treatment for bacterial infection depends on which bacterium caused the infection; viral meningitis is less severe and normally does not require treatment.

**microbes:** living microorganisms, including bacteria, fungi, and protozoa.

**microbicides:** products designed to prevent the spread of HIV and other sexually transmitted diseases; these products are considered experimental.

**MMR:** measles, mumps, and rubella.

**molds.** See fungi.

*morph-, morpho-:* shape.

**mortality rate:** the number of deaths from a disease, divided by the total number of cases of the same disease.

**MRSA:** methicillin-resistant Staphylococcus aureus.

**mumps:** a highly contagious viral disease that leads to the swelling of the salivary glands; spread by airborne droplets; predominant among children between the age of two and twelve years who have not been vaccinated; no specific treatment exists for this disease.

**mutation:** a change in, for example a pathogen.

**myalgia:** generalized muscle aches and pain.

*my-, myo-:* muscle.

*myc-, myco-:* fungal, fungus.

*myx-, myxo-:* mucus.

*necr-, necro-:* death.

*nephr-, nephro-:* kidney.

**neurosyphilis:** infection of the central nervous system, brain, or spinal cord as a result of untreated syphilis.

**NSAID:** Nonsteroidal anti-inflammatory drug.

**nucleocapsid:** a viral structure including the capsid, or outer protein coat, and the nucleic acid of the virus.

*olig-, oligo-:* few, little.

*oo-:* egg.

**oophoritis:** inflammation of the ovaries.

**opportunistic infection:** an infection occurring under certain conditions.

**oral rehydration therapy:** the replacement of body fluids and salts lost during severe attacks of diarrhea.

*orchid-, orchit-, orchido-, orchio-:* testis.

**orchitis:** inflammation of one or both testicles caused by a bacterium or virus; symptoms include blood in the semen, testicle pain, fever, pain during intercourse, and pain with urination; bacterial infections are treated with antibiotics.

**organism:** a living thing.

**oropharyngeal squamous cell carcinoma:** cancer that forms in the middle tissues of the throat, including the soft palate, the base of the tongue, and the tonsils; caused by the human papillomavirus.

*-osis:* condition, usually abnormal.

*-ostomy:* opening.

**otitis media:** a middle-ear infection that normally develops as a result of throat infections; viral or bacterial; treatment depends upon the age and symptoms of the patient.

**ova and parasite test:** also known as fecal stool exam; used to identify the parasites causing abdominal illnesses.

*pan-, pant-, panto-:* all or everywhere.

**pancreatitis:** inflammation of the pancreas.

**pandemic:** a worldwide outbreak of a disease.

**papular:** a small, flat, rounded, pimple-like bump, about 0.5 centimeters in diameter; associated with genital warts.

**parameter:** a statistical term used to define population characteristics.

**parasite:** an organism that lives in or on a host and obtains its nutrients from that host; the relationship is potentially harmful to the host.

**pathogen:** a disease-causing agent, such as a bacterium or virus.

**pathogenesis:** the origin and chain of events that lead to the development of a disease.

**pathology:** the study of disease and its causes.

*-pathy, patho-, path-:* disease.

**pelvic inflammatory disease (PID):** infection of the uterus, Fallopian tubes, and other reproductive organs; often caused by complications from gonorrhea, chlamydia, or other sexually transmitted diseases; symptoms include fever, pelvic pain, painful urination, and unusual vaginal discharge with foul odor; scarring occurs, which can cause infertility and ectopic pregnancy; normally treated with antibiotics.

*-penia:* deficiency, lack of.

**percutaneous:** that which moves "through the skin."

**pertussis:** also referred to as whooping cough, a highly contagious disease that affects infants and young children; characterized by severe coughing spells, which make it difficult for the person to breath, eat, or sleep; a vaccine is available.

**phagocyte:** white blood cells that ingest microbes and antigens. See macrophage.

*pharmaco-:* drug, medicine.

*pharyng-, pharyngo-:* pharynx, throat.

**phlegm:** abnormal amount of mucus expectorated from the mouth.

**phylogeny:** the evolutionary history of genetically related organisms.

**PID:** See pelvic inflammatory disease (PID).

*-plasia, -plastic:* growth.

**plasmid:** a small, circular DNA molecule commonly found in bacteria and responsible for carrying various genes, such as antibiotic resistance genes.

*pleur-, pleura-, pleuro-:* rib, pleura (membrane that wraps around the outside of the lungs and lines the inside of the chest cavity).

**pleural effusion:** an abnormal collection of fluid between the layers of tissue that line the lungs and the chest wall.

**pleural space:** area between the lungs and chest wall.

*pneum-, pneuma-, pneumat-, pneumato-:* air, lung.

**pneumococcal infections:** caused by the bacterium Pneumococcus; account for 62 percent of invasive diseases worldwide; most common symptoms include fever, headache, chills, sweats, and malaise; normally treated with penicillin; vaccination is recommended for children and adults.

**poliomyelitis:** a highly contagious viral infection caused by various types of the poliovirus; spread person to person through airborne droplets and contaminated feces; affects the nervous system and can lead to paralysis; no treatment is available; vaccination is the best prophylactic measure.

**polymerase chain reaction (PCR):** a technical laboratory method for selecting and amplifying a section of DNA.

**prevalence:** the number of people living with a specific disease during a specific period of time.

**prevalence rate:** all new and preexisting cases of a disease during a specific period of time. See incidence rate.

**preventable diseases:** diseases that can be avoided or prevented through vaccination.

**primary immunodeficiency:** a genetic disorder involving a defect in the immune system leaving the affected individual prone to infection.

**prion:** an infectious agent composed solely of protein; thought to be the cause of various human and animal diseases characterized by neurological degeneration.

*proct-, procto-:* anus, rectum.

**prokaryote:** a cell that lacks a nuclear membrane (and therefore has no true nucleus) and membrane-bound organelles; bacteria are the only known prokaryotic organisms.

**prophylaxis:** preventive measures to avoid infection or disease.

**protozoa:** microscopic, single-celled, parasitic organisms. See organism, parasite.

*pyo-:* pus.

*pyro-:* fever.

**rabies:** a viral disease transmitted through the bite of an infected animal; attacks the central nervous system of both humans and animals; symptoms appear in stages and include fever and headaches, anxiety, confusion, hallucinations, and hypersalivation; advance symptoms are often followed by death; humans are treated with human rabies immune globulin.

**rehydration:** to restore lost water from the body.

*ren-, reno-:* kidney.

**renal failure:** also known as kidney failure; state in which kidneys stop filtering toxins from the blood because of chronic health problems.

**reportable disease:** a disease to be reported to public health authorities by health care providers.

**respiratory droplets:** small drops of moisture expelled from the upper respiratory tract.

**reverse transcriptase-polymerase chain reaction:** the reaction used by oncogenic viruses to form DNA from an RNA template.

*rhabd-, rhabdo-:* rod-shaped, striated.

*rhin-, rhino-:* nose.

**rhinovirus:** a virus that causes the common cold.

**rotavirus:** a virus that causes severe diarrhea in infants and children; the number one cause of severe dehydration and death from diarrhea in infants.

**Ritter disease:** See scalded skin syndrome.

*-rrhage, -rrhagic:* bleeding.

*-rrhea:* flow, discharge.

**rubella:** also known as German measles or three-day measles; an acute viral infection with symptoms similar to the flu, accompanied by a red rash; spread person-to-person through airborne droplets affecting both young and old; no treatment is available; vaccines are the recommended prophylactic treatment.

**rubeola:** See measles.

**Rx:** treatment, drug prescription.

**sanatoria (sanatorium, singular):** medical facilities for the chronically ill, in particular, persons with tuberculosis.

**sanitation:** the application of preventive measures to protect public health.

**SARS:** severe acute respiratory syndrome.

**scabies:** a contagious skin disease caused by mites; symptoms include itching, rashes, and sores; prescription medicated creams such as permethrin are used for treatment.

**scalded skin syndrome:** a severe form of staph infection that causes the skin to loosen from the body; treated with antibiotics.

**second-line drugs:** treatment or drugs used when standard therapy fails.

**sepsis:** the presence of multiple pathogens or toxins in the blood, also described as blood poisoning; characterized by elevated heart rate, a body temperature higher than 100.4° Fahrenheit or lower than 96.8° F, increased respiratory rate, and abnormal white blood cell count.

**sequelae:** any abnormal condition that develops as a result of a disease.

**sequencing:** determining the nucleotide order in a DNA strand.

**serology:** a blood test performed for antibody detection.

**seroprevalence:** prevalence measured by serologic testing.

**serum:** fluid portion of the blood.

**severe immunodeficiency:** a primary disorder of the immune system characterized by a severe defect in the T- and B-lymphocyte systems; infants born with this disorder commonly develop a severe, sometimes life-threatening infection, such as meningitis, pneumonia, or bloodstream infection, within the first few months of life.

**sexually transmitted disease (STD):** any contagious disease acquired during sexual contact; most common diseases include bacterial vaginosis, chlamydia, gonorrhea, viral hepatitis, genital herpes, human papillomavirus, human immunodeficiency virus, syphilis, trichomoniasis, and pelvic inflammatory disease.

**shigellosis:** infection caused by ingesting Shigella bacteria; in developed countries, it is transmitted by food handlers who have been infected and do not properly wash their hands after using the toilet; severe forms of the infection are treated with antibiotics; mild forms do not need treatment.

**shingles:** See herpes zoster.

*-sis:* condition.

*somat-, somatico-, somato-:* body, bodily.

**staph infection of the skin:** infection caused by the Staphylococcus aureus bacterium; most common type of staph infection; symptoms include abscesses, boils, or furuncles with draining pus, all accompanied by fever, chills, and low blood pressure; mild forms of the infection can be treated with antibiotics.

*-stasis:* level, unchanging.

**STD:** See sexually transmitted disease (STD).

*stom-, stoma-, stomat-, stomato-:* mouth.

**stomach flu:** See gastroenteritis.

**strain:** in bacteriology, a homogeneous bacterial population with the same genetic characteristics as its ancestors; if the genetic characteristics are different, then it is considered a different strain.

**strep throat:** infection caused by the streptococcal bacterium. Most common symptoms include sudden severe sore throat, pain when swallowing, fever, swollen tonsils, swollen lymph nodes, and spots on the back of the throat; infection lasts from three to seven days and disappears without medication.

**Streptococcus pneumonia:** a bacterium that is the leading cause of pneumonia and otitis media, or middle-ear infection.

**sulfamethoxazole:** an antibiotic used in the treatment of AIDS.

**swine flu:** See flu, H1N1.

**syncope:** loss of consciousness caused by the reduction of blood flow to the brain.

**syphilis:** a sexually transmitted disease caused by the bacterium Treponema pallidum; may affect the genital area, mouth, or anus and consists of three stages; if left untreated, the bacteria will become dormant and will return months or years later; treatment with antibiotics depends on the length of time the person has been infected.

**syphilis, congenital:** a severe infection seen in infants of syphilis-infected mothers; the bacterium is passed from woman to fetus or to the newborn at birth; most infected children die shortly after birth.

**TB:** See tuberculosis (TB), pulmonary.

**temephos:** an insecticide applied to lakes, wetlands, and ponds to control mosquitos, midges, and black larvae.

**tetanus:** Also referred to as lockjaw; caused by the bacterium Clostridium tetani, which enters the body through a cut from a contaminated object; affects the nervous system and causes severe spasms; treatment includes antibiotics, medicines to reverse the toxins, muscle relaxers, and surgery; a vaccine is available.

**therapy:** disease treatment.

*thorac-, thoracico-, thoraco-:* chest.

**thymus cell (T cell):** a type of white blood cell that develops in the thymus; essential to the body's immunologic response.

**toxin:** a poisonous substance.

**trachoma:** a condition resulting from an eye infection with Chlamydia trachomatis; common in areas with water shortages; can cause irreversible blindness.

**transboundary diseases:** diseases that can spread across international boundaries, affecting economies and disrupting international trade.

**translation inhibitory proteins:** proteins that block viruses from infecting healthy cells.

**transmission:** the means by which a disease spreads from one person to another or from a vector, such as a mosquito, to a person.

**transverse myelitis:** a neurological disorder caused by inflammation and swelling along the spinal cord; may lead to motor and sensory nerve dysfunction; cause is believed to be a result of viral infection, abnormal immune reaction, or insufficient blood flow in the blood vessels of the spinal cord.

**trimethoprim:** an antibiotic used in the treatment of AIDS.

**Truvada:** an experimental drug for treating HIV infection.

**tuberculin:** a tuberculosis skin test, also known as purified protein derivative test.

**tuberculosis (TB), pulmonary:** an infectious disease that was once a major killer worldwide; primarily affects the lungs but may spread to other parts of the body; the predominant TB organism is Mycobacterium tuberculosis, which is spread person-to-person in airborne droplets; early disease stages are asymptomatic; once the disease develops, the infected person may cough up blood, have excessive sweating, fever, fatigue, and difficulty breathing; treatment includes a combination of four different drugs, lasting longer than six months.

*ur-, uro-:* urinary, urine.

**UTI:** urinary tract infection.

**vaccination:** See immunization.

**vaccine:** a substance containing attenuated (weakened) or dead components of an organism; administered to a person to generate immunity to that specific disease; vaccines may be given orally or injected.

**vaccine, booster:** the second vaccination given for a

particular disease to increase or extend the effectiveness of the original vaccine.

**vaccine, conjugated:** a vaccine consisting of more than one antigen; an example is the measles, mumps, and rubella (MMR) vaccine.

**vaccine, DTaP:** a vaccine for diphtheria, tetanus, and pertussis (whooping cough), given to children.

**vaccine, inactivated:** a vaccine that contains a copy of the dead or weakened virus.

**vaccine, Td:** a booster vaccine for tetanus and diphtheria.

**varicella:** See chickenpox.

**VD:** See sexually transmitted disease (STD).

**vector:** a disease-carrying vehicle, or agent, such as a mosquito or tick.

**virion:** a mature, infectious virus particle.

**viraemia:** the presence of a virus in the blood.

**viral infection:** any type of infection or disease caused by a virus.

**virulence:** the ability of any organism to cause disease.

**virus:** a microscopic infectious agent, composed primarily of protein and nucleic acid; can replicate, or reproduce, only within host cells.

**viscus:** any internal organ of the body located in the chest cavity.

**West Nile virus:** a virus spread by a mosquito; indigenous to eastern Africa; symptoms include fever, headache, body aches, skin rash, and swollen lymph nodes; severe forms of the disease cause meningitis and can be life-threatening; no specific treatment is available.

**western equine encephalitis:** a viral disease spread by a mosquito that can infect both humans and horses; mild symptoms include fever and headache, while severe symptoms can lead to a coma; no specific treatment is available.

**wild type:** the phenotype of any organism that occurs freely in nature.

**yeasts.** See fungi.

**yersiniosis:** a disease caused by the bacterium Yersinia enterocolitica; transmitted to people through the ingestion of raw or undercooked pork products; symptoms include fever, abdominal pain, and bloody diarrhea; mild forms of the disease resolve on their own, and other forms are treated with antibiotics.

**zoonotic transmission:** transmission of a disease from animals to humans.

*K. Yurckak*

# Bibliography

## ACQUIRED IMMUNODEFICIENCY SYNDROME (AIDS). *SEE ALSO* SEXUALLY TRANSMITTED DISEASES (STDs)

Barnett, Tony, and Alan Whiteside. *AIDS in the Twenty-first Century: Disease and Globalization.* 2d ed. New York: Palgrave Macmillan, 2006.

Bartlett, John G., and Ann K. Finkbeiner. *The Guide to Living with HIV Infection: Developed at the Johns Hopkins AIDS Clinic.* 6th ed. Baltimore: Johns Hopkins University Press, 2007.

Buckley, R. Michael, and Stephen J. Gluckman, eds. *HIV Infection in Primary Care.* Philadelphia: W. B. Saunders, 2002.

Cichocki, Mark. *Living with HIV: A Patient's Guide.* Jefferson, N.C.: McFarland, 2009.

Clark, Rebecca A., Robert T. Maupin, Jr., and Jill Hayes Hammer. *A Woman's Guide to Living with HIV Infection.* Baltimore: Johns Hopkins University Press, 2004.

Fan, Hung Y., Ross F. Conner, and Luis P. Villarreal. *AIDS: Science and Society.* 5th ed. Sudbury, Mass.: Jones and Bartlett, 2007.

Gallant, Joel. *One Hundred Questions and Answers About HIV and AIDS.* Sudbury, Mass.: Jones and Bartlett, 2007.

Irwin, Alexander, and Joyce Millen. *Global AIDS: Myths and Facts.* Cambridge, Mass.: South End Press, 2003.

Jessen, Heiko, and Hans Jaeger, eds. *Primary HIV Infection: Pathology, Diagnosis, Management.* New York: Georg Thieme, 2005.

Masci, Joseph R. *Outpatient Management of HIV Infection.* 3d ed. Boca Raton, Fla.: CRC Press, 2001.

Matthews, Dawn D., ed. *AIDS Sourcebook.* 3d ed. Detroit: Omnigraphics, 2003.

Morse, Stephen A., Ronald C. Ballard, and King K. Holmes. *Atlas of Sexually Transmitted Diseases and AIDS.* 3d ed. Philadelphia: Mosby, 2003.

Princeton, Douglas C. *Manual of HIV/AIDS Therapy.* Rev. ed. Laguna Hills, Calif.: Current Clinical Strategies, 2002.

Sax, Paul E., and Calvin J. Cohen. *HIV Essentials 2010.* 3d ed. Sudbury, Mass.: Jones and Bartlett, 2009.

Shearer, William T., and I. Celine Hansen, eds. *Medical Management of AIDS in Children.* Philadelphia: W. B. Saunders, 2003.

Stine, Gerald J. *AIDS Update 2010.* New York: McGraw-Hill Higher Education, 2010.

Weeks, Benjamin, and Edward Alcamo. *AIDS: The Biological Basis.* 5th ed. Sudbury, Mass.: Jones and Bartlett, 2009.

Whiteside, Alan. *HIV/AIDS: A Very Short Introduction.* New York: Oxford University Press, 2008.

## BACTERIAL INFECTIONS

Aktories, K., and T. D. Wilkins, eds. *Clostridium difficile.* Current Topics in Microbiology and Immunology. New York: Springer, 2010.

*Bacteremia: Webster's Timeline History, 1901-2007.* San Diego, Calif.: Icon Group International, 2009.

Bartram, Jaime, et al., eds. *Legionella and the Prevention of Legionellosis.* Geneva: World Health Organization, 2007.

Brogden, K., et al. *Virulence Mechanisms of Bacterial Pathogens.* 4th ed. Washington, D.C.: ASM Press, 2007.

Carson-DeWitt, R. *Gale Encyclopedia of Medicine: Rat-Bite Fever.* Detroit: Thomson Gale, 2004.

Chang, Hernan R. *MRSA and Staphylococcal Infections.* 2d ed. Jacksonville, Fla.: Author, 2008.

Cunha, B. A. *Pneumonia Essentials 2010.* 3d ed. Sudbury, Mass.: Jones and Bartlett, 2010.

Duker, Alfred A., Françoise Portaels, and Martin Hale. "Pathways of Mycobacterium Ulcerans Infection: A Review." In *Environment International.* Philadelphia: Saunders/Elsevier, 2006.

Emmeluth, Donald. *Deadly Diseases and Epidemics: Botulism.* New York: Chelsea House, 2005.

*Epididymitis: A Medical Dictionary, Bibliography, and Annotated Research Guide to Internet References.* San Diego, Calif.: Icon Health, 2004.

Evans, A. S., and P. S. Brachman, eds. *Bacterial Infections of Humans: Epidemiology and Control.* 3d ed. New York: Plenum, 1998.

Fein, A., et al. *Diagnosis and Management of Pneumonia and Other Respiratory Infections.* 2d ed. Mathews, N.C.: Professional Communications, 2006.

Gilmore, M. S. *The Enterococci: Pathogenesis, Molecular Biology, and Antibiotic Resistance.* Washington, D.C.: ASM Press, 2002.

Graham-Lomax, K., and D. Y. Graham. *Contemporary Diagnosis and Management of "H. pylori"-Associated Gastrointestinal Diseases.* 3d ed. Newtown, Pa.: Handbooks in Health Care, 2005.

Guilfoile, Patrick. *Tetanus.* Deadly Diseases and Epidemics. New York: Chelsea House, 2008.

_____. *Whooping Cough.* Edited by Hillary Babcock.

Deadly Diseases and Epidemics. New York: Chelsea House, 2010.

Guillemin, Jeanne. *Anthrax*. Berkeley: University of California Press, 2001.

Icon Health. *Brucellosis: A Medical Dictionary, Bibliography, and Annotated Research Guide to Internet References*. San Diego, Calif.: Author, 2004.

_____. *Gas Gangrene: A Medical Dictionary, Bibliography, and Annotated Research Guide to Internet References*. San Diego, Calif.: Author, 2004.

_____. *The Official Parent's Sourcebook on "Haemophilus influenzae" Serotype B: A Revised and Updated Directory for the Internet Age*. San Diego, Calif.: Author, 2002.

_____. *The Official Patient's Sourcebook on Bacterial Vaginosis: A Revised and Updated Directory for the Internet Age*. San Diego, Calif.: Author, 2002.

_____. *The Official Patient's Sourcebook on Pertussis: A Revised and Updated Directory for the Internet Age*. San Diego, Calif.: Author, 2002.

_____. *The 2002 Official Patient's Sourcebook on Shigellosis: A Revised and Updated Directory for the Internet Age*. San Diego, Calif.: Author, 2002.

Internal Commission on Microbiological Specifications of Foods. *Microorganisms in Foods 5: Characteristics of Microbial Pathogens*. New York: Springer, 1996.

James, William D., Timothy Berger, and Dirk Elston. *Andrews' Diseases of the Skin: Clinical Dermatology*. Philadelphia: Saunders/Elsevier, 2006.

Kollar, Linda, and Brian R. Shmaefsky. *Gonorrhea*. Deadly Diseases and Epidemics. New York: Chelsea House, 2005.

*Listeria, Listeriosis, and Food Safety*. Food Science and Technology. 3d ed. Boca Raton, Fla.: CRC Press, 2007.

Marrie, Thomas J. *The Disease*. Vol. 1 in *Q Fever*. Boca Raton, Fla.: CRC Press, 1990.

Nachamkin, Irving, Christine M. Szymanski, and Martin J. Blaser, eds. *Campylobacter*. 3d ed. Washington, D.C.: ASM Press, 2008.

O'Donnell, Judith A. *Pelvic Inflammatory Disease*. Deadly Diseases and Epidemics. New York: Chelsea House, 2006.

Parker, James N., and Phillip M. Parker, eds. *The Official Patient's Sourcebook on Chlamydia*. San Diego, Calif.: Icon Health, 2002.

_____. *The Official Patient's Sourcebook on Conjunctivitis*. San Diego, Calif.: Icon Health, 2002.

Raviglione, M. C. *Tuberculosis: The Essentials*. Lung Biology in Health and Disease. 4th ed. London: Informa Healthcare, 2009.

Sansonetti, Phillippe, ed. *Bacterial Virulence: Basic Principles, Models and Global Approaches*. Hoboken, N.J.: Wiley-Blackwell, 2010.

Shmaefsky, Brian R. *Meningitis*. 2d ed. Edited by Hilary Babcock. Deadly Diseases and Epidemics. New York: Chelsea House, 2010.

_____. *Syphilis*. Edited by Hilary Babcock. Deadly Diseases and Epidemics. New York: Chelsea House, 2009.

Siderovski, Susan Hutton. *Tularemia*. New York: Chelsea House, 2006.

Singleton, K. B. *The Lyme Disease Solution*. Charleston, S.C.: BookSurge, 2009.

Smith, Tara C. *"Streptococcus" (Group A)*. Edited by Hilary Babcock. 2d ed. Deadly Diseases and Epidemics. New York: Chelsea House, 2010.

_____. *"Streptococcus" (Group B)*. Edited by I. Edward Alcamo. Deadly Diseases and Epidemics. New York: Chelsea House, 2007.

Sommers, Michael. *Yeast Infections, Trichomoniasis, and Toxic Shock Syndrome*. Girls Health. New York: Rosen, 2007.

Strasheim, C., et al. *Insights into Lyme Disease Treatment: Thirteen Lyme-Literature Health Care Practitioners Share Their Healing Strategies*. South Lake Tahoe, Calif.: BioMed, 2009.

Sutton, E., and A. Lee. *Sexually Transmitted Diseases Sourcebook: Basic Consumer Health Information About Chlamydial Infections, Gonorrhea, Hepatitis, Herpes, HIV/AIDS*. Health Reference Series. 3d ed. Detroit: Omnigraphics, 2006.

Walker, David H. *Rocky Mountain Spotted Fever*. Edited by I. Edward Alcamo. Deadly Diseases and Epidemics. New York: Chelsea House, 2007.

Yancey, Diane. *Tuberculosis*. Twenty-First Century Medical Library. Breckenridge, Colo.: Twenty-First Century Books, 2007.

## DIAGNOSIS/LABORATORY METHODS

Garcia, Lynne Shore. *Diagnostic Medical Parasitology*. 5th ed. Washington, D.C.: ASM Press, 2007.

Jessen, Heiko, and Hans Jaeger, eds. *Primary HIV Infection: Pathology, Diagnosis, Management*. New York: Georg Thieme, 2005.

Levinson, Warren. *Review of Medical Microbiology and*

*Immunology.* 11th ed. New York: McGraw-Hill Medical, 2010.

McPherson, Richard A., and Matthew R. Pincus, eds. *Henry's Clinical Diagnosis and Management by Laboratory Methods.* 21st ed. Philadelphia: Saunders/Elsevier, 2007.

Sacher, Ronald A., and Richard A. McPherson. *Widmann's Clinical Interpretation of Laboratory Tests.* 11th ed. Philadelphia: Davis, 2000.

Smith, Thomas, Edwin H. Lennette, and Keith Jerome, eds. *Laboratory Diagnosis of Viral Infections.* 3d ed. London: Informa Healthcare, 1999.

Wallach, Jacques. *Interpretation of Diagnostic Tests.* 8th ed. Philadelphia: Wolters Kluwer Health/Lippincott Williams & Wilkins, 2007.

Wilson, Walter, and Merle Sande. *Current Diagnosis and Treatment in Infectious Diseases.* New York: McGraw-Hill Medical, 2001.

Wu, Alan H. B., ed. *Tietz Clinical Guide to Laboratory Tests.* 4th ed. St. Louis, Mo.: Mosby/Elsevier, 2006.


## DICTIONARIES AND DIRECTORIES

Brown, Brandon P., et al., eds. *Salem Health: Magill's Medical Guide.* 6th ed. 6 vols. Pasadena, Calif.: Salem Press, 2011.

Leikin, Jerrold B., and Martin S. Lipsky, eds. *American Medical Association Complete Medical Encyclopedia.* New York: Random House Reference, 2003.

*McGraw-Hill Encyclopedia of Science and Technology.* 10th ed. 20 vols. New York: McGraw-Hill, 2007.

Marcovitch, Harvey, ed. *Black's Medical Dictionary.* 42d ed. Lanham, Md.: Scarecrow Press, 2010.

*Physicians' Desk Reference.* 64th ed. Montvale, N.J.: PDR Network, 2009.

*Professional Guide to Diseases.* 9th ed. Philadelphia: Lippincott Williams & Wilkins, 2008.

Singleton, Paul, and Diana Sainsbury. *Dictionary of Microbiology and Molecular Biology.* Rev. 3d ed. Hoboken, N.J.: John Wiley & Sons, 2006.

*Stedman's Medical Dictionary.* 28th ed. Philadelphia: Lippincott Williams & Wilkins, 2006.

Tibayrenc, Michel, ed. *Encyclopedia of Infectious Diseases: Modern Methodologies.* Hoboken, N.J.: Wiley-Blackwell, 2007.

Wagman, Richard J., ed. *The New Complete Medical and Health Encyclopedia.* 4 vols. Chicago: J. G. Ferguson, 2002.

*Webster's New World Medical Dictionary.* 2d ed. New York: John Wiley & Sons, 2003.


## EMERGING INFECTIOUS DISEASES

Ali, S. Harris, and Roger Kell, eds., *Networked Disease: Emerging Infections in the Global City.* Hoboken, N.J.: Wiley-Blackwell, 2008.

Beltz, Lisa A. *Emerging Infectious Diseases: A Guide to Diseases, Causative Agents, and Surveillance.* Hoboken, N.J.: Wiley-Blackwell, 2011.

Charney, William, ed. *Emerging Infectious Diseases and the Threat to Occupational Health in the U.S. and Canada.* Public Administration and Public Policy. Boca Raton, Fla.: CRC Press, 2006.

Fong, I. W., and Kenneth Alibeck, eds. *New and Evolving Infections of the Twenty-first Century.* New York: Springer, 2010.

Knobler, Stacey L., et al., eds. *The Resistance Phenomenon in Microbes and Infectious Disease Vectors: Implications for Human Health and Strategies for Containment.* Washington, D.C.: National Academies Press, 2003.

Kocik, Janusz, Marian Negut, and Marek Janiak, eds. *Preparedness Against Bioterrorism and Re-emerging Infectious Diseases.* NATO Science Series I: Life and Behavioural Sciences. Burke, Va.: IOS Press, 2004.

Lal, Sunil, ed. *Biology of Emerging Viruses: SARS, Avian and Human Influenza, Metapneumovirus, Nipah, West Nile, and Ross River Virus.* Hoboken, N.J.: Wiley-Blackwell, 2007.

Lashley, F. R., and J. D. Durham. *Emerging Infectious Diseases: Trends and Issues.* 2d ed. New York: Springer, 2007.

Pollack, Andrew. "A Rising Hospital Threat." *The New York Times,* February 27, 2010, p. 1.

Strickland, G. Thomas, ed. *Hunter's Tropical Medicine and Emerging Infectious Diseases.* 8th ed. Philadelphia: W. B. Saunders, 2000.


## EPIDEMIOLOGY

Cliff, A. D., et al. *Infectious Diseases: A Geographical Analysis: Emergence and Re-emergence.* Oxford Geographical and Environmental Studies. New York: Oxford University Press, 2009.

Evans, A. S., and P. S. Brachman, eds. *Bacterial Infections of Humans: Epidemiology and Control.* 3d ed. New York: Plenum, 1998.

Kramer, Alexander, Mirjam Kretzschmar, and Klaus Krickeberg, eds. *Modern Infectious Disease Epidemiology.* New York: Springer, 2010.

Magnus, Manya. *Essential Readings in Infectious Disease Epidemiology.* Essential Public Health. Sudbury, Mass.: Jones and Bartlett, 2008.

Nelson, K. E., and C. M. Williams. *Infectious Disease Epidemiology: Theory and Practice.* 2d ed. Sudbury, Mass.: Jones and Bartlett, 2007.

## ETHICS. *SEE ALSO* POLICY

Battin, Margaret P., et al. *The Patient as Victim and Vector: Ethics and Infectious Disease.* New York: Oxford University Press, 2008.

Lindler, Luther E., Frank J. Lebeda, and George Korch, eds. *Biological Weapons Defense: Infectious Disease and Counterbioterrorism.* New York: Humana Press, 2004.

Selgelid, Michael, Michael Battin, and Charles B. Smith, eds. *Ethics and Infectious Disease.* Hoboken, N.J.: Wiley-Blackwell, 2006.

## FUNGAL INFECTIONS

Diamond, Richard D. *Atlas of Infectious Diseases: Fungal Infections.* Vol. 7. Philadelphia: Current Medicine Group, 2000.

Icon Health. *The Official Patient's Sourcebook on Cryptococcosis: A Revised and Updated Directory for the Internet Age.* San Diego, Calif.: Author, 2002.

_____. *The Official Patient's Sourcebook on Sporotrichosis: A Revised and Updated Directory for the Internet Age.* San Diego, Calif.: Author, 2002.

Jameson, T. K. *Secrets of Ringworm Treatment: Everything You Ever Needed to Know About Ringworm, Athletes Foot, Jock Itch, Other Forms of Fungal Infections, and How to Treat Them.* Seattle: CreateSpace, 2010.

Maertens, Johan A., and Kieren A. Marr, eds. *Diagnosis of Fungal Infections.* Infectious Disease and Therapy. London: Informa Healthcare, 2007.

Richardson, Malcolm, and David W. Warnock. *Fungal Infections and Management.* 3d ed. Hoboken, N.J.: Wiley-Blackwell, 2003.

Rona, Zoltan P. *Complete Candida Yeast Guidebook: Everything You Need to Know About Prevention, Treatment, and Diet.* 2d ed. New York: Three Rivers Press, 2000.

Surhone, Lambert M., Mariam T. Tenroe, and Susan F. Henssonow, eds. *Histoplasmosis.* Mauritius: Beta-Script, 2010.

Van Den Bossche, Hugo, Geert Cauwenbergh, and Donald W. R. MacKenzie. *Aspergillus and Aspergillosis.* New York: Springer, 1988.

Walzer, Peter, and Melanie T. Cushion, eds. *Pneumocystis Pneumonia.* Lung Biology in Health and Disease. 3d ed. London: Informa Healthcare, 2004.

## GENERAL SOURCES ON INFECTIOUS DISEASE

Betts, Robert F., Stanley W. Chapman, and Robert L. Penn, eds. *Reese and Betts' A Practical Approach to Infectious Diseases.* 5th ed. Philadelphia: Lippincott Williams & Wilkins, 2003.

Cohen, Jonathan, William G. Powderly, and Steven E. Opal. *Infectious Diseases.* 3d ed. St. Louis, Mo.: Mosby/Elsevier, 2010.

Feigin, Ralph D., et al., eds. *Textbook of Pediatric Infectious Diseases.* 6th ed. Philadelphia: Saunders/Elsevier, 2009.

Fisher, Randall G., and Thomas G. Boyce. *Moffet's Pediatric Infectious Diseases: A Problem-Oriented Approach.* 4th ed. Philadelphia: Lippincott Williams & Wilkins, 2004.

Frank, Steven A. *Immunology and Evolution of Infectious Disease.* Princeton, N.J.: Princeton University Press, 2002.

Gershon, Anne A., Peter J. Hotez, and Samuel L. Katz, eds. *Krugman's Infectious Diseases of Children.* 11th ed. Philadelphia: Mosby, 2004.

Giesecke, Johan. *Modern Infectious Disease Epidemiology.* 2d ed. New York: Oxford University Press, 2002.

Gorbach, Sherwood L., John G. Bartlett, and Neil R. Blacklow, eds. *Infectious Diseases.* 3d ed. Philadelphia: W. B. Saunders, 2004.

Grace, Christopher, ed. *Medical Management of Infectious Disease.* New York: Marcel Dekker, 2003.

Hart, C. A. *MicroTerrors: The Complete Guide to Bacterial, Viral and Fungal Infections That Threaten Our Health.* Tonawanda, N.Y.: Firefly Books, 2004.

Heymann, David L., ed. *Control of Communicable Diseases Manual.* 19th ed. Washington, D.C.: American Public Health Association, 2008.

Kasper, Dennis, and Anthony Fauci. *Harrison's Infectious Diseases.* New York: McGraw-Hill Professional, 2010.

Mandal, B. K., et al. *Lecture Notes: Infectious Diseases.* 6th ed. Hoboken, N.J.: Wiley-Blackwell, 2004.

Mandell, Gerald L., John E. Bennett, and Raphael Dolin, eds. *Mandell, Douglas, and Bennett's Principles and Practice of Infectious Diseases.* 7th ed. New York: Churchill Livingstone/Elsevier, 2010.

Plotkin, Stanley A., and Walter A. Orenstein, eds. *Vaccines.* 4th ed. Philadelphia: W. B. Saunders, 2004.

Remington, Jack S., et al., eds. *Infectious Diseases of the Fetus and Newborn Infant.* 6th ed. Philadelphia: Saunders/Elsevier, 2006.

Schlossberg, David, ed. *Clinical Infectious Disease.* New York: Cambridge University Press, 2008.

Smolinski, M. S., M. A. Hamburg, and J. Lederberg. *Microbial Threats to Health.* Washington, D.C.: National Academies Press, 2003.

Southwick, Frederick. *Infectious Diseases: A Clinical Short Course.* 2d ed. New York: McGraw-Hill Professional, 2007.

Wirth, Stefan, ed. *Pediatric Infectious Diseases Revisited.* New York: Springer, 2007.

Yoshikawa, Thomas, and Dean Norman, eds. *Infectious Disease in the Aging: A Clinical Handbook.* 2d ed. New York: Humana Press, 2009.

## IMMUNOLOGY

Doughty, Lesley A., and Peter Linden, eds. *Immunology and Infectious Disease.* Norwell, Mass.: Kluwer Academic, 2003.

Frank, Steven A. *Immunology and Evolution of Infectious Disease.* Princeton, N. J.: Princeton University Press, 2002.

Janeway, Charles A., Jr., et al. *Immunobiology: The Immune System in Health and Disease.* 6th ed. New York: Garland Science, 2005.

Kaufman, S. H., A. Sher, and R. Ahmed. *Immunology of Infectious Diseases.* Washington, D.C.: ASM Press, 2002.

Ryan, Kenneth J., and C. George Ray. *Sherris Medical Microbiology: An Introduction to Infectious Diseases.* 5th ed. New York: McGraw-Hill Medical, 2010.

## MICROBIOLOGY

Brooks, G. F., et al. *Jawetz, Melnick, and Adelberg's Medical Microbiology.* 24th ed. New York: McGraw-Hill, 2007.

Engleberg, N. Cary, Victor DiRita, and S. Terence Dermody, eds. *Schaechter's Mechanisms of Microbial Disease.* 4th ed. Philadelphia: Lippincott Williams & Wilkins, 2007.

Gillespie, Stephen, and Kathleen B. Bamford. *Medical Microbiology and Infection at a Glance.* 2d ed. Malden, Mass.: Blackwell, 2003.

Gladwin, Mark, and Bill Trattler. *Clinical Microbiology Made Ridiculously Simple.* 4th ed. Miami: MedMaster, 2009.

Madigan, Michael T., and John M. Martinko. *Brock Biology of Microorganisms.* 12th ed. San Francisco: Pearson/Benjamin Cummings, 2009.

Murray, Patrick R., et al., eds. *Manual of Clinical Microbiology.* 8th ed. Washington, D.C.: ASM Press, 2007.

Murray, Patrick R., Ken S. Rosenthal, and Michael A. Pfaller. *Medical Microbiology.* 6th ed. Philadelphia: Mosby/Elsevier, 2009.

Pommerville, Jeffery C. *Alcamo's Fundamentals of Microbiology.* 9th ed. Sudbury, Mass.: Jones and Bartlett, 2010.

Winn, Washington C., Jr., et al. *Koneman's Color Atlas and Textbook of Diagnostic Microbiology.* 6th ed. Philadelphia: Lippincott Williams & Wilkins, 2006.

## PARASITIC DISEASES

*African Sleeping Sickness: A 3-in-1 Medical Reference.* San Diego, Calif.: Icon Health, 2004.

Bogitsh, Burton J., Clint Earl Carter, and Thomas N. Oeltmann. *Human Parasitology.* 3d ed. Boston: Academic Press/Elsevier, 2005.

Holland, Celia V., and Malcolm W. Kennedy, eds. *The Geohelminths: Ascaris, Trichuris, and Hookworm.* World Class Parasites. New York: Springer, 2010.

Ravdin, Jonathan I., ed. *Amebiasis.* Tropical Medical Series. Hackensack, N.J.: World Scientific, 1999.

Roberts, Larry S., and John Janovy, Jr. *Gerald D. Schmidt and Larry S. Roberts' Foundations of Parasitology.* 8th ed. Boston: McGraw-Hill, 2009.

Scott, Marilyn E., and Gary Smith, eds. *Parasitic and Infectious Diseases.* Burlington, Mass.: Academic Press, 1994.

*Sleeping Sickness and Other Parasitic Tropical Diseases.* New York: Rosen, 2002.

## PATHOGENESIS

Friedman, Herman, Noel R. Rose, and Mauro Bendinelli, eds. *Microorganisms and Autoimmune Diseases.* Infectious Agents and Pathogenesis. New York: Springer, 1996.

Mims, Cedric A., Anthony Nash, and John Stephen.

*Mims' Pathogenesis of Infectious Disease.* 5th ed. Burlington, Mass.: Academic Press, 2000.

Robinson, D. Ashley, Edward J. Feil, and Daniel Falush, eds. *Bacterial Population Genetics in Infectious Diseases.* Hoboken, N.J.: Wiley-Blackwell, 2010.

Shetty, Nandini, Julian W. Tang, and Julie Andrews. *Infectious Disease: Pathogenesis, Prevention, and Case Studies.* Hoboken, N.J.: Wiley-Blackwell, 2009.


## POLICY AND PUBLIC HEALTH. *SEE ALSO* ETHICS

Griffiths, Jeffrey, et al., eds. *Public Health and Infectious Diseases.* Philadelphia: Elsevier, 2010.

Heymann, David L., ed. *Control of Communicable Diseases Manual.* 19th ed. Washington, D.C.: American Public Health Association, 2008.

Lindler, Luther E., Frank J. Lebeda, and George Korch, eds. *Biological Weapons Defense: Infectious Disease and Counterbioterrorism.* New York: Humana Press, 2004.

Lombardo, Joseph S., and David L. Buckeridge. *Disease Surveillance: A Public Health Informatics Approach.* Hoboken, N.J.: Wiley-Blackwell, 2007.

M'ikanatha, Nkuchia M., et al., eds. *Infectious Disease Surveillance.* Hoboken, N.J.: Wiley-Blackwell, 2007.

Roberts, Jennifer A., ed. *The Economics of Infectious Disease.* New York: Oxford University Press, 2006.


## PREVENTION

American Academy of Orthopaedic Surgeons. *Preventing Infectious Diseases.* Edited by Jeffrey Lindsey. 5th ed. Sudbury, Mass.: Jones and Bartlett, 2007.

Aral, Sevgi O., and John M. Douglas, eds. *Behavioral Interventions for Prevention and Control of Sexually Transmitted Diseases.* New York: Springer, 2008.

Aronson, Susan S., and Timothy R. Shope. *Managing Infectious Diseases in Child Care and Schools: A Quick Reference Guide.* 2d ed. Elk Grove Village, Ill.: American Academy of Pediatrics, 2009.

Birch, Kate. *Vaccine-Free Prevention and Treatment of Infectious Contagious Disease with Homeopathy.* 2d ed. Bloomington, Ind.: Trafford, 2007.

Centers for Disease Control and Prevention. *Epidemiology and Prevention of Vaccine-Preventable Diseases.* 11th ed. Washington, D.C.: Public Health Foundation, 2009.

Conte, John E. *Manual of Antibiotics and Infectious Diseases: Treatment and Prevention.* 9th ed. Philadelphia: Lippincott Williams & Wilkins, 2002.

Fisher, Margaret C., ed. *Immunizations and Infectious Diseases: An Informed Parent's Guide.* Elk Grove Village, Ill.: American Academy of Pediatrics, 2005.

Hawker, Jeremy, et al. *Communicable Disease Control Handbook.* Malden, Mass.: Blackwell, 2005.

Heymann, David L., ed. *Control of Communicable Diseases Manual.* 19th ed. Washington, D.C.: American Public Health Association, 2008.

Hubley, John. *The AIDS Handbook: A Guide to the Prevention of AIDS and HIV.* 3d ed. New York: Macmillan, 2002.

Knobler, Stacey, et al., eds. *The Impact of Globalization on Infectious Disease Emergence and Control: Exploring the Consequences and Opportunities.* Washington, D.C.: National Academies Press, 2006.

Lemon, Stanley M., et al., eds. *Global Infectious Disease Surveillance and Detections: Assessing the Challenges, Finding Solutions.* Washington, D.C.: National Academies Press, 2007.

Shetty, Nandini, Julian W. Tang, and Julie Andrews. *Infectious Disease: Pathogenesis, Prevention, and Case Studies.* Hoboken, N.J.: Wiley-Blackwell, 2009.

Torrence, Paul F., ed. *Combating the Threat of Pandemic Influenza: Drug Discovery Approaches.* Hoboken, N.J.: Wiley-Blackwell, 2007.

Wallace, Robert B., ed. *Maxcy-Rosenau-Last Public Health and Preventive Medicine.* 15th ed. New York: McGraw-Hill, 2008.

Weinberg, Winkler G. *No Germs Allowed! How to Avoid Infectious Diseases.* Piscataway, N.J.: Rutgers University Press, 2004.


## PRIONS

Hoernlimann, Beat, and Detlev Riesner et al. *Prions in Humans and Animals.* Berlin: Walter de Gruyter, 2006.

Prusiner, Stanley B., ed. *Prion Biology and Diseases.* 2d ed. Woodbury, N.Y.: Cold Spring Harbor Laboratory Press, 2004.

Ridley, Rosalind M., and Harry F. Baker. *Fatal Protein: The Story of CJD, BSE, and Other Prion Diseases.* New York: Oxford University Press, 1998.

Yam, Philip. *The Pathological Protein: Mad Cow, Chronic Wasting, and Other Deadly Prion Diseases.* New York: Copernicus Books/Springer, 2003.

## PROTOZOA

*African Sleeping Sickness: A 3-in-1 Medical Reference.* San Diego, Calif.: Icon Health, 2004.

Gilles, Herbert M., ed. *Protozoal Diseases.* New York: Hodder Arnold, 2000.

Khan, Naveed Ahmed. *Emerging Protozoan Pathogens.* New York: Taylor & Francis, 2008.

Rogers, Kara. *Fungi, Algae, and Protists.* New York: Britannica Educational Press, 2011.

Smith, Deborah F., and Marilyn Parsons, eds. *Molecular Biology of Parasitic Protozoa.* Frontiers in Molecular Biology. New York: Oxford University Press, 1996.

Sterling, Charles R., and Rodney D. Adam, eds. *The Pathogenic Enteric Protozoa: Giardia, Entamoeba, Cryptosporidium, and Cyclospora.* World Class Parasites. New York: Springer, 2004.

Wiser, Mark F. *Protozoa and Human Disease.* Oxford, England: Garland Science, 2010.

## SEXUALLY TRANSMITTED DISEASES (STDs). *SEE ALSO* ACQUIRED IMMUNODEFICIENCY SYNDROME (AIDS)

Centers for Disease Control and Prevention. *The National Plan to Eliminate Syphilis from the United States.* Atlanta: Department of Health and Human Services, 2006.

Faro, Sebastian. *Sexually Transmitted Diseases in Women.* Philadelphia: Lippincott Williams & Wilkins, 2003.

Hansfield, H. *Color Atlas and Synopsis of Sexually Transmitted Diseases.* 2d ed. New York: McGraw-Hill Professional, 2000.

Klausner, J., and E. Hook III. *Current Diagnosis and Treatment of Sexually Transmitted Diseases.* New York: McGraw-Hill Medical, 2007.

Larsen, Laura. *Sexually Transmitted Diseases Sourcebook.* Detroit: Omnigraphics, 2009.

McCance, Dennis J., ed. *Human Papilloma Viruses.* New York: Elsevier Science, 2002.

Morse, Stephen A., Ronald C. Ballard, and King K. Holmes. *Atlas of Sexually Transmitted Diseases and AIDS.* 3d ed. Philadelphia: Mosby, 2003.

Nardo, Don. *Human Papillomavirus.* San Diego, Calif.: Lucent, 2007.

Parker, James N., and Phillip M. Parker, eds. *The Official Patient's Sourcebook on Chlamydia.* San Diego, Calif.: Icon Health, 2002.

Shoquist, Jennifer, and Diane Stafford. *Encyclopedia of Sexually Transmitted Diseases.* New York: Facts On File, 2003.

Stanberry, Lawrence R., and David I. Bernstein, eds. *Sexually Transmitted Diseases: Vaccines, Prevention, and Control.* San Diego, Calif.: Academic Press, 2000.

Stine, Gerald J. *AIDS Update 2010.* New York: McGraw-Hill Higher Education, 2010.

Sutton, E., and A. Lee. *Sexually Transmitted Diseases Sourcebook: Basic Consumer Health Information About Chlamydial Infections, Gonorrhea, Hepatitis, Herpes, HIV/AIDS.* Health Reference Series. 3d ed. Detroit: Omnigraphics, 2006.

## TRANSMISSION

Apostolopoulos, Yorghos, and Sevil Sonmez, eds. *Population Mobility and Infectious Disease.* New York: Springer, 2010.

Busvine, James. *Disease Transmission by Insects: Its Discovery and Ninety Years of Effort to Prevent It.* New York: Springer, 1993.

Glesecke, Johan. *Modern Infectious Disease Epidemiology.* 2d ed. New York: Hodder Arnold, 2001.

Krasner, Robert. *The Microbial Challenge: Science, Disease, and Public Health.* 2d ed. Sudbury, Mass.: Jones and Bartlett, 2009.

Link, Kurt. *Understanding New, Resurgent, and Resistant Diseases: How Man and Globalization Create and Spread Illness.* Santa Barbara, Calif.: Praeger, 2007.

Mayer, Kenneth H., and H. F. Pizer, eds. *The Social Ecology of Infectious Diseases.* New York: Academic Press, 2007.

National Academy of Sciences. *Infectious Diseases in an Age of Change: The Impact of Human Ecology and Behavior on Disease Transmission.* Edited by Bernard Roizman. Washington, D.C.: National Academies Press, 1995.

Peters, C. J., and Charles H. Calisher, eds. *Infectious Diseases from Nature: Mechanisms of Viral Emergence and Persistence.* Archives of Virology. New York: Springer, 2005.

Wilson, Mary E., R. Levins, and A. Spielman. *Disease in Evolution: Global Changes and Emergence of Infectious Diseases.* New York: New York Academy of Sciences, 1995.

## TREATMENT

Baddour, Larry M., and Sherwood Gorbach. *Therapy of Infectious Diseases.* London: Saunders, 2003.

Bartlett, John G. *The Johns Hopkins Hospital 2005-6 Guide to Medical Care of Patients with HIV Infection.* 12th ed. Philadelphia: Lippincott Williams & Wilkins, 2005.

Bartlett, John G., Paul G. Auwaerter, and Paul A. Pham. *Johns Hopkins ABX Guide: Diagnosis and Treatment of Infectious Diseases.* 2d ed. Sudbury, Mass.: Jones and Bartlett, 2010.

Centers for Disease Control and Prevention. "Sexually Transmitted Diseases Treatment Guidelines 2010." Atlanta: Department of Health and Human Services, 2010.

Chin, Rachel L., ed. *Emergency Management of Infectious Diseases.* New York: Cambridge University Press, 2008.

Conte, John E. *Manual of Antibiotics and Infectious Diseases: Treatment and Prevention.* 9th ed. Philadelphia: Lippincott Williams & Wilkins, 2002.

Cunha, Burke A. *Tickborne Infectious Diseases: Diagnosis and Management.* Infectious Disease and Therapy. London: Informa Healthcare, 2000.

Elmer, Gary W., Lynne McFarland, and Christine Surawicz, eds. *Biotherapeutic Agents and Infectious Diseases.* New York: Springer, 1999.

Gallagher, Jason. *Antibiotics Simplified.* Sudbury, Mass.: Jones and Bartlett, 2008.

Gilbert, David N., et al., eds. *The Sanford Guide to Antimicrobial Therapy 2010.* 40th ed. Sperryville, Va.: Antimicrobial Therapy, 2010.

_____. *The Sanford Guide to HIV/AIDS Therapy 2010.* 18th ed. Sperryville, Va.: Antimicrobial Therapy, 2009.

Hopkins, Donald. *The Eradication of Infectious Diseases.* Edited by W. R. Dowdle. New York: John Wiley & Sons, 1998.

Jacobson, Jeffrey M., ed. *Immunotherapy for Infectious Diseases.* New York: Springer, 2002.

Klausner, J., and E. Hook III. *Current Diagnosis and Treatment of Sexually Transmitted Diseases.* New York: McGraw-Hill Medical, 2007.

Lacy, Charles F., et al. *The Drug Information Handbook.* 17th ed. Hudson, Ohio: Lexi-Comp, 2008.

Liska, Ken. *Drugs and the Human Body, with Implications for Society.* 8th ed. Upper Saddle River, N.J.: Pearson/Prentice Hall, 2009.

McCormack, Rango, et al., eds. *Drug Therapy: Decision Making Guide.* Philadelphia: Saunders/Elsevier, 2007.

Mainous, Arch G., III, and Claire Pomeroy, eds. *Management of Antimicrobials in Infectious Diseases.* New York: Springer, 2010.

Mandell, Gerald L., John E. Bennett, and Raphael Dolin, eds. *Mandell, Douglas, and Bennett's Principles and Practice of Infectious Diseases.* 7th ed. New York: Churchill Livingstone/Elsevier, 2010.

*Physicians' Desk Reference.* 64th ed. Montvale, N.J.: PDR Network, 2009.

Piscitelli, Stephen C., and Keith A. Rodvold, eds. *Drug Interactions in Infectious Diseases.* 2d ed. New York: Humana Press, 2005.

Princeton, Douglas C. *Manual of HIV/AIDS Therapy.* Rev. ed. Laguna Hills, Calif.: Current Clinical Strategies, 2002.

Washington University School of Medicine. *Infectious Diseases Subspecialty Consult.* Edited by Richard Starlin et al. Philadelphia: Lippincott Williams & Wilkins, 2005.

Welder, R. *Viral Infections and Treatments.* Infectious Disease and Therapy. London: Informa Healthcare, 2003.

## TROPICAL DISEASES

Berger, Stephen A., Charles H. Calisher, and Jay S. Keystone. *Exotic Viral Diseases: A Global Guide.* Shelton, Conn.: PMPH USA, 2003.

Cook, Gordon C., and Alimuddin I. Zumla, eds. *Manson's Tropical Diseases.* 22d ed. Philadelphia: Saunders/Elsevier, 2009.

Eddleston, M., et al. *Oxford Handbook of Tropical Medicine.* 3d ed. New York: Oxford University Press, 2008.

Feldman, Charles, and George A. Sarosi, eds. *Tropical and Parasitic Infections in the Intensive Care Unit.* New York: Springer, 2005.

Gill, Geoff, and Nick Beeching, eds. *Lecture Notes on Tropical Medicine.* 5th ed. Malden, Mass.: Blackwell, 2004.

Guerrant, R., D. Walker, D., and P. Weller. *Tropical Infectious Diseases: Principles, Pathogens, and Practice.* 3d ed. Philadelphia: Elsevier, 2011.

Jong, Elaine C., and Russell McMullen, eds. *Travel and Tropical Medicine Manual.* 4th ed. Philadelphia: Saunders/Elsevier, 2008.

Kwan-Gett, Tao Sheng Clifford, Charles Kemp, and

Carrie Kovarik. *Infectious and Tropical Diseases: A Handbook for Primary Care.* Philadelphia: Mosby/Elsevier, 2006.

Lorenzo Saviol. *Working to Overcome the Global Impact of Neglected Tropical Diseases.* Geneva: World Health Organization, 2010.

Lutz, Harald T., and Hassen A. Gharbi, eds. *Manual of Diagnostic Ultrasound in Infectious Tropical Diseases.* New York: Springer, 2006.

Peters, Wallace. *Atlas of Tropical Medicine and Parasites.* 6th ed. Philadelphia: Mosby/Elsevier, 2006.

Schwartz, Eli. *Tropical Diseases in Travelers.* Hoboken, N.J.: Wiley-Blackwell, 2009.

Strickland, G. Thomas, ed. *Hunter's Tropical Medicine and Emerging Infectious Diseases.* 8th ed. Philadelphia: W. B. Saunders, 2000.

## VIRAL INFECTIONS

Berger, Stephen A., Charles H. Calisher, and Jay S. Keystone. *Exotic Viral Diseases: A Global Guide.* Shelton, Conn.: PMPH USA, 2003.

Boss, John, and Margaret Esiri. *Viral Encephalitis in Humans.* Washington, D.C.: ASM Press, 2003.

Colligan, L. H. *Measles and Mumps.* New York: Benchmark Books, 2010.

Eccles, Ronald, and Olaf Weber, eds. *Common Cold.* Boston: Birkhäuser, 2009.

Fagan, Elizabeth Ann. *Viral Hepatitis.* New York: Garland Science, 2000.

Khalill, Kamel, and Kuan-Teh Jeang. *Viral Oncology: Basic Science and Clinical Applications.* Hoboken, N.J.: Wiley-Blackwell, 2009.

Klenk, H. D. *Ebola and Marburg Viruses: Molecular and Cellular Biology.* Horizon Bioscience. New York: Taylor & Francis, 2004.

*Novel and Re-emerging Respiratory Viral Diseases.* Hoboken, N.J.: Wiley-Blackwell, 2008.

Rothman, Alan. *Dengue Virus.* Current Topics in Microbiology and Immunology. New York: Springer, 2009.

Shenk, Thomas E. *Human Cytomegalovirus.* Edited by Mark F. Stinski. Current Topics in Microbiology and Immunology. New York: Springer, 2008.

Shors, Teri. *Understanding Viruses.* Sudbury, Mass.: Jones and Bartlett, 2008.

Smith, Tara C. *Ebola.* Deadly Diseases and Epidemics. New York: Chelsea House, 2005.

Sompayrac, Lauren M. *How Pathogenic Viruses Work.* Sudbury, Mass.: Jones and Bartlett, 2002.

Stanberry, Lawrence R. *Understanding Herpes.* Understanding Health and Sickness Series. 2d ed. Jackson: University Press of Mississippi, 2006.

Strauss, James, and Ellen Strauss. *Viruses and Human Disease.* 2d ed. Boston: Academic Press/Elsevier, 2008.

Swayne, David E., ed. *Avian Influenza.* Hoboken, N.J.: Wiley-Blackwell, 2008.

Wagner, Edward K., and Martinez J. Hewlett. *Basic Virology.* 3d ed. Malden, Mass.: Blackwell Science, 2008.

Welker, Reinhold, ed. *Viral Infections and Treatment.* Infectious Disease and Therapy. London: Informa Healthcare, 2003.

Wilshut, Jan, Janet Mcelhaney, and Abraham Palache. *Rapid Reference to Influenza.* 2d ed. Philadelphia: Mosby, 2006.

*Brandy Weidow, M.S.*

# Resources

## NATIONAL AND INTERNATIONAL HEALTH ORGANIZATIONS

### Centers for Disease Control and Prevention (CDC)
1600 Clifton Rd.
Atlanta, GA 30333
800-CDC-INFO (800-232-4636)
TTY: 888-232-6348
E-MAIL: cdcinfo@cdc.gov
WEB SITE: http://www.cdc.gov

The CDC provides tools and information in an effort to protect public health. Its Division of Foodborne, Bacterial, and Mycotic Diseases is a resource on foodborne illness and on bacterial and mycotic (fungal) diseases. Its Travelers' Health branch provides information on specific destinations, vaccinations, travel notices and health warnings, and infectious diseases related to travel. Its National Center for Emerging and Zoonotic Infectious Diseases provides information on infectious diseases that are spreading, whether through travel, natural- or human-made disasters, person-to-person contact, or health care settings.

### Health Canada
Address Locator 0900C2
Ottawa, Ontario, K1A 0K9
866-225-0709
TTY: 800-267-1245 (Health Canada)
FAX: 613-941-5366
E-MAIL: info@hc-sc.gc.ca
WEB SITE: http://www.hc-sc.gc.ca

Health Canada is the federal body responsible for helping Canadians maintain and improve health.

### Health Protection Agency (HPA)
7th Floor, Holborn Gate
330 High Holborn
London, England WC1V 7PP
020-7759-2700/2701
FAX: 020-7759-2733
E-MAIL: hpa.enquiries@hpa.org.uk
WEB SITE: http://www.hpa.org.uk

This independent organization set up by the British government is designed to protect the public from health threats, including infectious diseases and environmental hazards.

### The Joint Commission
One Renaissance Blvd.
Oakbrook Terrace, IL 60181
630-792-5000
FAX: 630-792-5005
WEB SITE: http://www.jointcommission.org

This organization sets standards for and accredits hospitals and associated organizations and advocates patient safety, including infection control.

### National Digestive Diseases Information Clearinghouse
2 Information Way
Bethesda, MD 20892–3570
800–891–5389
TTY: 866–569–1162
FAX: 703–738–4929
E-MAIL: nddic@info.niddk.nih.gov
WEB SITE: www.digestive.niddk.nih.gov

This service of the National Institute of Diabetes and Digestive and Kidney Diseases provides information on health and research for the public related to digestive and kidney diseases, and diabetes.

### National Health Service (U.K.)
0845-4647 (24-hour advice and support)
E-MAIL: http://www.nhs.uk/aboutnhschoices/pages/contactus.aspx (send messages via Web site)
WEB SITE: http://www.nhs.uk

This U.K. Department of Health arm provides publicly funded health care in the United Kingdom. Also provides medical advice and health education to the public.

### National Institute of Allergy and Infectious Diseases (NIAID)
Office of Communications and Government Relations
6610 Rockledge Dr., MSC 6612
Bethesda, MD 20892-6612
866-284-4107
TDD: 800-877-8339
FAX: 301-402-3573
E-MAIL: ocpostoffice@niaid.nih.gov
WEB SITE: http://www.niaid.nih.gov

This division of the U.S. Department of Health and Human Services lists allergy and infectious disease-related information and research by topic.

## World Health Organization (WHO)

Avenue Appia 20
1211 Geneva 27
FAX: + 41-22-791-31-11
WEB SITE: http://www.who.int

WHO is the authority for health within the United Nations system. It provides international leadership on health matters. The Web site includes an alphabetical index of health topics and updates on the status of global diseases.

## FOUNDATIONS AND SUPPORT/ADVOCACY GROUPS

### American Autoimmune Related Disease Association (AARDA)

22100 Gratiot Ave.
East Detroit, MI 48021
586-776-3900
FAX: 586-776-3903
WEB SITE: http://www.aarda.org

This organization offers patient information on a variety of conditions and newsletter articles relevant to autoimmune disease.

### American Leprosy Missions (ALM)

1 ALM Way
Greenville, SC 29601
800-543-3135
864-271-7040
FAX: 864-271-7062
E-MAIL: amlep@leprosy.org
WEB SITE: http://leprosy.org

This organization provides medical, rehabilitative, and social care, and information about leprosy. Also refers callers to treatment centers.

### American Lyme Disease Foundation

P.O. Box 466
Lyme, CT 06371
WEB SITE: http://www.aldf.com

This foundation offers information on prevention, diagnosis, and treatment of Lyme disease and other tickborne infections.

### American Social Health Association (ASHA)

Herpes Resource Center
P.O. Box 13827

Research Triangle Park, NC 27709
800-227-8922
FAX: 919-361-8425
WEB SITE: http://www.ashastd.org/herpes/herpes_overview.cfm

This association provides support and information for persons with recurring genital herpes infections and referrals to self-help groups in the United States and Canada.

### Creutzfeldt-Jakob Disease (CJD) Foundation

P.O. Box 5312
Akron, OH 44334
800-659-1991
WEB SITE: http://www.cjdfoundation.org

This foundation offers information and support for family members of persons with CJD.

### Cystic Fibrosis.com

WEB SITE: http://www.cysticfibrosis.com

This online social-health community includes online forums and chat rooms for people affected by cystic fibrosis, information about clinical trials, newsletters, and a search tool for finding a local cystic fibrosis center.

### Cystic Fibrosis Foundation

6931 Arlington Rd., 2d Floor
Bethesda, MD 20814
800-FIGHT-CF (344-4823)
FAX: 301-951-6378
E-MAIL: info@cff.org
WEB SITE: http://www.cff.org

This foundation funds and accredits cystic fibrosis care centers. Its Web site includes frequently asked questions about cystic fibrosis and a Living with Cystic Fibrosis section.

### Encephalitis Society

7B Saville St.
Malton, North Yorkshire, YO17 7LL
United Kingdom
+44-0-1653-699-599 (support line)
FAX: +44-0-1653-604-369
WEB SITE: http://www.encephalitis.info

The society provides information on encephalitis, conducts research, raises awareness, and maintains an online register of affected persons.

**Foundation for Sarcoidosis Research**
122 South Michigan Ave.
Suite 1700
Chicago, IL 60603
866-358-5477
FAX: 312-322-9808
WEB SITE: http://www.stopsarcoidosis.org
The foundation Web site includes a disease overview, research news, information for patients about talking to their doctors and finding specialists, and links to support groups.

**Gay Men's Health Crisis**
The Tisch Building
119 W. 24th St.
New York, NY 10011
800-AIDS-NYC
212-367-1000
WEB SITE: http://www.gmhc.org
This organization provides support and therapy groups for persons with AIDS and their families. It offers volunteer crisis counselors, a buddy program for assistance with tasks, and an HIV/AIDS prevention program.

**Hepatitis Foundation International (HFI)**
504 Blick Dr.
Silver Spring, MD 20904
800-891-0707
301-622-4200
FAX: 301-622-4702
E-MAIL: info@hepatitusfoundation.org
WEB SITE: http://www.hepfi.org
This foundation provides education and information about viral hepatitis. It maintains a database of support groups.

**Herpes Viruses Association (HVA)**
41 North Road
London N7 9DP
0845-123-2305 (helpline)
E-MAIL: info@herpes.org.uk
WEB SITE: http://www.herpes.org.uk
This association provides information and runs trials related to the herpes virus.

**Immune Deficiency Foundation**
40 West Chesapeake Ave.
Suite 308
Towson, MD 21204

800-296-4433
E-MAIL: idf@primaryimmune.org
WEB SITE: http://www.primaryimmune.org
This foundation provides information for persons with inherited immunodeficiency diseases and their families and for medical professionals.

**Kawasaki Disease Foundation**
9 Cape Ann Cir.
Ipswich, MA 01938
978-356-2070
FAX: 978-356-2079
E-MAIL: info@kdfoundation.org
WEB SITE: http://www.kdfoundation.org
This nonprofit partnership of parents, patients, and professionals provides education and support. The Web site includes a discussion forum.

**National Necrotizing Fasciitis Foundation**
WEB SITE: http://www.nnff.org
This foundation provides online fact sheets, links to a discussion group, and a state-by-state list of contacts for support.

**National Organization for Rare Disorders**
55 Kenosia Ave.
P.O. Box 1968
Danbury, CT 06813-1968
203-797-9590
FAX: 203-798-2291
WEB SITE: http://rarediseases.org
This nonprofit federation of voluntary health organizations helps people with rare diseases, and the organizations that serve them.

**Project Inform**
1375 Mission St.
San Francisco, CA 94103-2621
800-822-7422
415-558-8669
FAX: 415-558-0684
WEB SITE: http://www.projinf.org
This clearinghouse and hotline provides AIDS and HIV treatment information and advocacy and information on current drugs and where they can be obtained.

**WORLD: An Information and Support Network by, for, and About Women with HIV-AIDS**
414 13th St.
2d Floor
Oakland, CA 94612
510-986-0340
FAX: 510-986-0341
WEB SITE: http://www.womenhiv.org
This network offers support and information for women infected with or affected by AIDS or HIV. It also sponsors retreats and classes.

## GENERAL SUPPORT WEB SITES

**Daily Strength**
http://www.dailystrength.org/support-groups/
infectious-diseases
This Web site provides a forum for discussion and an "Ask an Expert" feature on a variety of infectious diseases.

**Drugs.com Support Groups**
http://www.drugs.com/answers/support-group
This Web site provides opportunities to ask questions and includes links to blogs with topic-specific information.

**iMedix.com**
http://www.imedix.com/support_groups
This site hosts support groups and also provides links to other resources.

## PROFESSIONAL ORGANIZATIONS

**Alliance for the Prudent Use of Antibiotics (APUA)**
75 Kneeland St.
P.O. Box 4014
Boston, MA 02111-1901
617-636-0966
FAX: 617-636-3999
WEB SITE: http://www.tufts.edu/med/apua
E-MAIL: apua@tufts.edu
This international alliance advocates for the cautious and knowledgeable use of antibiotics through activities focused on education, advocacy, research, and surveillance.

**American Academy of Dermatology (AAD)**
930 E. Woodfield Rd.
P.O. Box 4014
Schaumburg, IL 60168-4014
866-503-SKIN (7546)
FAX: 847-240-1859
WEB SITE: http://www.aad.org
This organization represents practicing dermatologists in the United States and provides fact sheets for the public on skin conditions.

**Infectious Diseases Society of America (IDSA)**
1300 Wilson Blvd.
Suite 300
Arlington, VA 22209
703-299-0200
FAX: 703-299-0204
WEB SITE: http://www.idsociety.org
This society represents infectious disease specialists and promotes excellence in patient care through education, research, and prevention efforts.

**National Foundation for Infectious Diseases (NFID)**
4733 Bethesda Ave.
Suite 750
Bethesda, MD 20814
301-656-0003
FAX: 301-907-0878
E-MAIL: info@nfid.org
WEB SITE: info@nfid.org
This nonprofit organization educates the public and health care professionals on causes, prevention, and treatment of infectious diseases.

## GENERAL ONLINE INFORMATION

**Drugs.com**
http://www.drugs.com
This searchable site provides information on prescription drugs.

**Health Hotline: National Institutes of Health (NIH)**
http://healthhotlines.nlm.nih.gov
This is a searchable index of toll-free health hotlines.

**Health Topics: Medline**
http://www.nlm.nih.gov/medlineplus/healthtopics.
html

This is the National Library of Medicine's health information site.

## Infections: Merck Manuals, Online Medical Library

http://www.merck.com/mmhe/sec17.html

This searchable, patient-oriented medical manual is published by Merck Research Laboratories. The Infections page includes explanations about various types of infections, treatments, and vaccinations, and includes general biology information.

## KidsHealth.org

http://kidshealth.org/parent/infections

Sponsored by Nemours, a large nonprofit organization devoted to children's health. Provides information for parents on how infections affect children.

## Mayo Clinic

http://www.mayoclinic.com

Physicians, scientists, and researchers from the Mayo Clinic contribute to this searchable Web site on various diseases and conditions.

## Organized Wisdom

http://organizedwisdom.com

This searchable, patient-oriented site provides "wisdom cards" that feature links provided by experts on specific topics.

## PDR Health

http://www.pdrhealth.com

This site from the publishers of the Physicians' Desk Reference provides searchable information on diseases and medications.

## WebMD

http://www.webmd.com

This Web site provides searchable drug and disease information reviewed regularly by a medical review board.

## ONLINE FACT SHEETS/QUICK REFERENCES

### "Acanthamoeba Infection": Centers for Disease Control and Prevention

http://www.cdc.gov/acanthamoeba

This site includes information on risk, diagnosis, treatment, and prevention of acanthamoeba infection.

### "Acute Cholecystitis": American Medical Association

http://jama.ama-assn.org/cgi/reprint/289/1/124. pdf

This patient education page contains information on the symptoms and diagnosis of acute cholecytistis.

### "Antibiotic Awareness Campaign": National Health Service (U.K.)

http://www.nhs.uk/nhsengland/arc

This NHS article reviews responsible antibiotic use to help prevent resistance to antibiotics.

### "Biological Threats": Ready America

http://www.ready.gov/america/beinformed/ biological.html

This page, sponsored by the U.S. Federal Emergency Management Agency (FEMA), provides an overview of biological threats and actions to take in the event of biological threat exposure or risk for exposure.

### "Body Lice": Centers for Disease Control and Prevention

http://www.cdc.gov/lice/body/factsheet.html

This fact sheet covers the identification, spread, diagnosis, and treatment of body lice.

### "Campylobacteriosis": Centers for Disease Control and Prevention

http://www.cdc.gov/healthypets/diseases/ campylobacteriosis.htm

This section provides information on the transmission and prevention of campylobacteriosis.

### "Cancer Vaccines": National Cancer Institute

http://www.cancer.gov/cancertopics/factsheet/ therapy/cancer-vaccines

This fact sheet reviews approved preventive vaccines, treatment vaccines, and ongoing research.

### "CDC Says 'Take 3' Actions to Fight the Flu": Centers for Disease Control and Prevention

http://www.cdc.gov/flu/protect/preventing.htm

This publication outlines key recommendations for influenza prevention.

### "Cholera": World Health Organization

http://www.who.int/topics/cholera

This section includes a collection of resources on

cholera prevention and treatment, and on worldwide organizations.

**"Consumer Fact Sheet on MRSA": Alliance for the Prudent Use of Antibiotics**

http://www.tufts.edu/med/apua/consumers/personal_home.shtml

This fact sheet for health consumers discusses MRSA spread and risk reduction.

**"Coxsackievirus Infections": KidsHealth**

http://kidshealth.org/parent/infections/bacterial_viral/coxsackie.html

This resource provides information for parents on the spread, symptoms, and treatment of coxsackie virus infections.

**"Defenses Against Infection": Merck Manuals**

http://www.merck.com/mmhe/sec17/ch188/ch188d.html

This brief chapter features a basic explanation of the body's defenses against infection.

**"Facts About Pneumococcal Disease": National Foundation for Infectious Diseases**

http://www.nfid.org/factsheets/pneumofacts.shtml

This fact sheet informs patients about risk, prevention, and treatment of pneumococcal infection.

**"Get Smart: Know When Antibiotics Work": Centers for Disease Control and Prevention**

http://www.cdc.gov/features/getsmart

This article guides patients on appropriate antibiotic use and the dangers of misuse.

**"Graft-Versus-Host Disease (GVHD)": National Institutes of Health**

http://www.cc.nih.gov/ccc/patient_education/pepubs/gvh.pdf

This fact sheet for patients and families describes GVHD prevention, symptoms, and treatment.

**"H. pylori and Peptic Ulcers": National Institute of Digestive and Diabetes and Kidney Diseases**

http://digestive.niddk.nih.gov/ddiseases/pubs/hpylori

This information page explains the connection between H. pylori and ulcers and how ulcers are diagnosed and treated.

**"Healthcare-Associated Infections": Centers for Disease Control and Prevention**

http://www.cdc.gov/hai/infectiontypes.html

This section focuses on key hospital-acquired infections and steps for protecting both patients and health care workers.

**"Household Water Treatment and Safe Storage": World Health Organization**

http://www.who.int/household_water

This page provides, among other tips, guidance on water treatment to combat contamination.

**"Human Papillomavirus (HPV) Vaccine": Infectious Diseases Society of America**

http://www.idsociety.org/content.aspx?id=6532

This statement summarizes the position of the Infectious Diseases Society of America on the HPV vaccine and provides recommendations.

**"Immune System": KidsHealth**

http://kidshealth.org/parent/general/body_basics/immune.html

This "body basics" feature provides a review of how the immune system works.

**"Immunization Schedule": Centers for Disease Control and Prevention**

http://www.cdc.gov/vaccines/recs/schedules

This page includes links to child, adolescent, and adult schedules for recommended immunizations.

**"The Impact of Infectious Diseases": Global Health Council**

http://www.globalhealth.org/infectious_diseases

This summary describes the impact of infectious diseases worldwide.

**"Infectious Disease Specialist": Infectious Diseases Society of America**

http://www.idsociety.org/content.aspx?id=3956

This resource describes the training and roles of infectious disease specialists.

**"Kaposi's Sarcoma": National Cancer Institute**

http://www.cancer.gov/cancertopics/pdq/treatment/kaposis

This fact sheet provides general information on Kaposi's sarcoma.

**"Kuru Information Page": National Institute of Neurological Diseases and Stroke**

http://www.ninds.nih.gov/disorders/kuru

This site provides information on kuru causes, prognosis, and research.

**"Lyme Disease": Infectious Diseases Society of America**

http://www.idsociety.org/lymediseasefacts.htm

This fact sheet by infectious disease specialists covers transmission, symptoms, and treatment of Lyme disease.

**"Lymphatic Filariasis (Elephantiasis)": World Health Organization**

http://www.who.int/mediacentre/factsheets/fs102

This information page discusses the cause, symptoms, diagnosis, and treatment of elephantiasis.

**"Meningococcal Meningitis": World Health Organization**

http://www.who.int/mediacentre/factsheets/fs141

This patient fact sheet reviews prevention, symptoms, diagnosis, treatment, and public health response to meningococcal meningitis.

**"Monitoring Surgical Wounds for Infection": Health Protection Agency (U.K.)**

http://www.hpa.org.uk/web/hpawebfile/hpaweb_c/1203084356092

This page describes the risks for and development and treatment of surgical wound infections.

**"Mosquito-Borne Diseases": American Mosquito Control Association**

http://www.mosquito.org/mosquito-information/mosquito-borne.aspx

This page describes specific mosquito-borne diseases, the regions affected, and the impact of these diseases.

**"Necrotizing Fasciitis": National Necrotizing Fasciitis Foundation**

http://www.nnff.org/nnff_factsheet.htm

This patient fact sheet discusses disease prevention and treatment and outcomes of necrotizing fasciitis.

**"NINDS Encephalitis Lethargica": National Institute of Neurological Disorders and Stroke**

http://www.ninds.nih.gov/disorders/encephalitis_lethargica/encephalitis_lethargica.htm

This information page reviews treatment, prognosis, and research related to encephalitis lethargica.

**"Pancreatitis": National Institute of Diabetes and Digestive and Kidney Diseases**

http://digestive.niddk.nih.gov/ddiseases/pubs/pancreatitis

This patient fact sheet reviews diagnosis, treatment, and complications of pancreatitis.

**"Parasites": Centers for Disease Control and Prevention**

http://www.cdc.gov/ncidod/dpd/parasites

This page features an alphabetical index of parasites and the diseases they cause.

**"Prion Diseases": Centers for Disease Control and Prevention**

http://www.cdc.gov/ncidod/dvrd/prions

This page provides an overview of prion diseases and links to additional resources.

**"Progressive Multifocal Leukoencephalopathy Information Page": National Institute of Neurological Disorders and Stroke**

http://www.ninds.nih.gov/disorders/pml

This fact sheet summarizes risk, prevention, and treatment of progressive multifocal leukoencephalopathy.

**"Rabies Vaccine": Centers for Disease Control and Prevention**

http://www.cdc.gov/vaccines/pubs/vis/downloads/vis-rabies.pdf

This fact sheet provides patient information on the rabies vaccine, including who qualifies and details of vaccination.

**"Removing Obstacles to Healthy Development": World Health Organization**

http://www.who.int/infectious-disease-report/index-rpt99.html

This report covers the impact of infectious diseases in developing countries.

**"Rotavirus": Centers for Disease Control and Prevention**

http://www.cdc.gov/rotavirus

This site provides information on protecting children from rotavirus infection.

**"Seasonal Influenza (Flu)": Centers for Disease Control and Prevention**

http://www.cdc.gov/flu

This page includes basic facts for the public on seasonal influenza.

**"Sepsis: What You Should Know": Surviving Sepsis Campaign**

http://www.survivingsepsis.org/what_you_should_know

This review by the European Society of Critical Care Medicine, the International Sepsis Forum, and the Society of Critical Care Medicine includes information on transmission, course, and treatment of sepsis.

**"Sexually Transmitted Diseases (STDs)"**

http://www.avert.org/std.htm

Sponsored by an international AIDS charity, this page reviews diagnosis, treatment, and prevention of common STDs.

**"Strep Throat": KidsHealth**

http://kidshealth.org/parent/infections/bacterial_viral/strep_throat.html

This page provides information for parents on prevention, detection, and treatment of strep throat in children.

**"Surgical Site Infections": Institute for Healthcare Improvement**

http://www.ihi.org/ihi/topics/patientsafety/surgicalsiteinfections

This fact sheet focuses on preoperative and postoperative steps for preventing surgical site infections.

**"Trachoma": International Trachoma Initiative**

http://www.trachoma.org

This summary provides an overview of trachoma, its global impact, and the public health strategies to prevent and treat it.

**"Understand Quarantine and Isolation": Centers for Disease Control and Prevention**

http://www.bt.cdc.gov/preparedness/quarantine

As part of its Emergency Preparedness and Response Education, the CDC provides information for the public on situations that warrant quarantine and isolation.

**"Vaccines": Centers for Disease Control and Prevention**

http://www.cdc.gov/vaccines/vpd-vac/vaccines-list.htm

This index page includes links to information for parents about vaccines.

**"Viral Hemorrhagic Fever": Centers for Disease Control and Prevention**

http://www.cdc.gov/ncidod/dvrd/spb/mnpages/dispages/vhf.htm

This resource includes an overview and fact sheet on types, transmission, prevention, symptoms, and treatment of hemorrhagic fever viral infections.

**"Warts": American Academy of Dermatology**

http://www.aad.org/public/publications/pamphlets/common_warts.html

This patient pamphlet explains common warts and their treatment.

**"What Is Antibiotic Resistance and Why Is It a Problem?": Alliance for the Prudent Use of Antibiotics**

http://www.tufts.edu/med/apua/patients/patient.html

This overview provides information for patients on using antibiotics responsibly.

*Katherine Hauswirth, M.S.N., R.N.*

# Web Sites

## GENERAL INFORMATION

### A.D.A.M Medical Encyclopedia
http://www.nlm.nih.gov/medlineplus/
encyclopedia.html

The content of A.D.A.M's Medical Encyclopedia is offered as a service of the National Library of Medicine (NLM) and the National Institutes of Health (NIH). The Medical Encyclopedia covers a range of topics that include many diseases, conditions, and medical tests and procedures. Accompanying many of the entries are clear illustrations with informative captions.

### Centers for Disease Control and Prevention (CDC)
http://www.cdc.gov

The CDC Web site has extensive information about all aspects of health and healthy living, from diseases and conditions to vaccinations and workplace safety.

### Healthy Children
http://www.healthychildren.org

The American Academy of Pediatrics children's health Web site. It includes a "Symptom Checker" tool.

### Mayo Clinic
http://www.mayoclinic.com

The Mayo Clinic Web site offers a wealth of information and advice on topics ranging from diseases and conditions, medications, and medical tests to healthy living.

### National Foundation for Infectious Diseases (NFID)
http://www.nfid.org

The NFID is "dedicated to educating the public and healthcare professionals about the causes, treatment and prevention of infectious diseases." The Web site includes news and fact sheets about many infectious diseases.

### Organization of Teratology Information Specialists (OTIS)
http://www.otispregnancy.org

OTIS is dedicated to the education of expectant parents about exposure during pregnancy to infections, medications, illegal substances, vaccines, and more.

### RxList
http://www.rxlist.com

A comprehensive information source for prescription drugs, supplements, and diseases and conditions. It also contains a pill identifier. The site includes prescribing information for physicians and patients.

## ONLINE SUPPORT

Note that online support groups should not take the place of a physician's advice.

### DailyStrength
http://www.dailystrength.org/support-groups

This Web site offers online support forums for a variety of life's challenges, including diseases, conditions, and treatments. In addition to gaining support, people can share experiences or ask questions and generally interact with other persons in similar situations.

### MDJunction
http://www.mdjunction.com/support-groups

This site is for people with certain medical conditions who want to exchange support and advice.

## TRAVEL MEDICINE

### Centers for Disease Control and Prevention (CDC)
Traveler's Health
http://wwwnc.cdc.gov/travel

Travel to foreign countries can expose a person to uncommon infectious diseases. The CDC's Traveler's Health Web site has everything from outbreak alerts for various countries to help in finding a local travel medicine clinic. The site covers diseases and specific destinations with their particular health concerns, as well as information about vaccinations needed before travel.

### University of Pennsylvania Health System
Penn Travel Medicine
http://www.pennmedicine.org/travel

The University of Pennsylvania's Travel Medicine site includes information on several common travel diseases and tips to stay healthy when traveling.

## BACTERIAL DISEASES

### BACTERIAL MENINGITIS
**National Meningitis Association (NMA)**
http://www.nmaus.org

NMA is a nonprofit organization dedicated to curbing meningitis through education and vaccination.

### BOTULISM
**FoodSafety.gov**
Botulism
http://www.foodsafety.gov/poisoning/causes/bacteriaviruses

Information about botulism illness, with links to additional resources. FoodSafety.gov is the U.S. government's food safety information site.

### DIPHTHERIA
**DTaP Vaccine Information Statement**
http://www.cdc.gov/vaccines/pubs/vis

A site containing the mandatory Vaccine Information Statement, which is given to people who get the DTaP (diphtheria, tetanus, acellular pertussis) vaccine.

**Immunization Action Coalition (IAC)**
Diphtheria: Questions and Answers
http://www.immunize.org/catg.d/p4203.pdf

A printable three-page handout on diphtheria from the IAC.

**National Library of Medicine (NLM)**
Diphtheria
http://www.nlm.nih.gov/medlineplus/diphtheria.html

The NLAM's diphtheria portal, with links to many resources about the disease and related topics.

### GROUP A STREPTOCOCCAL INFECTIONS
**National Institute of Allergy and Infectious Diseases (NIAID)**
Group A Streptococcal Infections
http://www.niaid.nih.gov/topics/streptococcal

This NIAID site contains information about topics that include complications, research, and surveillance. There are also links to the major diseases caused by group A Streptococcus.

### HAEMOPHILUS INFLUENZAE TYPE B (HIB) INFECTION
**The Hib Initiative**
http://www.hibaction.org/aboutdisease.php

The Hib Initiative seeks to reduce global Hib disease rates and Hib-related deaths through the use of the Hib vaccine.

### HELICOBACTER PYLORI INFECTION
**H. Pylori Learning Center**
http://www.hpylorilearningcenter.com

The Learning Center provides information about *H. pylori*, associated infection, and treatments. The site is maintained by Meridian Bioscience and has sections for patients and health care professionals.

**The Helicobacter Foundation**
http://www.helico.com

The Helicobacter Foundation was started by Barry Marshall, who codiscovered the bacteria. The Web site includes information about *H. pylori* and its history and treatments and provides a chat forum.

### MRSA INFECTION
**American Academy of Pediatrics (AAP)**
Information for Schools/Parents/Students on Community-Acquired Methicillin-Resistant *Staphylococcus aureus*
http://www.aap.org/new/mrsa.htm

Information from the AAP regarding methicillin-resistant *Staphylococcus aureus* (MRSA) infection in community settings and how to reduce the risk.

**MRSA Survivors Network**
http://www.mrsasurvivors.org

A survivors' support and advocacy organization whose mission is to stop MRSA infections and death.

**National Library of Medicine (NLM)**
MRSA
http://www.nlm.nih.gov/medlineplus/mrsa.html

The MRSA portal of the NLM, with links to many resources about the disease and related topics.

**WebMD**
DTaP and Tdap Vaccines
http://children.webmd.com/vaccines/dtap-and-tdap-vaccines

The difference between the initial diphtheria,

tetanus, acellular pertussis (DTaP) vaccine and the adolescent booster vaccine (Tdap) is discussed in easy-to-understand terms.

### WebMD

Tetanus: Topic Overview

http://children.webmd.com/vaccines/tc/tetanus-topic-overview

Tetanus and tetanus vaccine information from a trusted site.

## FUNGAL INFECTIONS

### KidsHealth

Fungal Infections

http://kidshealth.org/kid/health_problems

Aimed at children, this page gives an overview of fungal infections of the skin, how to manage them, and, most important, how to avoid them.

### HISTOPLASMOSIS
### National Eye Institute (NEI)

Facts About Histoplasmosis

http://www.nei.nih.gov/health/histoplasmosis/histoplasmosis.asp

Frequently asked questions about all aspects of histoplasmosis, prepared by the NEI.

## PARASITIC DISEASES

### Centers for Disease Control and Prevention (CDC)

Parasitic Diseases

http://www.cdc.gov/ncidod/dpd

The CDC's portal to information on parasitic diseases. The site includes links to specific diseases and links for special groups, such as blood donors. Also included are special topics, such as parasites in drinking water.

### HEAD LICE
### HeadLice.org

http://www.headlice.org

News, information, and a comment forum about head lice and head lice infestations.

### KidsHealth

Head Lice

http://kidshealth.org/parent/infections/common/lice.html

The head lice section of this Web site offers information in English and Spanish and separate supplemental information for parents, kids, and teens.

### TOXOPLASMOSIS
### March of Dimes

Toxoplasmosis Fact Sheet

http://www.marchofdimes.com/complications_toxoplasmosis.html

The March of Dimes is dedicated to the fight against birth defects and disorders. This fact sheet, aimed at pregnant women, discusses the risks for and prevention of toxoplasmosis infections in the newborn.

## VACCINE-PREVENTABLE DISEASES

### Centers for Disease Control and Prevention (CDC)

Immunization Schedules

http://cdc.gov/vaccines/recs/schedules

This page contains the CDC's vaccination schedules for children, teenagers, and adults.

### Centers for Disease Control and Prevention (CDC)

Vaccines and Preventable Diseases

http://cdc.gov/vaccines/vpd-vac

The CDC portal on vaccines and vaccine-preventable diseases. Also includes links to updated information about vaccine shortage and vaccine safety and to information for specific groups.

### Immunization Action Coalition (IAC)

Vaccine Information Statements

http://www.immunize.org/vis

Though the IAC is geared toward health care professionals, this part of its Web site contains the Vaccine Information Statements (VIS), the mandatory information handouts that every person receives upon being vaccinated. The statements provide excellent, concise overviews of diseases, the benefits of vaccines, and possible side effects from vaccines. The statements are available in English and other languages (the page has a languages tab).

## Viral Diseases

**AIDS.** *See* **HIV/AIDS**

### Anthrax
**National Library of Medicine (NLM)**
Anthrax Tutorial
http://www.nlm.nih.gov/medlineplus/tutorials
   This tutorial from the NLM's Patient Education Institute can be read, run as a self-playing module, or used interactively. Includes basic information about anthrax, including its potential as an agent of bioterrorism.

### Avian Influenza. *See* Influenza.

### Chickenpox
**KidsHealth**
Chickenpox
http://kidshealth.org/parent/infections/skin/chicken_pox.html
   This Web page provides information about chickenpox and its treatment, prevention, and complications. Also includes links to related topics. The text is available in Spanish and in audio.

**Mayo Clinic**
Chickenpox
http://www.mayoclinic.com/health/chickenpox/ds00053
   Detailed disease information from the Mayo Clinic.

### Hantavirus
**National Center for Infectious Diseases (NCID)**
"Tracking a Mystery Disease"
http://www.cdc.gov/ncidod/diseases/hanta/hps/noframes/history.htm
   This page details the history of hantavirus infection that first appeared in the Four Corners area of the United States in 1993 and covers the disease itself.

### Hepatitis (General)
**American Liver Foundation (ALF)**
http://www.liverfoundation.org
   The ALF is dedicated to supporting people affected by liver disease, to educating the public, and to promoting research. This Web site contains information on hepatitis A, B, and C and on related topics such as liver transplant, cirrhosis, and clinical trials.

**Centers for Disease Control and Prevention (CDC)**
Division of Viral Hepatitis
http://www.cdc.gov/hepatitis
   The CDC's Division of Viral Hepatitis has information for the public and for health care professionals. The site contains news and statistics and links to the CDC's pages for hepatitis A through E.

**Hepatitis Foundation International (HFI)**
http://www.hepfi.org
   HFI is dedicated to promoting healthy living and hepatitis prevention and to supporting research and education. The site has support information for persons living with hepatitis.

### Hepatitis A
**FoodSafety.gov**
Hepatitis A
http://www.foodsafety.gov/poisoning/causes/bacteriaviruses/hepatitisa.html
   FoodSafety.gov is the U.S. government's food safety information site. This page provides basic information about hepatitis A, with links to additional resources.

**National Library of Medicine (NLM)**
Hepatitis A
http://www.nlm.nih.gov/medlineplus/hepatitisa.html
   The NLM's hepatitis A portal, with links to many resources about the disease and related topics.

### Hepatitis B
**eMedicineHealth**
Hepatitis B
http://www.emedicinehealth.com/hepatitis_b/article_em.htm
   This site has comprehensive coverage of hepatitis B. It includes a user forum and provides links to related topics, such as the anatomy of the digestive system, liver transplants, and sexually transmitted diseases.

**Hepatitis B Foundation**
http://www.hepb.org
   The Hepatitis B Foundation engages in advocacy, education, research funding, and more. This site is filled with links to resources, news, and other information.

**Immunization Action Coalition (IAC)**
Hepatitis B: Questions and Answers
http://www.immunize.org/catg.d/p4205.pdf

The IAC provides this seven-page booklet about hepatitis B that includes information on the basics ("What is hepatitis B?" "How is it spread?") and detailed information ("What blood tests are available?" "What are the complications of chronic hepatitis B infection?").

**HEPATITIS C**
**Hepatitis Central**
http://www.hepatitis-central.com

A clearinghouse Web site, Hepatitis Central contains information on living with hepatitis C, treatments, research, and support.

**National Institute of Diabetes and Digestive and Kidney Diseases (NIDDK)**
What I Need to Know About Hepatitis C
http://digestive.niddk.nih.gov/ddiseases/pubs/hepc_ez

This site provides a detailed fact sheet from the NIDDK covering all aspects of hepatitis C.

**U.S. Department of Veterans Affairs (VA)**
Hepatitis C
http://www.hepatitis.va.gov

This VA site provides hepatitis C information, from testing through clinical trials.

**HEPATITIS D.** *See* **HEPATITIS B (HEPATITIS D OCCURS ONLY IN PEOPLE WHO ARE ALSO INFECTED WITH THE HEPATITIS B VIRUS)**

**HEPATITIS E**
**Everyday Health**
Hepatitis E: The Basics
http://www.everydayhealth.com/hepatitis/hepatitis-e-basics.aspx

Offers an overview, including information about statistics, transmission, prevention, symptoms, and treatment.

**HERPES SIMPLEX INFECTION**
**America Social Health Association (ASHA)**
Herpes Resource Center
http://www.ashastd.org/herpes/herpes_overview.cfm

The ASHA runs this resource site, which focuses on genital herpes (herpes simplex 2) infections. The site includes a topic overview, discussion of emotional issues, support group listings by state, and text in Spanish.

**HerpesDiagnosis**
http://www.herpesdiagnosis.com

This site answers important questions about herpes simplex infections. It also includes a section for physicians.

**HIV/AIDS**
**Elizabeth Glazer Pediatric AIDS Foundation**
http://www.pedaids.org

Children infected with HIV face different issues and burdens than adults. The Elizabeth Glazer Pediatric AIDS Foundation supports research, prevention, and treatment programs aimed at eradicating HIV infection in children. The foundation sponsors programs across the globe, and the Web site contains issue briefs, program information, and ways to get involved.

**U.S. Department of Health and Human Services (DHHS)**
AIDS.gov
http://aids.gov

The U.S. government's AIDS information site. Covers AIDS basics and the latest news concerning HIV science and HIV/AIDS policies, among other topics. The site is managed by the DHHS.

**U.S. Department of Health and Human Services (DHHS)**
AIDSinfo.gov
http://www.aidsinfo.nih.gov

This DHHS site focuses on all health aspects of HIV infection and AIDS and includes information about clinical trials for treatments and vaccination research and trials.

**INFLUENZA**
**Centers for Disease Control and Prevention (CDC)**
Influenza
http://www.cdc.gov/flu

This CDC site includes extensive influenza information for the public and for health care professionals. Topics include influenza basics, treatments, vaccines, and news alerts.

## Flu.gov

http://flu.gov

This site contains news and information about the flu and its treatment and prevention. Information is available for specific groups such as the elderly, travelers, and expectant parents.

## World Health Organization (WHO)

Influenza

http://www.who.int/topics/influenza

This WHO site has links to fact sheets and information about vaccinations, H1N1 influenza, avian influenza, and more.

## MEASLES

### Measles Initiative

http://measlesinitiative.org

The Measles Initiative is a partnership between the American Red Cross, the Centers for Disease Control and Prevention, the United Nations Foundation, United Nations Children's Fund, and the World Health Organization. This partnership aims "to reduce global measles mortality through mass vaccination campaigns and by strengthening routine immunization."

## World Health Organization (WHO)

Measles Fact Sheet

http://www.who.int/mediacentre/factsheets/fs286

A concise fact sheet about measles worldwide.

## RABIES

### World Health Organization (WHO)

Rabies

http://www.who.int/rabies

WHO's portal to rabies information, with links to a rabies fact sheet and other links to specific issues associated with rabies.

## RESPIRATORY SYNCYTIAL VIRUS

### Centers for Disease Control and Prevention (CDC)

Respiratory Syncytial Virus Infection

http://www.cdc.gov/rsv

The CDC's respiratory syncytial virus infection portal, with information, statistics, and resources for health consumers and professionals.

## KidsHealth

RSV (Respiratory Syncytial Virus Infection)

http://kidshealth.org/parent/infections/lung/rsv.html

This site, run by the Nemours Foundation, contains a summary of RSV that is also available in Spanish and in audio versions. It is written in friendly, easy-to-understand terms and contains links to related topics.

## YELLOW FEVER

### World Health Organization (WHO)

Yellow Fever Fact Sheet

http://www.who.int/mediacentre/factsheets/fs100

WHO's fact sheet on yellow fever summarizes information about all aspects of the disease.

## ZOONOTIC DISEASES

### King County, Washington, Department of Health

Zoonotic Disease Program

http://www.kingcounty.gov/healthservices/health/ehs/zoonotics.aspx

This King County Department of Health site has links and information about zoonoses in general and a comprehensive list of specific diseases, with links to further information. Also includes links for people in higher-risk groups.

### World Health Organization (WHO)

Zoonoses and Veterinary Public Health

http://www.who.int/zoonoses

WHO's zoonoses and veterinary public health division engages in the surveillance, control, and prevention of zoonotic diseases.

## OTHER DISEASES

### Creutzfeldt-Jakob Disease Foundation

http://cjdfoundation.org

This foundation provides education, support, and advocacy for and by people affected by Creutzfeldt-Jakob disease.

### GBS/CIDP Foundation International

http://www.gbs-cidp.org

Information and support for people affected by Guillain-Barré syndrome and chronic inflammatory demyelinating polyneuropathy.

*Adi R. Ferrara, ELS*

# Medical Journals

**American Family Physician**
American Academy of Family Physicians (AAFP)
Biweekly
American Academy of Family Physicians
  Publishes articles on primary care with some articles about infectious diseases.

**American Journal of Critical Care**
American Association of Critical Care Nurses (AACCN)
Bimonthly
American Association of Critical Care Nurses/Inno-
  Vision Group
  Publishes clinical studies, basic research studies, case reports, and reviews related to the care of the critically ill patient. Issues often feature articles on infectious diseases, especially pulmonary infections.

**American Journal of Epidemiology**
Johns Hopkins School of Hygiene and Public Health
Biweekly
Oxford University Press
  Publishes articles on the epidemiology of all types of medical conditions, including infection.

**American Journal of Infection Control**
Association for Professionals in Infection Control and
  Epidemiology (APIC)
Monthly
Mosby
  Contains articles on infections and infection control in healthcare settings.

**American Journal of Medicine**
Association of Professors of Medicine (APM)
Monthly
Elsevier
  Publishes original clinical research on topics of interest to physicians in internal medicine. Some articles concern infectious diseases.

**American Journal of Obstetrics and Gynecology**
Monthly
Mosby/Elsevier
  Publishes articles on the latest diagnostic procedures and research in obstetrics and gynecology, in

cluding maternal-fetal medicine. Some articles concern obstetric and gynecological infections.

**American Journal of Public Health**
American Public Health Association (APHA)
Monthly
American Public Health Association
  Publishes articles on all aspects of public health, including infectious diseases.

**American Journal of Respiratory and Critical Care
  Medicine**
American Thoracic Society (ATS)
Biweekly
American Thoracic Society
  Publishes articles on diseases of the lung, including infections. A section is devoted to tuberculosis and mycobacteria disease.

**American Journal of Tropical Medicine and
  Hygiene**
American Society of Tropical Medicine and Hygiene
  (ASTMH)
Monthly
American Society of Tropical Medicine and Hygiene
  The leading international journal of tropical medicine. Publishes articles covering new research in tropical medicine, parasitology, immunology, infectious diseases, epidemiology, molecular biology, virology, and international medicine.

**Annals of Emergency Medicine**
American College of Emergency Physicians (ACEP)
Monthly
Elsevier
  A leading international journal of emergency medicine. Publishes articles on both adult and pediatric emergency medicine, and most issues contain one or more articles related to infectious diseases.

**Annals of Internal Medicine**
American College of Physicians (ACP)
Monthly
American College of Physicians
  General medical topics are covered with meta-anal-

ysis articles often being featured. Articles on infections and epidemiology are included in many issues.

### Annals of Surgery

American Surgical Association (ASA) and European Surgical Association (ESA)
Monthly
Wolters Kluwer Health/Lippincott Williams & Wilkins
An international journal with articles on clinical research related to surgical technique and practice. Some of the articles concern surgical infections.

### Antimicrobial Agents and Chemotherapy

American Society for Microbiology (ASM)
Monthly
American Society for Microbiology
The leading research journal devoted to new antimicrobial agents.

### Archives of Virology

Virology Division of the International Union of Microbiological Societies (IUMS)
Monthly
Springer Wien
Publishes articles on viruses, viruslike agents, and virus infections of humans, animals, plants, insects, and bacteria.

### British Journal of Surgery

Association of Surgeons of Great Britain and Ireland (ASGBI) and other European surgical societies
Monthly
John Wiley & Sons
The journal publishes articles on all aspects of surgery, with occasional articles related to surgical infection.

### British Medical Journal

British Medical Association (BMA)
Weekly
BMJ Group
This distinguished journal publishes original research and reviews on a wide variety of medical topics, including infectious diseases.

### Bulletin of the World Health Organization

World Health Organization (WHO)
Monthly
World Health Organization
An international journal with news and original research articles on public health topics, most of which are related to infectious diseases.

### Canadian Journal of Infectious Diseases and Medical Microbiology

Association of Medical Microbiology and Infectious Disease Canada (AMMI Canada)
Bimonthly
Pulsus
Publishes articles on all aspects of infectious diseases and medical microbiology.

### Canadian Medical Association Journal

Canadian Medical Association (CMA)
Biweekly
Canadian Medical Association
A general medical journal featuring articles on clinical research and on case reports, practice updates, and clinical guidelines. A few of the articles concern infectious diseases.

### Chest

American College of Chest Physicians (ACCP)
Monthly
American College of Chest Physicians
Publishes articles on cardiopulmonary diseases, including infections such as pneumonia and tuberculosis. Infections diseases associated with COPD, asthma, chronic bronchitis, and cystic fibrosis are also featured in articles and reviews.

### Clinical Infectious Diseases

Infectious Diseases Society of America (IDSA) and the HIV Medicine Association (HIVMA)
Biweekly
University of Chicago Press
The leading journal on the clinical aspects of infectious diseases, including HIV, for the United States and around the world. Also publishes IDSA guidelines on the diagnosis and treatment of infectious diseases.

### Clinical Microbiology and Infection

European Society of Clinical Microbiology and Infectious Diseases (ESCMID)
Monthly
Wiley-Blackwell
Publishes original research in clinical microbiology, infectious diseases, virology, and parasitology.

## Clinical Microbiology Reviews
American Society for Microbiology (ASM)
Quarterly
American Society for Microbiology

Publishes reviews of new developments in clinical microbiology and immunology. Topics include pathogenic mechanisms, specific microbial pathogens, new antimicrobial agents, and new diagnostic techniques.

## Critical Care Medicine
Society of Critical Care Medicine (SCCM)
Monthly
Wolters Kluwer Health/Lippincott Williams & Wilkins

This leading journal in critical care medicine often publishes clinical investigations, laboratory investigations, or case reports related to infectious diseases.

## Diagnostic Microbiology and Infectious Diseases
Monthly
Elsevier

Publishes articles on clinical microbiology and the diagnosis and treatment of infections.

## Emerging Infectious Diseases
Centers for Disease Control and Prevention (CDC)
Monthly
Centers for Disease Control and Prevention

Publishes articles on new infectious diseases and new aspects of existing infectious diseases with a global scope. All issues are available free at http://www.cdc.gov/eid.

## European Journal of Clinical Microbiology and Infectious Diseases
Monthly
Springer Berlin/Heidelberg

Publishes articles on the epidemiology, diagnosis, clinical research, molecular biology, and animal studies of infectious diseases of bacterial, fungal, viral, or parasitic origin.

## Heart and Lung
American Association of Heart Failure Nurses (AAHFN)
Bimonthly
Elsevier

Publishes articles in the areas of acute and critical care and in respiratory and heart-failure nursing. Some articles concern infection control and cardiopulmonary infections.

## HIV Medicine
British HIV Association (BHIVA) and European AIDS Clinical Society (EACS)
Ten times per year
Wiley-Blackwell

A journal devoted to both the research and clinical aspects of HIV disease that also contains invited review articles.

## Infection and Immunity
American Society for Microbiology (ASM)
Monthly
American Society for Microbiology

A highly respected journal that publishes articles on all aspects of research on infection-producing organisms and on host interactions.

## Infectious Control and Hospital Epidemiology
Society for Healthcare Epidemiology of America (SHEA)
Monthly
University of Chicago Press

Publishes studies focused on the epidemiology of hospital infections. Publishes SHEA guidelines on hospital-acquired infections.

## Infectious Disease Clinics of North America
Quarterly
Saunders/Elsevier

Each issue focuses on a specific infectious disease topic with a guest editor and articles by selected experts.

## Influenza and Other Respiratory Viruses
International Society for Influenza and Other Respiratory Viruses (ISIRV)
Bimonthly
Wiley-Blackwell

The journal contains articles on the prevention, detection, treatment, and control of influenza and other respiratory viruses.

## International Journal of Antimicrobial Agents
International Society of Chemotherapy (ISC)
Monthly
Elsevier

The journal publishes original research and reviews on the physical, pharmacological, in vitro and clinical properties of antimicrobial agents.

### International Journal of Parasitology

Australian Society for Parasitology (ASP)
Monthly
Elsevier

The journal contains articles on basic and applied parasitology. Parasites, host-parasite relationships, and the socioeconomic impact of parasitic infections represent the range of topics covered.

### International Journal of STD and AIDS

British Association for Sexual Health & HIV (BASHH) and the International Union Against Sexually Transmitted Infections (IUSTI)
Monthly
Royal Society of Medicine Press

The journal publishes articles on original research, case reports, and reviews concerning the investigation and treatment of sexually transmitted infections, HIV and AIDS.

### Journal of Antimicrobial Chemotherapy

British Society of Antimicrobial Chemotherapy (BSAC)
Monthly
Oxford University Press

This international journal publishes original research articles on antibacterial, antiviral, antifungal, and antiprotozoal agents. Both the laboratory and clinical use of antimicrobial agents are reported.

### Journal of Bacteriology

American Society for Microbiology (ASM)
Monthly
American Society for Microbiology

Articles published relate to both human and plant bacteria and are research oriented. Mini reviews are featured along with reviews of scientific meetings.

### Journal of Bone and Joint Surgery

Monthly (both American and British volumes)
Journal of Bone and Joint Surgery and British Editorial Society of Bone and Joint Surgery

A leading journal of orthopedics that publishes articles on research, case reports, and reviews related to orthopedics. Some of these articles concern orthopedic infections.

### Journal of Clinical Microbiology

American Society for Microbiology (ASM)
Monthly

American Society for Microbiology

Clinical and research articles on all aspects of clinical microbiology are published.

### Journal of Clinical Pharmacology

American College of Clinical Pharmacology (ACCP)
Monthly
Sage

Publishes articles on the pharmacokinetics and pharmacodynamics of drugs. Each issue usually contains at least one article on an antimicrobial agent.

### Journal of Clinical Virology

Monthly
Elsevier

This international journal publishes articles on the epidemiology, pathogenesis, diagnosis and detection, and prevention and treatment of human viral infections.

### Journal of Emergency Medicine

American Academy of Emergency Medicine (AAEM)
Eight times per year
Elsevier

The journal publishes research papers and clinical studies pertinent to emergency medicine and infectious diseases are often included.

### Journal of Hospital Infection

Hospital Infection Society (HIS)
Monthly
Elsevier

The journal contains articles on hospital-acquired infections and related subjects.

### Journal of Infection

British Infection Society (BIS)
Monthly
Saunders/Elsevier

This journal publishes articles on infectious diseases, epidemiology, and clinical microbiology.

### Journal of Infectious Diseases

Infectious Diseases Society of America (IDSA) and the HIV Medicine Association (HIVMA)
Biweekly
University of Chicago Press

The journal includes both clinical and research articles on viral, bacterial, fungal, and parasitic infections.

**Journal of Medical Virology**
Monthly
Wiley-Liss

Articles on basic and applied research on human viruses are published. The journal includes reports on the characterization, diagnosis, epidemiology, immunology, and pathogenesis of human virus infection.

**Journal of Parasitology**
American Society of Parasitologists (ASP)
Bimonthly
American Society of Parasitologists

The journal contains research articles in the field of parasitology.

**Journal of the American College of Surgeons**
American College of Surgeons (ACS)
Monthly
Elsevier

The journal publishes original research and reviews on all aspects of surgery. Some of the articles concern the diagnosis, prevention, and treatment of surgical infections.

**Journal of the American Medical Association**
American Medical Association (AMA)
Weekly
American Medical Association

The journal contains articles on a wide variety of medical topics, but often publishes important and timely articles on infectious diseases.

**Journal of Travel Medicine**
International Society of Travel Medicine (ISTM)
Bimonthly
Wiley-Blackwell

Travel medicine related articles are published and the majority concern infectious diseases.

**Journal of Urology**
American Urological Association (AUA)
Monthly
American Urological Association

The journal publishes clinically relevant research and practice-oriented reports in the field of urology. There is a section devoted to infection and inflammation.

**Journal of Virology**
American Society for Microbiology (ASM)
Monthly

American Society for Microbiology

The journal publishes research articles on viruses, response to viral infections, vaccines, and antivirals.

**Lancet Infectious Diseases**
Monthly
Elsevier

Articles on research, opinion, news, and clinical cases concerning infectious diseases are published.

**Mayo Clinic Proceedings**
Mayo Clinic
Monthly
Mayo Foundation for Medical Education and Research

This journal publishes on a wide scope of medical topics, including infectious diseases and antibiotics.

**Medical Journal of Australia**
Australian Medical Association (AMA)
Biweekly
Australasian Medical

A general medical journal that sometimes publishes articles on infectious diseases and parasitology.

**Microbiology and Molecular Biology Reviews**
American Society for Microbiology (ASM)
Quarterly
American Society for Microbiology

This journal publishes state-of-the-art reviews of various topics concerning microbiology and microbial molecular biology.

**Morbidity and Mortality Weekly Report**
Centers for Disease Control and Prevention (CDC)
Weekly
Centers for Disease Control and Prevention

Articles are published on epidemiological aspects of illnesses, that are most often infections, from the United States and worldwide. Surveillance, recommendations, and advisories are covered. Issues are available free online at www.cdc.gov/mmwr.

**New England Journal of Medicine**
Massachusetts Medical Society (MMS)
Weekly
Massachusetts Medical Society

A leading medical journal that publishes articles on medical research, reviews, and case studies all of which may include infectious diseases.

## Obstetrics and Gynecology

American Congress of Obstetricians and Gynecologists (ACOG)

Monthly

Wolters Kluwer Health/Lippincott Williams & Wilkins

A leading journal that publishes articles on original research and commentaries concerning the field of obstetrics and gynecology.

## Pediatric Infectious Disease Journal

Pediatric Infectious Diseases Society (PIDS) and the European Society for Paediatric Infectious Diseases (ESPID)

Monthly

Wolters Kluwer Health/Lippincott Williams & Wilkins

Articles are published on all aspects of infections in children.

## Pediatrics

American Academy of Pediatrics (AAP)

Monthly

American Academy of Pediatrics

This is the most widely circulated pediatrics journal and contains a large percentage of articles about pediatric infections and vaccines.

## Proceedings of the National Academy of Sciences

National Academy of Sciences of the United States of America (NAS)

Weekly

National Academy of Sciences of the United States of America

This is a leading journal of the sciences and includes cutting-edge articles in the areas of medical sciences and microbiology.

## Scandinavian Journal of Infectious Diseases

Monthly

Informa Healthcare

Articles devoted to the clinical and microbial aspects of infectious diseases are published in English

## Science

American Association for the Advancement of Science (AAAS)

Weekly

American Association for the Advancement of Science

Cutting-edge research articles on all types of scientific topics are published with many on infectious diseases and microbes.

## Sexually Transmitted Diseases

American Sexually Transmitted Disease Association (ASTDA), International Union Against Sexually Transmitted Infections (IUSTI), and Scandinavian Society for Genitourinary Medicine (SSGM)

Monthly

Wolters Kluwer Health/Lippincott Williams & Wilkins

Articles are published on the epidemiological and clinical aspects of sexually transmitted diseases, including HIV.

## Southern Medical Journal

Southern Medical Association (SMA)

Monthly

Wolters Kluwer Health/Lippincott Williams & Wilkins

The journal publishes articles on all aspects of medicine. Original research and case reports of infectious diseases are occasionally featured.

## Surgical Infections

Surgical Infection Society (SIS)

Bimonthly

Mary Ann Lieber

Articles concern the biology, prevention, and treatment of postoperative infections.

## Transactions of the Royal Society of Tropical Medicine and Hygiene

Royal Society of Tropical Medicine and Hygiene (RSTMH)

Monthly

Elsevier

The journal publishes original articles and invited reviews across a broad range of topics including tropical medicine, infectious diseases, microbiology, epidemiology, and chemotherapy.

## Vaccine

Weekly

Elsevier

This journal publishes articles on vaccines and vaccination for diseases associated with viruses, bacteria, mycoplasmas, protozoa, helminths, arthropods, and prions.

## Virology

Biweekly

Academic Press/Elsevier

This journal publishes basic research in all branches of virology.

*H. Bradford Hawley, M.D.*

# Pharmaceutical List

## ANTIBIOTICS

### AMINOGLYCOSIDES

#### Amikacin
PRINCIPAL USES: Serious bacterial infections, meningitis
ROUTE OF ADMINISTRATION: Intramuscular, intravenous
SITE OF METABOLISM: Kidneys
POTENTIAL SIDE EFFECTS: Neurotoxicity, nephrotoxicity, ototoxicity
TRADE NAMES: Amikin

#### Gentamicin
PRINCIPAL USES: Osteomyelitis, skin infections, endocarditis, meningitis, sepsis, conjunctivitis, peritonitis, urinary tract infection
ROUTE OF ADMINISTRATION: Intramuscular, intravenous
SITE OF METABOLISM: Kidneys
POTENTIAL SIDE EFFECTS: Neurotoxicity, nephrotoxicity, ototoxicity, teratogenic
TRADE NAMES: Garamycin

#### Streptomycin
PRINCIPAL USES: Tuberculosis, brucellosis, chancroid, tularemia, urinary tract infection, granuloma inguinale
ROUTE OF ADMINISTRATION: Intramuscular
SITE OF METABOLISM: Kidneys
POTENTIAL SIDE EFFECTS: Neurotoxicity, nephrotoxicity, ototoxicity, eosinophilia, facial paresthesias
TRADE NAMES: None

#### Tobramycin
PRINCIPAL USES: Meningitis, cystic fibrosis, conjunctivitis, skin infections, pneumonia, osteomyelitis
ROUTE OF ADMINISTRATION: Intramuscular, intravenous, solution for nebulization
SITE OF METABOLISM: Kidneys
POTENTIAL SIDE EFFECTS: Neurotoxicity, nephrotoxicity, ototoxicity
TRADE NAMES: Nebcin, TOBI (nebulized solution)

### CARBAPENEMS

#### Ertapenem
PRINCIPAL USES: Prophylaxis for colorectal surgery, community-acquired pneumonia, diabetic foot infections, urinary tract infections
ROUTE OF ADMINISTRATION: Intramuscular, intravenous
SITE OF METABOLISM: Kidneys
POTENTIAL SIDE EFFECTS: Gastrointestinal upset, headache, vaginitis
TRADE NAMES: Invanz

#### Imipenem/cilastatin
PRINCIPAL USES: Sepsis, osteomyelitis, skin infections, infective endocarditis
ROUTE OF ADMINISTRATION: Intravenous
SITE OF METABOLISM: Kidneys
POTENTIAL SIDE EFFECTS: Gastrointestinal upset, thrombophlebitis
TRADE NAMES: Primaxin

#### Meropenem
PRINCIPAL USES: Skin infections, intra-abdominal infections, meningitis
ROUTE OF ADMINISTRATION: Intravenous
SITE OF METABOLISM: Kidneys
POTENTIAL SIDE EFFECTS: Gastrointestinal upset, headache, Stevens-Johnson syndrome
TRADE NAMES: Merrem

### CEPHALOSPORINS: FIRST GENERATION
Provide gram-positive and some gram-negative coverage

#### Cefadroxil
PRINCIPAL USES: Streptococcal pharyngitis/tonsillitis, urinary tract infection, skin infections
ROUTE OF ADMINISTRATION: Oral
SITE OF METABOLISM: Kidneys
POTENTIAL SIDE EFFECTS: Rash, gastrointestinal upset
TRADE NAMES: Duricef

#### Cefazolin
PRINCIPAL USES: Bacterial endocarditis prophylaxis, surgical prophylaxis, cholangitis, genital infections, osteomyelitis, skin infections, pneumococcal pneumonia, urinary tract infection
ROUTE OF ADMINISTRATION: Intramuscular, intravenous

SITE OF METABOLISM: Kidneys

POTENTIAL SIDE EFFECTS: Gastrointestinal upset, eosinophilia, Stevens-Johnson syndrome

TRADE NAMES: Ancef

## Cephalexin

PRINCIPAL USES: Bacterial endocarditis prophylaxis, otitis media, osteomyelitis, skin infections, streptococcal pharyngitis, urinary tract infection

ROUTE OF ADMINISTRATION: Oral

SITE OF METABOLISM: Kidneys

POTENTIAL SIDE EFFECTS: Gastrointestinal upset, increased liver enzymes

TRADE NAMES: DisperDose, Keflex, Panixine

## CEPHALOSPORINS: SECOND GENERATION

Less gram-positive, increased gram-negative coverage in comparison with first-generation agents; some anaerobic coverage

## Cefaclor

PRINCIPAL USES: Otitis media, group A streptococcal pharyngitis/tonsillitis, COPD exacerbation, bronchitis, urinary tract infection

ROUTE OF ADMINISTRATION: Oral

SITE OF METABOLISM: Kidneys

POTENTIAL SIDE EFFECTS: Gastrointestinal upset, erythema multiforme, fever

TRADE NAMES: Ceclor, Raniclor

## Cefoxitin

PRINCIPAL USES: Gonorrhea, osteomyelitis, skin infections, pelvic inflammatory disease, surgical prophylaxis, urinary tract infection

ROUTE OF ADMINISTRATION: Intramuscular, intravenous

SITE OF METABOLISM: Kidneys

POTENTIAL SIDE EFFECTS: Thrombophlebitis

TRADE NAMES: Mefoxin

## Cefprozil

PRINCIPAL USES: Otitis media, group A streptococcal pharyngitis/tonsillitis, bronchitis, sinusitis

ROUTE OF ADMINISTRATION: Oral

SITE OF METABOLISM: Kidneys

POTENTIAL SIDE EFFECTS: Gastrointestinal upset, increased liver enzymes, dizziness, vaginitis, Stevens-Johnson syndrome

TRADE NAMES: Cefzil

## Cefuroxime

PRINCIPAL USES: COPD exacerbation, otitis media, bronchitis, gonorrhea, impetigo, Lyme disease, pharyngitis/tonsillitis, sinusitis, urinary tract infection, meningitis, surgical prophylaxis

ROUTE OF ADMINISTRATION: Intramuscular, intravenous, oral

SITE OF METABOLISM: Kidneys

POTENTIAL SIDE EFFECTS: Gastrointestinal upset, vaginitis, Stevens-Johnson syndrome, eosinophilia

TRADE NAMES: Ceftin, Kefurox, Zinacef

## CEPHALOSPORINS: THIRD GENERATION

Less gram-positive, increased gram-negative in comparison with second-generation agents; some *Pseudomonas* coverage

## Cefdinir

PRINCIPAL USES: Otitis media, bronchitis, community-acquired pneumonia, sinusitis, pharyngitis/tonsillitis

ROUTE OF ADMINISTRATION: Oral

SITE OF METABOLISM: Kidneys

POTENTIAL SIDE EFFECTS: Gastrointestinal upset, vaginitis, headache

TRADE NAMES: Omnicef

## Cefditoren

PRINCIPAL USES: Bronchitis, community-acquired pneumonia, pharyngitis/tonsillitis, skin infections

ROUTE OF ADMINISTRATION: Oral

SITE OF METABOLISM: Kidneys

POTENTIAL SIDE EFFECTS: Gastrointestinal upset, vaginitis

TRADE NAMES: Spectracef

## Cefixime

PRINCIPAL USES: Gonorrhea, COPD exacerbation, otitis media, bronchitis, pharyngitis/tonsillitis, urinary tract infection

ROUTE OF ADMINISTRATION: Oral

SITE OF METABOLISM: Kidneys, bile

POTENTIAL SIDE EFFECTS: Gastrointestinal upset, urticaria

TRADE NAMES: Suprax

## Cefoperazone

PRINCIPAL USES: Gonorrhea, endometritis, skin infec-

tions, pelvic inflammatory disease, peritonitis, urinary tract infection
ROUTE OF ADMINISTRATION: Intramuscular, intravenous
SITE OF METABOLISM: Bile, kidneys
POTENTIAL SIDE EFFECTS: Gastrointestinal upset, Disulfiram-like reaction with alcohol
TRADE NAMES: Cefobid

**Cefotaxime**
PRINCIPAL USES: Pneumococcal meningitis, sepsis, cesarean section prophylaxis, gonorrhea, osteomyelitis, pneumonia, pelvic inflammatory disease, surgical prophylaxis, urinary tract infection
ROUTE OF ADMINISTRATION: Intramuscular, intravenous
SITE OF METABOLISM: Kidneys, liver
POTENTIAL SIDE EFFECTS: Rash, gastrointestinal upset, Stevens-Johnson syndrome, agranulocytosis
TRADE NAMES: Claforan

**Cefpodoxime**
PRINCIPAL USES: Otitis media, bronchitis, community-acquired pneumonia, gonorrhea, sinusitis, pharyngitis/tonsillitis, urinary tract infection
ROUTE OF ADMINISTRATION: Oral
SITE OF METABOLISM: Kidneys
POTENTIAL SIDE EFFECTS: Gastrointestinal upset
TRADE NAMES: Vantin

**Ceftazidime**
PRINCIPAL USES: Meningitis, sepsis, cystic fibrosis, osteomyelitis, skin infections, urinary tract infection
ROUTE OF ADMINISTRATION: Intramuscular, intravenous
SITE OF METABOLISM: Kidneys
POTENTIAL SIDE EFFECTS: Phlebitis, gastrointestinal upset, encephalopathy
TRADE NAMES: Ceptaz, Fortaz, Tazicef

**Ceftibuten**
PRINCIPAL USES: Otitis media, chronic bronchitis exacerbation, pharyngitis/tonsillitis
ROUTE OF ADMINISTRATION: Oral
SITE OF METABOLISM: Kidneys
POTENTIAL SIDE EFFECTS: Gastrointestinal upset, headache, elevated serum blood urea nitrogen, Stevens-Johnson syndrome, psychiatric disturbances
TRADE NAMES: Cedax

**Ceftizoxime**
PRINCIPAL USES: Gonorrhea, osteomyelitis, skin infec-

tions, septic arthritis, meningitis, pelvic inflammatory disease, sepsis, urinary tract infection
ROUTE OF ADMINISTRATION: Intravenous
SITE OF METABOLISM: Kidneys
POTENTIAL SIDE EFFECTS: Rash, increased liver enzymes, fever
TRADE NAMES: Cefizox

**Ceftriaxone**
PRINCIPAL USES: Meningitis, gonorrhea, otitis media, epididymitis, pelvic inflammatory disease, bacterial endocarditis prophylaxis, surgical prophylaxis, urinary tract infection
ROUTE OF ADMINISTRATION: Intramuscular, intravenous
SITE OF METABOLISM: Kidneys, bile
POTENTIAL SIDE EFFECTS: Gastrointestinal upset, increased liver enzymes, Stevens-Johnson syndrome, kernicterus in newborns
TRADE NAMES: Rocephin

**CEPHALOSPORINS: FOURTH GENERATION**
Increased *Pseudomonas* coverage in comparison with third-generation agents

**Cefepime**
PRINCIPAL USES: Neutropenic fever prophylaxis, skin infections, pneumonia, urinary tract infection
ROUTE OF ADMINISTRATION: Intramuscular, intravenous
SITE OF METABOLISM: Kidneys
POTENTIAL SIDE EFFECTS: Gastrointestinal upset, headache, rash, encephalopathy
TRADE NAMES: Maxipime

**MACROLIDES**

**Azithromycin**
PRINCIPAL USES: Streptococcal pharyngitis, otitis media, sinusitis, chronic bronchitis exacerbation, Chlamydia, gonorrhea, chancroid, disseminated Mycobacterium avium complex disease prevention, prophylaxis for contacts of pertussis-infected persons, cervicitis/urethritis, bacterial endocarditis prophylaxis, community-acquired pneumonia, pelvic inflammatory disease
ROUTE OF ADMINISTRATION: Oral, intravenous
SITE OF METABOLISM: Liver
POTENTIAL SIDE EFFECTS: Gastrointestinal upset, headache
TRADE NAMES: Zithromax, Zmax

## Clarithromycin

PRINCIPAL USES: Prophylaxis of bacterial endocarditis, Mycobacterium avium complex disease prevention, component of *H. pylori* disease treatment regimen, COPD exacerbation, otitis media, community-acquired pneumonia, sinusitis, streptococcal pharyngitis

ROUTE OF ADMINISTRATION: Oral

SITE OF METABOLISM: Kidneys, liver

POTENTIAL SIDE EFFECTS: Gastrointestinal upset, changes in taste, headache, Stevens-Johnson syndrome

TRADE NAMES: Biaxin, Biaxin XL

## Erythromycin

PRINCIPAL USES: Chlamydia, pro-motility agent, acne, rheumatic fever prophylaxis, endocarditis prophylaxis, conjunctivitis, diphtheria, gonorrhea, neonatal gonococcal/chlamydial conjunctivitis prophylaxis, Legionnaires' disease, listeriosis, prophylaxis for contacts of pertussis-infected persons, syphilis

ROUTE OF ADMINISTRATION: Oral

SITE OF METABOLISM: Liver

POTENTIAL SIDE EFFECTS: Gastrointestinal upset, liver dysfunction, arrhythmias, ototoxicity, reports of association with pyloric stenosis

TRADE NAMES: E-mycin, EES, Ery-tab, Eryc, Erypred

## PENICILLINS: FIRST GENERATION

Natural penicillins; covers streptococci, anaerobes

## Benzathine penicillin

PRINCIPAL USES: Syphilis, bejel, pinta, rheumatic fever, streptococcal pharyngitis, yaws

ROUTE OF ADMINISTRATION: Intramuscular

SITE OF METABOLISM: Kidneys

POTENTIAL SIDE EFFECTS: Urticaria, rash, gastrointestinal upset, fever, eosinophilia, pseudomembranous colitis, psychiatric disturbances

TRADE NAMES: Bicillin L-A

## Penicillin G

PRINCIPAL USES: Pneumococcal pneumonia, pneumococcal meningitis, Actinomyces, anthrax, syphilis, clostridial infections, diphtheria, gonorrhea, infective endocarditis, Pasteurella, rat bite fever, pericarditis

ROUTE OF ADMINISTRATION: Intravenous

SITE OF METABOLISM: Kidneys

POTENTIAL SIDE EFFECTS: Hyperkalemia, hemolytic anemia, seizures, interstitial nephritis

TRADE NAMES: None

## Penicillin V

PRINCIPAL USES: Bacterial pharyngitis, infective endocarditis, erysipelas, skin infections, otitis media, pneumococcal pneumonia, rheumatic fever, scarlet fever, streptococcal pharyngitis

ROUTE OF ADMINISTRATION: Oral

SITE OF METABOLISM: Kidneys

POTENTIAL SIDE EFFECTS: Rash, gastrointestinal upset

TRADE NAMES: Nadopen-V, Veetids

## Procaine penicillin

PRINCIPAL USES: Group A streptococcal infections, anthrax, bejel, pinta, yaws, syphilis, diphtheria, bacterial endocarditis, erysipelas, rat bite fever, scarlet fever

ROUTE OF ADMINISTRATION: Intramuscular

SITE OF METABOLISM: Kidneys

POTENTIAL SIDE EFFECTS: Rash, urticaria

TRADE NAMES: Wycillin

## PENICILLINS: SECOND GENERATION

Penicillinase-resistant; covers streptococci, *Staphylococcus aureus*

## Dicloxacillin

PRINCIPAL USES: Methicillin/oxacillin-sensitive *S. aureus* infections

ROUTE OF ADMINISTRATION: Oral

SITE OF METABOLISM: Kidneys, liver

POTENTIAL SIDE EFFECTS: Gastrointestinal upset

TRADE NAMES: Dynapen

## Nafcillin

PRINCIPAL USES: Methicillin/oxacillin-sensitive *S. aureus* infections

ROUTE OF ADMINISTRATION: Intramuscular, intravenous

SITE OF METABOLISM: Liver

POTENTIAL SIDE EFFECTS: Hypokalemia, interstitial nephritis

TRADE NAMES: None

## Oxacillin

PRINCIPAL USES: Methicillin/oxacillin-sensitive *S. aureus* infections

ROUTE OF ADMINISTRATION: Intramuscular, intravenous

SITE OF METABOLISM: Kidneys, liver
POTENTIAL SIDE EFFECTS: Rash, gastrointestinal upset
TRADE NAMES: Bactocill

**PENICILLINS: THIRD GENERATION**
Aminopenicillins; covers streptococci, some gram-negatives

**Amoxicillin**
PRINCIPAL USES: Acute sinusitis, community-acquired pneumonia, Lyme disease, Chlamydia, otitis media, bacterial endocarditis prophylaxis, gonorrhea, H. pylori, streptococcal pharyngitis/tonsillitis
ROUTE OF ADMINISTRATION: Oral
SITE OF METABOLISM: Kidneys
POTENTIAL SIDE EFFECTS: Rash, gastrointestinal upset
TRADE NAMES: Amoxil, DisperMox, Polymox, Trimox

**Amoxicillin-clavulinic acid**
PRINCIPAL USES: Otitis media, sinusitis, pneumonia, urinary tract infection
ROUTE OF ADMINISTRATION: Oral
SITE OF METABOLISM: Kidneys
POTENTIAL SIDE EFFECTS: Rash, gastrointestinal upset, vaginitis, candidiasis, Stevens-Johnson syndrome
TRADE NAMES: Augmentin, Augmentin ES-600, Augmentin XR

**Ampicillin**
PRINCIPAL USES: Sepsis, meningitis, bacterial endocarditis prophylaxis, gonorrhea, digestive tract infections
ROUTE OF ADMINISTRATION: Intravenous
SITE OF METABOLISM: Kidneys
POTENTIAL SIDE EFFECTS: Rash, urticaria, gastrointestinal upset
TRADE NAMES: Principen

**Ampicillin-sulbactam**
PRINCIPAL USES: Skin infections, intra-abdominal infections, pelvic inflammatory disease
ROUTE OF ADMINISTRATION: Intramuscular, intravenous
SITE OF METABOLISM: Kidneys
POTENTIAL SIDE EFFECTS: Rash, gastrointestinal upset, pseudomembranous enterocolitis
TRADE NAMES: Unasyn

**PENICILLINS: FOURTH GENERATION**
Extended spectrum; added *Pseudomonas* coverage

**Carbenicillin**
PRINCIPAL USES: Urinary tract infection, prostatitis
ROUTE OF ADMINISTRATION: Oral
SITE OF METABOLISM: Kidneys
POTENTIAL SIDE EFFECTS: Rash, urticaria, hypokalemia, gastrointestinal upset, pseudomembranous enterocolitis
TRADE NAMES: Geocillin

**Piperacillin**
PRINCIPAL USES: Gonorrhea, skin infections, intra-abdominal infections, surgical prophylaxis, sepsis, urinary tract infection
ROUTE OF ADMINISTRATION: Intramuscular, intravenous
SITE OF METABOLISM: Kidneys, bile
POTENTIAL SIDE EFFECTS: Thrombophlebitis, rash, gastrointestinal upset, headache, fever
TRADE NAMES: None

**Piperacillin-tazobactam**
PRINCIPAL USES: Appendicitis, peritonitis, community-acquired and nosocomial pneumonia, skin infections, pelvic inflammatory disease, endometritis
ROUTE OF ADMINISTRATION: Intravenous
SITE OF METABOLISM: Kidneys
POTENTIAL SIDE EFFECTS: Rash, gastrointestinal upset, candidiasis, headache, insomnia, agitation, fever, neutropenia
TRADE NAMES: Zosyn

**Ticarcillin**
PRINCIPAL USES: Skin infections, intra-abdominal infections, sepsis, urinary tract infection
ROUTE OF ADMINISTRATION: Intramuscular, intravenous
SITE OF METABOLISM: Kidneys
POTENTIAL SIDE EFFECTS: Thrombophlebitis, rash, coagulation abnormalities
TRADE NAMES: Ticar

**Ticarcillin-clavulinic acid**
PRINCIPAL USES: Endometritis, osteomyelitis, intra-abdominal infections, sepsis, urinary tract infection
ROUTE OF ADMINISTRATION: Intravenous
SITE OF METABOLISM: Kidneys
POTENTIAL SIDE EFFECTS: Thrombophlebitis, headache, seizure
TRADE NAMES: Timentin

## Quinolones: First generation

Covers gram-negative; no *Pseudomonas* coverage

### Nalidixic acid

Principal uses: Urinary tract infection

Route of administration: Oral

Site of metabolism: Kidneys, liver

Potential side effects: Rash, photosensitivity, gastrointestinal upset, headache, somnolence, dizziness, prolonged QT interval, neuropathy, psychiatric disturbances

Trade names: NegGram

## Quinolones: Second generation

Covers gram-negative, *Pseudomonas*, *S. aureus*, some atypicals

### Ciprofloxacin

Principal uses: Urinary tract infection, pyelonephritis, prostatitis, sinusitis, bronchitis, neutropenic fever, gonorrhea, osteomyelitis, intra-abdominal infections, nosocomial pneumonia, pneumococcal disease, anthrax

Route of administration: Oral, intravenous

Site of metabolism: Liver, kidneys

Potential side effects: Gastrointestinal upset, dizziness, eye pain, Stevens-Johnson syndrome, hematologic disturbances, neuropathy, tendonitis

Trade names: Cipro, Cipro-XR, ProQuin XR

### Lomefloxacin

Principal uses: Chronic bronchitis exacerbation, prostate surgery prophylaxis, urinary tract infection

Route of administration: Oral

Site of metabolism: Liver, kidneys

Potential side effects: Photosensitivity, gastrointestinal upset, dizziness, headache

Trade names: Maxaquin

### Norfloxacin

Principal uses: Urinary tract infection, conjunctivitis, gonorrhea, prostatitis

Route of administration: Oral

Site of metabolism: Liver, kidneys

Potential side effects: Gastrointestinal upset, dizziness, headache, prolonged QT interval, Stevens-Johnson syndrome, thrombocytopenia, tendonitis, seizure, interstitial nephritis

Trade names: Noroxin

### Ofloxacin

Principal uses: Chlamydia, epididymitis, otitis media/externa, conjunctivitis, chronic bronchitis exacerbation, community-acquired pneumonia, corneal ulcers, cystitis/urethritis, gonorrhea, pelvic inflammatory disease, prostatitis

Route of administration: Oral

Site of metabolism: Liver, kidneys

Potential side effects: Rash, gastrointestinal upset, dizziness, insomnia, headache, eye pain, prolonged QT interval, Stevens-Johnson syndrome, hematologic disturbances, tendonitis

Trade names: Floxin

## Quinolones: Third generation

Covers gram-negative, *Pseudomonas*, gram-positive, *S. aureus*, pneumococcus, increased atypicals

### Levofloxacin

Principal uses: Chlamydia, epididymitis, conjunctivitis, prostatitis, sinusitis, chronic bronchitis exacerbation, community-acquired/nosocomial pneumonia, urinary tract infection/pyelonephritis, corneal ulcers, skin infections, anthrax

Route of administration: Oral, intravenous

Site of metabolism: Kidneys, liver

Potential side effects: Gastrointestinal upset, headache, prolonged QT interval, Stevens-Johnson syndrome, tendonitis, seizure

Trade names: Levaquin

## Quinolones: Fourth generation

Increased pneumococcus and decreased *Pseudomonas* coverage compared to first, second, and third generations

### Gatifloxacin

Principal uses: Urinary tract infection/pyelonephritis, conjunctivitis, chronic bronchitis exacerbation, gonorrhea, skin infections, sinusitis

Route of administration: Oral, intravenous

Site of metabolism: Kidneys

Potential side effects: Taste disorders, eye irritation

Trade names: None

### Gemifloxacin

Principal uses: Chronic bronchitis exacerbation, community-acquired pneumonia

Route of administration: Oral

SITE OF METABOLISM: Feces, kidney

POTENTIAL SIDE EFFECTS: Rash, gastrointestinal upset, increased liver enzymes, tendonitis, neuropathy

TRADE NAMES: Factive

## Moxifloxacin

PRINCIPAL USES: Chronic bronchitis exacerbation, intra-abdominal infection, skin infections, acute sinusitis, community-acquired pneumonia, conjunctivitis, sinusitis

ROUTE OF ADMINISTRATION: Oral, intravenous

SITE OF METABOLISM: Liver, kidneys

POTENTIAL SIDE EFFECTS: Tendonitis, gastrointestinal upset, eye irritation, prolonged QT interval, Stevens-Johnson syndrome, hematologic disturbances

TRADE NAMES: Avelox

## Sulfonamides

PRINCIPAL USES: Sulfadiazine

ROUTE OF ADMINISTRATION: CNS toxoplasmosis, otitis media, chancroid, conjunctivitis, meningitis, malaria, nocardiosis, rheumatic fever, trachoma, urinary tract infection

SITE OF METABOLISM: Oral

POTENTIAL SIDE EFFECTS: Kidneys gastrointestinal upset, crystalluria

TRADE NAMES: None

## Trimethoprim-sulfamethoxazole

PRINCIPAL USES: Treatment and prophylaxis of Pneumocystis, urinary tract infection, MRSA skin infection, COPD exacerbation, otitis media, shigellosis, traveler's diarrhea

ROUTE OF ADMINISTRATION: Oral

SITE OF METABOLISM: Kidneys

POTENTIAL SIDE EFFECTS: Urticaria, gastrointestinal upset, Stevens-Johnson syndrome, *C. difficile* diarrhea, aplastic anemia, hepatic necrosis

TRADE NAMES: Bactrim, cotrimoxazole, Sepra, Sulfatrim

## TETRACYCLINES

## Demeclocycline

PRINCIPAL USES: Acne, Actinomyces infection, amebic infection, anthrax, Bartonella, brucellosis, chancroid, cholera, clostridial infection, rickettsial disease, gonorrhea, granuloma inguinale, conjunctivitis, Campylobacter, Listeria, lymphogranuloma vene-

reum, Mycoplasma pneumonia, urethritis, plague, psittacosis, Q fever, syphilis, trachoma, tularemia, urinary tract infection, yaws

ROUTE OF ADMINISTRATION: Oral

SITE OF METABOLISM: Kidneys, feces

POTENTIAL SIDE EFFECTS: Photosensitivity, gastrointestinal upset, monilial superinfection, hepatotoxicity

TRADE NAMES: Declomycin

## Doxycycline

PRINCIPAL USES: Chlamydia, gonorrhea, syphilis, Lyme disease, periodontitis, acne rosacea, acne vulgaris, malaria prophylaxis, epididymitis, pelvic inflammatory disease, Acinetobacter, actinomycosis, amebic infection, anthrax, Bartonella, brucellosis, chancroid, cholera, clostridial infection, granuloma inguinale, conjunctivitis, Campylobacter, Listeria, lymphogranuloma venereum, plague, psittacosis, Q fever, Rocky Mountain spotted fever, shigellosis, skin infections, tularemia, rickettsial typhus, urinary tract infection, yaws

ROUTE OF ADMINISTRATION: Oral, intravenous

SITE OF METABOLISM: Liver, kidneys

POTENTIAL SIDE EFFECTS: Photosensitivity, gastrointestinal upset, elevated serum blood urea nitrogen, staining of teeth in children

TRADE NAMES: Adoxa, Doryx, Monodox, Oracea, Periostat, Vibramycin, Vibra-Tabs

## Minocycline

PRINCIPAL USES: Acne vulgaris, Listeria, actinomycosis, clostridial infections, amebic infections, anthrax, Chlamydia, cholera, Campylobacter, brucellosis, Bartonella, shigellosis, Acinetobacter, rickettsial disease, gonorrhea, conjunctivitis, Mycobacterium marinum, skin infections, meningococcal carrier state eradication, periodontitis, syphilis, Ureaplasma, urinary tract infection

ROUTE OF ADMINISTRATION: Intravenous, oral

SITE OF METABOLISM: Liver, kidneys

POTENTIAL SIDE EFFECTS: Dizziness

TRADE NAMES: Dynacin, Minocin, Solodyn

## Tetracycline

PRINCIPAL USES: Acne, Actinomyces, anthrax, syphilis, amebic infection, Bartonella, brucellosis, chancroid, Chlamydia, cholera, clostridial infection, rickettsial disease, gonorrhea, granuloma inguinale, *H. pylori* infection, conjunctivitis, Campylobacter,

skin infections, Listeria, lymphogranuloma venereum, Mycoplasma, Ureaplasma, periodontitis, plague, psittacosis, shigellosis, trachoma, tularemia, urinary tract infection, yaws
ROUTE OF ADMINISTRATION: Oral
SITE OF METABOLISM: Liver, kidneys
POTENTIAL SIDE EFFECTS: Photosensitivity, gastrointestinal upset
TRADE NAMES: Sumycin

## OTHER ANTIBIOTICS

### Aztreonam
PRINCIPAL USES: Cystic fibrosis, endometritis, skin infections, intra-abdominal infections/peritonitis, sepsis, urinary tract infection
ROUTE OF ADMINISTRATION: Intramuscular, intravenous
SITE OF METABOLISM: Kidneys
POTENTIAL SIDE EFFECTS: Chest pain, gastrointestinal upset, elevated liver enzymes, elevated serum creatinine, upper respiratory symptoms, fever, erythema multiforme, C. difficile colitis, hematologic disturbances, ototoxicity, nephrotoxicity, angioedema
TRADE NAMES: Azactam

### Chloramphenicol
PRINCIPAL USES: Meningitis, cystic fibrosis, rickettsial disease, H. influenzae, lymphogranuloma venereum, otitis externa, Salmonella, typhoid
ROUTE OF ADMINISTRATION: Intravenous
SITE OF METABOLISM: Liver, kidneys
POTENTIAL SIDE EFFECTS: Gray baby syndrome, aplastic anemia, headache, confusion
TRADE NAMES: Chloromycetin

### Clindamycin
PRINCIPAL USES: MRSA infections, bacterial vaginosis, bacterial endocarditis prophylaxis, intra-abdominal infections, empyema, pneumonitis, pelvic inflammatory disease, sepsis
ROUTE OF ADMINISTRATION: Oral, intramuscular, intravenous
SITE OF METABOLISM: Liver
POTENTIAL SIDE EFFECTS: Pseudomembranous colitis, rash, gastrointestinal upset, jaundice
TRADE NAMES: Cleocin

### Daptomycin
PRINCIPAL USES: Skin infections, S. aureus bacteremia/endocarditis, intravascular-line infection
ROUTE OF ADMINISTRATION: Intravenous
SITE OF METABOLISM: Kidneys
POTENTIAL SIDE EFFECTS: Gastrointestinal upset, throat pain, rhabdomyolysis, renal failure
TRADE NAMES: Cidecin, Cubicin

### Fosfomycin
PRINCIPAL USES: Urinary tract infection
ROUTE OF ADMINISTRATION: Oral
SITE OF METABOLISM: Kidneys
POTENTIAL SIDE EFFECTS: Gastrointestinal upset, headache
TRADE NAMES: Monurol

### Linezolid
PRINCIPAL USES: Skin infections, community-acquired/nosocomial pneumonia, vancomycin-resistant Enterococcus infection
ROUTE OF ADMINISTRATION: Oral, intravenous
SITE OF METABOLISM: Oxidation, kidneys
POTENTIAL SIDE EFFECTS: MAO inhibition, myelosuppression, rash, gastrointestinal upset, headache, fever, neuropathy, serotonin syndrome
TRADE NAMES: Zyvox

### Metronidazole
PRINCIPAL USES: Bacterial vaginosis, H. pylori eradication, anaerobic infections, C. difficile infection, trichomoniasis, Giardia, pelvic inflammatory disease, urethritis, amebic disease, meningitis, colorectal surgery prophylaxis, acne rosacea
ROUTE OF ADMINISTRATION: Oral, intravenous
SITE OF METABOLISM: Kidneys, liver
POTENTIAL SIDE EFFECTS: Gastrointestinal upset, dizziness, headache, vaginal candidiasis, Stevens-Johnson syndrome, neuropathy, seizure, ototoxicity
TRADE NAMES: Flagyl

### Nitrofurantoin
PRINCIPAL USES: Urinary tract infection treatment and prophylaxis
ROUTE OF ADMINISTRATION: Oral
SITE OF METABOLISM: Kidneys, liver
POTENTIAL SIDE EFFECTS: Gastrointestinal upset, neuropathy, hemolytic anemia, pulmonary disease
TRADE NAMES: Furadantin, Macrobid, Macrodantin

## Rifaximin

PRINCIPAL USES: Traveler's diarrhea, hepatic encephalopathy prophylaxis

ROUTE OF ADMINISTRATION: Oral

SITE OF METABOLISM: Feces

POTENTIAL SIDE EFFECTS: Peripheral edema, gastrointestinal upset, ascites, dizziness, headache, fatigue

TRADE NAMES: Xifaxan

## Quinupristin/dalfopristin

PRINCIPAL USES: Infection secondary to ampicillin-
and vancomycin-resistant Enterococcus, skin infections,

ROUTE OF ADMINISTRATION: Intravenous

SITE OF METABOLISM: Bile

POTENTIAL SIDE EFFECTS: Thrombophlebitis, injection site reactions, gastrointestinal upset, obstructive jaundice, arthralgias

TRADE NAMES: Synercid

## Tigecycline

PRINCIPAL USES: Skin infections, intra-abdominal infections, community-acquired pneumonia

ROUTE OF ADMINISTRATION: Intravenous

SITE OF METABOLISM: Bile, kidneys

POTENTIAL SIDE EFFECTS: Gastrointestinal upset, pancreatitis

TRADE NAMES: Tygacil

## Vancomycin

PRINCIPAL USES: *C. difficile*/*S. aureus* enterocolitis,
MRSA infection, infective endocarditis

ROUTE OF ADMINISTRATION: Intravenous, oral

SITE OF METABOLISM: Kidneys

POTENTIAL SIDE EFFECTS: Gastrointestinal upset, eryth-
roderma, thrombocytopenia, ototoxicity, nephrotoxicity, Red Man syndrome

TRADE NAMES: Vancocin

## ANTIVIRALS

## Abacavir

PRINCIPAL USES: HIV

ROUTE OF ADMINISTRATION: Oral

SITE OF METABOLISM: Liver

POTENTIAL SIDE EFFECTS: Hypersensitivity, rash, gastrointestinal upset, headache, fever, fatigue, Stevens-Johnson syndrome, hepatomegaly, hepatotoxicity

TRADE NAMES: Ziagen, ABC

## Acyclovir

PRINCIPAL USES: Acute treatment of and daily chronic
suppressive therapy for genital herpes, varicella
zoster, chickenpox, HSV encephalitis, neonatal HSV
infection

ROUTE OF ADMINISTRATION: Oral, intravenous

SITE OF METABOLISM: Kidneys

POTENTIAL SIDE EFFECTS: Contact dermatitis, gastrointestinal upset, headache, malaise, Stevens-Johnson syndrome, thrombotic thrombocytopenic purpura, renal failure

TRADE NAMES: Zovirax

## Adefovir

PRINCIPAL USES: Chronic hepatitis B

ROUTE OF ADMINISTRATION: Oral

SITE OF METABOLISM: Kidneys

POTENTIAL SIDE EFFECTS: Nephrotoxicity, lactic acidosis, hepatic steatosis, asthenia, pancreatitis

TRADE NAMES: Hepsera

## Amantadine

PRINCIPAL USES: Influenza treatment and prophylaxis,
extrapyramidal syndrome, Parkinsonism

ROUTE OF ADMINISTRATION: Oral

SITE OF METABOLISM: Kidneys

POTENTIAL SIDE EFFECTS: Peripheral edema, ortho-
static hypotension, gastrointestinal upset, headache, confusion, insomnia, fatigue, psychiatric disturbances, congestive heart failure, hematologic
disturbances, neuroleptic malignant syndrome

TRADE NAMES: Symmetrel

## Atazanavir

PRINCIPAL USES: HIV

ROUTE OF ADMINISTRATION: Oral

SITE OF METABOLISM: Liver

POTENTIAL SIDE EFFECTS: Rash, gastrointestinal upset,
headache, hyperbilirubinemia, cardiac abnormalities, Stevens-Johnson syndrome

TRADE NAMES: Reyataz, ATV

## Cidofovir

Principal uses: CMV retinitis in persons with AIDS

Route of administration: Intravenous

Site of metabolism: Kidneys

Potential side effects: Nephrotoxicity, rash, gastrointestinal upset, headache, neutropenia

Trade names: Vistide

## Darunavir

Principal uses: HIV

Route of administration: Oral

Site of metabolism: Liver

Potential side effects: Elevated serum cholesterol/triglycerides, gastrointestinal upset, headache, hyperglycemia

Trade names: Prezista

## Didanosine

Principal uses: HIV

Route of administration: Oral

Site of metabolism: Liver, kidneys

Potential side effects: Rash, gastrointestinal upset, headache, elevated liver enzymes, myocardial infarction, Stevens-Johnson syndrome, pancreatitis, thrombocytopenia, hepatomegaly, rhabdomyolysis, optic neuritis, nephrotoxicity

Trade names: Videx, Videx EC, ddI

## Efavirenz

Principal uses: HIV

Route of administration: Oral

Site of metabolism: Liver

Potential side effects: Rash, elevated liver enzymes/triglycerides, gastrointestinal upset, dizziness, headache, depression, fever, prolonged QT interval, depression

Trade names: Sustiva, EFV

## Emtricitabine

Principal uses: HIV

Route of administration: Oral

Site of metabolism: Kidneys

Potential side effects: Hyperpigmentation, rash, gastrointestinal upset, dizziness, headache, depression, cough, hepatomegaly

Trade names: Emtriva, FTC

## Enfuvirtide

Principal uses: HIV

Route of administration: Subcutaneous

Site of metabolism: Serum

Potential side effects: Gastrointestinal upset, peripheral neuropathy, conjunctivitis, fatigue, pancreatitis, pneumonia

Trade names: Fuzeon, T-20

## Entecavir

Principal uses: Chronic hepatitis B

Route of administration: Oral

Site of metabolism: Kidneys

Potential side effects: Nausea, dizziness, headache, fatigue, lactic acidosis, hepatomegaly

Trade names: Baraclude

## Famciclovir

Principal uses: Acute treatment of and daily chronic suppressive therapy for genital herpes, oral herpes, varicella zoster

Route of administration: Oral

Site of metabolism: Kidneys

Potential side effects: Headache, gastrointestinal upset, dysmenorrheal, erythema multiforme

Trade names: Famvir

## Fosamprenavir

Principal uses: HIV

Route of administration: Oral

Site of metabolism: Liver

Potential side effects: Rash, gastrointestinal upset, headache, myocardial infection, Stevens-Johnson syndrome, neutropenia, nephrolithiasis, angioedema

Trade names: Lexiva, 908

## Foscarnet

Principal uses: CMV retinitis, HSV infection

Route of administration: Intravenous

Site of metabolism: Kidneys

Potential side effects: Nephrotoxicity, reduced seizure threshold, gastrointestinal upset, anemia, headache, fever, electrolyte disturbances

Trade names: Foscavir

## Ganciclovir

Principal uses: CMV infection/retinitis, HSV keratitis

Route of administration: Intravenous, oral

Site of metabolism: Kidneys

POTENTIAL SIDE EFFECTS: Myelosuppression, carcinogenic, teratogenic, decreased fertility, pruritus, sweating, gastrointestinal upset, ophthalmologic disturbances, fever, cardiac abnormalities, Stevens-Johnson syndrome, rhabdomyolysis, renal failure
TRADE NAMES: DHPG

## Indinavir
PRINCIPAL USES: HIV
ROUTE OF ADMINISTRATION: Oral
SITE OF METABOLISM: Liver, kidneys
POTENTIAL SIDE EFFECTS: Nephrolithiasis, gastrointestinal upset, lipodystrophy, hyperbilirubinemia, backache, hyperglycemia
TRADE NAMES: Crixivan, IDV

## Interferon-2b
PRINCIPAL USES: Chronic hepatitis B, chronic hepatitis C, Kaposi's sarcoma, condyloma acuminatum, follicular lymphoma, hairy cell leukemia, malignant melanoma
ROUTE OF ADMINISTRATION: Subcutaneous, intramuscular
SITE OF METABOLISM: Kidneys
POTENTIAL SIDE EFFECTS: Alopecia, rash, gastrointestinal upset, neutropenia, elevated liver enzymes, musculoskeletal pain, headache, asthenia, depression, fatigue, Stevens-Johnson syndrome, pancreatitis, cardiomyopathy, hepatotoxicity, rhabdomyolysis, pneumonitis
TRADE NAMES: Intron A

## Lamivudine
PRINCIPAL USES: HIV, chronic hepatitis B
ROUTE OF ADMINISTRATION: Oral
SITE OF METABOLISM: Kidneys
POTENTIAL SIDE EFFECTS: Gastrointestinal upset, lipodystrophy, headache, fatigue, lactic acidosis, pancreatitis, hepatomegaly
TRADE NAMES: Epivir, Epivir-HBV, 3TC

## Maraviroc
PRINCIPAL USES: HIV
ROUTE OF ADMINISTRATION: Oral
SITE OF METABOLISM: Liver, kidneys
POTENTIAL SIDE EFFECTS: Hepatotoxicity, rash, bacterial superinfection, dizziness, cough, fever, cardiac disturbances, myositis, seizure, secondary neoplasm
TRADE NAMES: Selzentry

## Nelfinavir
PRINCIPAL USES: HIV
ROUTE OF ADMINISTRATION: Oral
SITE OF METABOLISM: Liver
POTENTIAL SIDE EFFECTS: Lipodystrophy, diarrhea, prolonged QT interval, hyperglycemia
TRADE NAMES: Viracept, NFV

## Nevirapine
PRINCIPAL USES: HIV
ROUTE OF ADMINISTRATION: Oral
SITE OF METABOLISM: Liver, kidneys
POTENTIAL SIDE EFFECTS: Hepatotoxicity, rash, lipodystrophy, Stevens-Johnson syndrome, gastrointestinal upset, hematologic disturbances, rhabdomyolysis
TRADE NAMES: Viramune, NVP

## Oseltamivir
PRINCIPAL USES: Treatment and prophylaxis for influenza
ROUTE OF ADMINISTRATION: Oral
SITE OF METABOLISM: Liver, kidneys
POTENTIAL SIDE EFFECTS: Gastrointestinal upset, dysrhythmia, Stevens-Johnson syndrome, hepatitis, seizures, delirium
TRADE NAMES: Tamiflu

## Palivizumab
PRINCIPAL USES: RSV prophylaxis in high-risk infants
ROUTE OF ADMINISTRATION: Intramuscular
SITE OF METABOLISM: Liver
POTENTIAL SIDE EFFECTS: Upper respiratory tract infection, thrombocytopenia
TRADE NAMES: Synagis

## Peginterferon alfa-2a
PRINCIPAL USES: Chronic hepatitis C, chronic hepatitis B
ROUTE OF ADMINISTRATION: Subcutaneous
SITE OF METABOLISM: Liver, kidneys
POTENTIAL SIDE EFFECTS: Alopecia, dermatitis, weight loss, gastrointestinal upset, thrombocytopenia, myalgias, dizziness, headache, insomnia, anxiety, irritability, cough, fatigue, rigors, Stevens-Johnson syndrome, hematologic disturbances, neuropathy, myositis
TRADE NAMES: Pegasys

**Peginterferon alfa-2b**
Principal uses: Chronic hepatitis C
Route of administration: Subcutaneous
Site of metabolism: Kidneys
Potential side effects: Alopecia, hyperuricemia, gastrointestinal upset, myalgias, dizziness, headache, insomnia, pharyngitis, fever, rigors, pancreatitis, visual disturbances, psychiatric disturbances
Trade names: PEG-Intron

**Ribavirin**
Principal uses: Severe RSV infections, hepatitis C
Route of administration: Aerosol, oral
Site of metabolism: Lung, cellular, kidneys
Potential side effects: Rash, gastrointestinal upset, neutropenia, headache, fatigue, cardiac/hematologic/electrolyte disturbances, suicidal ideation
Trade names: Virazole, Rebetol, Copegus, Ribasphere

**Ritonavir**
Principal uses: HIV
Route of administration: Oral
Site of metabolism: Liver
Potential side effects: Elevated cholesterol, gastrointestinal upset, parasthesias, Stevens-Johnson syndrome, cardiac abnormalities, pancreatitis, neutropenia, nephrotoxicity
Trade names: Norvir, RTV

**Saquinavir**
Principal uses: HIV
Route of administration: Oral
Site of metabolism: Liver
Potential side effects: Lipodystrophy, gastrointestinal upset, cardiac arrhythmias
Trade names: Invirase, SQV

**Stavudine**
Principal uses: HIV
Route of administration: Oral
Site of metabolism: Liver, kidneys
Potential side effects: Rash, gastrointestinal upset, headache, neuropathy, anemia, pancreatitis, hepatomegaly, Guillain-Barré syndrome
Trade names: Zerit, d4T

**Telbivudine**
Principal uses: Chronic hepatitis B
Route of administration: Oral
Site of metabolism: Kidneys
Potential side effects: Elevated creatine kinase/liver enzymes, headache, cough, fatigue
Trade names: Tyzeka

**Tenofovir**
Principal uses: HIV, chronic hepatitis B
Route of administration: Oral
Site of metabolism: Kidneys
Potential side effects: Rash, gastrointestinal upset, asthenia, hepatomegaly, osteopenia, nephrotoxicity
Trade names: Viread, TDF

**Tipranavir**
Principal uses: HIV
Route of administration: Oral
Site of metabolism: Feces
Potential side effects: Hepatotoxicity, rash, hyperlipidemia, gastrointestinal upset, fatigue, fever, pancreatitis
Trade names: Aptivus

**Valacyclovir**
Principal uses: Acute treatment of and daily chronic suppressive therapy for genital herpes, oral herpes, varicella zoster, varicella
Route of administration: Oral
Site of metabolism: Kidneys
Potential side effects: Rash, gastrointestinal upset, headache, fatigue, seizure
Trade names: Valtrex

**Valganciclovir**
Principal uses: CMV retinitis, CMV prophylaxis in persons at high risk
Route of administration: Oral
Site of metabolism: Kidneys
Potential side effects: Myelosuppression, carcinogenic, teratogenic, decreased fertility, gastrointestinal upset, fever
Trade names: Valcyte

**Zidovudine**
Principal uses: HIV treatment and post-exposure prophylaxis
Route of administration: Oral
Site of metabolism: Liver, kidneys
Potential side effects: Gastrointestinal upset, headache, insomnia, malaise, neutropenia
Trade names: Retrovir, AZT, ZDV

# ANTIFUNGALS

## Amphotericin B

PRINCIPAL USES: Mucocutaneous leishmaniasis, aspergillosis, blastomycosis, candidiasis, coccidioidomycosis, cryptococcal meningitis, histoplasmosis, mucormycosis, sporotrichosis

ROUTE OF ADMINISTRATION: Intravenous

SITE OF METABOLISM: Tissue

POTENTIAL SIDE EFFECTS: Weight loss, gastrointestinal upset, headache, malaise, dysrhythmias, hypokalemia, thrombocytopenia, seizure, nephrotoxicity

TRADE NAMES: Amphotec, Abelcet, AmBisome, Fungizone

## Anidulafungin

PRINCIPAL USES: Candidemia, esophageal candidiasis

ROUTE OF ADMINISTRATION: Intravenous

SITE OF METABOLISM: Chemical

POTENTIAL SIDE EFFECTS: Hypokalemia, diarrhea, DVT

TRADE NAMES: Eraxis

## Caspofungin

PRINCIPAL USES: Aspergillosis, candidal infection, neutropenic fever prophylaxis

ROUTE OF ADMINISTRATION: Intravenous

SITE OF METABOLISM: Kidney, liver

POTENTIAL SIDE EFFECTS: Hypotension, rash, diarrhea, elevated liver enzymes, fever, shivering, Stevens-Johnson syndrome, pancreatitis, nephrotoxicity

TRADE NAMES: Cancidas

## Clotrimazole

PRINCIPAL USES: Vaginal candidiasis, oropharyngeal candidiasis, pityriasis versicolor, tinea infections

ROUTE OF ADMINISTRATION: Oral

SITE OF METABOLISM: Liver

POTENTIAL SIDE EFFECTS: Gastrointestinal upset, elevated liver enzymes

TRADE NAMES: Clotrimaderm, Mycelex

## Fluconazole

PRINCIPAL USES: Vaginal, oropharyngeal, esophageal, and systemic candidiasis, cryptococcal meningitis

ROUTE OF ADMINISTRATION: Oral, intravenous

SITE OF METABOLISM: Kidney

POTENTIAL SIDE EFFECTS: Nausea, increased liver enzymes, headache, Stevens-Johnson syndrome

TRADE NAMES: Diflucan

## Flucytosine

PRINCIPAL USES: Candidiasis, cryptococcal infections

ROUTE OF ADMINISTRATION: Oral

SITE OF METABOLISM: Kidney

POTENTIAL SIDE EFFECTS: Myelosuppression, gastrointestinal upset, headache, confusion, hallucinations, thrombocytopenia

TRADE NAMES: Ancobon

## Griseofulvin

PRINCIPAL USES: Tinea infections, onychomycosis

ROUTE OF ADMINISTRATION: Oral

SITE OF METABOLISM: Skin

POTENTIAL SIDE EFFECTS: Photosensitivity, rash, gastrointestinal upset, headache

TRADE NAMES: Grisactin 500, Grifulvin V

## Itraconazole

PRINCIPAL USES: Onychomycosis, oropharyngeal/esophageal candidiasis, empiric treatment of suspected fungal infection in persons with neutropenia, aspergillosis, blastomycosis, histoplasmosis

ROUTE OF ADMINISTRATION: Oral, intravenous

SITE OF METABOLISM: Liver

POTENTIAL SIDE EFFECTS: Many drug interactions, negative inotropic agent, hypokalemia, rash, gastrointestinal upset, Stevens-Johnson syndrome, congestive heart failure, neutropenia

TRADE NAMES: Sporanox

## Ketoconazole

PRINCIPAL USES: Blastomycosis, candidal infections, chromoblastomycosis, coccidioidomycosis, seborrheic dermatitis, histoplasmosis, pityriasis versicolor, tinea infections

ROUTE OF ADMINISTRATION: Oral

SITE OF METABOLISM: Liver

POTENTIAL SIDE EFFECTS: Hepatotoxicity, many drug interactions, pruritis, gastrointestinal upset

TRADE NAMES: Nizoral

## Micafungin

PRINCIPAL USES: Candidal infections, prophylaxis for candida in bone marrow transplant recipients

ROUTE OF ADMINISTRATION: Intravenous

SITE OF METABOLISM: Liver, feces

POTENTIAL SIDE EFFECTS: Rash, gastrointestinal upset,

anemia, headache, hematologic disturbances
TRADE NAMES: Mycamine

### Nystatin
PRINCIPAL USES: Oral thrush, vaginal candidiasis
ROUTE OF ADMINISTRATION: Oral
SITE OF METABOLISM: None
POTENTIAL SIDE EFFECTS: Gastrointestinal upset
TRADE NAMES: Mycostatin, Nyaderm, Candistatin

### Posaconazole
PRINCIPAL USES: Prophylaxis for disseminated Aspergillus or Candida, candidal infections
ROUTE OF ADMINISTRATION: Oral
SITE OF METABOLISM: Glucuronidation
POTENTIAL SIDE EFFECTS: Hypokalemia, gastrointestinal upset, headache, fever, prolonged QT syndrome
TRADE NAMES: Noxafil

### Terbinafine
PRINCIPAL USES: Onychomycosis, dermal mycosis, tinea capitis
ROUTE OF ADMINISTRATION: Oral
SITE OF METABOLISM: Liver, kidney
POTENTIAL SIDE EFFECTS: Diarrhea, headache, Stevens-Johnson syndrome, neutropenia, systemic lupus erythematosis
TRADE NAMES: Lamisil

### Voriconazole
PRINCIPAL USES: Candidiasis, aspergillosis, mycosis
ROUTE OF ADMINISTRATION: Oral
SITE OF METABOLISM: Liver
POTENTIAL SIDE EFFECTS: Peripheral edema, rash, gastrointestinal upset, headache, hallucinations, fever, prolonged QT interval, Stevens-Johnson syndrome, pancreatitis, encephalopathy, optic neuritis
TRADE NAMES: Vfend

## ANTIMALARIALS

### Atovaquone/proguanil
PRINCIPAL USES: Antimalarial prophylaxis and treatment
ROUTE OF ADMINISTRATION: Oral
SITE OF METABOLISM: Feces, liver, kidney
POTENTIAL SIDE EFFECTS: Gastrointestinal upset, increased liver enzymes, dizziness, headache, cough, Stevens-Johnson syndrome, neutropenia
TRADE NAMES: Malarone

### Chloroquine
PRINCIPAL USES: Antimalarial prophylaxis and treatment in regions with malaria still sensitive to chloroquine, amebic infections
ROUTE OF ADMINISTRATION: Oral
SITE OF METABOLISM: Kidney, liver
POTENTIAL SIDE EFFECTS: Cardiac disturbances, gastrointestinal upset, seizure, retinopathy
TRADE NAMES: Aralen

### Mefloquine
PRINCIPAL USES: Antimalarial prophylaxis and treatment in areas resistant to chloroquine
ROUTE OF ADMINISTRATION: Oral

SITE OF METABOLISM: Liver
POTENTIAL SIDE EFFECTS: Bradycardia, gastrointestinal upset, dizziness, anxiety, depression, seizure, pneumonitis
TRADE NAMES: Lariam

### Primaquine
PRINCIPAL USES: Relapse-prevention of malaria
ROUTE OF ADMINISTRATION: Oral
SITE OF METABOLISM: Liver
POTENTIAL SIDE EFFECTS: Hemolysis in G6PD-deficient persons, gastrointestinal upset
TRADE NAMES: None

### Quinine
PRINCIPAL USES: Given malaria, nocturnal leg cramps
ROUTE OF ADMINISTRATION: Oral
SITE OF METABOLISM: Liver
POTENTIAL SIDE EFFECTS: Cinchonism, hemolysis in G6PD-deficient persons, thrombocytopenia, prolonged QT interval, gastrointestinal upset
TRADE NAMES: Qualaquin

## ANTIMYCOBACTERIALS

### Dapsone
PRINCIPAL USES: Leprosy, prophylaxis and treatment for Pneumocystis, acne, dermatitis herpetiformis
ROUTE OF ADMINISTRATION: Oral
SITE OF METABOLISM: Liver, kidneys
POTENTIAL SIDE EFFECTS: Erythema multiforme, gastrointestinal upset, hemolysis in persons with G6PD deficiency, hepatitis
TRADE NAMES: None

### Ethambutol
PRINCIPAL USES: Tuberculosis
ROUTE OF ADMINISTRATION: Oral
SITE OF METABOLISM: Liver, kidneys
POTENTIAL SIDE EFFECTS: Hyperuricemia, mania, gastrointestinal upset, neutropenia, thrombocytopenia, neuropathy, optic neuritis
TRADE NAMES: Myambutol

### Isoniazid
PRINCIPAL USES: Active/inactive tuberculosis treatment and prophylaxis
ROUTE OF ADMINISTRATION: Oral
SITE OF METABOLISM: Liver, kidneys
POTENTIAL SIDE EFFECTS: Hepatotoxicity
TRADE NAMES: INH

### Pyrazinamide
PRINCIPAL USES: Tuberculosis
ROUTE OF ADMINISTRATION: Oral
SITE OF METABOLISM: Liver, kidneys
POTENTIAL SIDE EFFECTS: Hepatotoxicity, neuropathy, psychiatric/hematologic disturbances
TRADE NAMES: PZA

### Rifabutin
PRINCIPAL USES: Mycobacterium avium-intracellulare prophylaxis
ROUTE OF ADMINISTRATION: Oral
SITE OF METABOLISM: Liver
POTENTIAL SIDE EFFECTS: Rash, gastrointestinal upset, uveitis, body fluid discoloration, neutropenia
TRADE NAMES: Mycobutin

### Rifampin
PRINCIPAL USES: Active/inactive tuberculosis, eradication of Neisseria meningitidis carrier state
ROUTE OF ADMINISTRATION: Oral, intravenous
SITE OF METABOLISM: Liver
POTENTIAL SIDE EFFECTS: Skin color changes, nausea, body fluid discoloration, thrombocytopenia, hepatotoxicity
TRADE NAMES: Rimactane, Rifadin

## ANTIPARASITICS

### Albendazole
PRINCIPAL USES: Neurocysticercosis, echinococcosis
ROUTE OF ADMINISTRATION: Oral
SITE OF METABOLISM: Liver
POTENTIAL SIDE EFFECTS: Gastrointestinal upset, headache, Stevens-Johnson syndrome, hematologic disturbances
TRADE NAMES: Albenza

### Atovaquone
PRINCIPAL USES: Pneumocystis treatment and prophylaxis
ROUTE OF ADMINISTRATION: Oral
SITE OF METABOLISM: Feces
POTENTIAL SIDE EFFECTS: Rash, gastrointestinal upset, headache, insomnia, cough, dyspnea, fever, Stevens-Johnson syndrome
TRADE NAMES: Mepron

### Ivermectin
PRINCIPAL USES: Strongyloidiasis, scabies, onchocerciasis
ROUTE OF ADMINISTRATION: Oral
SITE OF METABOLISM: Liver
POTENTIAL SIDE EFFECTS: Pruritis, dizziness, seizure
TRADE NAMES: Stromectol

### Mebendazole
PRINCIPAL USES: Pinworm, roundworm, whipworm, and hookworm infections
ROUTE OF ADMINISTRATION: Oral
SITE OF METABOLISM: Liver
POTENTIAL SIDE EFFECTS: Rash, gastrointestinal upset, headache
TRADE NAMES: Vermox

## Nitazoxanide

PRINCIPAL USES: Diarrhea secondary to Cryptosporidium or Giardia infection
ROUTE OF ADMINISTRATION: Oral
SITE OF METABOLISM: Liver
POTENTIAL SIDE EFFECTS: Gastrointestinal upset, headache
TRADE NAMES: Alinia

## Paromomycin

PRINCIPAL USES: Amebic infection, hepatic coma
ROUTE OF ADMINISTRATION: Oral
SITE OF METABOLISM: Not absorbed
POTENTIAL SIDE EFFECTS: Gastrointestinal upset
TRADE NAMES: Humatin

## Pentamidine

PRINCIPAL USES: Prophylaxis and treatment of pneumocystis
ROUTE OF ADMINISTRATION: Intramuscular, intravenous, aerosol
SITE OF METABOLISM: Kidneys
POTENTIAL SIDE EFFECTS: Rash, nausea, nephrotoxicity, bronchospasm, dyspnea, dysrhythmias, hypotension, pancreatitis, thrombocytopenia
TRADE NAMES: Pentam, NebuPent

## Praziquantel

PRINCIPAL USES: Schistosomiasis, neurocysticercosis, chlonorchiasis
ROUTE OF ADMINISTRATION: Oral
SITE OF METABOLISM: Liver, kidneys
POTENTIAL SIDE EFFECTS: Gastrointestinal upset, dizziness, fever, dysrhythmias, seizure
TRADE NAMES: Biltricide

## Pyrantel

PRINCIPAL USES: Pinworm and roundworm infections
ROUTE OF ADMINISTRATION: Oral
SITE OF METABOLISM: Not absorbed
POTENTIAL SIDE EFFECTS: Gastrointestinal upset, dizziness, headache, somnolence
TRADE NAMES: Antiminth, Pin-X, Pinworm

## Pyrimethamine

PRINCIPAL USES: Central nervous system toxoplasmosis in persons with AIDS, malaria
ROUTE OF ADMINISTRATION: Oral
SITE OF METABOLISM: Liver
POTENTIAL SIDE EFFECTS: Rash, Stevens-Johnson syndrome, leucopenia
TRADE NAMES: Daraprim

## Thiabendazole

PRINCIPAL USES: Helminth infections, strongyloidiasis, cutaneous larva migrans, ascariasis, trichinosis
ROUTE OF ADMINISTRATION: Oral
SITE OF METABOLISM: Liver, kidneys
POTENTIAL SIDE EFFECTS: Gastrointestinal upset, dizziness, drowsiness, Stevens-Johnson syndrome
TRADE NAMES: Mintezol

## Tinidazole

PRINCIPAL USES: Trichomoniasis, giardiasis, amebiasis, bacterial vaginosis
ROUTE OF ADMINISTRATION: Oral
SITE OF METABOLISM: Kidneys, liver
POTENTIAL SIDE EFFECTS: Nausea, vaginal candidiasis, parasthesias, neuropathy
TRADE NAMES: Tindamax

*Jennifer Birkhauser, M.D.*

# HISTORICAL RESOURCES

# Time Line of Major Developments in Infectious Disease

| YEAR | EVENT |
| --- | --- |
| **1700 B.C.E.** | The unknown writers of an ancient Egyptian text on trauma surgery known as the Edwin Smith Papyrus emphasize the importance of keeping wounds clean to prevent infection. They suggest applying such remedies as honey and moldy bread as anti-infectives. |
| **420 B.C.E.** | Hippocrates of Cos classifies diseases as acute, chronic, endemic, or epidemic–terms still used in the diagnosis and management of infectious disease. Hippocrates also introduces the notion that human health is based on balancing four bodily fluids (blood, yellow bile, black bile, and phlegm) that he calls humors and that disease results from imbalance among the humors rather than infectious organisms. |
| **c. 350 B.C.E.** | Aristotle, philosopher-tutor of Alexander the Great, writes a treatise on zoology translated into Latin as the *Historia animalium*, in which he synthesizes the opinions of earlier Greek philosophers to outline the notion of spontaneous generation. Aristotle's theory holds that life (including disease organisms) can emerge from nonliving matter that contains "vital heat." |
| **36 B.C.E.** | Marcus Terentius Varro, a Roman librarian, publishes *Rerum rusticarum* (*On Agriculture*), a treatise that enunciates an early version of the germ theory of disease. Varro warns against developing farms in swamps or marshes because "such locations breed certain minute creatures which cannot be seen by the eyes, but which float in the air and enter the body through the mouth and nose and cause serious diseases." |
| **25 B.C.E.** | Vitruvius, a Roman architect and engineer, dedicates his book on architecture to Augustus Caesar. Explaining why cities should not be built on or near wetlands, Vitruvius outlines what is called the miasmatic theory of infectious disease–namely, that disease is caused and spread by a miasma, or foul air, emanating from rotting plant and animal matter. The miasmatic theory of disease will hold sway throughout the Middle Ages and last until the 1850's. Although it will be disproved by the germ theory of disease, the miasmatic theory does lead to improvements in sanitation and water purification that reduce the severity of epidemics. |
| **169 C.E.** | Claudius Galen, personal physician to three successive Roman emperors, describes the plague that decimates the Empire during the reign of Marcus Aurelius in sufficient detail to allow it to be identified by modern epidemiologists as smallpox. Galen's emphasis on the importance of observation and keeping records of patients' symptoms to guide treatment becomes a major legacy to Western medicine. Galen, however, also hands Hippocrates' humoral theory of disease to the Middle Ages and to Islamic medicine. |
| **1025** | Ibn Sīnā (known in the West as Avicenna), a Persian physician, completes a fourteen-volume medical encyclopedia known as the *Canon of Medicine*. Based on the surviving works of Galen and Hippocrates, the *Canon* will be used in European medical schools as late as 1650. In the field of infectious disease, Ibn Sīnā identifies sexually transmitted diseases, recognizes tuberculosis as a contagious illness, and notes that infectious diseases can be spread by contaminated soil and water. |
| **1346** | In one of the earliest known episodes of germ warfare, the Mongol army besieging Kaffa (now Feodosiya) in the Crimea throws the corpses of Mongol soldiers who had died of bubonic plague over the city walls. This tactic is thought to have introduced the plague, or Black Death, to medieval Europe. |

| YEAR | EVENT |
|------|-------|
| 1545 | Ambroise Par, a French surgeon considered the founder of battlefield medicine, publishes an essay recommending the application of topical antiseptics, rather than boiling oil (which was standard practice at the time), to prevent infection in soldiers' wounds. Par's preferred antiseptic is a mixture of turpentine, egg yolk, and rose oil. |
| 1546 | Girolamo Fracastoro, an Italian physician, writes a treatise on infectious diseases in which he introduces the concept of fomites–inanimate objects or substances that can be contaminated and can transfer disease organisms from one person to another. Fracastoro also identifies typhus for the first time and gives syphilis its present name. |
| 1578 | Li Shihzen, an eminent Chinese physician and pharmacologist, completes the first draft of the *Bencao Gangmu*, usually translated into English as the *Compendium Materia Medica*. Li not only compiles the largest reference work on anti-infective plants and prescriptions in Chinese medicine until its replacement in 1959 but also introduces the use of steam and fumigation to prevent the spread of infectious disease. |
| 1668 | Francesco Redi, an Italian physician, publishes an account of experiments with covered and uncovered jars containing pieces of meat and fish that disprove the commonly accepted belief that maggots arise spontaneously from decaying food. Redi's experiments are the first step toward disproving Aristotle's theory of spontaneous generation. |
| 1680 | Antoni van Leeuwenhoek, a Dutch tradesman and scientist, is elected a fellow of the English Royal Society for his observations of single-celled organisms conducted with his handmade microscopes. Leeuwenhoek refers to these microorganisms as "animalcules," or tiny animals. |
| 1796 | Edward Jenner, an English scientist, inoculates an eight-year-old boy with material from a milkmaid's cowpox blisters and then goes on to demonstrate that the inoculation produced immunity to smallpox. By 1840, Jenner's vaccine is so widely accepted that the British government provides vaccination to its citizens free of charge. |
| 1847 | Ignaz Semmelweis, a Hungarian physician working in Vienna, reduces maternal mortality from puerperal fever from 35 percent to less than 1 percent by insisting that doctors and medical students disinfect their hands (at that time, by using a solution of chlorinated lime) before attending to patients in childbirth. |
| 1855 | John Snow, an English physician, publishes the second edition of his essay *On the Mode of Communication of Cholera* following an 1854 outbreak in the Soho neighborhood of London. Although the germ theory of disease has not yet been fully elaborated, Snow is skeptical of the prevailing miasmatic theory. He traces the Soho outbreak to a public water pump on Broad Street by interviewing residents and mapping clusters of cholera cases. Snow's study marks the beginning of modern epidemiology. |
| 1857 | A controversy begins between Justus von Liebig, an eminent German chemist, and Louis Pasteur, a French bacteriologist, over the nature of fermentation. Liebig maintains that fermentation (and by extension human disease) can be explained as chemical changes taking place in the presence of oxygen without the involvement of microscopic organisms–sometimes called the mechanistic theory of disease. Pasteur argues that fermentation requires the presence of living (yeast) cells. Over the next two decades, Pasteur's view slowly gains acceptance. |
| 1862 | Pasteur conducts the first test of the process eventually known as pasteurization to prevent the spoilage of milk, beer, and wine by bacterial or fungal contamination. His experiments with |

| YEAR | EVENT |
|------|-------|
| **1862 (cont.)** | boiled broths in vessels containing filters or long swan-shaped necks that trap dust particles follow up on Redi's earlier experiments in disproving spontaneous generation. Pasteur's 1870 experiments with yeasts growing in the absence of oxygen succeed in disproving Liebig's mechanistic theory. |
| **1867** | Joseph Lister, an English surgeon, publishes a paper in the *British Medical Journal*, "On the Antiseptic Principle of the Practice of Surgery," describing his use of carbolic acid to disinfect surgical instruments as well as practitioners' hands inside the operating theater. Lister is one of only two British surgeons honored with a public statue. |
| **1877** | Robert Koch, a German physician, identifies the bacterium that causes anthrax. This discovery is followed by the identification of the tuberculosis bacterium in 1882 and the successful isolation of *Vibrio cholerae* in 1883. Koch is awarded the 1905 Nobel Prize in Physiology or Medicine for his work on tuberculosis. |
| **1884** | Robert Koch and his colleague Friedrich Loeffler work out a set of four postulates for establishing a causal relationship between a specific microorganism and a specific disease. Published in 1890, Koch's postulates stipulate the following: The suspected microorganism must be found in large numbers in all organisms with the disease but should not be found in healthy ones; the microorganism must be isolated from a diseased subject and grown in a pure culture; the cultured microorganism should cause disease when injected into a healthy subject; and the microorganism must be isolated from the diseased experimental subject and shown to be identical to the original causative microorganism. Koch eventually abandons the first postulate when he identifies asymptomatic carriers of cholera and typhoid fever. |
| **1885** | Louis Pasteur successfully treats a nine-year-old boy bitten by a rabid dog with a vaccine that he had developed but had tested only on animals. The success of Pasteur's vaccine leads to the foundation of Pasteur Institute in 1887, a research institution that has produced many leaders in the field of infectious diseases. |
| **1892** | Dimitri Ivanovsky, a Russian biologist, identifies a virus as the cause of tobacco mosaic. The new type of infectious organism is given its name by Martinus Beijerinck, a Dutch microbiologist, in 1898. Beijerinck, however, mistakenly identifies viruses as liquid in nature, a theory later disproved by Wendell Stanley. |
| **1894** | Alexandre Yersin, a researcher at the Pasteur Institute, and Kitasato Shibasaburō, a Japanese bacteriologist, discover the bacterium that causes bubonic plague during an outbreak of the disease in Hong Kong. The plague bacterium, originally named *Pasteurella pestis*, is renamed *Yersinia pestis* in Yersin's honor in 1967. |
| **1897** | Ronald Ross, a British physician working in India, works out the entire life cycle of the malaria parasite and its transmission by mosquitoes from sick animals or humans to healthy ones. He is awarded the 1902 Nobel Prize in Physiology or Medicine for his work on malaria. |
| **1900** | Walter Reed, a U.S. military physician, and Carlos Finlay, a Cuban public health specialist, show that yellow fever is transmitted to humans by a mosquito vector rather than by direct contact. Their proof of Finlay's hypothesis, first outlined in 1881, gives further impetus to the new field of epidemiology. UNESCO's biennial prize in microbiology is named in honor of Finlay. |
| **1909** | Paul Ehrlich, a German researcher who had already been awarded the 1908 Nobel Prize in Physiology or Medicine for his work in immunology, discovers Salvarsan, an arsenic compound |

| YEAR | EVENT |
|------|-------|
| **1909 (cont.)** | that is more effective in treating syphilis than the mercury compounds then in use. Salvarsan becomes the most frequently prescribed drug in the world from 1910 until the emergence of penicillin as a treatment for syphilis in the 1940's. |
| **1932-1972** | The Tuskegee Public Health Service Syphilis Study, a forty-year study of African American sharecroppers diagnosed with syphilis, becomes the most infamous study of infectious disease in U.S. history. It was revealed that the researchers failed to treat the infected men with penicillin after the antibiotic was shown to be effective against syphilis in the 1940's. The scandal leads to the establishment of the Office for Human Research Protections (OHRP) and new regulatory safeguards to protect human subjects participating in clinical research. |
| **1937-1945** | The Imperial Japanese army operates Unit 731, a covert biological research unit that conducts lethal experiments on humans and develops methods of germ warfare for use on Chinese civilians. Experiments involve injecting women, infants, and the elderly as well as prisoners of war with disease organisms and vivisecting them to study the effects of the diseases on internal organs. The number of people estimated to have died as a result of Unit 731's research is 580,000. |
| **1942** | The Office of National Defense Malaria Control Activities is founded in Atlanta as a branch of the U.S. Public Health Service. The organization is renamed several times: the National Communicable Disease Center (NCDC) in 1967, the Centers for Disease Control (CDC) in 1980, and the Centers for Disease Control and Prevention in 1992. It is still known as the CDC. |
| **1945** | Sir Alexander Fleming shares the Nobel Prize in Physiology or Medicine with Baron Florey, an Australian pathologist, and Ernst Boris Chain, a German-born British biochemist, for the discovery of penicillin. Penicillin is credited with permanently changing the treatment of bacterial infections. |
| | The U.S. Army introduces the first influenza vaccine made from inactivated viruses to protect soldiers against the epidemic expected during the upcoming winter. |
| **1948** | The World Health Organization (WHO) is constituted by the General Assembly of the United Nations as the successor organization of the League of Nations Health Organization. WHO's mandate includes not only controlling outbreaks of infectious diseases but also distributing vaccines, diagnostic equipment, and drugs to prevent or treat these diseases. |
| **1952** | Dorothy Horstmann, an American epidemiologist, demonstrates that the polio virus reaches the brain through the bloodstream rather than growing within the nervous system itself, as was previously thought. Horstmann's work makes possible the development of both the Salk and the Sabin polio vaccines. Horstmann becomes the first female full professor of medicine at Yale in 1961. |
| | Selman Waksman, a Russian-born American biochemist, is awarded the Nobel Prize in Physiology or Medicine for his discovery of streptomycin, the first drug that proves able to cure tuberculosis. Waksman also coins the term "antibiotic." |
| **1955** | The killed-virus polio vaccine developed by Jonas Salk at the University of Pittsburgh passes its field trials and is publicly announced as safe and effective. Salk is honored in 1956 with a gold medal presented by U.S. president Dwight D. Eisenhower. |
| **1962** | The oral live-virus polio vaccine developed by Albert Sabin at the University of Cincinnati is licensed for public distribution. |

| YEAR | EVENT |
|------|-------|
| 1967 | The discovery of the first filovirus, Marburg virus, followed by the identification of Ebola virus in 1976, intensifies concern about previously unknown zoonoses–infectious diseases transmitted to humans by nonhuman animals. |
| 1969 | The retroviral disease later known as acquired immunodeficiency syndrome (AIDS) enters North America through a single infected immigrant from Haiti. |
| 1979 | Robert Gallo, an American virologist, successfully isolates the first human retrovirus, HTLV-1, which causes T cell leukemia and lymphoma in adults. |
| 1980 | The World Health Organization declares smallpox to have been eradicated–the only infectious disease affecting humans to have been eradicated. |
| 1982 | Stanley B. Prusiner, an American neurologist, coins the term "prion," from the words "protein" and "infectious," to describe the causative agents of bovine spongiform encephalopathy and Creutzfeldt-Jakob disease. Prusiner is awarded the Nobel Prize in Physiology or Medicine in 1997 for his work on prions. |
| | The CDC renames an emerging retroviral disease called gay-related immune deficiency (GRID) as AIDS. |
| 1988 | The World Health Organization, United Nations Children's Fund (UNICEF), and the Rotary Foundation begin a global campaign to eradicate polio. |
| 1993 | Terry Yates, a biologist at the University of New Mexico, identifies a hantavirus as the cause of a mysterious respiratory illness killing people in the Four Corners region of the United States and identifies the deer mouse as the vector of the disease. |
| 1994 | The CDC certifies that the Americas are polio-free; in 2002, the World Health Organization certifies that Europe is polio-free. |
| 1996 | Maurice Hilleman, an American microbiologist, introduces the first vaccine against hepatitis A. Hilleman develops more than three dozen vaccines in the course of his career and is credited with saving more lives than any other twentieth-century scientist. Eight of Hilleman's vaccines are still routinely administered; in addition to the hepatitis A vaccine, they include vaccines against chickenpox, *Haemophilus influenzae*, hepatitis B, measles, meningitis, mumps, and pneumonia. |
| 2001 | Two sets of letters containing anthrax spores are mailed to various U.S. politicians and American news organizations not long after the terrorist attacks of September 11. The Amerithrax case, as the Federal Bureau of Investigation names it, reawakens widespread fears of biological warfare and triggers one of the most complicated investigations in the history of American law enforcement. |
| 2008 | Luc Montagnier and Françoise Barré-Sinoussi of the Pasteur Institute share the Nobel Prize in Physiology or Medicine for their discovery of the human immunodeficiency virus (HIV) as the cause of AIDS with Harald zur Hausen, a German virologist who discovered the role of human papillomavirus (HPV) infection in cervical cancer. |
| 2010 | A malaria vaccine developed by the pharmaceutical company GlaxoSmithKline begins late-stage clinical testing at eleven sites in seven African nations. It was hoped that the vaccine could be submitted for approval by regulatory bodies as early as 2011. |

*Rebecca J. Frey, Ph.D.*

# Biographical Dictionary of Scientists in Infectious Disease

**al-Rāzī (c. 864-c. 925):** Also known as Rhazes or Bakr Muhammad ibn Zakariyā, Arabic physician who developed the first clinical description differentiating measles and smallpox. He also was a noted pediatrician, among the first physicians emphasizing that field.

**Avery, Oswald (1877-1955):** Canadian-born American physician who with his colleagues Colin MacLeod and Maclyn McCarty determined that deoxyribonucleic acid (DNA) is the genetic material in cells. Avery was also noted for his pioneering work on the biochemistry of the pneumococcus, the etiological agent for most forms of bacterial pneumonia.

**Baltimore, David (1938-    ):** American molecular biologist and Nobel laureate (1975) who was a co-discoverer of reverse transcriptase, the enzyme found in ribonucleic acid (RNA) tumor virus and human immunodeficiency virus (HIV), which copies RNA into deoxyribonucleic acid (DNA).

**Bancroft, Edward (1744-1821):** American physician who, in 1769, observed that yaws, an infectious disease common in hot, humid climates, is transmitted by flies. The agent was later determined to be *Treponema pertenue*, a spirochaete similar to that which causes syphilis.

**Bang, Bernhard Lauritz Frederik (1848-1932):** Danish veterinarian who discovered *Brucella abortus*, the agent causing Bang's disease in nonhuman animals and undulant fever (brucellosis) in humans.

**Barr, Yvonne (1932-    ):** British virologist who, with Michael Epstein, identified the etiological agent of infectious mononucleosis and Burkitt's lymphoma. The agent was later named the Epstein-Barr virus.

**Bassi, Agostino (1773-1856):** Italian entomologist who applied his study of silkworm disease to the theory that human diseases too are caused by microscopic agents.

**Bayle, Gaspard Laurent (1774-1816):** French physician who described the pathological distinctions among different forms of tuberculosis.

**Behring, Emil von (1854-1917):** German physician and Nobel laureate (1901) honored for his discovery of the etiological agent of diphtheria and the role played by the toxin it produces in development of the disease.

**Beijerinck, Martinus (1851-1931):** Dutch microbiologist who demonstrated that cell-free filtrates, which he called contagium vivum fluidum, could be used to transmit tobacco mosaic disease. Because he published this work, Beijerinck is often credited with the discovery of viruses. He is better known for his studies of nitrogen and sulfur cycling in nature.

**Bergey, David Hendricks (1860-1937):** American physician and microbiologist who developed the modern taxonomic classification scheme for bacteria. Each updated edition of *Bergey's Manual of Systemic Bacteriology* remains the bible of microbiology into the twenty-first century.

**Billroth, Theodor (1829-1894):** German physician noted for his innovations in abdominal surgery. In 1874, he described several forms of coccal-shaped bacteria in pus-filled infections, coining the term "strepto" (chains) and "coccus" (berries).

**Bishop, J. Michael (1936-    )** American molecular biologist and Nobel laureate who proposed that mutations in cellular oncogenes, first discovered in ribonucleic acid (RNA) tumor viruses, are the molecular basis for some forms of cancer.

**Bittner, John J. (1904-1961):** American biologist credited with the first isolation of a mammalian tumor virus, the mouse mammary tumor virus.

**Blumberg, Baruch S. (1925-    ):** American physician and Nobel laureate (1976) who isolated hepatitis B virus (HBV) and was instrumental in the development of the HBV vaccine.

**Bordet, Jules (1870-1961):** Belgian physician and Nobel laureate (1919) who developed serological techniques used to diagnose infectious diseases. Bordet also isolated the pertussis (whooping cough) bacillus, which received the genus name *Bordetella* in his honor.

**Boylston, Zabdiel (1679-1766):** American physician who introduced variolation into Boston during the 1720's as a means to immunize against smallpox.

**Bretonneau, Pierre (1778-1862):** French physician who was the first to identify typhoid fever and diphtheria. His description of the pseudo-membrane in the throats of persons with diphtheria improved the ability to diagnose the disease.

**Brill, Nathan Edwin (1860-1925):** American physician who first described the form of typhus called Brill's disease (Brill-Zinsser disease), an illness associated with louse or flea-borne transmission of *Rickettsia prowazekii*.

**Bruce, David (1855-1931):** Australian physician whose investigation of Malta fever among British forces on the island of Malta during the 1880's led to his determination of the bacterial cause of the disease. The agent was later named *Brucella*, while the disease became known as brucellosis. Bruce later determined the disease African sleeping sickness was the result of a trypanosome infection transmitted by the tsetse fly.

**Budd, William (1811-1880):** British physician who was among the first advocates of the theory that infectious diseases such as cholera and typhoid fever are transmitted through sewage-contaminated water.

**Buist, John Brown (1846-1915):** British microbiologist who, while staining lymphatic fluid from a cowpox vessel, was the first to observe pox viruses. Brown mistook the particles for spores.

**Burgdorfer, Willy (c. 1925-    ):** Swiss-born American scientist who discovered the etiological agent for Lyme disease in 1981, with the organism named *Borrelia burgdorferi* in his honor.

**Burnet, Frank Macfarlane (1899-1985):** Australian physician and Nobel laureate (1960) known primarily for his contributions to immunology. Burnet identified the staphylococcal toxin in a contaminated diphtheria vaccine associated with an outbreak in Bundaberg, Australia, in 1928. In 1933, he was a member of the team that isolated the influenza virus, proving that the disease was of viral and not bacterial origin. Burnet also contributed to the understanding of the epidemiology of herpesviruses.

**Carroll, James (1854-1907):** British-born American physician who, as a member of the Walter Reed Commission in Cuba in 1900, helped confirm the role of the mosquito in transmission of yellow fever.

**Chamberland, Charles (1851-1908):** French microbiologist and colleague of Louis Pasteur who developed a porcelain filter that could be used to size microorganisms. The ability of infectious material small enough to pass the filter led to the discovery of viruses. Chamberland helped develop a vaccine against chicken cholera using an attenuated form of the bacillus.

**Chanock, Robert M. (1924-2010):** American physician and virologist who discovered respiratory syncytial virus, a common cause of sometimes serious respiratory infections in children, and also isolated parainfluenza viruses.

**Cohn, Ferdinand Julius (1828-1898):** German microbiologist who developed the first classification system for microorganisms. Working with Robert Koch, Cohn discovered certain bacteria are capable of surviving environmental challenges in a spore state.

**Coley, William Bradley (1862-1936):** American surgeon who in the 1890's discovered that the induction of erysipelas, a streptococcal infection, in persons with cancer sometimes resulted in regression of the disease. Subsequent injection of *Streptococcus* produced similar results. In the late twentieth century, it was determined that the likely explanation for this regression was induction of tumor necrosis factor by the infectious agent in the person with cancer.

**Crick, Francis (1916-2004):** British X-ray crystallographer and Nobel laureate (1962) who, with colleague American molecular biologist James Watson and with the work of X-ray crystallographer Rosalind Franklin, produced the first accurate model of deoxyribonucleic acid (DNA) structure.

**Dalldorf, Gilbert (1900-1997):** American physician who discovered and classified coxsackie viruses, agents that cause an illness similar to that of a mild polio infection. Coxsackie viruses were the first of numerous human viruses isolated in fecal material. Dalldorf also demonstrated the effects of virus interference, that coinfection by different viruses may result in modifying the infection by each.

**Davaine, Casimir (1812-1882):** French physician who first discovered the presence of bacteria in the blood of animals sick with anthrax. While Davaine was unable to definitively prove these were the etiological agents, he did demonstrate that in their absence the blood from the animal was not infectious.

**Dochez, Alphonse (1882-1964):** American physician who, with his colleague Oswald Avery, observed the presence of antibodies in the blood of persons with pneumococcal pneumonia. Dochez and Avery used the purified antibody to establish passive immunity in treating the disease. Dochez later applied the same procedures to demonstrate scarlet fever is a streptococcal infection.

**Domagk, Gerhard (1895-1964):** German physician and Nobel laureate (1939) whose discovery of the sulfa drugs (sulfanilamide) led to the first effective broad-spectrum antibiotic.

**Douglass, William (1691-1752):** Scottish physician who, in 1736 in New England, provided the first clinical description of scarlet fever, a streptococcal infection.

**Dulbecco, Renato (1914-    ):** Italian American physician, virologist, and Nobel laureate (1975) who, in 1952, reported a plaque assay for quantifying the number of virus particles in a sample. The method was first adapted for growth of polio and equine encephalitis virus and later applied to numerous animal viruses.

**Eberth, Karl Joseph (1835-1926):** German pathologist who in the 1880's discovered the etiological agent of typhoid fever. The organism was originally assigned the genus name *Eberthella*; the name later changed to *Salmonella*.

**Ehrlich, Paul (1854-1915):** German physician and immunologist whose side-chain theory became the model for antibody production. Ehrlich developed a method for standardization of diphtheria antiserum, work that in part led to him being awarded the 1908 Nobel Prize in Physiology or Medicine. Ehrlich's "magic bullet," an arsenic derivative known as Salvarsan used to treat syphilis, was among the first antimicrobial drugs synthetically developed.

**Elford, William Joseph (1900-1952):** British chemist who developed a method for measuring the size of viruses using a membrane filtration system.

**Enders, John Franklin (1897-1985):** American virologist and Nobel laureate (1954) who, with his colleagues Thomas Weller and Frederick Robbins, demonstrated the ability of poliovirus to grow in nonneural tissue, providing an opening for development of polio vaccines.

**Epstein, Michael Anthony (1921-    ):** British pathologist who, with Yvonne Barr, isolated the etiological agent for infectious mononucleosis and Burkitt's lymphoma. The agent was named the Epstein-Barr virus.

**Escherich, Theodor (1857-1911):** German pediatrician who discovered the intestinal organism *Bacterium coli*, later renamed *Escherichia coli*. Because the organism is found only in the colon, it was adapted as a surrogate marker for sewage contamination of water.

**Fenner, Frank (1914-2010):** Australian physician who, as chair of the Global Commission for the Certification of Smallpox Eradication, confirmed the worldwide eradication of the disease. Fenner had previously participated in a project introducing rabbit myxoma virus into the rabbit population of Australia as a means to control their numbers.

**Finlay, Carlos (1833-1915):** Cuban physician who proposed that the vector for the transmission of yellow fever was a mosquito. Walter Reed later provided definitive proof for Finlay's theory.

**Fleming, Alexander (1881-1955):** British microbiologist who discovered the antibacterial enzyme lysozyme in body fluids and the antibiotic penicillin, produced by a mold, *Penicillium*, that had contaminated one of his laboratory cultures. He was awarded the 1945 Nobel Prize in Physiology or Medicine for his fortuitous discovery.

**Fracastoro, Girolamo (c. 1478-1553):** Italian physician and the founder of epidemiology. He proposed the existence of "spores" that could transmit disease from person to person, a theory that predated the nineteenth century germ theory of disease. Fracastoro's writings include the poem "Syphilis: Or, The French Disease," about a shepherd boy Syphilius who blamed the loss of his sheep on the gods, resulting in him being punished with the disease named for him.

**Francis, Edward (1872-1957):** American physician who after repeated exposure to tularemia determined that infection confers a lifelong immunity. The etiological agent, *Francisella tularensis*, was named for him.

**Francis, Thomas, Jr. (1900-1969):** American physician and virologist who was among the first to isolate the influenza virus. In 1945, he helped produce the first influenza vaccine.

**Franklin, Rosalind (1920-1958):** British X-ray crystallographer whose analysis of deoxyribonucleic acid (DNA) and viral protein structures contributed to an understanding of their structures.

**Gaffky, Georg Theodor August (1850-1918):** German physician who was among the first to isolate *Salmonella* from persons with typhoid. The genus *Gaffkya* was named for him. As a colleague of Robert Koch, Gaffky was among the members of commissions sent by the German government to investigate the cholera epidemic in Egypt in 1883 and the plague epidemic in India in 1897.

**Gajdusek, D. Carleton (1923-2008):** American physician, virologist, and Nobel laureate (1976) whose study of kuru, a slow neurological disease transmitted by cannibalism within the Fore tribe on New Guinea in the 1950's, led to the discovery of prions.

**Gallo, Robert Charles (1937-    ):** American biochemist who, with Luc Montagnier, isolated the human immunodeficiency virus (HIV) and developed a diagnostic tool for its identification.

**Goodpasture, Ernest William (1886-1960):** American physician who developed methods for growing viruses and rickettsia in embryonated eggs. The procedure proved critical in the production of vaccines against smallpox and influenza. Use of embryonated eggs for production of influenza vaccine has continued into the twenty-first century.

**Gorgas, William Crawford (1854-1920):** American physician and member of the U.S. Army Medical Corps. In his role as chief sanitary officer in Cuba, he demonstrated that control of mosquito breeding areas resulted in the near eradication of yellow fever. Gorgas's application of these methods on the Isthmus of Panama made it possible to build the Panama Canal.

**Gram, Hans Christian (1853-1938):** A Danish physician and pharmacologist who developed the staining method known as the Gram stain, which is routinely used in the identification of bacteria.

**Gregg, Norman (1892-1966):** Australian physician and ophthalmologist who observed the link in pregnant women between rubella infection during the first trimester of the pregnancy and development of birth disorders known as rubella syndrome.

**Griffith, Frederick (1881-1941):** British biologist who observed that a transforming principle could transfer genetic material between avirulent and virulent pneumococci; the material was subsequently shown to be deoxyribonucleic acid (DNA).

**Halsted, William Stewart (1852-1922):** American physician who pioneered the use of rubber gloves during surgery as a means to reduce the threat of infection.

**Hansen, Gerhard Armauer (1841-1912):** Norwegian physician who, in 1873, identified the organism later known as *Mycobacterium leprae* as the etiological agent of leprosy. Leprosy is also known as Hansen's disease.

**Henle, Friedrich (1809-1885):** German physician and anatomist who developed an early version of the germ theory of disease. His studies of renal structure resulted in a portion of the renal tubules being named the loop of Henle.

**Hilleman, Maurice (1919-2005):** American physician who developed vaccines against many significant childhood diseases, including measles, mumps, rubella, and chickenpox.

**Hippocrates (c. 460-c. 370 B.C.E.):** Greek physician considered to be the founder of Western medicine. In a large number of writings, Hippocrates and his students compiled an extensive clinical description of diseases. He also described the possible role of factors such as diet and environmental conditions in the development of illness.

**Hoffmann, Erich (1868-1959):** German physician who, with his colleague Fritz Schaudinn in 1905, isolated the etiological agent of syphilis, naming it *Spirochaeta pallida*.

**Holmes, Oliver Wendell, Sr. (1809-1894):** American physician who determined that the transmission of puerperal fever among women who recently gave birth was the result of unhygienic practices among attending physicians. A similar conclusion was reached independently by the Hungarian physician Ignaz Semmelweis.

**Huebner, Robert (1914-1998):** American physician and virologist who isolated the etiological agent for rickettsialpox as well as the first of numerous adenoviruses associated with respiratory infections of humans. Huebner's work also provided evidence for the role of oncogenes, first discovered in viruses, in the transformation of normal cells into cancer cells.

**Isaacs, Alick (1921-1967):** British physician and virologist who discovered interferon, an antiviral agent produced by cells infected with viruses.

**Ivanovski, Dmitri (1864-1920):** Russian biologist who in the 1890's discovered that what is now recognized as a virus is the agent of tobacco mosaic disease, the first demonstration that such submicroscopic particles exist. Ivanovski's failure to report his work led to others being credited for the discovery.

**Jenner, Edward (1749-1823):** English physician who developed the first effective smallpox vaccine.

**Jenner, William (1815-1898):** British physician and physician to Queen Victoria who described the clinical distinctions between typhoid fever and typhus.

**Kahn, Reuben Leon (1887-1974):** American physician who developed the Kahn test, a precipitin test for the presence of syphilis.

**Kauffmann, Fritz (1899-1978):** German physician and microbiologist who, with Philip Bruce White, developed the first classification scheme for identification of strains of *Salmonella* in 1934. The Kauffmann-White system remains the current method of classification.

**Kendrick, Pearl (1890-1980):** American physician who developed the first effective vaccine against pertussis (whooping cough). She also suggested that the childhood vaccination against pertussis should be combined with that against diphtheria, producing the forerunner of the DTaP vaccine that included the inactivated tetanus toxin.

**Kircher, Athanasius (1601-1680):** Jesuit priest who, after observation of microorganisms using primitive microscopes, suggested that diseases such as plague could be associated with these agents.

**Kitasato, Shibasaburō (1852-1931):** Japanese physician credited with the isolation of tetanus toxin and the isolation, with Alexandre Yersin, of the plague bacillus.

**Klebs, Edwin (1834-1913):** German pathologist who, with his colleague Friedrich Loeffler, identified *Corynebacterium diphtheria* as the etiological agent of diphtheria in 1883.

**Klemperer, Georg (1865-1946):** German physician who, in 1891, first introduced the use of patient's serum for the treatment of pneumococcal (*Streptococcus pneumoniae*) infections.

**Koch, Robert (1843-1910):** German physician and Nobel laureate (1905) credited with confirming the role of the anthrax bacillus as the etiological agent of that disease and with isolation of the tuberculosis bacillus (1882). In 1883, Koch isolated the etiological agent of cholera while investigating an outbreak in Egypt. Koch and his colleague Friedrich Loeffler developed what became known as Koch's postulates, a series of experimental procedures linking a disease with a specific etiological agent.

**Koplik, Henry (1858-1927):** American physician whose observation of a characteristic rash known as Koplik's spots became a diagnostic tool for identifying measles.

**Koprowski, Hilary (1916-    ):** Polish born American physician and virologist who developed the first attenuated polio vaccine. The vaccine was later superseded by the more effective Sabin vaccine.

**Lancefield, Rebecca (1895-1981):** American microbiologist who developed the first classification system for the streptococci. The Lancefield system remains the modern classification scheme.

**Landsteiner, Karl (1868-1943):** Austrian physician and Nobel laureate (1930) noted for his discovery of both ABO and Rhesus (Rh) blood groups and, with his colleague Erwin Popper, for the isolation of poliovirus in 1908.

**Lazear, Jesse William (1866-1900):** American physician who, as a member of the Walter Reed Commission in 1900, helped confirm the role of mosquitoes in the transmission of yellow fever. Lazear exposed himself to a mosquito that had recently fed on a person with yellow fever and then developed the disease, from which he died.

**Leeuwenhoek, Antoni van (1632-1723):** Dutch tradesman and lensmaker whose development and improvement of microscopes led to the discovery of microorganisms. His observations and drawings of microscopic organisms have resulted in the designation of Leeuwenhoek as the founder of microscopy.

**Lewis, Sinclair (1885-1951):** American writer, novelist, and Nobel laureate in literature (1930) whose novel *Arrowsmith* (1925) described a fictional American physician, Martin Arrowsmith, who used the recently discovered bacteriophages as agents to control a plague epidemic in the Caribbean. Lewis anticipated similar applications as a clinical measure by a decade.

**Lister, Joseph (1827-1912):** British physician and surgeon who developed antiseptic surgery.

**Loeffler, Friedrich (1852-1915):** German physician who, with colleague Edwin Klebs, isolated the etiological agent for diphtheria now known as *Corynebacterium diphtheriae*. Loeffler also helped develop what became known as Koch's postulates with colleague Robert Koch.

**McCoy, George Walter (1876-1952):** American physician associated with the U.S. Plague Laboratory in San Francisco who, in 1911, described tularemia, a plaguelike disease carried primarily by rodents that can infect other animals, including humans. McCoy later isolated the agent, now known as *Francisella tularensis.*

**Mahoney, John F. (1889-1957):** American physician who, in 1943, began the use of penicillin for the treatment of syphilis. His research also involved the mechanism of infection by the spirochaete. Mahoney established the Venereal Disease Research Center on Staten Island, New York, for the study of sexually transmitted diseases.

**Marshall, Barry J. (1951-    ):** An Australian physician and Nobel laureate (2005) who discovered that stomach ulcers are likely the result of infection by the bacterium *Helicobacter pylori*. Marshall's discovery led to the use of antibiotics as a means to cure ulcers and to prevent their recurrence.

**Maxcy, Kenneth Fuller (1889-1966):** American physician and epidemiologist who, in 1926, determined that the transmission of endemic typhus (murine typhus) was by lice and fleas. The etiological agent of the disease was later determined to be *Rickettsia typhi*.

**Metchnikoff, Élie (1845-1916):** Russian microbiologist and Nobel laureate (1908) whose discovery of phagocytosis by white blood cells led to cellular theories of immunity.

**Montagnier, Luc (1932-    ):** French biochemist and Nobel laureate (2008) who isolated the human immunodeficiency virus (HIV).

**Mooser, Hermann (1891-1971):** Swiss microbiologist who was the first to differentiate the characteristics and means of transmission of epidemic typhus from endemic typhus.

**Negri, Adelchi (1876-1912):** Italian physician whose report of inclusion bodies in neurons of persons who died from rabies resulted in a postmortem diagnosis tool for the disease. The term "Negri bodies" was coined to describe the structures.

**Neisser, Albert L. (1855-1916):** German physician who identified the etiological agent causing the sexually transmitted disease gonorrhea. The organism was later named *Neisseria gonorrheae*. Neisser is sometimes credited as a codiscoverer, with Gerhard Hansen, of the leprosy bacillus.

**Nicolle, Charles (1866-1936):** French physician and Nobel laureate (1928) who demonstrated the role of lice in transmitting epidemic typhus.

**Noguchi, Hideyo (1876-1928):** Japanese physician who discovered the role of the syphilis agent, *Treponema pallidum*, in paresis (neurological disorders) associated with the tertiary state of the disease. Noguchi also conducted research in tropical diseases such as Oroya fever.

**Obermeier, Otto (1843-1873):** German bacteriologist who first observed the presence of the spirochaete *Borrelia* in the blood of persons with relapsing fever, publishing his observations from the previous decade in 1873.

**Pacini, Filippo (1812-1883):** Italian anatomist who, in 1854, first reported the presence of *Vibrio cholerae* in persons with cholera. Pacini's observation was not recognized until Robert Koch's isolation of the same organism thirty years later.

**Paracelsus (Philippus von Hohenheim; 1493-1541):** Swiss physician who introduced the use of mercury for the treatment of syphilis.

**Pasteur, Louis (1822-1895):** French chemist considered one of the founders of microbiology for his role in developing the germ theory of disease. Noted for developing vaccines against anthrax and rabies and for the use of pasteurization for preserving milk.

**Pettenkofer, Max von (1818-1901):** German physician considered a founder of modern hygiene. Pettenkofer rejected the idea of germs as the cause of disease, going so far as to swallow a culture of cholera bacilli to demonstrate his belief. His groundwater theory argued that the earth emitted miasmas that were the agents of disease. Though in error, his theory did contribute to improved hygiene and the building of sewage systems, which led to reduction of disease.

**Pfeiffer, Emil (1846-1921):** German physician who provided the first description of infectious mononucleosis. An alternative name for mononucleosis was Pfeiffer's disease.

**Pfeiffer, Richard Friedrich Johannes (1858-1945):** German physician who, in 1892, isolated a bacterium from persons with influenza that he named *Bacterium influenza*, mistakenly believing that "Pfeiffer's bacillus" was the etiological agent. The organism, subsequently named *Haemophilus influenzae*, was later shown to be associated with other childhood diseases.

**Plenčič, Marcus Antonius (1705-1786):** Austrian physician referred to as the Slovene Pasteur. In 1762, he proposed that contagium animatum, tiny seeds or "animals" found in diseased persons, were actually the agents of the illness. Plencic's theory predated the germ theory of disease by more than one century.

**Prowazek, Stanislaus von (1875-1915):** Czech parasitologist who, with his colleague Henrique da Rocha Lima in 1915, discovered the etiological agent of epidemic typhus, later named *Rickettsia prowazekii*. Prowazek succumbed to typhus acquired while investigating an outbreak in a German prison.

**Prusiner, Stanley B. (1942-    ):** American physician and Nobel laureate (1997) whose discovery of prions contributed to understanding their role in slow neurological diseases.

**Ramon, Gaston (1886-1963):** French biologist who developed modern methods for the inactivation of diphtheria and tetanus toxins for use in vaccines.

**Reed, Walter (1851-1902):** American physician who proved Carlos Finlay's hypothesis that yellow fever is transmitted by the mosquito *Aedes aegypti*.

**Ricketts, Howard T. (1871-1910):** American physician who discovered the role of ticks in the transmission of Rocky Mountain spotted fever. While investigating an outbreak of typhus fever in Mexico, Ricketts concluded that the two diseases could have similar causes. Shortly after demonstrating the role of the body louse in its spread, Ricketts became infected and died.

**Rocha Lima, Henrique da (1879-1956):** Brazilian physician who was codiscoverer of the etiological agent of epidemic typhus. He named the agent *Rickettsia prowazekii* for two scientists who died from the disease.

**Ross, Ronald (1857-1932):** British physician and Nobel laureate (1902) who discovered the etiological agent of malaria, *Plasmodium*, and its life cycle in the *Anopheles* mosquito vector.

**Rous, Peyton (1879-1970):** American biologist and Nobel laureate (1966) who demonstrated that a virus could transmit tumors in chickens. Subsequently named the Rous sarcoma virus, the agent was the first of the ribonucleic acid (RNA) tumor viruses to be discovered.

**Roux, Pierre-Paul-Émile (1853-1933):** French physician who demonstrated the agent of rabies travels along nerves to the brain. His later work clarified the role of diphtheria toxin in the disease and demonstrated that syphilis can be studied in nonhuman primates.

**Rush, Benjamin (1746-1813):** American physician and a signer of the Declaration of Independence. Rush's views on medical treatment (he was an advocate of bleeding and purging) reflected the knowledge of the period. His description of the yellow fever outbreak in Philadelphia in 1793 is considered a definitive account of the event.

**Sabin, Albert (1906-1993):** American physician whose research into poliomyelitis led to an understanding of its means of transmission. Sabin's development of the oral poliovirus vaccine played a major role in the control of the disease.

**Salk, Jonas (1914-1995):** American physician and virologist who developed the first effective (killed) vaccine against poliomyelitis.

**Salmon, Daniel Elmer (1850-1914):** American veterinary surgeon who established the Bureau of Animal Industry within the U.S. Department of Agriculture. In collaboration with his assistant Theobald Smith, Salmon isolated the etiological agent for hog cholera, the genus name becoming *Salmonella* in his honor.

**Schaudinn, Fritz (1871-1906):** German zoologist who, with his colleague Erich Hoffman in 1905, discovered the etiological agent of syphilis, which they called *Spirochaeta pallida*. The agent later became known as *Treponema pallidum*. Schaudinn also described the role of *Entamoeba histolytica* as the agent of amebic dysentery.

**Schottmüeller, Hugo (1867-1936):** German physician who observed the variations in red blood cell hemolysis (a, b, and g) produced by various types of streptococci, applying these observations to an early classification system. He also distinguished various streptococcal fevers, including paratyphoid fever.

**Semmelweis, Ignaz (1818-1865):** Hungarian physician who determined that puerperal fever, a highly virulent infection common in women shortly after giving birth in hospitals, was the result of contamination by attending physicians. By enforcing among his colleagues the procedure of handwashing between patient visits, Semmelweis was able to largely control infection. The etiological agent was later shown to be *Streptococcus*.

**Sennert, Daniel (1572-1637):** German physician who, in 1619, coined the term "roteln," or "rubella," to describe the rash associated with the illness. Sennert also distinguished the disease from measles, which produces a similar rash.

**Shiga, Kiyoshi (1871-1957):** Japanese physician who isolated the etiological agent of bacterial dysentery during an 1897 epidemic. The bacillus was named *Shigella* in his honor.

**Shope, Robert Ellis (1929-2004):** American physician and virologist who isolated Rift Valley fever virus during an epidemic in Egypt in 1977. Shope provided the first description of Lyme disease in the United States that same year. He also contributed to studies of viral hemorrhagic fevers and other newly emerging diseases.

**Smith, Theobald (1859-1934):** American physician

who demonstrated the role played by ticks in transmitting disease. Smith and his mentor, Daniel Salmon, isolated the agent of hog cholera, the bacterium that became *Salmonella cholera-suis*.

**Snow, John (1813-1858):** British physician whose epidemiological study of two cholera outbreaks in London during the early 1850's illustrated the role of sewage contamination of water supplies as the primary source of the epidemics. Snow also was physician to Queen Victoria. His administration of chloroform during the births of two of her children opened the way for more common use of anesthesia.

**Stanley, Wendell Meredith (1904-1971):** American biochemist and Nobel laureate (1946) for his crystallization of the tobacco mosaic virus. Stanley's conclusion, later proven inaccurate, was that viruses consist entirely of protein.

**Sternberg, George Miller (1838-1915):** American physician who simultaneously, with Louis Pasteur, reported the presence of pneumococcus in persons with pneumonia. Sternberg also was among the first to observe that the course of a viral infection may be followed by antibody production in the infected person.

**Sydenham, Thomas (1624-1689):** British physician who was known as the English Hippocrates because of his use and recording of observations in describing the progression of disease. He also pioneered the use of cooling patients for treating disease, treated malaria with quinine, and used opium for treating pain.

**Temin, Howard M. (1934-1994):** American molecular biologist and Nobel laureate (1975) who was a co-discoverer of reverse transcriptase, the enzyme found in ribonucleic acid (RNA) tumor virus and human immunodeficiency virus (HIV) that copies RNA into deoxyribonucleic acid (DNA). The role of the enzyme provided an explanation for the subsequent discovery that such viruses integrate within the chromosome of infected cells.

**Theiler, Max (1899-1972):** South African-born American physician and Nobel laureate (1951) who, in 1930, introduced the first vaccine against yellow fever.

**Twort, Frederick (1877-1950):** British physician who discovered bacteriophages, viruses that infect bacteria, while studying a culture of *Staphylococcus*. Twort also demonstrated the vitamin requirement

of *Mycobacterium leprae*, the etiological agent of leprosy, and determined the cause of Johne's disease, an intestinal infection of ruminants, to be *Mycobacterium avium*, a variant of the tuberculosis and leprosy agents.

**Varmus, Harold E. (1939-    ):** American molecular biologist and Nobel laureate (1989) who, with J. Michael Bishop, proposed that oncogenes found in ribonucleic acid (RNA) tumor viruses originate in the host cell and normally play a role in regulation of cell replication.

**Virchow, Rudolf (1821-1902):** German physician and pathologist who applied the concept of *omnis cellula e cellula* ("all cells come from cells"). In his argument that even if bacteria were discovered in a diseased animal, it did not necessarily follow that the organism was the etiological agent, Virchow suggested the role of toxins in causing disease.

**Waksman, Selman Abraham (1888-1973):** Ukraine-born American soil microbiologist and Nobel laureate (1952) who isolated more than twenty antibiotics from soil organisms; the term "antibiotic" was coined by Waksman to illustrate the function of these agents. Among these isolates was streptomycin, the first effective treatment for tuberculosis, and neomycin.

**Wassermann, August von (1866-1925):** German microbiologist who developed the first diagnostic test for syphilis.

**Watson, James D. (1928-    ):** American molecular biologist and Nobel laureate (1962) who, with his colleague Francis Crick, produced the first accurate model of deoxyribonucleic acid (DNA) structure.

**Welch, William Henry (1850-1934):** American physician and a founder of the modern field of scientific pathology. Welch demonstrated the role of *Staphylococcus aureus* in infected abscesses and the role of *Clostridium welchii*, named in his honor, as a cause of gas gangrene.

**White, Philip Bruce (1891-1949):** British microbiologist who, during the 1920's, developed an early classification procedure for *Salmonella*. The system was modified during the 1930's by Fritz Kauffmann and became known as the Kauffmann-White classification.

**Wilkins, Maurice (1916-2004):** British physicist whose analysis of deoxyribonucleic acid (DNA) contributed to an understanding of its structure.

**Wright, Almroth Edward (1861-1947):** British physician and immunologist who developed the first typhoid vaccine.

**Yersin, Alexandre (1863-1943):** French microbiologist credited with isolating *Yersinia pestis*, the etiological agent of plague.

**Zinsser, Hans (1878-1940):** American physician who authored numerous books for general readers on the subject of medical outbreaks. Zinsser developed the first vaccine targeting endemic typhus and was considered the world's authority on the disease.

**Zur Hausen, Harald (1936-    ):** German virologist and Nobel laureate (2008) who discovered the role played by human papillomaviruses (HPV) as etiological agents of cervical cancer.

*Richard Adler, Ph.D.*

# Nobel Prizes for Discoveries in Infectious Diseases

## 1902
### Ronald Ross (Great Britain)

Ross's studies of malaria, showing how it enters organisms and how its life cycle manifests in mosquitoes, laid the foundation for combating this disease.

## 1903
### Niels Ryberg Finsen (Denmark)

Finsen developed treatments for diseases using concentrated light therapy for lupus vulgaris, a disease from which he himself suffered. He also devised light therapy for the treatment of other diseases, including smallpox, using concentrated red light.

## 1905
### Robert Koch (Germany)

Koch was cited by the Nobel Foundation for his work on tuberculosis. However, he worked on many infectious diseases, including cholera, malaria, typhus, and several diseases of cattle. He is probably best known for the method Koch's postulates, used for identifying infectious agents.

## 1907
### Alphonse Laveran (France)

Laveran was awarded the prize for his work on the role of protozoa in causing disease, especially his work on malaria and trypanosomiasis.

## 1908
### Élie Metchnikoff (Ukraine) and Paul Ehrlich (Germany)

The award was given for studies on immunity. Metchnikoff 's work concerned the role of phagocytosis and of cellular responses in immunity. Ehrlich developed staining methods for blood cells, the quantification and standardization of sera, and searched for new antipathogen agents, especially those effective against syphilis. Ehrlich was one of the founders of chemotherapy.

## 1919
### Jules Bordet (Belgium)

Bordet was awarded the prize for his discoveries relating to immunity. He developed methods to diagnose microbes using sera from recovered victims. His work on what would later be called Bordetella pertussis laid the foundation for determining the cause of whooping cough.

## 1928
### Charles Nicolle (France)

Nicolle worked at the Pasteur Institute in Tunis. His work on typhus showed that it is spread by body lice. He developed laboratory animal models for typhus and showed that when the contaminating parasites were eliminated, the disease died out.

## 1939
### Gerhard Domagk (Germany)

Domagk discovered the antibiotic effects of prontosil, a derivative of sulphanilamide, effective against staphylococci and hemolytic streptococci. This work laid the foundation for the development of other sulphonamide drugs.

## 1945
### Sir Alexander Fleming (Great Britain), Ernst Boris Chain (Germany), and Baron Florey (Australia)

Fleming was awarded the prize for the discovery of penicillin and Chain and Florey received the prize for discovering penicillin's curative effects in various infectious diseases.

## 1948
### Paul Müller (Switzerland)

Müller was cited for his work on the synthesis and use of the contact poison dichloro-diphenyl-trichloro-ethane (DDT) against arthropods. This work helped to combat such arthropod-borne diseases as typhus and malaria.

## 1951
### Max Theiler (South Africa)

Theiler showed that yellow fever is caused by a filterable virus. He developed a mouse model and worked on a vaccine against the disease.

## 1952
### Selman Abraham Waksman (Ukraine/United States)

Waksman was awarded the prize for his discovery of streptomycin, the first antibiotic effective against tuberculosis. He went on to discover many other antibiotics.

## 1954

### John Franklin Enders, Thomas Huckle Weller, and Frederick Chapman Robbins (United States)

Enders, Weller, and Robbins developed methods to grow poliomyelitis virus in cultured cells, methods that would eventually lead to the development of vaccines by Jonas Salk and Albert Sabin.

## 1966

### Peyton Rous (United States)

Rous was awarded the prize for his discovery of tumor-inducing viruses, including the Rous sarcoma virus that bears his name.

## 1972

### Gerald M. Edelman (United States) and Rodney Robert Porter (Great Britain)

Edelman and Porter elucidated the chemical structure of antibodies, an important step in understanding how the immune system fights infectious agents.

## 1975

### David Baltimore (United States), Renato Dulbecco (Italy), and Howard M. Temin (United States)

The prize was given for work with tumor viruses. Dulbecco developed methods to quantitate animal viruses and showed how oncogenic viruses induce cancer. Temin and Baltimore independently discovered reverse transcriptase, the enzyme that synthesizes a deoxyribonucleic acid (DNA) copy of the ribonucleic acid (RNA) viral genome found in retroviruses.

## 1976

### Baruch S. Blumberg and Carleton Gajdusek (United States)

Blumberg and Gajdusek were cited for their discoveries concerning new mechanisms for the origin and dissemination of infectious diseases. Blumberg worked on filiariad diseases, including elephantiasis, while Gajdusek worked on kuru, eventually leading to the discovery of prions by Stanley B. Prusiner.

## 1980

### Baruj Benacerraf (Venezuela), Jean Dausset (France), and George D. Snell (United States)

The prize was given to Benacerraf, Dausset, and Snell for understanding how surface antigens play a role in the body's immune response in relation to infections, cancer immune surveillance, and in tissue transplantation.

## 1984

### Niels K. Jerne (Great Britain), Georges J. F. Köhler (Germany), and César Milstein (Argentina)

Jerne was cited for his theoretical work on cellular immunity, which has been used in the diagnosis and treatment of disease. Köhler and Milstein developed the technique of monoclonal antibody production in hybridomas. Monoclonal antibodies have been used extensively in disease diagnosis and treatment and as a research reagent.

## 1987

### Susumu Tonegawa (Japan)

Tonegawa was awarded the prize for his discovery of the generation of antibody diversity in an organism.

## 1996

### Peter C. Doherty (Australia) and Rolf M. Zinkernagel (Switzerland)

Doherty and Zinkernagel were cited for their work on how the immune system recognizes virus-infected cells. This research led to understanding cell-mediated immune responses.

## 1997

### Stanley B. Prusiner (United States)

Prusiner was awarded the prize for his discovery of prions, a new biological principle of infection. Prions, proteinaceous infectious particles, are responsible for kuru and bovine spongiform encephalopathy (BSE) and Creutzfeldt-Jakob disease, its variant in humans.

## 2005

### Barry J. Marshall and J. Robin Warren (Australia)

The prize was given for the discovery that the bacterium *Helicobacter pylori* is a cause of chronic gastritis and peptic ulcer disease. Marshall had observed the frequent presence of *H. pylori* in gastric biopsies and proposed it as the cause of gastritis and peptic ulcers. His hypothesis was not accepted by the scientific community, however, until Marshall infected himself with the organism, developed the disease, and then cured it with antibiotics.

**2008**

**Harald zur Hausen (Germany), Françoise Barré-Sinoussi (France), and Luc Montagnier (France)**

Hausen received the prize for his discovery that human papillomaviruses are a cause of cervical cancer in humans. Barré-Sinoussi and Montagnier were the original discoverers of the human immunodeficiency virus (HIV), the cause of acquired immunodeficiency syndrome (AIDS).

*Ralph R. Meyer, Ph.D.*

# INDEXES

# Entries by Anatomy or System Affected

# Category Index

**Fungal Infections**

**Immune Response**

**Parasites**

# Subject Index